The Modern Hospital

Rifat Latifi
Editor

The Modern Hospital

Patients Centered, Disease Based, Research Oriented, Technology Driven

Springer

Editor
Rifat Latifi
New York Medical College, School of Medicine
Department of Surgery and Westchester Medical Center
Valhalla, NY
USA

ISBN 978-3-030-01393-6 ISBN 978-3-030-01394-3 (eBook)
https://doi.org/10.1007/978-3-030-01394-3

Library of Congress Control Number: 2018965615

This Springer imprint is published by the registered company Springer Nature Switzerland AG
The registered company address is: Gewerbestrasse 11, 6330 Cham, Switzerland

To my wife Drita and our children, Kalterina, Qendresa, Kushtrim, Fortesa, and Lulejeta, and to our grandchildren, Zana, Adelina, Norik, and Ellis, with love and affection. Thank you for making my life so meaningful and beautifully substantial.

Foreword

The task assigned to *The Modern Hospital: Patient-Centered, Disease-Based, Research-Oriented, Technology-Driven* was to describe and analyze, and critically appraise all elements of the hospitals of the past, the current modern hospitals and the attempts to predict the future of these complex institutions. It is brilliantly written by experts and students of this ever-changing field and will serve well all those who train in, practice in, lead individual departments, or manage an entire hospital, alone, or as part of a complex corporation or healthcare system. The editor and the authors of this tome are to be commended on successfully accomplishing this major challenge.

While there is an outstanding and comprehensive chapter herein on the history of the American hospital transformation written by Professor Halperin, this foreword will add my personal involvement in witnessing the metamorphosis of the house for the sick and injured into a modern hospital over half century, as a student, house officer, practicing surgeon, and leader of several major departments of surgery. The necessity for a facility in which to provide healthcare for the sick and injured indigent, poor, and often homeless population of colonial America was perceived by Dr. Thomas Bond, a physician who enlisted the influential support of Benjamin Franklin to help him establish the first hospital in the New World in 1751 in Philadelphia. Its purpose was to provide a place where physicians, nurses, and other healthcare providers could serve the needs of those who did not possess the resources nor the homes in which physicians could visit and care for them, as they did for the more affluent and gentrified citizens of the community. "House calls" were the standard of healthcare at that time. Shortly thereafter, it became apparent that a large proportion of hospitalized patients had predominantly mental and/or neurological problems which required special attention, and after a dark period of inhumane treatment, the hospital established the Pennsylvania Institute, a subsidiary facility exclusively for the mentally ill and functionally impaired patients about 4 miles west of the main hospital. It was here that Dr. Benjamin Rush became the "Father of Psychiatry" in America and advanced this neophyte specialty for the rest of his career. Obstetrics and Gynecology were the next specialties established in the hospital and quickly became prominent as the "Lying-In" branch of Pennsylvania Hospital. By the time of the Civil War, the specialty of Surgery advanced with the building of the surgical amphitheater on the top floor. The Hospital also served as the major clinical teaching facility for the School of Medicine of the University of Pennsylvania, which was the first medical school in America, established in

1744. By the turn of the nineteenth century, the first hospital, planned specifically as a teaching hospital, was built in West Philadelphia on the main campus of the University and subsequently served together with Pennsylvania Hospital to educate and train thousands of physicians. The Children's Hospital of Philadelphia, established near Pennsylvania Hospital, was designed and equipped to meet the special needs of children and was relocated in the mid-twentieth century to the University Medical Center in West Philadelphia, where it functions as part of the most spectacular and comprehensive medical complex in the world.

In 1957, as a neophyte medical student, I first set foot in the Hospital of the University of Pennsylvania, where I was taught physical diagnosis and was first exposed to hospitalized patients with a wide variety of medical problems. The hospital had 960 beds, mostly organized primarily by specialty into the classical Florence Nightingale open-ward configuration of 40 beds that favored efficiency of patient care and teaching functions, but offered little to no patient privacy. No intensive care units, intermediary care units, step-down units, or other specialty care units existed. As an intern in 1962, I was the first house officer assigned to the first surgical ICU, which consisted of four beds in a converted three-room corner of the hospital in which the two dividing walls were removed to create an open area for four beds, each with an assigned, around-the-clock nurse, who actually provided and comprised the intensive care. A small EKG monitor, a suction pump, and an oxygen line were available at each bed, and I was physically present 36 h on, 12 h off, each 2-day shift, to provide physician and other services. Oxygen was supplied, usually via an oxygen tent, sometimes via nasal cannula. There were no ventilators available, and if a patient required ventilation assistance, it was provided via a mask or endotracheal tube attached to a rubber Ambu bag which was squeezed manually for hours or days by anesthesia personnel, surgical residents, medical students, nurses, and others in valiant efforts to save lives. Nasogastric tubes were connected to Wangensteen three-bottle suction, chest tubes were attached to water-seal drainage, and blood gas determinations were tedious, time-consuming, and expensive complex procedures carried out intermittently as needed.

During the 6 years of my general/cardiothoracic surgical training ending in 1967, the Nightingale wards were all replaced by private and semiprivate patient rooms, and multiple specialty and special care areas emerged to change extensively the way medicine was practiced in the hospital, including a 20-bed coronary care unit, a 12-bed surgical intensive care unit, an 8-bed cardiac surgery unit, a 4-bed neurosurgical intensive care unit, a 4-bed hemodialysis unit, neonatal intensive care and premature infant care units, and a 12-bed extramural NIH-supported research critical care unit. Additionally, special areas were created to serve gynecologic oncology, orthopedic surgery, ENT and head and neck surgery, infectious disease and immunology, trauma, burns, plastic/reconstructive/oral-maxillofacial surgery, vascular surgery, transplantation, psychiatry, etc. The hospital was obviously a dynamic institution which continuously modified, remodeled, or reinvented itself in accordance with patient needs and medical/surgical advances. Such will continue to occur unabated in the future as indicated for optimal patient care. The major anticipated changes will be tied to the technological and therapeutic advances as they occur, and ultimately, hospitals will essentially become highly specialized intensive care institutions; and all other care will be provided in outpatient facilities or at home. Super-specialty hospitals, such as children's hospitals, designated specific cancer centers for adults or children, transplantation centers, gene therapy and stem cell therapy centers, and other needs and special services, as they arise or become evident, will be created or morphed, as will be described and discussed extensively and comprehensively by the many experts who have been assembled to address the current and future of hospital-related healthcare in this unique volume conceived, organized, and edited by the visionary Dr. Rifat Latifi.

I have chosen to introduce this important and timely tome by relating a minimal glimpse of my knowledge and experiences of hospital-based medical practice in this country during the past two and a half centuries, together with a brief personal description of the changes that I have lived through during the 60 years of my active career in medicine and surgery. As described in this book, what has transpired during those years in hospital-based practice has been truly phenomenal, and the changes which can be expected in the future defy the imagination but will transform the practice of medicine in an exciting, mind-boggling manner for the benefit of the profession and humanity. I greatly appreciate the opportunity to participate in this challenging undertaking, and I eagerly look forward to the publication of this landmark educational endeavor.

New Haven, CT, USA
Scranton, PA, USA
Stanley J. Dudrick

Dallas, PA, USA
Waterbury, CT, USA
Edward S. Anderson

Foreword

There is perhaps no industry today as complex as the healthcare industry. *The Modern Hospital: Patient-Centered, Disease-Based, Research-Oriented, Technology-Driven* explores that complexity in all its grandeur and grit, because it is written from a variety of perspectives by a number of authorities, including clinicians, administrators, researchers, and students of today's hospital, and addresses all aspects of the modern hospital, which is, as the title of the text suggests, patient-centered, research-oriented, technology-driven, and disease-based from an organizational, functional, architectural, ergonomics, and patient-flow standpoint.

A hot-button topic for decades, healthcare leaders find themselves perched, yet again, on a new frontier as our nation works to balance the importance of an industry (that accounts for 18.9% of the GDP and more than 150 million jobs) and its proper place in dueling national, regional, and local priorities for revenues, reimbursement dollars, regulatory reform, and oversight. This is no small order, because, in our opinion, there are elements of the business of healthcare that are seriously complicating, and perhaps even adversely impacting, healthcare, and very few in our nation, outside of healthcare organizations themselves, seemed to be concerned. The list of challenges is lengthy. As an example, currently hospitals are in some way incentivized or disincentivized, and very publicly so, to keep people healthy, happy, satisfied, feeling less pain, and receiving more information, in the hospital less (or at least for less than two midnights) or out of the hospital more, or altogether. The layers and level of regulatory fervor have reached not only a fever pitch but have pitched regulatory agencies against one another, catching healthcare in the middle. Recently, a hospital replaced hundreds of doorknobs in a mental health institution in order to comply with a national-level regulator, only to be told a few weeks later by a state-level regulator to replace all the new doorknobs with the old ones. Perhaps the most visible example of the complexity of healthcare is the patient bill. Patients don't like them, not because they don't want to pay them but because they are difficult to understand. Well, hospitals don't like them either. But, with a Medicare billing manual that today is measured in feet, when it was once measured in inches, hospitals are required to prepare bills in a certain way, if they are to get paid. Finally, tops among clinician complaints are that they would like to spend less time documenting care, as required by multiple layers of regulatory oversight, and more time actually caring for people.

But, this complexity has brought brilliant solutions as well. The field of telemedicine is a game changer and, in our opinion, will overhaul the way care is delivered at every level. And, it will impact not only access to and quality of care but who provides and who receives care. Layering artificial intelligence that constantly monitors patients, data, and trends with a telemedicine backbone quickly reduces hundreds of data points for thousands of patients into immediate and often actionable information. As an example, studies have shown that using a well-structured telemedicine program in ICUs in the United States can dramatically reduce morbidity and mortality. This same backbone brings trauma surgeons electronically to remote areas to provide "care" to a severely injured person hundreds of miles from the closest trauma center and helps seniors stay in their homes longer with regular "visits" with their family physician making "house calls." The implications on quality and cost alone for the entire healthcare system are remarkable, to say the least.

Just a decade or so ago, most healthcare leaders were managing one hospital or a small affiliate network at most. Today, we are overseeing highly competitive, comprehensive networks of hospitals, physician groups, and vast ambulatory and outpatient feeder systems, along with post-acute services, rehabilitation centers, and nursing and assisted living facilities, if not more. Yes, it is complex, but it doesn't have to be complicated. Most simply stated, if you invest your resources in quality, this will attract volume, which generates revenue, which enables you to reinvest dollars back into quality (Fig. 1). In other words, these three elements are crucial to the success of modern hospital that the current and future healthcare leaders should focus on: quality, volume, and revenue.

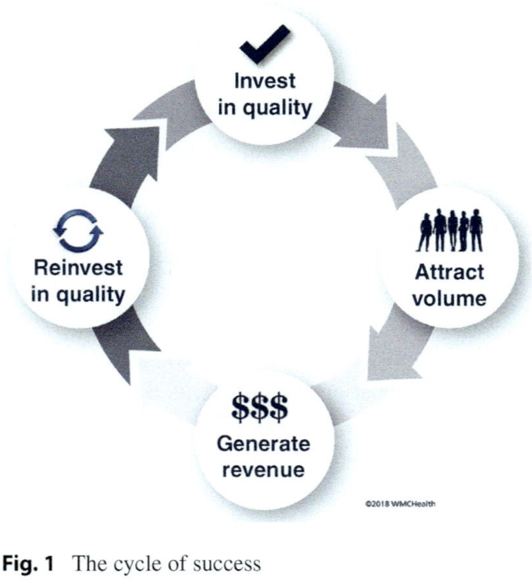

Fig. 1 The cycle of success

It is our opinion that hospitals will play a vital, lifesaving role in our lives for generations. Many inside, and now from far outside the healthcare industry, are looking at how to reduce the cost of the US healthcare system. But their focus on the easiest marks in the healthcare chain, hospital revenues, is misguided. It would make much more sense to focus on those unregulated but mandatory expenses that hospitals bear, such as unchecked malpractice costs, which are driven by those outside of the healthcare delivery system.

By providing a comprehensive, state-of-the art review of the modern hospital, this text serves as a valuable resource for those hospital leaders, physicians, surgeons, nurses, and researchers of today and the future, interested in all aspects of hospital organizational issues and our industry as a whole. Finally, this textbook provides a concise, yet comprehensive, summary of the current status of the field that will help understand the transformation and management of this challenging phenomenon called the modern hospital.

Michael Israel
Valhalla, NY, USA
Gary Brudnicki

Preface

It is difficult to imagine how a professor of surgery living in the twentieth century would react if he were told that one day, surgeons would be removing the appendix through the vagina or the mouth. What would he say if we told him we would be using nanotechnology to deliver tiny tubes in places that only the greatest anatomist would know existed? Or if he knew that we would provide the most complex and exact care imaginable?

Well, this is today's hospital. This is the modern hospital with all its beauty, complexities, developments, and flaws. Through the triumphs and setbacks, we have been fortunate to be a part of it. Science has made unimaginable progress, and the hospitals have both pushed that progress forward and reaped the rewards of it. This book is about the progress that we have made.

So why did I want to write this book? It would seem that books on hospitals should be written by administrators, not by clinicians who spent their days and nights there. But on the other hand, maybe not. Our deep, personal knowledge of the modern hospitals lends us a unique point of view. I've spent my career in hospitals – some were poor, some were rich, and some were the mecca of modern medicine and surgery.

As a medical student, a resident, a fellow, and a staff surgeon, basically, I have lived in the hospital. Yet, for most of my career, I didn't understand the complexities of the modern hospital. Nor did I really have any "interest" in learning them. And why would I? I thought that administrators make possible for the hospital to function and my job as a surgeon was simply to take care of patients.

I came early in the morning to do rounds or the morning report and went to the ICU, hospital ward, trauma room, or operating room. I spent my day taking care of patients. If I needed anything, I spoke with my chief or my departmental chair and then I went home, collapsed into bed, and started it all over again the next morning. Weekends, weekdays, and holidays. It didn't matter. As a trauma attending, I wanted to be on call during major holidays because they tended to be the busiest days and I would have the chance to operate on and care for the sickest of the sick and most injured patients.

Both as a trainee and as faculty, for days I did not see the light outside of the hospital. I came home after dark and left before dawn. My wife and kids thought it was normal for the life of a trauma and academic surgeon. I did too, and still do.

I didn't know how hospitals ran or what was required to lead them. It didn't matter to me who was at the helm. As the Director of Department of surgery at one of the premier American hospitals, the Westchester Medical Center Health Network, I thought that the best way for me to learn about the hospital was to write and edit a comprehensive, state-of-the art review of the modern hospital that will serve as a valuable resource to all of us: hospital administrators, clinicians, surgeons, nurses, researchers, and the public who has an interest in the hospital as an industry. In addition, this textbook will serve as a useful resource for current and future researchers dealing with, and interested in, this challenging phenomenon called the modern hospital in all aspects of the hospital organizational issues. Finally, after 2 years of working on it, I can say that this textbook provides a concise, yet comprehensive, summary of the current status of the field that will help understand the transformation and management of the modern hospital. All chapters are written by practicing experts in their fields and will include the most current scientific and clinical information. I hope that the reader will share my view after reading this book.

Valhalla, NY, USA Rifat Latifi
August, 2018

Acknowledgment

To all those who contributed to this tome – authors, coauthors, research fellows, administrative assistants, and Springer team led by Richard Hruska.

Thank you for your sacrifice, dedication, and selflessness with your time. I hope we have succeeded to create a great book that others will enjoy and will help us understand all the complexities and intricacies of the modern hospital that, in the words of Paul Starr, "continue to have three separate centers of authority—the trustees, physicians, and administrators—posing a great puzzle to students of formal organizations."[1]

[1] Paul Starr: *The Social Transformation of American Medicine*. Basic Book, Inc. Publishers, New York, 1984.

Contents

Contributors

Russell J. Andrews, MD Department of Nanotechnology & Smart Systems, NASA Ames Research Center, Moffett Field, CA, USA

Peter S. Arno, PhD Political Economy Research Institute, University of Massachusetts, Amherst, Amherst, MA, USA

Eden Avishai, BSc Department of Immunology, Department of Neuroscience, The Ruth and Bruce Rappaport Faculty of Medicine, Technion-Israel Institute of Technology, Haifa, Israel

David K. Barnes, MD Department of Emergency Medicine, UC Davis Health, UC Davis Medical Center, UC Davis School of Medicine, Sacramento, CA, USA

Collin L. Beers, AIA Stantec Architecture, Philadelphia, PA, USA

Kara Bennorth, BA, MBA Department of Administration, WMCHealth, Valhalla, NY, USA

Vincenzo Costigliola, MD European Association for Predictive, Preventive and Personalised Medicine, EPMA, Brussels, Belgium

Rachel Cyrus, MD Department of Internal Medicine, Northwestern Feinberg School of Medicine, Chicago, IL, USA

Colene Yvonne Daniel The Bonne Sante Group, LLC, Washington, DC, USA

Michael J. Demeure, MD, MBA Hoag Family Cancer Institute, Hoag Memorial Hospital Presbyterian, Newport Beach, CA, USA

Translational Genomics Research Institute, Phoenix, AZ, USA

Thomas Diflo, MD, FACS Department of Surgery, Section of Intra-abdominal Organ Transplantation, Westchester Medical Center, New York Medical College, Valhalla, NY, USA

Charles R. Doarn, MBA Family and Community Medicine, University of Cincinnati, College of Medicine, Cincinnati, OH, USA

Xiang Da (Eric) Dong, MD, FACS New York Medical College, School of Medicine, Department of Surgery, Surgical Oncology, Westchester, Medical Center, Valhalla, NY, USA

Maureen Doran, MS, MBA Center for Regional Healthcare Innovation, WMCHealth, Hawthorne, NY, USA

Andrew M. Eisen, MD Graduate Medical Education, The Valley Health System, Las Vegas, NV, USA

James M. Feeney, MD, FACS Department of Surgery, Westchester Medical Center, Valhalla, NY, USA

John J. Fildes, MD Department of Surgery, UNLV School of Medicine, Las Vegas, NV, USA

Abe Fingerhut, MD, FACS, FRCPS, FRCS Surgical Research, Surgical Department, University of Graz, Graz, Austria

Leslie S. Forrest, MHA Graduate Medical Education, The Valley Health System, Las Vegas, NV, USA

William H. Frishman, MD, MACP Department of Medicine, Westchester Medical Center, New York Medical College, Valhalla, NY, USA

Renee Garrick, MD, FACP Department of Medicine, New York Medical College, Westchester Medical Center, Valhalla, NY, USA

Shekhar Gogna, MD Department of Surgery, Westchester Medical Center, Valhalla, NY, USA

Joshua B. Goldberg, MD Department of Surgery, Westchester Medical Center, Valhalla, NY, USA

Olga Golubnitschaja, PhD, MD Radiological Clinic, Rheinische Friedrich-Wilhelms-Universität Bonn, Bonn, Germany

Breast Cancer Research Centre, Rheinische Friedrich-Wilhelms-Universität Bonn, Bonn, Germany

Centre for Integrated Oncology, Cologne-Bonn, Rheinische Friedrich-Wilhelms-Universität Bonn, Bonn, Germany

European Association for Predictive, Preventive and Personalised Medicine, EPMA, Brussels, Belgium

Priya Goyal, MD Department of Surgery, Westchester Medical Center, Valhalla, NY, USA

Gabriel Gruionu, PhD Division of Trauma, Emergency Surgery and Surgical Critical Care, Massachusetts General Hospital/Harvard Medical School, Boston, MA, USA

Lucian Gheorghe Gruionu, PhD Medical Engineering Laboratory, Faculty of Mechanics and the INCESA Institute, University of Craiova, Craiova, Dolj, Romania

Alejandro Guerrero, MD, MSc, FACS Acute Care Surgery, InterTrauma Medical, New York, NY, USA

Edward C. Halperin, MD, MA New York Medical College, Valhalla, NY, USA

Amy Joseph, MSN, NP Graduate Medical Education, The Valley Health System, Las Vegas, NV, USA

Bellal Joseph, MD, FACS Division of Trauma, Critical Care, Emergency Surgery, and Burns, Department of Surgery, University of Arizona, Tucson, AZ, USA

Saju Joseph, MD Graduate Medical Education, The Valley Health System, Las Vegas, NV, USA

Masashi Kai, MD Department of Surgery, Westchester Medical Center, Valhalla, NY, USA

June Keenan, MS, MPH Center for Regional Healthcare Innovation, WMCHealth, Hawthorne, NY, USA

Martha M. Kennedy, PhD, CRNP, RN Department of Surgery, The Johns Hopkins Hospital, Baltimore, MD, USA

Steven L. Lansman, MD, PhD Department of Surgery, Westchester Medical Center, Valhalla, NY, USA

Rifat Latifi, MD, FACS, FICS New York Medical College, School of Medicine, Department of Surgery and Westchester Medical Center, Valhalla, NY, USA

Zvi Lefkovitz, MD Department of Radiology, Westchester Medical Center, Valhalla, NY, USA

Ramin Malekan, MD Department of Surgery, Westchester Medical Center, Valhalla, NY, USA

Allison G. McNickle, MD UNLV School of Medicine, Las Vegas, NV, USA

Ronald C. Merrell, MD Department of Surgery, Virginia Commonwealth University, Richmond, VA, USA

Christopher Nabors, MD, PhD Department of Medicine, Westchester Medical Center, New York Medical College, Valhalla, NY, USA

Kevin J. O'Leary, MD, MS Department of Internal Medicine, Northwestern Feinberg School of Medicine, Chicago, IL, USA

Angelo Ortiz, BS, AAS Department of Radiology, Westchester Medical Center, Valhalla, NY, USA

Hunter M. Pattison, MD Department of Emergency Medicine, UC Davis Medical Center, Sacramento, CA, USA

Stephen J. Peterson, MD Department of Medicine, New York Presbyterian Brooklyn Methodist Hospital, Brooklyn, NY, USA

Jake Poore Integrated Loyalty Systems, Orlando, FL, USA

Kartik Prabhakaran, MD, MHS, FACS Department of Surgery, Westchester Medical Center, Valhalla, NY, USA

David J. Samson, MS, Epidemiology Department of Surgery, Westchester Medical Center, Valhalla, NY, USA

John A. Savino, MD, FACS Westchester Medical Center Health Network, New York Medical College, Valhalla, NY, USA

Michael J. Seiler, RT, CLLP Department of Radiology, Westchester Medical Center, Valhalla, NY, USA

Jane C. Shivnan, MScN, RN, AOCN Health Care Consultant, Glen Burnie, MD, USA

David Spielvogel, MD Department of Radiology, Westchester Medical Center, Valhalla, NY, USA

Janet (Jessie) Sullivan, MD Center for Regional Healthcare Innovation, WMCHealth, Hawthorne, NY, USA

Elizabeth H. Tilley, PhD Department of Surgery, Westchester Medical Center, Valhalla, NY, USA

James A. Unti, MD, MS, FACS Department of Surgery, Saint Joseph Hospital, Chicago, IL, USA

Selman Uranues, MD Department of Surgery, Section for Surgical Research, Medical University of Graz, Graz, Austria

Lara Stolzenburg Veeser, MBiotech, MSc Department of Business Administration, Carlos III University, Getafe, Madrid, Spain

Gregory Veillette, MD, FACS New York Medical College, Westchester Medical Center, Valhalla, NY, USA

George C. Velmahos, MD, PhD, MSEd Division of Trauma, Emergency Surgery, and Surgical Critical Care, Massachusetts General Hospital, Boston, MA, USA

Deborah Viola, MBA, PhD Data Management and Analytics, Westchester Medical Center Health Network, Valhalla, NY, USA

James Elvis Waha, MD Department of Surgery, Division of General Surgery, Medical University of Graz, Graz, Austria

Nabil Wasif, MD, MPH Department of Surgery, Mayo Clinic Arizona, Phoenix, AZ, USA

Jane S. Wey, MD Department of Surgery, Riverside Health System, Newport News, VA, USA

Vaughn Whittaker, MB, MPH Department of Surgery, Westchester Medical Center and New York Medical College, School of Medicine, Valhalla, NY, USA

Muhammad Zeeshan, MD Division of Trauma, Critical Care, Emergency Surgery, and Burns, Department of Surgery, University of Arizona, Tucson, AZ, USA

Part I

Hospital Transformation and Academic Health Systems

1 The New Medical World Order: Not So Flat

Rifat Latifi

Introduction

A few decades ago, the medical world did not have any particular major order. Each country took care of people the way they thought it would be best and they could afford or knew how to do it. With some exceptions, hospitals for the most part existed and worked in silos, and isolated each from other (hospital for the lungs, hospital for the heart, hospital for infectious diseases, etc.), and all of them were separated from other industries. Now, technological advances have established a new medical order which, when combined with hospital and corporate leadership, is responsible for new developments that are accessible to millions of people. This new medical order has transformed the healthcare industry into a web-linked interdependent, complex, competitive industry, with the philosophy of domination, takeover of hospitals and creating large corporation of healthcare industry for the most part. This world order is with full of contrast and dichotomy, growing the wider gap between the hospitals of western world and third world countries and between hospitals of rural and urban America. So, the medical world, after all, may not be so flat.

How does one see the world? It depends – on where you stand, what stage of life you're in, your socioeconomic status, your educational achievements, where you live, and where you grew up. As a child, the world is different from the world that adults see. When I was a child, the world seemed small as I looked from the hills of the village I grew up in. I grew up without technology or electricity. My only connection to the outside world was the library in the village and the books that I read. As a child, I always wondered if the moon and the stars, the sun and the rain, and the tears and the laughter that happened in my village were the same around the world. My world was different then. It was small, contained to my village and the books I read. But as I grew older, the world grew, too, yet for some reason becomes smaller.

Like most physicians, I have spent my entire adult life in the hospital. I was educated in Prishtina, Kosovo. I worked as a researcher at Texas Medical Center in Houston and Pennsylvania Hospital in Philadelphia as a fellow to Dr. Stanley J. Dudrick and later did surgical residencies at Cleveland Clinic Foundation and Yale University and a trauma and critical care fellowship at Lincoln Medical Center in the Bronx. I was a staff surgeon at Virginia Commonwealth in Richmond; University Medical Center in Tucson; Hamad General Hospital in Doha, Qatar; and finally Westchester Medical Center in Valhalla, New York.

R. Latifi (✉)
New York Medical College, School of Medicine, Department of Surgery and Westchester Medical Center, Valhalla, NY, USA
e-mail: rifat_latifi@nymc.edu; rifat.latifi@wmchealth.org

R. Latifi (ed.), *The Modern Hospital*, https://doi.org/10.1007/978-3-030-01394-3_1

So, like most surgeons and physicians, I grew up in the hospitals. Moreover, I had the honor over the years to work as a volunteer, lecture as visiting professor, rebuild healthcare system through telemedicine, or simply had an opportunity to visit 75 countries. This has given me the opportunity to understand the new medical world order. Of course, my perspective is colored by my upbringing and biases, and this introductory chapter to this book on modern hospital is a personal perspective.

Is the Medical World Flat?

"The world is flat," cried Tom Friedman in his famous book [1] describing workflow software, open sourcing, outsourcing, off-shoring, supply chaining, in-sourcing, and information. Subsequently, one of the best known trauma surgeons in the world, Donald Trunkey, said "the medical world is flat too" [2] and effectively described many of the processes that demonstrate the de facto new medical world order. However, I don't think that's the case when it comes to medical care worldwide. Or maybe, the question should be asked, how flat is flat? Despite the considerable progress that has been made, the medical world is still divided into those who have everything and those who barely get by. In other words, there have never been wider differences between hospitals in rich and poor countries in providing care for their populations, despite many processes, guidelines, and other progress made worldwide.

Yet, "few institutions have undergone as radical metamorphosis as have hospitals in their modern history," writes Paul Star in his classic and must-read book for anyone who works in medicine, *The Social Transformation of American Medicine* [1]. He continues to say that "in developing from places of dreaded impurity and exiled human wreckage into awesome new moral identity," hospitals have simply undergone an amazing transformation. The metamorphosis of hospitals has been a result of metamorphosis of the medical field overall. Surgeons and physicians and with that hospitals have combined intuition, ingenuity, and courage to advance medical technologies around the world. The industry is developing in multiple facets. Patients are becoming better educated consumers and expecting better outcomes, and hospitals are undergoing major transformations by embracing and integrating technological advances. These are just a few of the factors which provide evidence that surgery, trauma, and critical care medicine and all other fields of the medicine have undergone an amazing evolution. The best consequence of this evolution is that the care of the patient has been greatly improved, outcomes are significantly better, and the development and appreciation of surgical science have progressed immensely. To be a student of surgery and medicine today requires that one must embrace the technological advances and the "new surgery and medicine world order" in addition to becoming a master of the anatomy, physiology, and pathology of the disease. Following and understanding all the attempts of countries around the world to reform their healthcare system have become a profession on its own [3], some of which are politically based, wealth-based, and based on other factors.

The transition from death houses to kitchen surgery to modern, scientifically based, evidence-based hospitals is a reflection of the collective contribution of human development, various scientific achievements, and advances in every field of medicine and surgery through technological revolution. But, in this social transformation, modern hospitals have become an industry on their own. Hospitals now attract the interest of other businesses and industries which didn't used to pay attention to the medical industry. The small community hospital no longer belongs to the community, but is a part a major healthcare conglomerate, often geographically far apart.

The merger, acquisition, and scaling (MAS) or frankly takeover was prevalent mostly among pharmaceutical industries [4]. However, this practice now is very common among healthcare institutions and thus creation of hospital chains. Thus, while old hospital has evolved and transformed into the "modern hospital," this new modern hospital in fact is no longer "independent" but part of major corporations, for the most part. The hospital as we know it today exists in a new era – the era of major business conglomerates and managed care organization swallowing small and large hospitals, buying their own health insurance plans, and dominating the market of medicine. The competition is fiercer then ever and only the best of the best will survive. There is a prevailing thought that in a very short time, there will be around 20–25 major healthcare systems in the USA that will dictate how physicians take care of patients, what hospitals look like, and even which patients get what kind of procedures or surgical operations. While studies by Burns et al. [4] address many questions that have to do with MAS of pharmaceutical industry, all these questions can be adopted and asked to address the MAS of hospitals. One has to wonder though, does merger and acquisition (not sure about scaling) of hospitals by new mega chains actually offer more leverage? What kind of challenges and opportunities can be created? Will this lead to more innovations and improvement on processes, or will it create unfortunate situations where faculty will be leaving the institution because of these new acquisitions and new bosses and new corporate rules? There are still few unknown issues: which acquisitions and mergers will be best for the future of medicine? When academic hospital takes over smaller nonacademic hospitals with hope that they will create a new academic network, will this improve healthcare of that community, or, as many from the business world may believe, can the corporate world "teach" academic medical institutions how to run themselves more businesslike? Will this translate to better medicine, better healthcare, and more research and development for humankind? These and other questions perhaps will be answered in in the future by historian of healthcare reforms and students of healthcare.

While examples of both of these scenarios are plenty around us, it has become clear that medicine and hospitals are no longer only have to see themselves as treatment centers for the sick and injured, but have to look after the bottom (business) line. Moreover, it is a complex and competitive business that is being watched and managed by government agencies on the federal and state level, insurance companies, social media, patients, and patients' advocates, to the point that it may not be fun anymore going into the business of medicine for young generation.

Another major trend in recent years is planting major medical franchise or medical schools in the countries that are medically not well developed but can afford western-type care and education. While this is not the main theme of this chapter and the book in your hand, the question remains as to the effectiveness of providing care to those who perhaps could not afford such expensive care and the long-term sustainability of such operations.

Two Faces of Medical World

There are at least two major faces of the medical world [5]. In the first, we have everything we need. We waste money by duplicating and sometimes tripling the expenses for excessive testing. This face begs the question: are we really making a major difference in outcomes?

The other face of the medical world often lacks even the most basic elements of care. In order to understand and address these major gaps created between the rich and poor countries, the Lancet Commission on Global Surgery was launched in January 2014 [5].

The commission brought together an international, multidisciplinary team of 25 commissioners, supported by advisors and collaborators in more than 110 countries and 6 continents, and focused on the domains of healthcare delivery and management; workforce, training, and education; economics and finance; and information management. In 2015, the commission published the report in which it presented the following five key messages as a set of indicators and recommendations to improve access to safe, affordable surgical and anesthesia care in LMICs and a template for a national surgical plan:

1. Five billion people do not have access to safe, affordable surgical and anesthesia care when needed. Access is worst in low-income and lower-middle-income countries, where nine of ten people cannot access basic surgical care.

2. One hundred and forty-three million additional surgical procedures are needed in LMICs each year to save lives and prevent disability. Of the 313 million procedures undertaken worldwide each year, only 6% occur in the poorest countries, where over a third of the world's population lives. Low operative volumes are associated with high case-fatality rates from common, treatable surgical conditions. Unmet need is greatest in eastern, western, and central sub-Saharan Africa and South Asia.
3. Thirty-three million individuals face catastrophic health expenditure due to payment for surgery and anesthesia care each year. An additional 48 million cases of catastrophic expenditure are attributable to the nonmedical costs of accessing surgical care. A quarter of people who have a surgical procedure will incur financial catastrophe as a result of seeking care. The burden of catastrophic expenditure for surgery is highest in low-income and lower-middle-income countries and, within any country, lands most heavily on poor people.
4. Investing in surgical services in LMICs is affordable, saves lives, and promotes economic growth. To meet present and projected population demands, urgent investment in human and physical resources for surgical and anesthesia care is needed. If LMICs were to scale-up surgical services at rates achieved by the present best-performing LMICs, two-thirds of countries would be able to reach a minimum operative volume of 5000 surgical procedures per 100,000 population by 2030. Without urgent and accelerated investment in surgical scale-up, LMICs will continue to have losses in economic productivity, estimated cumulatively at US $12.3 trillion (2010 US$, purchasing power parity) between 2015 and 2030.
5. Surgery is an "indivisible, indispensable part of health care." Surgical and anesthesia care should be an integral component of a national health system in countries at all levels of development. Surgical services are a prerequisite for the full attainment of local and global health goals in areas as diverse as cancer, injury, cardiovascular disease, infection, and reproductive, maternal, neonatal, and child health. Universal health coverage and the health aspirations set out in the post-2015 Sustainable Development Goals will be impossible to achieve without ensuring that surgical and anesthesia care.

This is the "other world" described on this report by Lancet Commission on Global Surgery [5] and others [6]. Alkire et al. [6] modeled access to surgical services using the commission's definition of access, which includes capacity, safety, timeliness, and affordability, and used a mathematical modeling approach to answer the following question: How many people worldwide lack access to safe, affordable, and timely surgical care in 196 countries with respect to four dimensions: timeliness, surgical capacity, safety, and affordability? They found that at least 4.8 billion people of the world's population do not have access to surgery. This is higher, in fact more than double than previous estimates [7]. The proportion of the population without access varied widely when stratified by epidemiological region: greater than 95% of the population in South Asia and central, eastern, and western sub-Saharan Africa do not have access to care, whereas less than 5% of the population in Australasia, high-income North America, and Western Europe lack access [6].

There are plenty of reasons why this is such a dismal situation, but insufficient surgical infrastructure including lack of surgeons, space, and technology is the main one. Moreover, millions of people each year face ruinous financial hardship when they are forced to pay for their own surgery and anesthesia. For example, low-income and lower-middle-income countries, representing 48% of the global population, have 20% of this workforce or 19% of all surgeons, 15% of anesthesiologists, and 29% of obstetricians. Africa and Southeast Asia are particularly underserved. In terms of density, low-income countries have 0.7 providers per 100,000 population

(IQR 0.5–1.9), compared with 5.5 (1.8–28.2) in lower-middle-income countries, 22.6 (11.6–56.7). These parts of the world struggle to take care of their populations [8].

So, while a large portion of the world struggles to provide basic healthcare services to their population, such as essential surgery (basic ventilator support), many hospitals rely on volunteers or organizations from the developed world to serve these populations.

In contrast, we in the western part of the world mostly (with some exceptions – see below care in rural America) have access to modern, highly technical and scientific medical and surgical care.

About 3.7 billion people risk catastrophic expenditure if they need surgery [9]. Every year, 33 million of them are driven to financial catastrophe from the costs of surgery alone, and 48 million from nonmedical costs, leading to 81 million cases worldwide [10]. The burden of catastrophic expenditure is highest in low- and middle-income countries; within any country, it falls on the poor. Estimates are sensitive to the definition of catastrophic expenditure and the costs of care. The inequitable burden distribution is robust to model assumptions.

On the other hand, in our western world, we use the most advanced medical and surgical technologies from nanotechnologies and genomics to robotic-assisted surgery. As a result of significant medical advances, many diseases that were deadly until just few years ago, today, are fully treatable. Yes, the cost is astronomical but the cure is possible.

A number of examples are summarized by Burns on his book [3] that illustrate technological convergence including examples of the use of pharmacodynamics and pharmacokinetics that pharmaceutical companies use to deliver drugs; radiological and minimally invasive techniques to access neurovascular, cardiovascular, and molecular system; and finally neuron-based pharmacotherapy.

This unprecedented development has made the dichotomy in the medical world even wider. A baby born in Andes of Peru, where the Amazon River begins to flow, will live less than 40 years, which is less than half the life expectancy of people living in the western world. Only in the last 20–30 years has life expectancy increased significantly among western countries. For example, the largest increase in our trauma population admission at the Westchester Medical Center Health Network Level I Trauma Center has been among patients greater than 85 years old. These dramatic changes are due to many factors but mostly due to technological advances. The dynamic of technological evolution is interdependent with many factors, including creating and proving complex clinical research, navigating through science and intellectual property, working on competitive environment, and adopting to and redefining or reconfiguring the business platform based on preclinical and clinical information [4].

Can LIC and LMI countries afford such investment to ensure all the above factors which will eventually lead to mega expenses to cure their population? The simple answer is no or at least not yet.

Even in the western world, there is a similar lack of quality of care. In the rural western world, the quality of care is often low, and there is a lack of basic medical access, let alone access to expert medical care. While this introductory chapter was not meant to delve into detailed data analysis of the new medical world order, it is clear that the discrepancies between rich, middle-income and low-income countries are tremendous. How to reduce this gap is a matter of debate, but I believe hospitals should be the same everywhere in the world. Care should be the same in the rich countries and in poor countries, and in the city and in rural regions. We do not accept quality of agriculture technologies in the rural region to be inferior to the one near the city, right? Why should accept a lesser quality hospital, less experienced surgeon, and lack of anesthesia and medication?

Finally, the Lancet Commission on Global Surgery has produced a "wish list" or target to reduce the major gap in global surgery. This wish list, while noble, is very ambitious and includes a minimum of 80% coverage of essential surgical and anesthesia services per country; 100% of countries with a least 20 surgical, anesthetic, and obstetric physicians per 100,000 population; 80% of countries by 2020 and 100% of countries by 2030 tracking surgical volume; a minimum of 5000 procedures per 100,000 population; 80% of countries by 2020 and 100% of countries by 2030 tracking perioperative mortality; in 2020 assess global data and set national targets; 100% protection against impoverishment from out-of-pocket payments for surgical and anesthesia care; and 100% protection against catastrophic expenditure from out-of-pocket payments for surgical and anesthesia care by 2030.

There is no question that these are great "marching orders" and goal for all of us. Perhaps, if and when all these goals and objectives are met, the hospitals of the world will resemble one another, and the world may be flat as seen by few other authors.

In summary, the new medical world order has created gaps that are difficult to reduce or erase between the rich and poor countries and between the urban and rural world and will need serious investment in human capacities, infrastructure, and policies from lawmakers and philanthropists. The gap is even more pronounced between the rural and urban region in LIC and MICs. Pharmaceutical and medical industry companies have made great progress in their scientific and financial bottom line but still have work to do when it comes to reducing and hopefully eliminating this gap. Maybe then the world will look a bit flat.

Summary

There are no questions that our world has become smaller and maybe flatter. Yet, I think that there is plenty for us to do to make sure that the concept of equal care and similar outcomes around the world be achieved, and there is much more that every one of us can and must do.

References

1. Starr P. The social transformation of American medicine: the rise of a sovereign profession and the making of a vast industry. New York: Basics Books; 1984.
2. Trunkey D. The medical world is flat too. World J Surg. 2008;32(8):1583–604. https://doi.org/10.1007/s00268-008-9522-z.
3. Raffel MW. Healthcare and reform in industrialized countries. Pennsylvania: The Pennsylvania State Press, University Park; 1997.
4. Burns LR. The business of healthcare innovation. Cambridge: Cambridge University Press; 2005.
5. Meara JG, Leather AJM, Hagander L, et al. Global surgery 2030: evidence and solutions for achieving health, welfare, and economic development. Lancet. 2015;386(9993):569–624.
6. Alkire BC, Raykar NP, Shrime MG, et al. Global access to surgical care: a modelling study. Lancet Glob Health. 2015;3(6):e316–e23.
7. Funk LM, Weiser TG, Berry WR, et al. Global operating theatre distribution and pulse oximetry supply: an estimation from reported data. Lancet. 2010;376:1055–61.
8. Holmer H, et al. Global distribution of surgeons, anaesthesiologists, and obstetricians. Lancet Glob Heal. 2015;3:S9–S11.
9. Casey KM. The global impact of surgical volunteerism. Surg Clin North Am. 2007;87(4):949–60.
10. Shrime MG, Dare AJ, Alkire BC, O'Neill K, Meara JG. Catastrophic expenditure to pay for surgery: a global estimate. Lancet Glob Health. 2015;3(02):S38–44. https://doi.org/10.1016/S2214-109X(15)70085-9.

2 Five Transformative Episodes in the History of the American Hospital

Edward C. Halperin

An Arrogant First Year Medical Student

In 1975, as a first year student at the Yale University School of Medicine, I was required to take a course in "Behavioral Medicine." The syllabus ranged over a variety of subjects at the intersection of psychiatry, psychology, and social medicine. The instructors were two senior psychiatry residents. Our class was required to read two books which had been published in 1969: *People in Pain* by Mark Zborowski has since acquired the status of a classic in medical anthropology and Philip Roth's novel *Portnoy's Complaint*, which was considered highly controversial at the time [1, 2]. I denounced the latter in class as salacious self-hating anti-Semitic tripe. My teachers, in turn, criticized me as being close-minded and unwilling to explore new and challenging ideas.

Eventually the course turned its attention to what a hospital was and was not. The teachers were advocating the point of view that a hospital was a generalized "healing or therapeutic community" – a social institution of great complexity and nuance. When I was called upon by the teachers to offer my opinion, I confirmed my teacher's indictment of being close-minded with all the arrogance and self-righteousness of youth by declaiming that a hospital was a glorified hotel that needed to be efficiently managed by paid managers so that the doctors could practice medicine within it. Perhaps this chapter is my opportunity to make amends for my youthful arrogance. Far wiser individuals than I, in the last four decades, have devoted considerable time and attention to studying the history, organization, performance, strengths, and weaknesses of American hospitals [3, 4]. In this chapter I will strive to make a small contribution to the conversation about the place of the American hospital.

What Is a Hospital?

The etymology of the English noun *hospital* is from the Old French *hospital* and Latin *hospitale*, a place of reception for guests. The first usage in English of the word *hospital* to describe an institution or establishment for the care of the sick or wounded, or for those requiring medical treatment, dates from the fifteenth and sixteenth centuries. The words *hotel* and *hostel* are doublets of hospital. Other contemporary and obsolete words closely related in origin to hospital are *hospice*, *hospitably* (adverb, in a hospitable manner), *hospitable*, *hospitage* (the position of a guest), *hospitality*, *hospitaller* (in a religious house or hospice, the person who receives guests), *host*, *hosteler* (one who receives guests), *hostelry* (an inn or guest house), *hoster* (innkeeper), and *hostess* [5].

E. C. Halperin (✉)
New York Medical College, Valhalla, NY, USA
e-mail: Edward_halperin@nymc.edu

R. Latifi (ed.), *The Modern Hospital*, https://doi.org/10.1007/978-3-030-01394-3_2

Our fundamental idea of a hospital as a physical place of, at least, hospitable refuge and, at most, a place for the provision of scientifically skilled and compassionate care for the sick has evolved. Hospitals are now linked to outpatient care, health professions education, and biomedical research. They are major employers in their local communities – indeed, in some parts of the United States, they are *the* major employer. Hospitals have been characterized as part of a medical-industrial food chain in which patients/customers enter via the outpatient clinic, are admitted into hospitals for procedures and discharged to post-hospital care systems, and throughout the process, are direct or indirect purchasers of professional care, drugs, and medical procedures. Simply stated, the hospital business is a big business. By the onset of the twenty-first century, the simple definition of hospital as an institution for the care of the sick or wounded, or for those who require medical treatment, has been subsumed into a long list of adjectival modifications or alternative words or phrases. Here is a partial list: academic medical center, army medical center, cancer center, children's hospital, community hospital, health center, health system, heart center, heart hospital, medical center, naval hospital, research hospital, teaching hospital, and university hospital.

For some massive hospital systems, the word *hospital* has been deemed too confining and too restrictive. Thus the former North Shore-Long Island Jewish Hospital system has shed any nomenclature associations with Long Island and Judaism and has been rebranded as *Northwell Health*; Duke University Medical Center has been dubbed *Duke Health*; Johns Hopkins Hospital is *Johns Hopkins Medicine*; and the University of Pittsburgh Medical Center is now *UPMC: Life Changing Medicine, an integrated global health-care company*.

Writing history is all about making choices. No historian can cite all sources, explore all avenues, and cover every event. To do so would not be history, it would be chronology. A historian has to pick and choose what events to focus upon. For this chapter, I will focus on what I believe are five transformative episodes in the history of the American hospital.

Episode 1: The Creation of Public Poor Houses in the United States and How They Evolved into Tax-Supported Hospitals

Many of America's public hospitals came into existence not as institutions for care of the sick but, rather, as institutions for the care of the poor [3]. This is one of the initial transformative episodes in the history of the American hospital.

The Dutch and British colonial governments on the east coast of what is now the United States quickly had to deal with the provision of food, clothing, and shelter for indigents. It was ascertained that those cared-for in so-called *poor houses* consisted of two general populations: those who were poor and those who were poor because they were too physically or mentally ill to work. Colonial public hospitals were created for the care of this latter group [6]. Let's consider three examples.

The City Almshouse of Philadelphia was founded in 1730–1731. By 1751 a group of physicians and leading citizens of Philadelphia petitioned the Pennsylvania Provincial Assembly to establish an institution for the care of "the insane and indigent sick." Benjamin Franklin worked actively for the hospital's creation and was named the founding clerk of the new Pennsylvania Hospital (Fig. 2.1). The hospital's Board of Managers petitioned Thomas and Richard Penn in England to donate a site. Through a combination of land purchase and gifts, a site was obtained, and the country's oldest hospital, older than the country itself, was established [6].

At the 1769 graduation ceremonies of the medical department of Kings College of New York, now Columbia University, conducted at Trinity Church at the southern tip of Manhattan, the graduation speaker, Dr. Samuel Bard, told the assembly that New York City was in dire need of a general hospital both for the care of the sick and the education of new physicians. In 1771 a royal charter was granted to "The Society of the Hospital, in the City of New York." The time required for acquisition of land, the destruction of the newly constructed building by fire, and the Revolutionary War prevented the hospital from opening until 1791 [6].

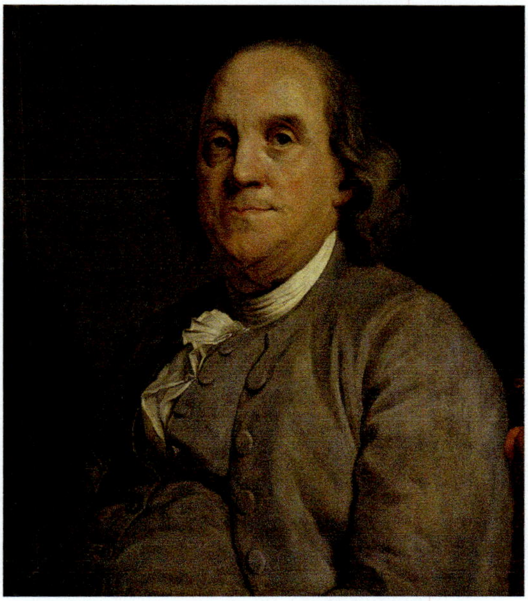

Fig. 2.1 Benjamin Franklin (1706–1790) was one of the founders of the Pennsylvania Hospital designed "to care for the sick-poor and insane who were wandering the streets of Philadelphia." (Reprinted from Benjamin Franklin by Joseph Siffred Duplessis. Wikipedia. Retrieved from: https://commons.wikimedia.org/wiki/File:Benjamin_Franklin_by_Joseph_Siffred_Duplessis_left.jpg)

A third example of the creation of the public hospital out of a poor house is to be found in one of the Dutch settlements across the East River from New Amsterdam, later New York: the seventeenth-century Dutch village of Breuckelen on the eastern tip of Long Island. Breuckelen was dubbed Brooklyn and shared Kings County in the colony of New York with other settlements called Flatbush, New Utrecht, Flatlands, Bushwick, and Gravesend. Eventually the name Brooklyn was adopted for the entire settlement, and the names of the other towns were incorporated as the names of the individual neighborhoods of Brooklyn. In 1898 Brooklyn merged with Manhattan, parts of the Bronx, and some rural areas of Kings County, Queens, and Staten Island and formed the modern city of New York [7]. Brooklyn remains the most populous of New York's five boroughs.

In British colonial Brooklyn, the care of the poor was done by a system of contracts. Needy individuals were placed with a family for room and board at public expense. The system was expensive. Eventually the burden of cost combined with a desire to consolidate the care of the poor within a more humane system led to the creation of public almshouses.

Within Brooklyn's almshouse "able-bodied and infirm paupers, the sick, the crippled and helpless, idiots, lunatics, criminals and persons suffering with contagious diseases were all housed in the one building...the lot of the first recorded physician [of the Brooklyn almshouse] could not have been a happy one" [8]. In 1835 Brooklyn's Superintendent of the Poor along with physicians working at the county almshouse proposed making a distinction between the indigent and those in the almshouse who were both indigent and in need of medical care. They proposed the creation of a public hospital "for lunatics" and for "paupers laboring under infectious disease" [8]. In 1837 the public hospital of Brooklyn, Kings County Hospital, was established and remains in operation today.

The New York City newspaper editor, poet, author, and public figure William Cullen Bryant, in an 1876 speech, articulated the role of the hospital in providing care for the indigent sick. By the time Bryant spoke the role of the hospital for meeting a societal obligation was well entrenched in America:

> In all the centuries that preceded the hospital era, and while the Greek and Roman civilizations were are their height, there were no institutions…no retreated where the friendless, sick, the old man consumed at once by age and illness, and the poor man wounded and mangled by accident could be received and kindly treated. It was the religion of love and sympathy that brought in the hospital and gathered into its friendly wards, and laid on its comfortable beds, waited upon by experienced nurses, those who otherwise might have perished. [9]

Episode 2: The Rise of Roman Catholic Hospitals in the United States

The Origins of Roman Catholic Hospital in the United States

In the Middle Ages in Europe, communities grappled with the problem of how to deal with coreligionists who became ill while traveling. Christian and Jewish communities developed social and physical structures to house and care for these itinerants. The tradition of faith-based health care continued in the New World. There was a strong tradition in the Anglican/Episcopal, Baptist, Lutheran, Methodist, Presbyterian, and Seventh-Day Adventist communities of creating hospitals. Faith-based fraternal organizations also played a role [3, 10].

American Roman Catholic hospitals were founded in the mid-nineteenth century to respond to epidemics, the growing numbers of Roman Catholic European immigrants, and the social problems inherent to the concentration of these immigrants in urban centers [3] (Fig. 2.2). Throughout the nineteenth century and well into the twentieth century, there was a strong anti-Catholic sentiment among American Protestants. The presidential nominations of Alfred Smith in 1928 and John F. Kennedy in 1960 provoked public hostility toward Roman Catholics and "Creeping Papism." Many Roman Catholic hospitals were located in densely populated urban areas to provide services to Catholics who lived in their parishes. Strong attachments were formed between the local Catholic population and "their hospital" [11].

What Is a Roman Catholic Hospital?

There are three general types of American Roman Catholic hospitals. *Archdiocesan hospitals* are under the immediate control of the local bishop or cardinal. *Order hospitals* are owned by a particular religious order such as the Jesuits or the Sisters of Charity. *Public juridical hospitals* are public corporations which operate hospitals under guidelines of the church. Examples of the latter in the United States include Ascension Healthcare and Catholic Health West.

The United States Conference of Catholic Bishops periodically publishes a printed and online booklet titled *Ethical and Religious Directives for Catholic Health Care Services* [12]. It contains specific directives for the operation of a Roman Catholic hospital including lists of prohibited medical services. Observance of these directives varies, to some extent, among American Roman Catholic hospitals.

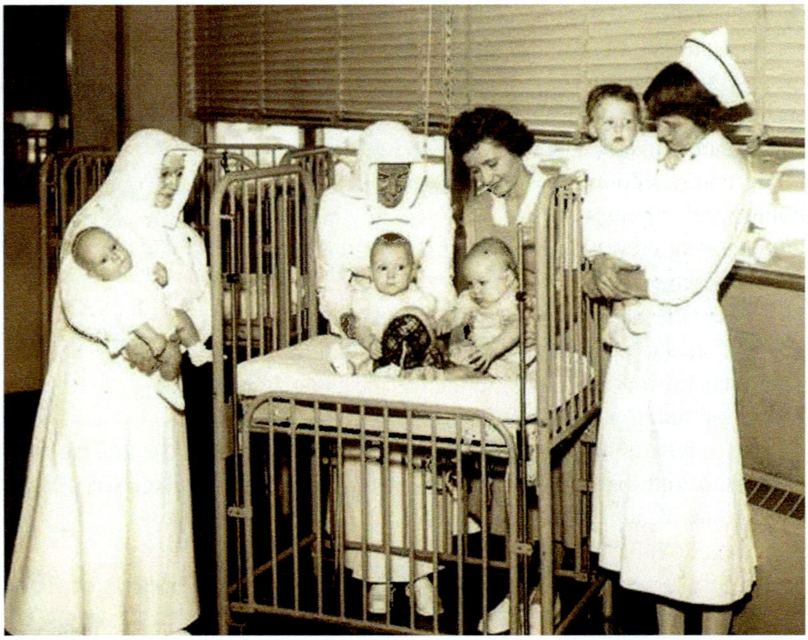

Fig. 2.2 St. Vincent's Nursery and Babies Hospital of Montclair, New Jersey, traced its origins to the late 1800s when the Sisters of Charity of Saint Elizabeth opened the Saint Vincent Foundling Asylum in Immaculate Conception parish in Montclair to care for abandoned children. St. Vincent's ultimately merged into what is now called the St. Joseph's Healthcare System based in Paterson, New Jersey. (Courtesy of St. Joseph's Health, Paterson, NJ)

The Impact of the Expansion of the Market Share of Roman Catholic Hospitals on US Health Care

In 2013 it was estimated that one in ten acute-care hospital beds in the United States were in a Roman Catholic-owned or Roman Catholic-affiliated hospital. By 2017 that number had risen to one in six acute-care hospital beds. The increasing presence of Roman Catholic hospitals is a result both of the explosion of hospital mergers and acquisitions in the United States and the growth of management contracts. With the increasing number of public and other hospitals either signing management contracts with Roman Catholic hospital systems or being acquired by them, the number of hospital beds being operated in accordance with the *Ethical and Religious Directives* has grown [13]. In 46 regions of the United States, the sole local community hospital is a Roman Catholic hospital [13].

The implications of this expansion of the presence of Catholic hospitals have proven to be most controversial in the realm of women's reproductive health services. If they are fully compliant with the *Ethical and Religious Directives*, Roman Catholic hospitals will not permit an abortion to be performed, will not provide "backup services" for outpatient abortion clinics, will not allow elective sterilization such as the performance of a tubal ligation on a woman at the same time as a Caesarean delivery, and will not promote or dispense contraception. Sexual assault victims are not to receive treatment that would destroy a fertilized egg or prevent it from implanting. Couples cannot receive sperm or egg donations from people other than their spouses. When a Roman Catholic hospital is the sole local provider, the full range of reproductive health services in an area is partially curtailed. Furthermore, the federal law protects the right of hospitals and doctors to refrain from conducting abortions or sterilization procedures if that is their wish.

Allegations have been made that the lives and safety of some women have been jeopardized by this situation. In 2013, the American Civil Liberties Union (ACLU) sued the United States Conference of Catholic Bishops on behalf of a Michigan woman who went to her county hospital when she was 18-week pregnant because her water broke. Instead of terminating the pregnancy to avoid infection, the complaint alleged, Mercy Health Partners discharged the patient with pain medication in accordance with the Catholic directives. She later miscarried after contracting a severe infection, according to the suit. A federal judge dismissed the case on jurisdictional grounds – saying it was not the role of the courts to interfere in religious matters. The case is under appeal [13, 14]. Multiple other suits of a similar nature have been filed.

We can expect that the story of the transformative role of Roman Catholic hospitals in the United States will continue to be written [15].

Episode 3: The Rise and Fall of the American Jewish Hospital

The Stuyvesant Pledge and the Colonial Origins of the American Jewish Hospital

In 1654 23 Jewish refugees from the Inquisition in Brazil boarded the French frigate *Sainte Catherine* and sailed to North America. In September the ship entered New Amsterdam's harbor [16]. The director-general of New Netherlands, Peter Stuyvesant, requested permission from his superiors at the Dutch West India Company in Amsterdam to refuse entry to these "deceitful...very repugnant...hateful enemies and blasphemers of the name of Christ" (Fig. 2.3). Stuyvesant was disappointed to receive a reply wherein his Board of Directors reminded him that some of the company's shareholders were Dutch Jews. He was ordered to admit the 23 refugees provided that "the poor among them shall not become a burden to the company or to the community but be supported by their own nation" [16].

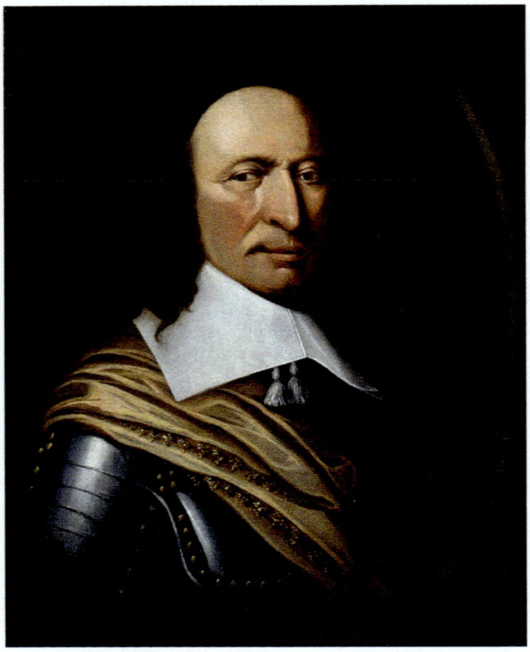

Fig. 2.3 Peter Stuyvesant (1610–1672), director-general of New Netherlands, participated in the setting of conditions associated with Jews entering New Amsterdam. (Collection of the New York Historical Society)

It is from the "Stuyvesant Pledge" that some historians trace the establishment of the network of American Jewish communal institutions. Hospitals, schools, and social service agencies were created to assure the ruling Christian classes of the Dutch and the English colonies and the eventually independent United States that American Jews would never represent a societal burden.

Other Causes for the Creation of American Jewish Hospitals

American Jews created hospitals in response to the indignity of Christians' attempts to convert them as they lay on their death beds. Evangelicals, sure that they had the "good news" that needed to be "carried to the Jews," attempted these conversions on individuals in no condition to resist.

A second motivating factor for the creation of American Jewish hospitals was, similar to the reason that immigrant urban Roman Catholics created hospitals, the desire for institutions which respected faith traditions. A Jewish hospital could be expected to show respect for the circumscribed views of Judaism on the indications for autopsy, to provide kosher food along with an on-site synagogue, a rabbi on the hospital chaplaincy service, and a mezuzah on the door post [16–18].

Probably the most powerful impetus for the creation of American Jewish hospital was pervasive American medical anti-Semitism. From the beginning of the twentieth century through the 1960s, almost all US medical schools, graduate medical education (GME) programs, and hospital credentialing systems employed a restrictive quota system. The system was designed to deny medical school admission to Jewish applicants, restrict the access of those Jews who did graduate from medical school to graduate medical education positions, and deny hospital staff privileges to Jewish physicians. Jewish hospitals offered Jewish medical students a place to obtain residencies and Jewish doctors a place to practice [18].

The Rise of the American Jewish Hospital

There were three waves of construction of Jewish hospitals in the United States. The first wave, from 1854 to 1880, was fostered by relatively secular German-Jewish immigrants. The first Jewish hospital was founded in 1854 by these immigrants in Cincinnati. During the Civil War, the Jews' Hospital of Manhattan opened its doors to all wounded Union soldiers, Jew and non-Jew alike. The hospital changed its name to the more inclusive-sounding Mount Sinai Hospital. By 1868 there were also Jewish hospitals in Baltimore, Chicago, and Philadelphia [18].

The second wave of Jewish hospital construction, from 1880 to 1945, was the product of relatively more religiously observant Eastern European Jewish immigrants. The third wave, from 1945 to 1960, was fueled by the financial support of the federal Hill-Burton Act. By 1966 the Jewish hospitals in the United States had a combined inpatient bed capacity of 25,000, admitted over 560,000 patients, delivered 75,800 babies, and provided 3.5 million outpatient visits [18].

I estimate that there have been, at one time or another, about 113 Jewish hospitals in the United States. These include 18 hospitals whose names include the word Jewish; 14 named Sinai or Mount Sinai; 8 named either Beth Abraham, Beth David, Beth El, or Beth Israel; 5 whose name includes the word Hebrew; 3 named Montefiore; and 2 named Menorah [18].

The Fall of the American Jewish Hospital

Of the 113 Jewish hospitals, less than one-fifth are still operating independently with a name and characteristics which, at least minimally, connote a Jewish heritage. The remainder have closed, been purchased by or merged into another hospital, or transitioned into a nursing home/extended care facility [16]. Almost none today meet the criteria of being a Jewish hospital: a name designed to identify the hospital as being under Jewish auspices, governance derived primarily from the Jewish community, a predominantly Jewish administrative and medical staff, philanthropic support obtained primarily from the Jewish community, a history of founding principally by Jews, and availability of Jewish religious practices [19].

Why Did They Disappear and Does It Matter?

American Jewish hospitals have largely disappeared for four reasons. First, independent, community-based small hospitals have a hard time surviving in the evolving health-care economy. Jewish hospitals are no different from their non-Jewish counterparts in being subjected to market pressures. Second, a decline in widespread medical anti-Semitism undercut a driving force for the creation and maintenance of Jewish hospitals. Third, the population of self-identifying Jews is declining as a percentage of the overall US population. Finally, as it has become more common for them to direct their philanthropic support to museums, opera companies, symphony orchestras, and secular universities, it has become less common for wealthy Jews to view it as their obligation to support Jewish hospitals [18].

Jewish hospitals institutionalized the Jewish community's commitment to the poor, fulfilled the Stuyvesant Pledge to provide care to members of the Jewish community, fostered the Jewish community's traditional commitment to education, and served as a public face of the Jewish community. The decline of these hospitals is a result of the American Jewish community's success. Indeed, they are institutions which so profoundly succeeded in aiding and abetting the success of the American Jewish community that they rendered themselves obsolete [18].

Episode 4: Litigation and the Desegregation of Southern Hospitals

By the end of World War II, southern US hospital racial segregation took two general forms. In some hospitals there were separate white and black inpatient wards and outpatient clinics, while the entire medical staff was white. In some communities separate hospitals were operated for white and blacks with white and black medical staffs, respectively. There were also variations where white physicians might practice part time in black hospitals. Other aspects of medical segregation included separate medical societies, separate medical schools for blacks, laws which prevented the transfusion of blood donated by blacks into whites and vice versa, and laws prohibiting anatomical dissection of the cadavers of whites in black medical schools [20, 21].

The first major southern hospitals to be desegregated were the Veterans Administration hospitals. On July 26, 1948, President Truman issued Executive Order 9981 by which it was "declared to be the policy of the President that there shall be equality of treatment and opportunity for all persons in the armed services without regard to race, color, religion or national origin. This policy shall be put into effect as rapidly as possible, having due regard to the time required to effectuate any necessary changes without impairing efficiency or morale." Following upon and consistent with the president's order, the Veterans Administration hospital system was desegregated in 1950 by a directive from the system's chief medical administrator. The desegregation of the vast majority of other hospitals was the result of other forms of federal action.

In 1946 the Hospital Survey and Construction Act, commonly called the Hill-Burton Act, became law. The law appropriated federal money to help build new public and nonprofit hospitals and expand existing hospitals. The act created intricate federal regulations and incorporated a "separate-but-equal" clause that permitted racially segregated hospitals [20].

The most important southern US hospital desegregation case originated in Greensboro, North Carolina [22–24]. L. Richardson Memorial Hospital served a predominantly black patient population where patients were often crowded several to a room or placed on stretchers in the hallway. The Moses H. Cone Memorial Hospital was a modern, well-equipped facility which had opened in 1953 and had received Hill-Burton money for its construction. It served a predominantly white patient population but admitted black patients who required medical services not available at Richardson. White doctors practiced at both hospitals, but Cone allowed no black doctors or dentists on its staff. A black patient with a black doctor who was admitted to Cone was required to transfer care to a white doctor.

In 1962 a test case was organized by George C. Simkins, Jr., a black Greensboro dentist and community leader. Simkins and eight other black physicians and dentists applied for staff privileges at Cone Hospital and were denied. The nine physicians and dentists sued, along with two patients, contending that the hospital had received Hill-Burton federal money in accordance with a North Carolina state plan to improve hospital services. The plaintiffs also sued another all-white Greensboro facility, Wesley Long Community Hospital, on similar grounds. By receiving government money, the plaintiffs contended, Cone and Long had become "instruments of the state." Furthermore, the plaintiffs asserted that the clause in the Hill-Burton Act allowing separate-but-equal hospital facilities was unconstitutional under the due process and equal protection provisions of the US Constitution.

Cone and Long countered that both white and black hospitals had been the beneficiaries of Hill-Burton money, that they were private institutions, and that they were not instruments of the state. Cone viewed itself as a paternalistic protector of L. Richardson Memorial Hospital because it supplemented services not provided at Richardson rather than trying to put Richardson and black physicians out of business by drawing black patients to a more modern and commodious facility staffed by white doctors and dentists.

The US District Court held for the defendants. The Court asserted that the acceptance of federal funds for hospital construction did not bind the hospitals to accept black patients or black physicians and dentists on their staffs. Simkins and his fellow plaintiffs appealed to the US Court of Appeals.

In 1963 the US Court of Appeals for the Fourth Circuit held for the black physicians, dentists, and patients by a three-to-two vote [22–24]. Chief Judge Simon Sobeloff wrote the decision for the majority (Fig. 2.4). Sobeloff's decision ruled that private hospitals that had participated in Hill-Burton programs were sufficiently bound to state and federal interests to be, in turn, bound by constitutional prohibitions against racial discrimination. Those portions of the Hill-Burton Act that tolerated separate-but-equal hospital facilities were ruled unconstitutional. The defendants appealed to the US Supreme Court which declined to hear the case and allowed the decision authored by Sobeloff to stand [20, 22–27].

Following the *Simkins* decision, the US Surgeon General issued nondiscrimination regulations applying to Hill-Burton funding. The federal Civil Rights Act of 1964 mandated the integration of almost all hospitals. President Lyndon Johnson's Department of Health, Education, and Welfare (HEW) pursued policies designed to enforce desegregation of hospital

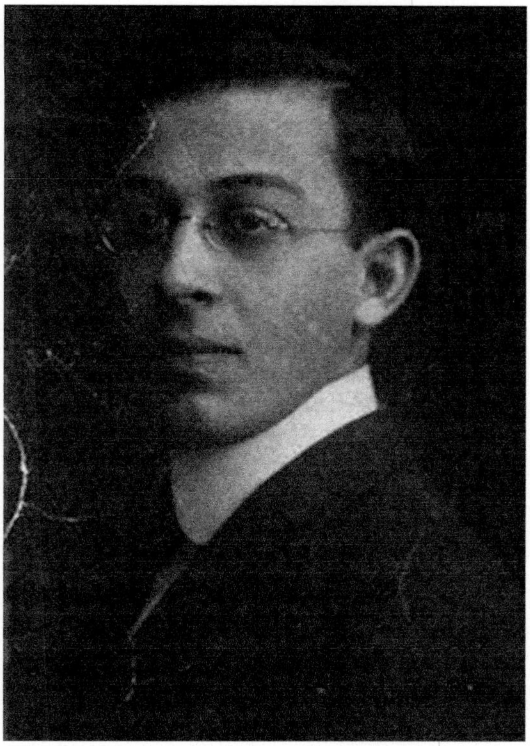

Fig. 2.4 Judge Simon E. Sobeloff of the US Court of Appeals, Fourth Circuit, wrote the decision for the majority in the *Simkins v. Cone* case. The *Simkins* decision has been called "the most significant battle for integration in hospitals" [20]. Sobeloff (1894–1973) had served as solicitor general of the United States early in the administration of President Dwight D. Eisenhower and had the responsibility of arguing the government's position in public school desegregation cases. (Provided courtesy of The University of Maryland Carey School of Law)

medical staffs and patient care. The central lever used to desegregate hospitals was Medicare money. HEW made it clear that segregated hospitals would be denied Medicare payments for inpatient care. As historian D.B. Smith observed, it was the golden rule. He who has the gold rules [23]. Rex Hospital in Raleigh, North Carolina, for example, was denied Medicare reimbursement in 1966 because of persistent racial discrimination [20].

Southern hospitals were as segregated as southern schools, lunch counters, buses, water fountains, waiting rooms, and bathrooms. With rare exceptions, white southern medical leaders were not at the forefront of desegregation but, instead, reacted to legal pressure and public demonstrations and desegregated their institutions only when forced to do so [20, 22–24].

Episode 5: Changes in the Relationship of the American Hospital to Undergraduate Medical Education

With the widespread acceptance of bedside teaching rounds as an essential component of medical education in the nineteenth century, the hospital became the focus of clinical undergraduate medical education (UME) leading to the M.D. degree.

Not all hospital leaders, however, were sympathetic to the needs of medical student education. In the late nineteenth century, the Ladies' Hahnemann Hospital Association of New York City assured its potential donors that no medical student education would be tolerated on the wards of its hospital.

We wish again to bring before our Association, and especially before those who are not familiar with our work, an important feature of our charity, which should justly claim for it the support of all women, viz., the freedom from clinical instruction. As this hospital is specifically designed to meet the wants of the refined class of poor who are unable to afford a private room and attendance, the managers offer the same kind of privacy of treatment which the more fortunate in private rooms are able to secure. This is a distinctive feature in this hospital and one that it would be well to remember in soliciting contributions from the public [9].

Critics of the participation of medical students in patient care were resoundingly answered by the Dean of the Johns Hopkins School of Medicine William Welch (1850–1934) in a 1907 speech wherein he argued for the role of medical education in improving the quality of care in hospitals:

> A main purpose of the kind of clinical training under consideration is precisely to teach students when and how to examine patients, and I am informed by my clinical colleagues that students

are, if anything, overcautious in their anxiety to refrain from any possibly injurious disturbance of the patient and that they carefully observe any directions which may be given regarding patients… Dr. Keen… expressed himself on this point of possible harm to the patient from bedside instructing in those forcible words: "I speak after experience of nearly forty years as a surgeon to a half dozen of hospitals and can confidently say that I have never known a single patient injured or his chances of recovery lessened by such teaching at the bedside."

So far from being detrimental, the teaching of physicians and students is distinctly advantageous to a hospital and its patients. The teaching hospital is in general more influential, more widely useful and more productive in contributions to medical knowledge than a hospital not concerned with teaching. Such a hospital is more attractive to physicians and surgeons of distinction and, therefore, more likely to be able to attach such men to its attending staff, and thereby secure the best medical service. The stimulating influence of eager alert students on the clinical teachers in hospitals has been so delightfully depicted by Dr. Keen, in the address just cited, and which should be widely read by trustees and physicians, that I cannot refrain from quoting his remarks on this point in full. He says: "Moreover, trustees may overlook one important advantage of a teaching hospital. Who will be least slovenly and careless in his duties, he who prescribes in the solitude of the sick chamber and operates with two of three assistants only, or he whose every movement is eagerly watched by hundreds of eyes, alert to detect every false step, the omission of an important clinical laboratory investigation, the neglect of the careful examination of the back, as well as the front of the chest, the failure to detect any important physical sign or symptom? Who will be most certain to keep up with the progress of medical science, he works alone with no one to discover his ignorance; or he who is surrounded by a lot of bright young fellows who have read the last 'Lancet' or the newest 'Annals of Surgery,' and can trip him up if he is not abreast of the times? I always feel at the Jefferson Hospital as if I were on the run with a pack of lively dogs at my heels. I cannot afford to have the youngsters familiar with operations, means of investigation or newer methods of treatment of which I am ignorant. I must perforce study, read, catalogue, and remember, or give place to others who will. Students are the best whip and spur I know." There is no teacher who will not subscribe to these words of Dr. Keen. It should furthermore be emphasized that the efficiency of the teaching hospital in its main functions of treating diseased and injured patients is increased not only by securing the most skilful medical staff, but the constant stimulus of their interest an activity and by the spirit pervading the institution, but also by the participation of advanced students in the work of the dispensary and wards in accordance with the system of clinical training which I am urging on your attention. It is really lamentable to contemplate the immense clinical material which exists in the public hospitals of our large cities and which could be made available for the education of students and physicians and for the advancement of medical knowledge, but which is utilized for these purposes either not at all or very inadequately. Medical schools of these cities do not begin to secure the advantages of location which rightfully belong to them and they allow themselves to be outstripped by schools less favorably situated and the hospitals themselves are less useful than would otherwise be the case. [28]

By the turn of the twentieth into the twenty-first century, the relationship of teaching hospitals to UME has been buffeted by powerful economic trends. They include:

1. Fewer and fewer physicians are in individual and small group private practices. The trend is increasingly toward physicians being employed either in very large group private practices or being directly employed by hospitals [29]. Medical school-associated faculty practice plans have been swept up in this change. Because of this transition, individual physicians have less control over their schedule. The teaching of medical students on the wards is increasingly becoming a work assignment rather than the semisacred duty codified in the Hippocratic Oath [30]. When a physician is being held to productivity standards for generating clinical billable units per hour, the leisurely imparting of knowledge to student-learners is viewed as an expense by some hospital administrators [31].
2. There have been significant changes in the use of hospitals for the provision of health care. Many procedures which, in the past, were thought to require hospitalization have now been converted to outpatient or day-surgery procedures. It is rare for someone to be admitted to the hospital for a diagnostic work-up. When patients are admitted to the hospital, the average length of stay has plummeted. These

factors all combine to reduce the amount of time that exists for a medical student to learn inpatient clinical medicine in a measured and methodical way.

3. The United States is in the midst of a wave of hospital mergers and acquisitions [32]. This has been driven by a power relationship between hospitals and third-party payers for health care. Striving to create a countervailing force to insurance companies, hospitals have combined to create control over the delivery of health care in geographic areas. This puts the hospital in a position of exerting force on insurance companies to improve reimbursement for clinical care.

There is an African proverb which states "When the elephants fight the only thing which is for certain is that the grass loses." As insurance companies, large hospital systems, and large group medical practices battle for dollars, power, and market share, few corporate executives are lying awake at night worrying about the education of medical students in hospital-based clinical clerkships.

4. For-profit medical schools, most often domiciled on Caribbean islands, have entered the medical education marketplace. These schools target young people who have been rejected for admission by US medical schools because their standardized test scores on the Medical College Admission Test (MCAT) and their undergraduate grade point average are too low. Holding out the promise that "you'll get to be a doctor anyway," entrepreneurs have created offshore medical schools with lower academic standards which offer admission in return for the ability of the applicant to either pay tuition out-of-pocket or obtain federally subsidized student loans. Doing no discovery research, having no system of tenure, owning no teaching hospitals or clinics, having a poor pass rate on licensing examinations, and having a high attrition rate while collecting substantial tuition, these schools are very profitable for their owners. Unfortunately for the full-of-hope students, a minority ever successfully graduate, pass licensing examinations, and match into a US graduate medical education (GME) program [33].

To generate third and fourth year medical student, clinical clerkships for their customers, for-profit offshore medical schools have turned these clerkships into a salable commodity. Offering hospitals $400–$1000 per student per week for clerkships, the for-profit sector is purchasing clerkships and "bumping" onshore nonprofit medical schools out of hospitals [34]. To a US hospital administrator who sees the opportunity to collect millions of dollars from a for-profit medical school in return for clinical clerkships slots, and who need not concern himself/herself with meeting US educational accreditation standards, the offer is seductive. US medical school deans in many sections of the country face the demand from hospital administrators that "I can make $3 million per year selling clinical clerkships slots to a Caribbean for-profit school. Either you match or exceed the offer or get your students out of my building." The once sacred duty to educate the next generation of physicians has become the Wild West of a laissez-faire marketplace.

Conclusions

Physicians and hospital leaders imagine that they are data-driven, evidence-based individuals who both "lead by the numbers" and recognize that in running an organization "the main thing is to keep the main thing the main thing." Among the things that the study of medical history teaches us is that this image is fanciful. We learn from history that medicine is fundamentally a social activity that takes place in the context of a particular time and place.

We also learn, from the study of medical history, how rarely medicine put itself at the forefront of social change. Neither organized medicine nor national hospital organizations were leaders in opposing medical or hospital racial discrimination or anti-Semitism. Similarly, organized medicine and hospital organizations have been relatively silent regarding the growing number of areas of the United States where women's reproductive health care is compromised by the lack of availability of hospitals operating outside the directives of the United States Conference of Catholic Bishops. Feeding at the financial trough of for-profit Caribbean medical schools, some US hospitals and their organizations have failed to denounce the transformation of UME into a marketable commodity.

I hope that the readers of this chapter, when they encounter their own transformative episodes in the management of their hospitals and hospital system, will be informed by the lessons of the past and act with vision and moral courage [35].

References

1. Zborowski M. People in pain. Hoboken: Wiley, Jossey-Bass; 1969.
2. Roth P. Portnoy's complaint. New York: Random House; 1969.
3. Rise GB. Mending bodies, saving souls: a history of hospitals. New York: Oxford University Press; 1999.
4. Stevens R. In sickness and in wealth: American hospitals in the twentieth century. New York: Basic Books, Inc; 1989.
5. The compact edition of the Oxford English Dictionary. Volume I. A-O. Oxford: Oxford University Press; 1985, p. 1336–1337.
6. Cutter JB. Early hospital history in the United States. California State Med J. 1922;20:272–4.
7. Ellis ER. The epic of New York City. New York: Carroll and Graf publishers; 1966.
8. Mortimer D. Jones collection on the Kings County Hospital, 1903–1930s. Call number 1994.008. Brooklyn Historical Society Library, 128 Pierrepont Street, Brooklyn NY 11201.
9. Greenberg SJ. Cor et Manus: a history of New York Medical College. Valhalla: New York Medical College. [In press, 2018].
10. Cunningham A, Grell OP. Health care and poor relief in Protestant Europe 1500–1700. London: Routledge; 1997.
11. White KR. When institutions collide: the competing forces of hospitals sponsored by the Roman Catholic Church. Religions. 2013;4:14–29.
12. United States Conference of Catholic Bishops. Ethical and religious directives for Catholic health care services. 5th ed. Washington, DC: United States Conference of Catholic Bishops; 2009.
13. Martin N. The growth of catholic hospitals, by the numbers. Propublica December 18, 2013. https://www.propublica.org/article/the-growth-of-catholic-hospitals-by-the-numbers. Accessed 12 Oct 2017.
14. Tamesha Means v. United States Conference of Catholic Bishops – complaint in the U.S. District Court for the Eastern District of Michigan, Southern Division. November 29, 2013.
15. Wall BM. American Catholic Hospitals: a century of changing markets and missions. Piscataway: Rutgers University Press; 2011.
16. Sarna JD. American Judaism: a history. New Haven: Yale University Press. p. 20–4.
17. Halperin EC. The Jewish problem in U.S. medical education 1920–1950. J Hist Med Allied Sci. 2001;56:140–67.
18. Halperin EC. The rise and fall of the American Jewish hospital. Acad Med. 2012;87:610–4.
19. Bridge DE. The rise and development of the Jewish hospital in America [thesis]. Cincinnati: Hebrew Union College-Jewish Institute of Religion; 1985.
20. Halperin EC. Special report: desegregation of hospitals and medical societies in North Carolina. New Eng J Med. 1988;318:58–63.
21. Halperin EC. The poor, the Black, and the marginalized as the source of cadavers in United States anatomical education. Clin Anat. 2007;20:489–95.
22. Beardsley EH. Good-bye to Jim Crow: the desegregation of southern hospitals. 1945–1970. Bull History Med. 1986;60:367–86.
23. Smith DB. The power to heal: civil rights, Medicare, and the struggle to transform America's health care system. Nashville: Vanderbilt University Press; 2016.
24. Smith DB. Forgotten heroes: remembering Dr. Alvin Blount who helped integrate America's hospitals. Health Affairs Blog, September 1, 2017. http://www.healthaffairs.org/doi 10.1377/hblog20170901.061774/full/. Accessed 12 Jan 2018.
25. Simkins V, Moses H. Cone Memorial Hospital. Federal Reporter, 2nd series. Vol. 323. St. Paul, Minn: West Publishing. 1964:959–977.
26. Simkins V, Moses H. Cone Memorial Hospital. Federal Supplement 628. Vol. 211. St. Paul, Minn: West Publishing, 1963:688–741.
27. Simkins V. Moses H. Cone Memorial Hospital. Supreme Court Reporter. Vol. 84. St. Paul, Minn: West Publishing. 1965:793.
28. Welch WH. Papers and addresses by William Henry Welch in three volumes, vol. III. Baltimore: The John Hopkins Press; 1920. p. 38–139.
29. Kletke PR, Emmons DW, Gillis KD. Current trends in physicians' practice arrangements: from owners to employees. JAMA. 1996;276:555–60.
30. Edelstein L. The Hippocratic oath: text, translation, and interpretation. Baltimore: Johns Hopkins Press; 1943.
31. Ludmerer K. Time to heal: American medical education from the turn of the century to the era of managed care. Oxford: Oxford University Press; 1999.

32. Hospital merger and acquisition activity continues upward trend, according to Kaufman Hall analysis. Health System Management. January 24, 2017. Accessed 6 Oct 2017. http://health-system-management.advanceweb.com/hospital-merger-and-acquisition-activity-continues-upward-trend-according-to-kaufman-hall-analysis/.
33. Halperin EC, Goldberg RB. Offshore medical schools are buying clinical clerkships in U.S. hospitals: the problem and potential solutions. Acad Med. 2016;91:639–44.
34. Rymer M. Offshore Med school's scholarship deal has city college's steamed: the Grenada invasion. The Village Voice. August 8, 2012.
35. Young KM, Kroth PJ. Chapter three: hospitals: origin, organization, and performance in Sultz and Young's health care USA. 9th ed. Burlington: Jones and Bartlett Learning; 2017. p. 69–119.

Hospital and Healthcare Transformation over Last Few Decades

3

John A. Savino and Rifat Latifi

Physician-Hospital Relationship

In his chapter on the historical transformation of the hospital, Halperin addresses five most important transformative episodes in the history of the American hospital (Chap. 2 of this book). In this chapter, we will address few other elements that have transformed the physician-hospital relationship and transformation of the hospital itself as a result of healthcare system transformation as a consequence of many competing factors, which have changed tremendously the balance of the relationship between physicians and hospitals. While there will always be a need for a collaborative effort between both, this relationship is interesting and often time competitive, yet synergistic. Managing diverse economic interests of medical staffs is very complex [1]. Hospitals rely on physicians to admit and care for patients to hospitals, and in return, physician's expectations are that hospital as an institution is able and willing to create an infrastructure that enables such services to be rendered by the physicians according to their skills and practice. And for the most part, this relationship has functioned in a synergistic fashion for a long period of time. But this relationship has changed over the years. Traditionally, physicians expended significant political capital to avoid being captured by the hospital in order to maintain both professional autonomy and control over their income without managerial interference. However, during the Clinton administration, the physician independence diminished significantly. The current healthcare model in the United States is focused on an antagonistic environment between health systems, hospitals, and physicians versus the health insurance companies' reimbursement paradigms [2].

While there may be examples of excessive billing practices which eventually impact patients who are obligated to pay for the uncovered costs, most physicians are honest and ultimately wish to recommend the appropriate treatments rather than abuse the system for their own benefit and gain. In order to avoid abuse, the health systems and hospitals need to create quality control initiatives and protocols which inevitably would diminish claims denials and best practices for the patients. There are rising costs in healthcare throughout the world and uneven quality despite the efforts of well-intentioned, well-trained clinicians. Healthcare leaders and policy makers have attempted to ameliorate the innumerable issues, specifically attacking fraud, reducing errors, enforcing practice guidelines, making patients better consumers, and implementing electronic medical records, but unfortunately without significant results [2].

J. A. Savino (✉)
Westchester Medical Center Health Network, New York Medical College, Valhalla, NY, USA
e-mail: John.savino@wmchealth.org

R. Latifi
New York Medical College, School of Medicine, Department of Surgery and Westchester Medical Center, Valhalla, NY, USA

R. Latifi (ed.), *The Modern Hospital*, https://doi.org/10.1007/978-3-030-01394-3_3

From Supply-Driven to Patient-Driven System

Several years ago a fundamental new strategy was recommended which would maximize value for patients focused on achieving the best outcomes at the lowest cost. The change moves away from a supply-driven healthcare system organized around what physicians do and toward a patient-centered system organized around what the patients need. The emphasis is placed around patient outcomes rather than volume and profitability of services provided such as physician visits, hospitalizations, procedures, and tests. Contrary to the current fragmented system in which every local provider offers a full range of services, there needs to be a change to a system in which services for particular medical conditions are concentrated in health delivery organizations and in the right locations to deliver high-value care. The transformation requires restructuring how healthcare delivery is organized, measured, and reimbursed. Healthcare organizations have never been opposed to improving outcomes, yet their central focus has been on growing volumes and maintaining margins in a system with erratic quality and unsustainable costs. In order to curtail costs, payers have reduced reimbursements based on performance rather than fee-for-service [3].

In the United States, an increasing percentage of patients are covered by Medicare and Medicaid, which reimburse at a fraction of commercial private-plan levels. These pressures continue to influence hospitals to join health systems and for physicians to leave private practice in group entities to become employed by hospitals. The hospital mergers and acquisitions have led to a decline from 3.0 beds per 1000 people in 1999 to 2.6 in 2010. Physician income has plateaued in some specialties but with progressively increasing expenses. National retailers, Walmart, CVS, and Walgreens, have entered the primary care market by offering in-store clinics that provide basic services at 40% below what physicians' offices charge [4]. In early 2018 CVS and the health insurer Aetna proposed a $70 billion merger which would be the largest deal ever in the healthcare sector outside pharmaceutical company mergers and among the 20 largest deals in history. CVS is a retail pharmacy and provider chain (CVS stores and Minute Clinics) of mostly acute care services, at prices below those of outpatient clinics, urgent care facilities, and certainly emergency departments. Episodes of care originating at retail clinics might also be cheaper if they entail fewer referrals for additional care and that additional care does not generate benefits that exceed cost. CVS is sustaining competition from other organizations, specifically Amazon, which are siphoning revenues from front-of-store sales and threatening to enter the lucrative prescription drug delivery market [4]. At the time of this publication, patients were accustomed to high-quality, digitally enabled services and were growing weary of the antiquated way they access primary care. Certainly, the inconveniences of difficulty to park at a doctor's office, inability to schedule an appointment online, and unpredictably long waiting time leave a room for improvement. Providers will have to provide better, more convenient, and less costly care to remain competitive. When Amazon, J.P. Morgan Chase &Company, and Berkshire Hathaway launched their partnership in healthcare, they left more questions than answers in early 2018 about the new venture. Fundamentally, the shared goal was to provide high-quality, lower-cost healthcare to the 2.4 million employees and families [5]. US government payers (Medicare and Medicaid) raise payment levels minimally each year, if at all. Providers recover losses by demanding higher payment rates from commercial insurance plans. Employers have decreased their healthcare costs by engaging in price negotiations, reducing benefits, raising deductibles, and encouraging the patients to go to providers that accept lower rates or provide better outcomes. Patients will be asked to pay more which inevitably will encourage the healthcare institutions to become transparent and communicate exactly what they are giving patients, employers, and insurers for their money [3].

The Core of Value Transformation

At the core of the value transformation is changing the way clinicians are organized to deliver care. A suggested structure is an integrated practice unit (IPU) [3], a dedicated team made up of both clinical and nonclinical personnel which provides the full care cycle for patient's condition. IPUs treat not only a disease but also related conditions, complications, and circumstances that commonly occur along with it, such as kidney and eye disorders for patients with diabetes, or palliative care for those with metastatic cancer. The team takes responsibility for the full cycle of care for the condition, encompassing outpatient, inpatient, and rehabilitative care and supporting services (nutrition, social work, and behavioral health). Patient education, engagement, and follow-up are integrated into care. The unit has a single administrative and scheduling structure with the care co-located in dedicated facilities. A physician team clinical manager oversees each patient's care process. The team measures outcomes, costs, and processes for each patient using a common measurement platform. The providers on the team meet formally and informally on a regular basis to discuss patients, processes, and results. Joint accountability is accepted for outcomes and costs. The end results include faster treatment, better outcomes, lower costs, and improved market share of the condition. The key to the measurement process is to focus on the functional parameters that matter to the patient. There are three categories of health outcomes. Level one involves the health status achieved, for example, in prostate cancer treatment, patients care about mortality rates, but they are concerned about functional status such as incontinence and sexual dysfunction, where variability among providers is much greater. Level two outcomes relate to the nature of the care cycle and recovery. Even when functional outcomes are equivalent, patients whose care process is timely and free of chaos, confusion, and unnecessary setbacks, readmissions, and returns to the ED experience much better care than those that encounter delays and problems along the way. Level three outcomes relate to the sustainability of health. A hip replacement that lasts 2 years is inferior to the one that lasts 15 years, from both the patient's perspective and the provider's. Innovative technologies such as tablet computers, web portals, and telephonic interactive systems for collecting outcomes data from patients allow providers to track progress as they interact with patients [3].

To determine value providers must measure costs at the medical condition level, tracking expenses involved in treating the condition over the full cycle of care. This requires understanding the resources used in a patient's care, including personnel, equipment, and facilities, the capacity costs of supplying each resource, and the support costs associated with care, such as information technology and administration. By understanding true costs, clinicians will be able to work with administrators to improve the value of care with better outcomes. The dominant payment models, global capitation, and fee-for-service do not improve the value of care. Global capitation provides a single payment to cover all the patient's needs. It rewards providers for spending less but not specifically for improving outcomes or value. Fee-for-service couples payment to something providers can control and the variety of services such as MRI scans they provide, but not the overall cost and outcomes. Providers are rewarded for increasing volume, but that does not necessarily increase the value [3]. The payment approach best aligned with value is a bundled payment that covers the full care cycle for acute medical conditions, the overall care for chronic conditions for a defined period, or primary or preventive care for a defined patient population (healthy children). Sound bundled payment models should include severity adjustments or eligibility only for qualifying patients; care guarantees that hold the provider responsible for avoidable complications, such as infections after surgery; stop-loss provisions that mitigate the risk of unusually high-cost events; and mandatory outcomes reporting. Bundled payments have become the norm for organ transplant care, hip and knee replacements, and other procedures in the future, specifically spine surgery and possibly cardiac procedures [3]. Walmart, General Electric, Boeing, and Lowes have embraced bundled payments by encouraging their employees to obtain care at providers which have high volume and track records of excellent outcomes [6]. The hospitals are reimbursed for single bundled payments that include all physician and hospital costs associated with inpatient and outpatient pre- and postoperative care. Employees bear no costs including travel expenses, hotel, and meals provided their surgery is performed at declared centers of excellence. Providers are obviously concerned that the patient heterogeneity will not be adequately reimbursed, but excellent outcomes will inevitably increase referral volume and improve value.

In a patient-centered, value-driven care model, the ability of patients to interact and engage with both their health data and the healthcare delivery system electronically is a key driver of high-quality healthcare. The American Hospital Association Annual Survey Information Technology for community hospitals collected from November 2016 to April 2017 published in a brief focusing on the state of patients' access to engagement with their health data through health information technology (IT) [7]. The results were grouped into three categories of activity: accessing health data, interacting with health data, and obtaining healthcare services. Community hospitals are defined as all nonfederal, short-term general, and other special hospitals. Excluded are hospitals not accessible by the general public, such as prison hospitals or college infirmaries. Ninety-three percent of hospitals and health systems enable patients to view information from their health record online, up from only 27% in 2012. Eighty-four percent allow patients to download information from their health record, up from only 16% in 2012. Eighty-three percent enable patients to designate a caregiver to access health information on the patient's behalf, a slight increase over 2015 (the first year the question was included in the AHA survey) [7]. While all hospitals and health systems have increased patients' access to their health information, a greater percentage of larger hospitals (those greater than 300 or more beds) report that patients can view and download their health information and designate a caregiver to access their information than small hospitals (those with fewer than 100 beds) [7]. Large hospitals are more likely to support functionality for interacting with their health data. Seventy-three percent of hospitals and health systems give patients the ability to electronically transmit summaries of care to a third party, up from only 13% in 2013. Seventy-nine percent of hospitals and health systems enable patients to electronically request amendment to update or otherwise change their health record, up from 32% in 2012. Thirty-nine percent of hospitals and health systems allow patients to submit patient-generated health data to their health records, up from 8% in 2012. Eighty percent of large hospitals enable patients to electronically transmit summaries of care to a third party (such as a specialist physician after a referral), compared to 67% of small hospitals. Eighty-eight percent of large hospitals enable patients to electronically request an amendment to update or otherwise change their health record, compared to 74% of small hospitals. Fifty-three percent of large hospitals enable patients to submit their patient-generated health data to their health records, compared to 30% of small hospitals [7].

Many hospitals and health systems, particularly the large hospitals, enable patients to electronically conduct administrative activities including securing messaging to providers through the EHR, online appointment scheduling, providing additional convenience for ambulatory services, paying bills online for inpatient services, and requesting refills for prescriptions online. Prospectively, hospitals and health systems will continue to expand these capacities as new care delivery and payment models that are more dependent on access to data and patient engagement become more prevalent. These activities support a patient-centered healthcare system in which patients are partners with their healthcare providers and share in decision-making. Electronic patient engagement will continue to grow as hospitals and health systems refine and expand their IT systems [7].

In recent years, hospitals and health systems have significantly expanded providers' ability to share and receive patient information from a variety of care sources, both inside their own hospital/health system and with unaffiliated hospitals, health systems, or other settings. However, barriers, such as a lack of interoperability, continue to prevent universal sharing and effective use of information. Interoperability refers to the ability of electronic systems to efficiently and correctly transmit and receive information without the need for manual entry or other intervention by an individual. Interoperability is critical to effective use of shared information for core hospital activities such as care coordination, patient engagement, quality improvement, and ensuring patient safety [8]. In a recent speech, Seema Verma, the CMS administrator, at the 2018 Healthcare Information and Management System Society (HIMSS) announced several new initiatives designed to give patients unfiltered access to their health records and punish organizations that engage in data blocking [9]. The Agency plans to overhaul the Meaningful Use program for hospitals. The organization is moving away from giving credit to physicians for just having an electronic health record to actually assuring that it is focused on interoperability and releasing to patients their medical data. Unfortunately, the EHR currently presents difficulty for providers to effectively coordinate care for their patients. The technology for data sharing occurs effectively within a given healthcare system with inpatient and outpatient doctors in the same provider system able to share and edit the same clinical record. However, it is extremely rare for different provider systems to share data beyond their network because it's in the financial interest of the provider systems to hold on to the data of their patients. Inevitably, tests are repeated if the patient enters another provider network which drives up costs in addition to placing the patient's safety at risk, as well as quality of care.

Unfortunately, providers often use faxes to send and receive patient data in an era of artificial intelligence, machine learning, and precision medicine. Patients still have difficulty obtaining health records, and if they are successful and receive them, the information is often incomplete and incomprehensible due to technical jargon [9]. CMS is launching two specific initiatives designed to give patients access to their records. MyHealthEData [10], which is led by the White House Office of American Innovation, incorporates agencies throughout the Department of Health and Human Services, as well as the Department of Veterans Affairs, which will focus on breaking down the barriers limiting access and improving interoperability. Digital technology will shift the power from the doctors to the patients, and patient-centric medicine, in which patients generate medical data using their own digital devices and communicating via their smartphones [10]. Ms. Verma clearly stated that the administration would pull the lever to create a healthcare ecosystem that allows and encourages the healthcare market to tailor products and services to compete for patients, which will increase quality, decrease costs, and promote healthier lives. Doctors and hospitals now use EHRs, and patients have a widespread access to the Internet, and nearly everyone has access to a smartphone, providing many access points for viewing healthcare data securely. Uniform standards are being drafted for 21st century Cures Act that will enable EHRs to share information. Ms. Verma stated that other government agencies, including the Veteran's Administration, the National Institute of Health, and the Office of the National Coordinator for Health Information (ONC), are aligned with CMS regarding the confidentiality of patient records. CMS will be announcing a complete overhaul of Meaningful Use programs for hospitals and the Advancing Care Information performance category of the Quality Payment Program. Ensuring the security of healthcare data will be an absolute requirement in order to avoid negative payment adjustments or to receive an incentive payment.

These initiatives will not only reduce costs but will also increase interoperability and provide patients complete access to their data across all of the government programs [9].

CMS finalized requirements for certain programs that providers begin using the 2015 edition certified EHR technology starting in 2019. This version allows systems to share information with patients and care teams via open application programming interfaces, APIs, which will enable patients to transfer their data to other providers and permit access to their data to app developers. APIs are software that allow other software to connect to one another and are a primary way that data is shared electronically. CMS believes that the future of healthcare data interoperability centers on the development and implementation of open APIs. More clinical and payment data needs to be exchanged via APIs and that data will be sent to the provider and consumer [10]. The administration is serving as a convener by joining with patients, clinicians, and innovators to develop more open-source APIs for use across the entire digital health information system. The vision of the administration is to go beyond APIs not only to include EHRs but also the entire digital health information ecosystem. The administration will not allow providers and hospitals to engage in data blocking but will ensure that every patient and doctor has the opportunity to access their electronic data. CMS will overhaul the documentation requirements of Evaluation and Management codes which are codes that doctors use to bill Medicare for patient visits which will be updated in order to have doctors spend more time with the patient rather than having them spend time on the EHR. Medicare beneficiaries will have Blue Button 2.0 [10] which is a developer-friendly standards-based API that enables them to connect to their claims data to secure applications, services, and research programs that they trust. Blue Button 2.0 uses the same cloud infrastructure that supports a number of CMS IT systems. Blue Button 2.0 will create an ecosystem where tech innovators will be competing to serve Medicare beneficiaries and their caregivers to find better opportunities to use their claims data. The CMS administrator admonished the commercial insurers and others in the healthcare industry that all will be expected to create the tools to allow patients to control their information and be protected from unauthorized use. CMS will be re-examining its expectations for Medicare Advantage plans and qualified health plans (QHPs) offered through the federally facilitated exchanges and calling on all health insurers to release their data. CMS believes that the private plans that contract through Medicare Advantage and exchanges should provide the same benefit that is being provided through Medicare's Blue Button 2.0 [10].

Summary

The transformation of hospitals is the result of major advances in education, science, technology, and policies that have led to the creation of major healthcare systems, both nationally and internationally.

References

1. The Tangled Hospital-Physician Relationship/ Goldsmith J, Kaufman N, Lawton B @www.HealthAffairs.org May 9,2016. Accessed 4 June 2018.
2. Dowling M. Michael Dowling: Payers, providers and the long road from contention to cooperation. Becker's Hospital Review. February 16th, 2018. Retrieved from: https://www.beckershospitalreview.com/hospital-management-administration/michael-dowling-payers-providers-and-the-long-road-from-contention-to-cooperation.html.
3. Porter ME, Lee TH. The strategy that will fix health care. Harv Bus Rev October 2013. Retrieved from: https://hbr.org/2013/10/the-strategy-that-will-fix-health-care.
4. Dafny LS. Does CVS–Aetna spell the end of business as usual? NEJM. February 15, 2018;378(7):593–5.
5. Nosta J. Healthcare's Tipping Point: Amazon, Berkshire And JPMorgan Take On Care And Cost. Forbes.com. January 30th, 2018. Retrieved from: https://www.forbes.com/sites/johnnosta/2018/01/30/healthcares-tipping-point-amazon-berkshire-hathaway-and-jp-morgan-chase-take-on-care-and-cost/#49946f9a5af2.
6. Slotkin JR. Why GE, Boeing, Lowe's, and Walmart Are Directly Buying Health Care for Employees. Harv

Bus Rev June 8th, 2017. Retrieved from: https://hbr.org/2017/06/why-ge-boeing-lowes-and-walmart-are-directly-buying-health-care-for-employees.
7. American Hospital Association. Expanding electronic patient engagement. March 2018. Retrieved from: https://www.aha.org/system/files/2018-03/expanding-electronic-engagement.pdf.
8. eHealth Initiative. American Hospital Association Annual Survey IT Supplement Brief #2. March 2nd 2018. Retrieved from: https://www.ehidc.org/resources/american-hospital-association-annual-survey-it-supplement-brief-2.
9. CMS.gov. Centers for Medicare and Medicaid Services. Trump Administration Announces MyHealthEData Initiative to Put Patients at the Center of the US Healthcare System. March 6th, 2018. Retrieved from: https://www.cms.gov/Newsroom/MediaReleaseDatabase/Press-releases/2018-Press-releases-items/2018-03-06.html.
10. CMS.gov. Centers for Medicare and Medicaid Services. Trump Administration Announces MyHealthEData Initiative at HIMSS18. March 6th, 2018. Retrieved from: https://www.cms.gov/Newsroom/MediaReleaseDatabase/Fact-sheets/2018-Fact-sheets-items/2018-03-06.html.

4 Navigating and Rebuilding Academic Health Systems (AHS)

Colene Yvonne Daniel and Rifat Latifi

Introduction

Academic medical centers (AMC) also known as academic health systems (AHS) have become major and complex healthcare and business enterprises in the USA and around the world. The AHS also have the unique imperative to provide a complex mission of evidence-based clinical quality care, relevant teaching, and innovative research. To ensure completion of this mission, accomplished AHS have combined its teaching hospital(s) with teaching and research programs affiliated with medical schools and other colleges/universities, clinical faculty, and in some cases affiliated community physicians, or the AHS may own community physician group practices. In previous decades, healthcare organizations operated within fragmented governance, with financial and clinical practices that accounted for the overuse of care and unnecessary costs. Clinical care structures were set up and performed in silos with hospitals in most cases completely separate from the medical schools and universities. The governance of the teaching hospital(s) from the medical schools and universities was unaligned, which led to duplicative clinical practices – hence, reimbursements were based on volumes. In some cases, the clinical care objectives were in conflict with the teaching and research objectives. Hospitals funded teaching programs through traditional revenue streams, and research was funded through federal or nonprofit grants and traditional revenue streams. The C-Suite (clinical and administrative leaders) used monthly data to develop strategic plans based upon inpatient days. To prepare for the next decade, academic health systems will need to undergo significant changes to remain or become successful in today's challenging and competitive environment. Rebuilding AHS means to fundamentally realign the business and clinical principles and constantly adapt to the seismic shifts in healthcare. In this chapter, we will explore a number of aspects that will be required in the rebuilding process, always starting with the vison and strategy and ensuring that human capacities and all intricacies are met to achieve excellence in healthcare.

The description of the economic healthcare environment tends to use words as chaotic, challenging, or one that remains in flux. Mike Leavitt of the Leavitt Group urges hospital and health systems leaders to move beyond what is called the "fog of war" and to focus on the shift from fee-for-service to value-based reimbursement [1]. Rebuilding AHS while tackling the

C. Y. Daniel (✉)
The Bonne Sante Group, LLC,
Washington, DC, USA
e-mail: cdaniel@bonsantegrp.com

R. Latifi
New York Medical College, School of Medicine,
Department of Surgery and Westchester Medical
Center, Valhalla, NY, USA

R. Latifi (ed.), *The Modern Hospital*, https://doi.org/10.1007/978-3-030-01394-3_4

seismic changes in healthcare is complex in any environment. In the USA, however, the demographic challenges of baby boomers, the Affordable Care Act (ACA), and a myriad of new regulations compel AHS to pay careful attention to how they confront these challenges while providing quality care and teaching, state-of-the-art technology, and groundbreaking research. Even more complicating is that since 2017, the US Congress has dismantled parts of the ACA leaving the healthcare financing and regulatory environment in a more unsettling state. This situation has been difficult for all healthcare facilities, but it is especially difficult for AHS because of its unique mission, and AHS tend to care for more of the uninsured and underinsured patient populations.

In order for AHS to emerge successfully in today's environment and remain competitive, they will need to rebuild their business, educational, and scientific models. The first step to rebuilding the AHS was to restructure the governance. Over decades, many AHS integrated or more closely aligned its teaching hospital(s) with the medical, nursing, and allied health professional colleges/universities to provide excellence in teaching and innovative research, as well as to set common operational and financial goals. In the next decade as healthcare reimbursement continues toward the value-based models, AHS will realign resources to increase outpatient and home visits, technology care, and payer-provider partnerships. As stated, the complicating challenge of "rebuilding academic healthcare systems" is the fact that most of these systems provide a substantial amount of charity care to patients with the most complex social, behavioral, and health problems. AHS leaders will need to realign health networks, develop personalized patient-centered care, and incorporate technology with clinical practices, all under an integrated governance. The C-Suite will be undertaking a multitude of regulatory changes and new healthcare funding rules, so it will be essential to partner with their university partners and clinicians to maximize resources and to reduce the duplication of services, programs, and costs. Rebuilding AHS means that the leadership will need to enhance its expertise to ensure correct decision-making as it relates to health policy, modernizing the financial tools and implementing science and digital technology to achieve the mission and the margins.

Health Policy: Regulatory Challenges in Today's Environment

Academic health systems must be flexible to acclimate to the numerous regulatory and business challenges. According to Bloomberg Law, healthcare policy is one of the most important issues that AHS will need to tackle because of the instability of the Affordable Care Act [2]. Congressional legislation failed to repeal ACA, but the administration has been chipping away at key programs and taking actions, like refusing to make cost-sharing reductions (CSR) payments to insurers [3]. Congress also managed to repeal the individual mandate provision that required people to pay a penalty if they didn't have healthcare [4]. It is expected that without that incentive, healthy people most likely won't purchase insurance resulting in an increase in health insurance premiums. The slow dismantling of insurer offerings on federal and state health insurance exchanges has created uncertainty. According to Mike Leavitt, systems will need to study the policies and the payment systems emerging in both the public and private sectors, focusing specially on the role of Medicare Access and CHIP Reauthorization Act (MACRA), Medicare Advantage, Medicaid managed care, the integration of behavioral health, as well as, public and private ACAs to understand the reimbursement landscape [5].

The implementation of a quality payment program mandated by MACRA could be of a concern for academic healthcare systems. Under MACRA, providers can choose one of two methods for reimbursement in the value-based payment world. The first, Advanced Alternative Payment Model (AAPM), provides healthcare providers with incentive payments for taking on some risk related to their patients' outcomes. The second, the Merit-based Incentive Payment System (MIPS), adjusts a physician's payment based on an evaluation against four performance categories [6]. Rebuilding under the MACRA will necessitate a greater focus on quality metrics associated with preventive and primary care, Telehealth, and other technologies to correctly forecast reimbursements.

Medicaid will continue to be a prime payer for the uninsured, but the future shape of the program also is uncertain. CMS has indicated that Medicaid reforms are a high priority, and significant changes that includes allowing work requirements to be instituted [7]. One major way that Medicaid could be altered is if federal funding to states is provided via block grants and per capita caps [2]. Such financial changes could have a deleterious effect on the survival of the program. For academic health systems, Medicaid funds could be as high as one-third of its patient population. Also, if funds are interrupted, or materially decreased due to reforms, the solvency of AHS could be even more at jeopardy due to the high level of charity care.

From a health policy perspective, AHS encompass multiple care facilities and, thus, must be able to address all applicable regulations, for their facilities that are often geographically apart. This may present with some difficulties in the case of mergers or acquisitions with institutions across multiple states. Knowledge of the federal and each state regulation to maximize resources is modus operandi. Furthermore, to truly make a difference in the community that the AHS serve, the leadership must be adaptive, thoughtful, and creative to deal with constant turmoil, local cultures and sensitivities, and innovative technology. In summary, "innovative leaders who recognize the economic imperatives mandating change and engage with alternative payment, delivery models, and advanced technology will be rewarded" [1].

Healthcare Finance: Financial Modernization, Mergers and Acquisitions, and Cybersecurity

Academic health systems must modernize its approach to healthcare financing to rebuild its delivery systems for a future with limited resources. The healthcare financing situation in the USA is becoming critical. In 2018, health spending is projected to rise to 5.3%, reflecting rising prices of medical goods and services and higher Medicaid costs [8]. The increase represents a sharp uprise from 2017, which the US Centers for Medicare and Medicaid Services (CMS) now estimated to have a 4.6% climb to nearly $3.5 trillion [9]. As expected, the primary drivers of the increased spending include the aging baby boomer population that will increase enrollment in the Medicare and Medicaid health insurance program for the poor, elderly, and disabled. CMS projects on healthcare spending will on average rise 5.5% annually from 2017 to 2026 and will comprise 19.7% of the US economy in 2026, up from 17.9% in 2016 [10]. It is predicted that by 2026, healthcare spending is projected to reach $5.7 trillion [10]. Congress has declared that the projected levels of healthcare spending are unsustainable and are an undue burden on the US business economic to remain globally competitive. Congress and business executives are stating that there must be a major shift (meaning reduction) in the total cost of healthcare. There are multiple discussions on the end product, but there are many developed countries that have better health outcomes at a lower cost, and those countries' companies are not the primary sponsors supporting the healthcare business.

The US Congress has already started its journey to restructure healthcare financing by introducing the bipartisan MACRA (Medicare Access and CHIP Reauthorization Act) program [11]. MACRA incentivizes healthcare facilities to improve quality and efficiencies through collaboration, coordination, and the establishment of relationships with other healthcare organizations and payers. The emphasis on the MACRA program is the alternative payment models (APMs). The ultimate strategic and financial goals of AHS would be to move into advance alternative payment models (AAPMs). As AHS have implemented the MACRA program, they are dealing with multiple payment models, and all influence how care is delivered, teaching is reimbursed, and research overhead is covered leaving AHS to assume greater financial risk for quality and price [12]. Effective AHS that have transitions to MACRA also are grappling with the new payment models as they pertain to cost reductions, savings, and revenue growth. The paradigm shift to develop a totally integrated delivery and payment system focused on population health, care coordination, quality outcomes, reduced costs, and data reporting is moving forward and should begin to have real impact on AHS in 2020 [13]. Even the best AHS that are poised for the MACRA program must have the tools to make future determination of the organization's capacity. AHS are tertiary care centers with varied populations, and because of the complexities, it is not simple to select one value-based model from among the many options. Making the choice to move from a traditional reimbursement model to a value-based model requires tremendous care and planning. Therefore, due to the overwhelming range of value-based models (no-risk, low-risk, and high-risk) arrangements, AHS tend to negotiate with various payers, and they include:

- Pay for performance, wherein providers receive incentives for meeting quality targets.
- Shared-savings contracts, in which payers share with providers the cost savings achieved through value-based approaches to care.
- Bundled payments, in which healthcare facilities and providers agree to a single payment for all care and service associated with a specific condition or treatment.
- Shared risk, where payers and providers determine a budget and providers receive performance-based incentives when cost savings are realized; however, they cover a portion of the cost when savings targets are not achieved.
- Global capitation is a payment-per-person plan in which physicians accept members for a certain set price (without considering the number of visits).
- Provider-sponsored health plans are plans where providers assume 100% of the risk by directly collecting insurance premiums from members and providing care [14].

The US Department of Health & Human Services (HHS) has mandated that half of Medicare outlays shall be routed through alternative payment models (APMs) by the end of 2018. CMS is moving forward, and by 2020 the entire financial healthcare system will be based upon value not on volume [15]. Thus for AHS to achieve financial solvency in the future, they must have partnership with providers, consumers, and payers to achieve integration, improve access, and cost-effectiveness.

Rebuilding academic health systems will require modernizing the financial technology to enhance the capabilities needed for value-based reimbursement. Facing the ever shifting and numerous new regulations along with the rampant mergers and consolidations, the C-Suite of AHS must combine the financial predictive analysis and artificial intelligence with operational and strategic strategies to proactively make sound decisions. Therefore it is important that AHS apply technology to obtain and receive real-time data so that more accurate informed decisions can be made regarding clinical practices, teaching programs, or expanding research protocols [16]. The process of maintaining the academic edge or rebuilding the academic excellence must include evaluation of the uncertainty in the industry and predict financial models that will adapt to the ever-changing accounting rules or regulations. For example, current and future financial and regulatory operational processes must significantly include Big Data & Analytics, Predictive Analytics, and real-time data from digital technology regarding the population's health to efficiently amalgamate business and healthcare decisions. Modernizing financial technology will not only improve the value of clinical support and administrative services through efficiencies but will also improve academic productivity, teaching, and research [17]. Clinicians and administrators are being asked to achieve the (CMS) Five-Star Quality Rating, produce more clinical dollars, and continue to raise the academic edge in order to be competitive. The only way to accomplish set goals with the major changes on how providers are reimbursed will be to coordinate care practice models, target capital investments, embrace innovations, and have partnership with payers.

In an effort to be financially competitive, academic health systems are merging or acquiring systems. In 2016, hospital mergers and acquisitions totaled 102 deals, and many of those deals will close in 2018 depending upon federal and state regulatory review [18]. The most notable AHS to close mergers or acquisitions in 2018 were Advocate Health Care and Aurora Health Care, Beth Israel Deaconess Medical Center and Lahey Health, Carolinas Healthcare System and UNC Health Care, Dignity Health and Catholic Health Initiatives, Partners Healthcare and Care New England Health System, and Providence St. Joseph Health and Ascension Health. The merger of Dignity Health and Catholic Health Initiatives will create the US largest not-for-profit system, with 139 hospitals in 28 states [19].

The trend toward national or regional consolidation is to more align clinical, ambulatory, outpatient, home health, dental, behavioral, Telehealth, and senior living providers. Additionally, many AHS are announcing mergers to combine clinical, medical education, and research resources with the intent of increasing quality, engaging patients and becoming more effective across the continuum. Most of the mergers are focused on a stronger bargaining power with insurers, bolstering primary healthcare networks, telemedicine, and providing specialists procedures or therapeutics in a non-hospital/academic environment. The most common goals of these mergers and acquisitions are lowering the cost of clinical and support services, administration overhead including supply chain, and drugs costs so that the limiting resources can be redirected toward improving quality, patient experience, effective teaching, and beneficial research [20].

Cybersecurity investments are a "must" for rebuilding AHS. In healthcare, it is particularly central to meet HIPAA compliance and to address the dangers of data breaches. As healthcare providers are faced with the rapidly evolving technology-virtual visits, they are exposed to the ever-increasing risks of data breaches involving patient health information, civil penalties for violating the HIPAA privacy and security rules, potential lawsuits by affected patients, as well as a loss of consumer confidence. In the USA, data breaches have increased and become more diverse and severe. In 2017, healthcare systems reported 210 data breaches as defined by the US Department of Health & Human Services (HHS) [21]. As it relates to systems, 82% were providers, so more than 2.6 million individuals were collectively affected [22]. Thus it becomes difficult for healthcare systems to implement digital technology to monitor patient's health if clinicians and patients are concerned about confidentiality. Healthcare is especially attractive to cybercriminals because it is one of the few industries charged with handling valuable bulk data sets that combined personal health information (PHI), personally identifiable information, payment information, research, and intellectual properties [23]. Encouraging the use of scientific and digital technology for the betterment of patient care also leaves healthcare systems open to risks from multiple attackers because each avenue into the healthcare network is also an opportunity for a breach. Thus to protect clinicians, patients, and staff and to protect AHS reputations as "safe heavens," it is imperative to move forward with sharing clinical protocols and information across the continuum and to invest in advanced cybersecurity as a defense technology.

Building New or Rebuilding Clinical Department as Part of AHS

Creating new or rebuilding successful clinical programs is at the heart of rebuilding AHS. Progressive clinical and innovative programs are essential for the success of AHS. As a leaders, we have to concentrate on quality and volume, and financial aspect of the its services, which all start with the strategic vision and human capacities. The most important question that needs to be addressed is what kind of clinical services one has to concentrate and what the institution wishes to be known for. Major clinical programs, such as neurosurgical, transplant services, both chest (heart and lung) and intra-abdominal (liver, kidney, pancreas, intestines, uterus); cardiac services; thoracic surgical oncology; plastic, trauma, critical care and acute care surgical services; bariatric services; and others, are basic clinical programs of any academic healthcare system. Not all of them have to be in one campus (mothership), and some can be spread out through the various campuses of the AHS, based on the needs of community and strategic mission of the AHS.

Scientific and Digital Technology: The New Evolution in Virtual Clinical Services

Academic health systems will have to evolve and face new challenges with resourceful solutions, like virtual medicine. A new era of scientific and digital technology is providing patients with greater access to health information and resources through the Internet, not only driving revolutionary advancements in personalized medicine, teaching, and medical research but giving clinicians the ability to monitor patients' health status around the clock using data from sensors and devices. Using these sensors and devices will allow patients to be better educated about their health and to be trained to monitor themselves through clinical reminders, and when necessary, interventions can be introduced to stabilize the patient's health and reduce the need for unnecessary emergency room visits or inpatient admissions. Clinicians will have the ability to respond proactively in real time [24]. The ultimate goal for AHS is to meet the challenge to deliver high-quality and personalized care at a lower cost.

The requirements of MACRA force the focus on the approach of keeping its patient population healthy, i.e., as much as possible keeping the patients out of the hospital. Multidisciplinary teams should be informed to tailor patient's care plans so that the population can stay well. This requirement is a momentous task because, for decades, AHS business was built in inpatient beds. Now the AHS C-Suite has to study digital technology and data (Big Data & Analytics) to predict its patient population demands against the AHS supply and reassign staff, programs, and services to track clinical goals [25]. One example of success is the Banner Health Network model that has outlined the combining goals of reducing overall hospital admissions, reducing average length of stay (ALOS), avoiding hospital readmissions, utilizing high-tech imaging and digital services, and reducing CMS paid amounts per beneficiary [26].

Most AHS are at the forefront of using the technology such as the "Internet of Things." The "Internet of Things" is also known as "Industrial Internet," which is installing sensors everywhere and the sensor broadcast how it is feeling at any moment, allowing its performance to be immediately adjusted or predicted in response. This Internet of Things is creating a nervous system that will allow humans to keep up with the pace of change, make the information load more usable, and basically make everything intelligent [27]. Artificial intelligence, block chain, and cloud computing have matured and will continue to progress in medical devices, all feeding into Big Data & Analytics to help make predictive analytic decisions regarding population health. Research around genomics, health wearables, nanomedicine, robotics, and medical 3D printing is promising to deliver targeted, precised, and timely less costly healthcare services. The catalyst for AHS to implement scientific and digital transformation is to create more value for patients along the continuum of care. Scientific and digital technology provides an opportunity to coordinate single-step care providers into communities of care. Empowered and connected patients and the emergence of advanced medical devices, sensors, and wearables have allowed clinicians with their patients to make more fact-based care decisions. The goal is to ensure targeted and personalized responses across the spectrum of service providers. Systems are evolving from the optimization of single providers to building a community of specialists that collaborates in a wider ecosystem [24]. Scientific and digital technology allows AHS to harness cloud-based solutions and help professionals and consumers to jointly create more comprehensive, patient-centered, and cost-effective healthcare. AHS must help and encourage patients to navigate their healthcare needs, by fostering prevention, managing chronic diseases, and improving communications so that clinicians and researchers can make good real-time decisions. Academic healthcare systems are part of, and often led, the scientific and digital revolution where digital transformation creates more value in healthcare services within healthcare networks. Real-time digital platforms help eliminate inefficiencies in healthcare delivery, and stakeholders connect beyond traditional channels. The efficiencies are when the patient care strategies are matched with the overall patient experience and program so clinicians can coordinate supply and demand by closing the access gap, second opinions, specialist's appointments, medical equipment, and transport [28].

Telemedicine (Telehealth) is a part of the rebuilding and reshaping AHS, and it is growing exponentially because more and more states are passing laws to allow reimbursement for telemedicine providers. By the end of 2017, over 22 states had applied for license [29]. According to Bloomberg Law, it was noted that there had been a tremendous expansion of virtual medicine through practitioner visits made possible by Telehealth, but the reimbursement mechanisms are uncharted waters [30]. Worse for AHS, there is a lack of comprehensive federal coverage to reimburse for Telehealth. The C-Suite is struggling with the countless financial uncertainties and questions where to invest funding in so many pertinent clinical and administrative areas essential when rebuilding.

In summary, rebuilding academic health systems will be an ongoing, comprehensive, and complex challenge to accomplish as the leadership struggles to implement the "correct" value-based model(s) while achieving its unique mission. AHS will need to continue its integration, collaboration, coordination, and partnerships to collectively set provider/payer policy, provide strategic management – including human resource planning and quality metrics – and institute new financial models. Across the continuum of care, AHS will be required to enforce and adhere to the requisite the ever changing laws and govermental regulations. As AHS address the changing regulations, they also must contend with the fact that some reimbursement legislation has not been keeping pace with the most scientific and digital innovations. It will be important for AHS to utilize digital technology to collectively build community care systems and to promote virtual health services that is to develop a sustainable and equitable quality healthcare service, relevant teaching, and innovative research using data and technology to create a cost-effective financial model.

References

1. Leavitt M. Moving ahead on the long road toward value-based healthcare. FutureScan: trends and implications. 2018.
2. Loughran M, Paanaowski MA. Health Care Policy: Bloomberg Law. BNA's Health Law Reporter, 27 HLR 6, 1/4/2018. The Bureau of National Affairs, Inc. https://www.bna.com.
3. Hansard S, Pelham V, Yochelson M, Stankiewiz M, Swann J. Health industry faces uncertain regulatory landscape: Bloomberg Law. BNA Health Law Reporter, 27 HLR 6, 1/4/2018. The Bureau of National Affairs, Inc.
4. Schneider E, Squires D. From last to first – Could the U.S. health care system become the best in the world? The Commonwealth Fund. 5/10/2018.
5. Leavitt M. The value of perspective. FutureScan: trends and implications. 2018.
6. Centers for Medicare & Medicaid Services (CMS). 2017 Medicare advantage value-based insurance design model. Updated August 17. https://innovation.cms.gov/initiatives/vbid.
7. Medicaid. Gov. 2017. March 2017. March 2017 medicaid and CHIP enrollment data highlights. Accessed 19 June. www.medicaid.gov/medicaid/program-information/Medicaid-and-chip-enrollment-data/report-highlights.
8. Abutaleb Y. U.S. healthcare spending to climb 5.3 percent in 2018: agency [Reuters]. Health News. February 14, 2018.
9. U.S. Centers for Medicare & Medicaid Services. Gov. – Historical highlights of National Health expenditures. 8 Jan 2018 https://www.cms.gov/research-statistics-data-and systems/statistics-trends-andreports.
10. U.S. Centers for Medicare & Medicaid Services. Gov. – Projected NHE Fact Sheet. 2017–2026. https://www.cms.gov/research-statistics-data-andsystems/statistics-trends-and reports.
11. Medicare access and CHIP Reauthorization Act of 2015 & 2018 – Title XVIII of Social Security Act. Pub. L. 114–10. http://legislink.org/us/pl-114-10.
12. U.S. Department of Health Y Human Services. 2015. Better, smarter, healthier. In historic announcement, HHS sets clear goals and timeline for shifting medicare reimbursements from volume to value. Published Jan 26. www.hhs.gov/news/press/01/20150126a.html.

13. Baurngarten A. Analysis of integrated delivery systems and new providers-sponsored health plans. Robert-Wood Johnson Foundation; 2017. Published June. www.rwjf.org/content/dam/farm/reports/2017/rwjf437615.
14. Wagner K. The move toward value-based payment. Healthcare executive May/June 2015. American College of Healthcare Executives; 2015.
15. U.S. Centers for Medicare & Medicaid Services. Gov. – Alternative payment models & merit-based incentive payment systems in the quality payment program. Feb 2018. https://www.cms.gov/Medicare/Quality-Payment.../Comprehensive-List-of-APMs.pdf.
16. Healthcare financial reporting in the digital age: how new technologies are helping providers tackle challenges and uncertainty. Oracle_ERP_ White_Paper _2018. www.oracle.com.
17. NTT Data: thrive in a changing market with analytics as a core competency. NTT_ White_Paper_2018. Becker's Hospital Review. 2018. www.nttdataservices.com/healthplans.
18. Belliveau J. 6 major hospital merger deals making headlines in 2018: practice management news; 2018. https://revcycleintelligence.com.
19. Sanborn BJ. Merger and acquisition activity has record-breaking first quarter in 2018. Healthcare Finance News. http://www.healthcarefinancenews.com/
20. KPMG. The disruption challenge: as new entrants and cross-sector models abound, which direction should healthcare organizations turn? 2018. www.kpmg.com/us/healthcarelifesciences.
21. US Department of Health & Human Services Office of Civil Rights (OCR). Breach Portal: Notice to Secretary of HHS Breach of Unsecured Protected Health Information; 2017. Accessed July 14. https://ocrportal.hhs.gov/ocr/breach/breach_ report.jsf.
22. Riggi J, Pitch P. Healthcare's moment of cyber reckoning. FutureScan: healthcare trends and implications; 2018.
23. HFMA. Health leaders cite limited ability to share clinical information as key obstacle to value-based payment; 2018. https://www.hfma.org/Content.aspx?id=59416.
24. A future in digital health: transforming healthcare for patients and providers. SAP Digital Healthcare paper. 2017 Edition. https://www.sap.com.
25. How tech-enabled consumers are reordering the healthcare landscape. McKinsey & Company. November 2016. www.mckinsey.com/industries/healthcare-systems-and-services/our-insignts/how-tech-enabled-consumers-are-reordering-the-health-care-landscape.
26. Kuhn B, Lehn C. Value-based reimbursement: the banner health network experience. Front Health Serv Manag. 2015;32(2):17–31.
27. Friedman T. Thank you for being late. Chapter 3-Moore's Law. The Macmillan Corporation. Copyright 2016. Hardcopy ISBN: 978-0-374-27353-8.
28. American Hospital Association (AHA). Next generation of community health accessed; 2016. September 15, 2017. www.aha.org/content/17/committee-on-research-next-gen-community-health.pdf.
29. Loughran M, Paanaowski MA. Health care policy: Bloomberg Law. BNA's Health Law Reporter, 27 HLR 6, 1/4/2018. The Bureau of National Affairs, Inc.
30. The most exciting medical technologies of 2017. http://medicalfuturist.com/the-most-exciting-medical-technologies-of-2017.

5 Academic Mission of the New Hospital: More Than Just the Bottom Line

Abe Fingerhut and Rifat Latifi

Introduction

The academic mission of the hospitals and institutions affiliated with universities or medical faculties has been the key component to advancement in clinical science through education and research and training new generations of pupils who become the new leaders of this mission. However, in today's era of corporate domination, the academic mission of hospitals and hospitalists is in danger. Academic physicians have a quadruple mission: education, research, publication, but, above all, patient care. Although intertwined and related, sometimes one of these components enters into conflict with the others. Very often, in particular, the three first impact the fourth, the main principled mission, patient care. The reasons for these conflicts are multifactorial. The lion's share would be that all four are time- and effort-consuming, and there are only so many hours in 1 day. But the reality today is that other forces have come into play and shed difficulties on the performance as well as motivation of the academic mission. First and foremost, the reality today is that cost-effectiveness has become the prime goal for many institutions, and unlimited clinical spending is no longer an option. Secondly, as hospitals, and especially university hospitals, have become costly, mainly because they are high-technology and multidisciplinary enterprises, and reimbursement has declined, so have operating margins diminished [1]. The quest for balanced budgets and overconservative coding, the main reason for reduced operating margins, however, is not specific to the United States. The perils facing academic surgery today are widespread in all developed and developing countries. Currently, all four academic missions are equally and constantly in conflict with running the hospital, epitomized by the administrative and financial pressures that befall the academic surgeon. Indeed, as surgical services represent up to 75% of hospital net income [2], they have become one of the main targets for efforts to balance budgets and keep the bottom line above water. The problem is not new but more than ever, "academic centers cannot stand alone in the world as they did in the past. They need to be part of a network, health care system and a vision" [3].

With respect to their teaching mission, academic hospitalists face several challenges. First, the financial constraints and obligations emanating from the newly created entrepreneurial aspect of hospital administration discourage hospitalists from traditional academic pursuits. More and more often, clinical, operational, or administrative duties distract them from their educational role in academia. New and untrained for some of

A. Fingerhut, MD (✉)
Surgical Research, Surgical Department, University of Graz, Graz, Austria
e-mail: abefingerhut@aol.com

R. Latifi, MD
New York Medical College, School of Medicine, Department of Surgery and Westchester Medical Center, Valhalla, NY, USA

R. Latifi (ed.), *The Modern Hospital*, https://doi.org/10.1007/978-3-030-01394-3_5

the obligations that befall on the academic hospitalist, these new activities are time-consuming and divert time away from academic undertakings. Secondly, recent reductions in resident training hours and an increasing demand to provide safe and 24-h coverage have pushed the role of teachers beyond those of traditional teaching, requiring increasing participation in medical co-management of surgical patients and coverage of non-teaching services. Moreover, as working hour restrictions have axed the time necessary for patient contact, the gap separating what should be known and what is known has increased and so has intensified the teaching burden on academics.

The Cost of Teaching New Generations of Surgeons

The academic hospital is the training ground for future physicians, and especially surgeons, who by definition have to learn their trade in a specific environment, the operating room, the ward, and clinics. This process has become complex and multidimensional. While there is and always has been a great deal of faculty time dedicated to students, residents, and fellows teaching and education outside operating room or on rounds on the ward, the costs of teaching have been poorly studied but undoubtedly have a major impact on the academic mission in several ways.

Operating rooms have become the theater for complex and sometimes lengthy procedures, requiring longer setup time (e.g., robotic surgery), as well as time-consuming exchanges of information between senior and juniors for teaching purposes. Incremental costs related to longer operating times when residents and less experienced junior consultants operate as compared with senior consultants have been reported [4–6] (Straetmans personal communication (EAES 2005)). The reasons include slower progression compared with the more experienced operator and prolonged supervision in the operating room; both amputate the time necessary for the other components of the academic mission [4–6].

As a consequence, the money spent on surgeons' salaries does not directly contribute to hospital profits but still impacts on the budget. According to Harington et al., estimating that the average salary for an assistant professor of surgery is approximately $180,000 per year and based on a 60-h work per week, this is $45.52 in faculty costs (money lost) per anastomosis when a senior surgeon assists a junior surgeon performing an enteroenterostomy during laparoscopic Roux-en-Y gastric bypass [5].

Increased time spent in the OR to teach takes its toll on hospital budgets. The calculation varies from one institution to another and from one country (or healthcare system) to another, ranging from 300 US$/h [6] to 2000 US$ [5] or in Europe 12 euros/minute (720 euros/h) (Straetmans personal communication (EAES 2005)). If the cost of 1 h in the operating room is $2000 per hour, the cost for teaching one entero-enterostomy performed during laparoscopic Roux-en-Y gastric bypass is $1457 [5]. In their teaching program, they estimated that providing 15 senior residents an educational opportunity to perform just two laparoscopic enteroenterostomies a year would cost $45,061.

Conversion of laparoscopic to open procedures, another reason for increased procedural times [7] and increased costs (related to changes necessary in equipment (especially when disposable), in material, and sometimes in personnel), may be more frequently observed in teaching hospitals.

Moreover, Babineau et al. [5] estimated that "opportunity costs" for the teaching surgeon (money he or she could be earning if they were doing something else rather than teaching) were 1600 US$ lost per operation!

Dedicated Time for Academic Activities

The time necessary for and used for teaching has to be organized. In many countries, it is up to the senior doctors to determine who does what and to what degree. In France, for instance, it is the dean of the university and a specific educational committee for each university who set up the teaching program and agenda. The choice of who does what is distributed to the work force, but usually the tasks fall on the more junior staff. Teaching activities can be localized within the hospital but sometimes take place in the university facilities. As the teaching activities are daytime chores, the time necessary to teach means that the practitioners have to leave the wards, potentially creating conflicts with proper healthcare duties. There is no real time dedicated to research except those practitioners who have an appointment with the research unit (INSERM). In Austria, the university requires that 30% of academic staff's time be devoted to teaching and research (including publication). In the United States, however, there is no rule on this, with the exception of clerkship directors (in charge of medical student's education) or residency program directors (who are supposed to dedicate at least 30–40% of their time to this task). For the most part, there is no protected time for education or research and publication. There are some exceptions on the latter, however. For newly hired junior surgeons, some institutions may provide so-called seed money and lab support to start research projects for faculties, usually junior faculty. This, however, is expected to be productive and ensure future grants that may further support portions of their salaries.

Financial Constraints and Academic Mission

Today's financial constraints are often the result of one-sided administrative or hospital board decisions that derive from budget concerns rather than patient care. These constraints frequently amputate funding necessary for salaries of medical staff along with money necessary for medical devices and equipment.

In the first instance, these constraints can be responsible for not recruiting top-quality physicians or losing important faculty members, potentially leading to understaffing or sometimes shifting of responsibilities (the more senior surgeons often ask the more junior to replace them in the teaching role). Department chairs are more than ever under fire to maintain a high level of quality of the faculty they recruit but need to be able to propose financial compensation that will attract them and keep them [8]. In accordance to the UCSF mission statement [9], in order to continue its mission, most university hospitals "have to attract and educate the most promising students for future careers in the health sciences and health care professions, encourage and support research and scholarly activities in the relevant disciplines that will improve our basic understanding of the causes, mechanisms, treatment and prevention of disease, and the social interactions related to human health; bring to our patients the best in health care, from primary care to the most advanced available technologies" and finally "serve the community at large through education and service programs." This means that there have to be people dedicated to this cause. Not only the physicians but dedicated staff and office employees are needed to do the administrative work, an academic-geared recruiting service to find and attract the best students, on-site facilities that meet the standards of comfort that the students expect, expert guidance, and leadership.

With regard to the impact on academic mission, financial constraints that lead to not being able to buy the most effective device or outdated or run-down equipment slow the process of operations and therefore take away some of the precious time necessary for teaching or other academic mission components.

In addition to these financial constraints, more and more, there are major administrative constraints that hamper the academic mission of today's hospital. Rules and regulations, public perception on performing research, rules on translation of science from bench to clinical programs, and other permissions required for innovative procedures, pharmacovigilance, materiovigilance, and inter-hospital-one company buying procedures, which reduce the variability and customization of patient care, increase the learning period for rotating staff; this is characteristic of teaching hospitals.

Clinical Research

Running a research laboratory while building one's clinical practice is often seen as "mission impossible" to young surgeons [10, 11]. The future of basic science in academic surgery is identifying barriers to success for surgeon-scientists [11].

With such time and money constraints, the number of applications for grants has dwindled. Combined with a lower funding success rate, surgical research is imperiled [12].

Campbell et al. [13] conducted a survey of a subsample of department chairs and senior research administrators in US medical schools to assess the perceived quality and health of the clinical research enterprise related to the changing state of the US healthcare system. Slightly more than half (52%) of respondents rated the quality of research as good or excellent. They noted that pressure on clinical faculty to see patients, mandated by the hospital administrators to earn money, was largely responsible. Moreover, for clinically active staff to be able to be funded either intramurally or extramurally, there is a need for support staff to assist with grant writing. Lack of such support leads to lack of external support. They concluded that the concerns voiced frequently about clinical research are real, but strategies to deal with the problems are underdeveloped. Indeed, the leaders in this study felt that clinical research activities in academic centers were declining and because the policies established to correct this imbalance are lacking, they did not see a solution in the near future. Moreover, the problem is exaggerated today because of the rapid and sometime exponential increase in advances in basic research and technology.

The business-type exigencies of payers and administrative directives, along with declining reimbursement and communicating vessels of the existing, but dwindled funds for new clinical knowledge, make it difficult if not impossible to do clinical research today without changing the model [14, 15].

As nonacademic health systems get together with academic centers to create alliances, partnerships, or mergers, or even when they acquire these academic centers, profit-making should not cast a blind eye on the necessity of clinical research to find new knowledge to be used for the good of our patients.

According to Laret [16] of the San Francisco Medical School (University of California), academic medicine is in great peril from unprecedented budget cuts to education, flat budgets for research funding, and declining clinical income. In addition to ring-fenced funding, academic surgeons have been struck with an array of extra costs including higher contributions to personal liability insurance and pensions, pressure and time constraints due to increasing demands of patients and hospital employers related to patient safety concerns, and long working hours.

In his special communication to the annual meeting of the Association of American Medical Colleges, Laret [16] underlined that professional reimbursement from Medicare and Medicaid is so low that many physicians no longer provide care for Medicare or Medicaid patients. Moreover, Medicare and Medicaid reimbursement cannot cover the costs of providing care at most teaching hospitals. Notwithstanding, as measures are taken in every proposed plan to reduce federal and state spending and deficits, Medicare and Medicaid budgets are first in line for reductions. He outlined that indirect and direct medical education supplements are under heavy attack today, meaning that all too often, clinical income, although also dwindling in many hospitals, is increasingly used to cover the costs of education and underfunded research.

As clinical income falls, the entire academic enterprise is threatened as never before. In Japan, for instance, higher labor costs and increased ("consumption") taxes have taken their toll on hospital care as decreased salaries have led physicians to seek second jobs, decreasing the quality of care and academic missions [17].

According to Hauptman and colleagues [18], research in the present era of mergers between university and non-university units has a prospective of increasing the patient populations that can be included in clinical research but not necessarily under optimal scientific conditions.

Another problem particular to surgeons today is that although total National Institute of Health (NIH) funding has increased over the decade 2006–2016, the amount of funding allotted to surgical departments has declined. Increasing pressure by hospital administrators to devote more of surgeons' time on patient care, more financially beneficial to the hospital system, is certainly one of the reasons [12]. The complexity of application processes has also limited the number of institutions that get awarded such grants. In other words, only institutions and academic centers that have the necessary infrastructure (including research support staff) in place can successfully compete for those awards.

Industry Support and Research

As outlined in several studies, one negative consequence of decreasing funds for research and education is that practitioners are tempted to rely more and more on industry for teaching purposes. It is widely known that many training facilities worldwide are run by industry, even when they are located within academic centers. Extreme vigilance from the organizers and the instructors is necessary to avoid conflicts of interest in the pedagogical message, but as industry is the provider, this can indeed be problematic. Despite being the so-called "teaching" hospitals, the majority of community hospitals worldwide do not have even basic infrastructure in place and thus cannot compete successfully for grants and awards. This opens the possibility of industry to influence such activities, since they usually have support system to ensure the "result" or "qualities" of their products is published.

Publication

Publication, the vehicle of scientific discoveries, innovations, research, and clinical practice, is not limited to academic surgeons but has a predominant place in the academic mission. The motivation behind publication in the scientific world may be both egoistic and altruistic [19]. Among the egoistic motives for writing and publishing, academic and professional promotion is certainly in the minds of all surgeons aspiring an academic career [19, 20]. Among the "altruistic" motives is the main purpose of professional publishing: disseminate knowledge. In many academic settings, research, whether clinical or not, and its quality are measured, and, variably according to various countries, these metrics serve as the basis for funding [19]. However, there is no formal time allocated to this activity in most academic centers. Teaching medical writing and clinical methodology has been long neglected by medical schools, and most surgeons learn from experience. However, the quality of medical papers is highly reliant on the skills of critical appraisal that have to be taught somewhere along the careers of future academics [21]. This academic role has been neglected in many institutions, and when it does exist, the time and money necessary to accomplish this role have to be found, often at the expense of other activities or funding sources.

Solutions

Many of these activities have to be accomplished outside of hospital hours but then enter in conflict with hospital physician's personal and family life and activities [12], which may lead to personal problems such as burnout (see Chap. 41).

Notwithstanding the realities of the problems, on a more positive side, Laret [16] listed several central questions for leaders in academic medicine to think about and find solutions to. These include asking ourselves if we are genuinely open to hearing and accepting what society is saying to us about doing more, doing it better, and doing it at far lower cost; whether we have the courage to challenge, and retire, long-standing structures and academic cultures whose utility may have passed; and are we ready to embrace collaboration with entirely new partners and to use entirely new tools to achieve our missions. If the answer is to be yes, then there is some hope that solutions will be found. They conclude by stating that the moment for action is now. Maybe, we need to think differently about academic medicine to be able to continue our missions; we owe it to our students, our faculty and staff, our patients, our communities, and in fact our nation and the world. Because of decreasing resources and benefit-driven hospital policies, investment has to be considered from different sources to continue the academic mission and maintain the clinical value of past scientific discoveries and opportunities to improve care. Aside from accepting industry-related funding and to avoid the related conflict of interest [22], Moses et al. suggested that potential sources could include repatriation of foreign capital, new innovation bonds, administrative savings, patent pools, and public-private risk sharing collaborations [23].

In summary, while there are significant challenges that academic healthcare systems face today [10, 24–27] including training new healthcare professionals, disproportionate clinical care of complex and costly patients, charity care to uninsured and underinsured, and reduced research funding opportunities, there are a number of solutions proposed by these authors including new reimbursement methods, improvements in operational efficiency, price regulation, subsidization of education, improved decision-making and communication, utilization of industrial management tools, and increasing internal and external cooperation.

The academic mission of the modern hospital should be more than just the bottom line, as their true mission is training the new generations of healthcare providers and advancing the science of medicine and surgery. In this process, creative solutions need to be found and implemented to ensure such mission is not damaged or neglected even in the era of the corporate world.

References

1. Zelenock GB, Zambricki CS. The health care crisis. Impact on surgery in the community. Hospital Setting Arch Surg. 2001;136:585–91.
2. Zelenock GB, Stanley JC, More RA, et al. Differential clinical workloads among faculty at a major academic health center. Ann Surg. 1997;226:336–47.
3. Money J. Merger scuttled between OU Medical Center and St Anthony parent. Oklahoman. March 6, 2017. http://newsok.com/article/5540555. Accessed 11 June 2018.
4. Koperna T. How long do we need teaching in the operating room? The true costs of achieving surgical routine. Langenbeck's Arch Surg. 2004;389:204–8.
5. Harington DT, Roy GD, Ryder BA, Miner TJ, Richardson P, Cioffi WG. A time-cost analysis of teaching a laparoscopic entero-enterostomy. J Surg Edu. 2007;64:342–5.
6. Babineau TJ, Becker J, Gibbons G, Sentovich S, Hess D, Robertson S, Stone M. The "cost" of operative training for surgical residents. Arch Surg. 2004;139:366–70.
7. Gervaz P, Pikarsky A, Utech M, Secic M, Efron J, Belin B, Jain A, Wexner S. Converted laparoscopic colorectal surgery a meta-analysis. Surg Endosc. 2001;15:827–32.
8. Balser J, Lee TH. The danger and opportunity of leading a hospital interview NEJM Catalyst. August 7, 2017. https://catalyst.nejm.org/leading-academic-medical-center/. Accessed 11 June 2018.
9. University of California San Francisco Mission statement. https://www.ucsf.edu/sites/default/files/legacy_files/LRDP-Appendices-C.pdf. Consulted online March 2018.
10. Keswani SG, Moles CM, Morowitz M, Zeh H, Kuo JS, Levine MH, Cheng LS, Hackam DJ, Ahuja N, Goldstein AM, Basic Science Committee of the Society of University Surgeons. The future of basic science in academic surgery: identifying barriers to success for surgeon-scientists. Ann Surg. 2017;265:1053–9.
11. Ko CY, Whang EE, Longmire WP Jr, McFadden DW. Improving the surgeon's participation in research: is it a problem of training or priority? J Surg Res. 2000;91:5–8.
12. Narahari AK, Mehaffey JH, Hawkins RB, Charles EJ, Baderdinni PK, Chandrabhatla AS, Kocan JW, Jones RS, Upchurch GR, Kron IL, Kern JA, Ailawadi G. Surgeon scientists are disproportionately affected by declining NIH funding rates. J Am Coll Surg. 2018;226:474–81.
13. Campbell EG, Weissman JS, Moy E, Blumenthal D. Status of clinical research in Academic Health Centers views from the research leadership. JAMA. 2001;286:800–6.
14. Ioannidis JPA. Defending biomedical science in an era of threatened funding. JAMA. 2017;317(24):2483–4.
15. Katz IT, Wright AA. Scientific drought, golden eggs, and global leadership—why Trump's NIH funding cuts would be a disaster. N Engl J Med. 2017;376:1701–4.
16. Laret MR. Academic medicine in the 21st century. JAMA Intern Med. 2013;173:1739–41. https://doi.org/10.1001/jamainternmed.2013.7763.
17. Medical services in Tokyo area in danger of collapsing. Japan Times, Sept 21, 2015.
18. Hauptman PJ, Bookman RJ, Heinig S. Advancing the research mission in a time of mergers and acquisitions. JAMA. 2017;318:1321–2.
19. Schein M, Farndon JR, Fingerhut A. Why should a surgeon publish? Br J Surg. 2000;87:3–5.
20. Kron IL. Getting promoted. J Thorac Cardiovasc Surg. 2001;121:S17–8.
21. Fingerhut A, Lacaine F. Critical appraisal: an essential skill for all surgeons. Surg Innov. 2017:1–2. https://doi.org/10.1177/1553350617690311.

22. Galea S, Saltz R. Funding, Institutional conflicts of interest, and schools of public health realities and solutions. JAMA. 2017;317:17 1735–6.
23. Moses H, Matheson DHM, Cairns-Smith S, George BP, Palisch C, Dorsey R. The anatomy of medical research US and international comparisons. JAMA. 2015;313(2):174–89. https://doi.org/10.1001/jama.2014.15939.
24. Stimpson JP, Li T, Shiyanbola OO, Jacobson JJ. Financial sustainability of academic health centers: identifying challenges and strategic responses. Acad Med. 2014;89:853–7.
25. Goldman L. The academic health care system: preserving the missions as the paradigm shifts. JAMA. 1995;273:1549–52.
26. Jones RS, Debas HT. Research: a vital component of optimal patient care in the United States. Ann Surg. 2004;240:573–7.
27. Murphy B. Meeting the challenge of the academic mission: 3 strategies to improve efficiency in academic hospitals' ORs. Becker's Hospital Review, February 21st, 2017. Retrieved from: https://www.beckershospitalreview.com/hospital-management-administration/meeting-the-challenge-of-the-academic-mission-3-strategies-to-improve-efficiency-in-academic-hospitals-ors.html.

The Role of the Hospital in the Healthcare System

6

Renee Garrick, Janet (Jessie) Sullivan, Maureen Doran, and June Keenan

Introduction

According to Greek mythology, as long ago as 430 BCE, Asclepius, the god of medicine, was worshiped at early healing temples. Over time these temples became more elaborate, with specially designed healing spaces. The Asclepieion of Epidaurus which dates to 350 BCE contains marble tablets detailing the names, histories, and treatments of many of those ancient patients. In fact, according to the records, intra-abdominal surgical procedures were performed in these early settings under opium-like anesthesia [1]. The word "hospital" was later derived from the Latin *hospes*, signifying guest or foreigner, and expanded from the Old French *ospital* or "shelter for the needy." The term hospital, as a "charitable institution for sick and wounded people," came into use in the fifteenth century [2].

Over time, the settlement of villages, the injuries of war, and the spread of infectious illnesses lead to the development of infirmaries, and in 1751 the first hospital in the United States opened in Philadelphia [3]. During the next century, breakthroughs in the concepts of sterile technique, aseptic surgery, anesthesia, and radiographic imaging led to hospitals becoming sites for actual treatments and cure [4–6]. In the United States, the publication of the *Flexner Report* led to standardized medical training, and this coupled with improved therapeutics, such as antibiotics, and advances in technology made hospitals safer sites for care [7]. Over the ensuing years, ongoing remarkable advances in technology and medical therapeutics have stimulated public support for the financing and expansion of our current, largely hospital-based, healthcare infrastructure.

This chapter will initially focus on the recent history of the growth of the infrastructure of the hospital system in the United States and will then explore how the foundational pillar of inpatient care is changing, as a result of, and in response to, other pressures and changes that are occurring within the healthcare system. The co-variables and counterbalances of science, medicine, politics, and finances are discussed in greater detail in other parts of this edition; how elements of those forces will alter the role and focus of the hospital within the broader healthcare system will be reviewed here.

R. Garrick (✉)
Department of Medicine, New York Medical College, Westchester Medical Center, Valhalla, NY, USA
e-mail: Renee.Garrick@WMCHealth.org

J. Sullivan · M. Doran · J. Keenan
Center for Regional Healthcare Innovation, WMCHealth, Hawthorne, NY, USA

R. Latifi (ed.), *The Modern Hospital*, https://doi.org/10.1007/978-3-030-01394-3_6

The Rise of the Hospital-Based System of Healthcare

Several characteristics distinguish hospitals from other healthcare facilities such as clinics and ambulatory surgery centers. By definition, a hospital is able to provide overnight care and has qualified physicians and/or allied health providers, staff nurses, and other care providers available 24 hours a day 7 days a week. Typically, hospitals are able to provide higher levels of care than are ambulatory facilities. Recently, however, this distinction has become less clear, as some ambulatory care facilities are able to provide complex services including surgical and vascular interventions.

Several different types of hospitals are recognized in the United States. Two broad categories are federal (which includes the Veterans Administration hospitals and Army and Navy facilities) and nonfederal hospitals. Another classification is "for-profit vs. nonprofit" facilities. The split of these classes distinguishes the US system from most other countries, where the majority of healthcare is publicly funded. Hospitals may also be grouped by the types of services they provide: general acute care hospitals are geared to provide short-term medical and surgical care for a broad range of conditions and provide diagnostic imaging, laboratory services, and emergency department services. Most hospitals in the United States fall into this category and can be further identified by size (number of beds) and the intensity of services they provide. "Quaternary care" facilities provide more intensive and highly technical care, and "community hospitals" provide less complex "tertiary" and more basic "secondary" levels of inpatient care.

In addition to the general acute care hospitals, several types of single specialty hospitals have emerged in the US healthcare system. The most prevalent are specialized, free-standing psychiatric hospitals which care for patients who suffer from mental illness or substance use disorders. These patients often require extended inpatient stays and typically require treatment by highly specialized staff, including specialized nursing and social service staffs. Other specialty hospitals provide inpatient care with diagnostic and medical treatment for other specific diseases or conditions, such as specialized orthopedic or cardiovascular hospitals. These hospitals usually do not accept emergency care patients and cater to only elective admissions or patients specifically accepted in transfer from another institution. Some, but not all of these hospitals, are able to provide long-term inpatient care and follow-up for the chronically ill and rehabilitative and restorative services for physically challenged or disabled persons [8].

Two additional subcategories exist within acute care hospitals, teaching hospitals, and academic health centers. The terminology reference of "teaching hospital" typically implies that the hospital is engaged in the training of postgraduate medical students such as residents and fellows. In the United States, residency is the first level of postgraduate training after medical school and encompasses specific training in a broad area such as internal medicine, pediatrics, surgery, neurosurgery, obstetrics, family practice, anesthesiology, etc. Fellowship training, which is subspecialty training, begins following residency training. Fellows engage in subspecialty training in areas of medicine, such as cardiology, nephrology, rheumatology, etc., or in areas of surgery, such as cardiac surgery, trauma surgery, oncology surgery, etc. Many, but not all, teaching hospitals are also Academic Medical Centers. Academic Medical Centers are defined as those teaching hospitals that are linked to an academic center and must include a medical school and at least one additional school of health sciences, such as a school of nursing, or a graduate school of basic medical science which conveys doctorate (PhD) degrees. Academic Medical Centers are often defined by their tripartite mission of engagement in education of medical students and graduate residents and engagement in basic and translational research and in direct clinical care. Academic Medical Centers also participate in the training of other healthcare providers including nurses, nurse practitioners, physicians' assistants, respiratory therapists, physical and occupational therapists, speech and language therapists, and others. Although only 5% of all hospitals are

Academic Medical Centers, these hospitals occupy a unique place in the American healthcare system. Academic Medical Centers provide roughly 37% of all charity care, cover 26% of admissions covered by the publicly funded Medicaid program, and accept about 38% of all patients who need transfer to another facility to obtain a higher level of care [9].

The final classification of hospitals includes the “safety net” hospitals. These hospitals are legally mandated to provide all populations with care regardless of their ability to pay. Safety net hospitals typically provide care for a proportionally greater number of patients who are uninsured, underinsured, or covered by Medicaid Children’s Health Insurance Program (CHIP). In urban areas Academic Medical Centers with a mission of education and service often serve as safety net institutions. These safety net Academic Medical Centers are often the institutions that offer the most complex and costly care with the lowest margin of reimbursement such as trauma, burn, and high-intensity neonatal care. In more rural areas, private hospitals sometimes have a safety net function, and this is either typically specifically linked to their underlying mission or to the scarcity of alternative service providers. Because safety net hospitals are mandated to provide uncompensated care to many underserved and underinsured populations, the reimbursement for this care is financed through joint state and federal programs that are geared to reimburse these hospitals for the disproportionate share of free care provided [10].

US Trends in Size and Types of Hospitals

Over several decades the American Hospital Association has conducted an annual survey of hospitals in the United States. Aggregate data derived from this survey is published in *AHA Hospital Statistics*™ and allows an evaluation of trends [11].

Data from both the American Hospital Association and from the Centers for Medicare and Medicaid Services (CMS) demonstrate that there are fewer hospitals open for business in the United States in 2016 as compared to 2012 with almost all of this change (97%) due to a decrease in the number of hospitals in rural settings. During this period the number of very small (6–24 beds) hospitals and the number of very large (>500 beds) hospitals increased, while the number of hospitals in every other category diminished [11–13].

As shown in Fig 6.1a, b, which are derived from data available from survey data from the American Hospital Association, in 2016 fewer than 10% of US hospitals had over 400 beds, but these large hospitals accounted for 30–40% of all hospital services; 588 specialty hospitals accounted for 5% of inpatient days and primarily provided rehabilitative or long-term care [11].

The recent changes are a continuation of the trend of fewer hospitals providing shorter stays with a higher intensity of service. Since World War II, the number of hospitals and hospital beds relative to the US population has steadily declined, while the number of outpatient services provided and the total number of persons employed by hospitals have increased.

Figure 6.2 is a composite depiction of data derived from a number of sources and demonstrates the changes in bed number, utilization, and inpatient length of stay that have occurred during the past 70 years [14–17]. Adjusted for population growth, the number of patients admitted to the hospital each year increased from 1946 through 1980 and has since steadily declined. The fall in inpatient hospital admissions has been impressive. Based on American Hospital Association Survey, between 1980 and 2000 admissions fell on average 2% per year; there was a slight increase in admissions between 2000 and 2005 and then an 18% decline from 2005 to 2016. In 2016 a person in the United States was less likely to be admitted to hospital than at any time in the previous 70 years, and though this trend was true nationwide, a significant regional variation was present with fewer hospitalization days on the West Coast than the East (96.6 versus 127.9/1000 populations). During the same time interval, those who were admitted stayed fewer days in the hospital [18].

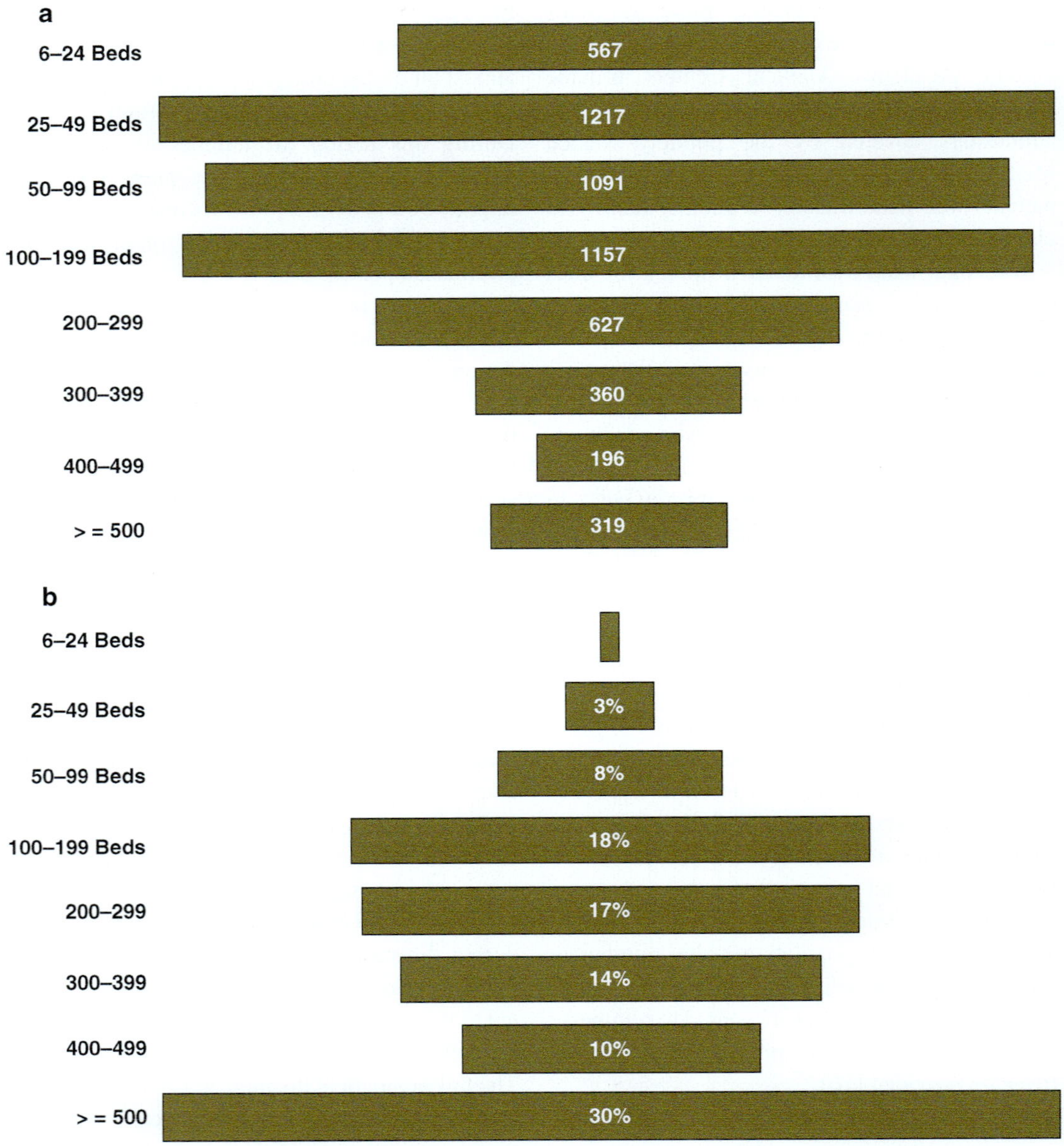

Fig. 6.1 (**a**) 2016 count of US hospitals classified by number of beds. (**b**) Percentage of 2016 inpatient days by size of hospital

This reduction in the hospital length of stay is, in part, linked to remarkable advancements in minimally invasive surgery which have dramatically altered the recovery time for medical procedures. For example, replacement of the aortic valve of the heart can now be done utilizing a minimally invasive procedure (transvenous aortic valve replacement) and be completed within a 2–3-day hospital stay. In the past, patients routinely required a 2–3-week hospital stay following aortic valve replacement. Moreover, many procedures, which previously required an inpatient stay, are now routinely done entirely in an outpatient setting at a lower cost and with increased convenience. Some of these outpatient centers are financially independent and compete with hospitals for patients and providers. Despite this competition, the data suggests a marked

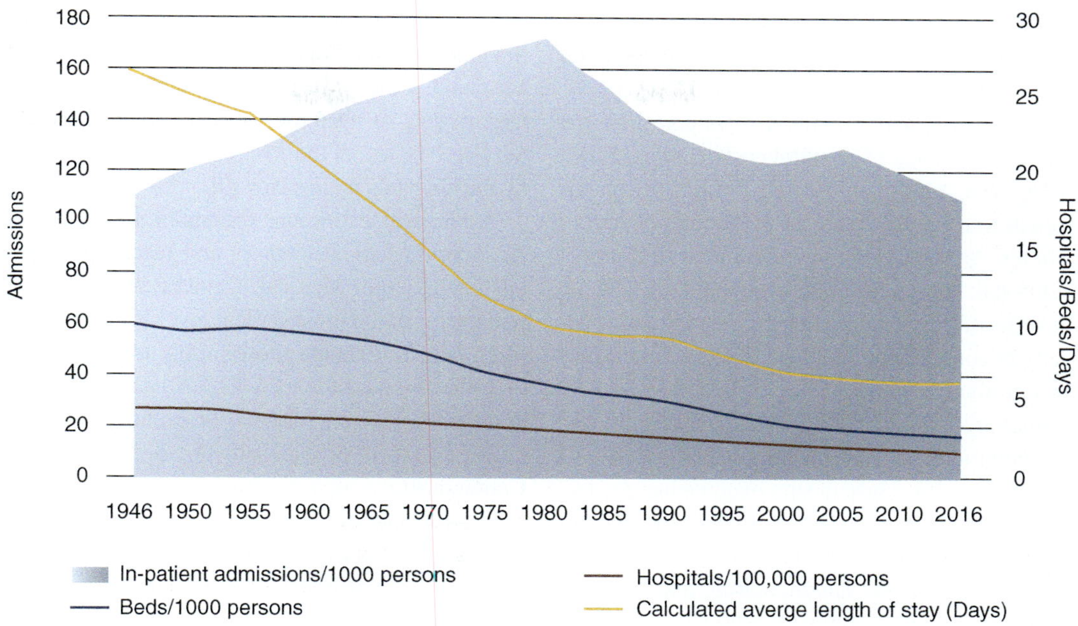

Fig. 6.2 Hospitals beds and admission per person 1946–2016

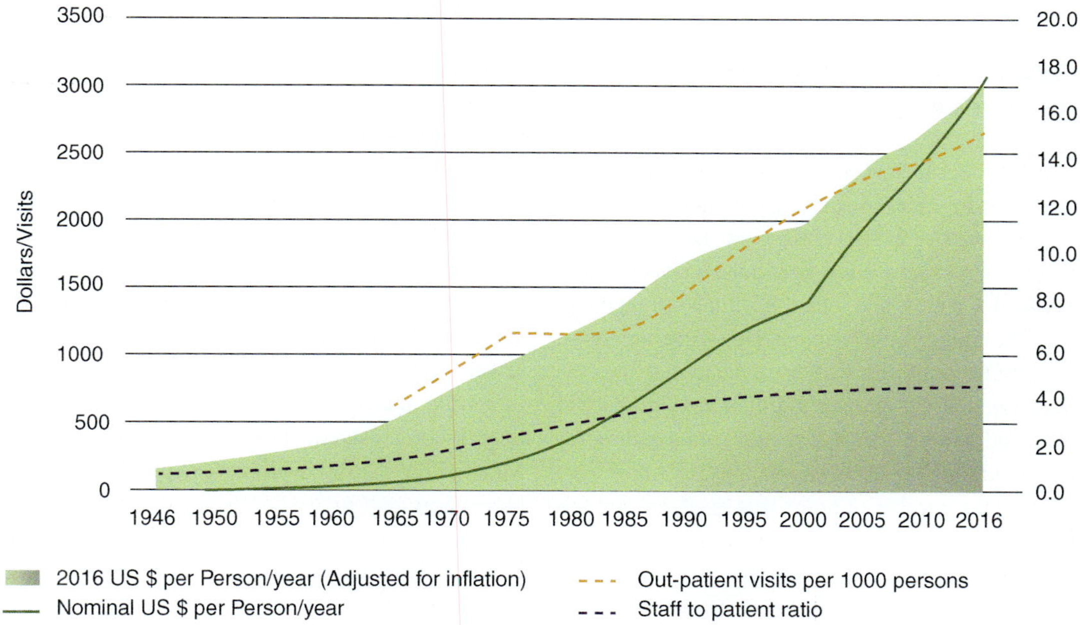

Fig. 6.3 US hospital expense per person 1946–2016; outpatient visits per person; staff to patient ratios

increase in the number of hospital outpatient services since 1965. In 2016 hospitals provided, on average, 2.7 outpatient services for every person in the United States, and outpatient services accounted for 49% of hospital revenue [19].

Figure 6.3 demonstrates data drawn from a number of sources and indicates the changes in several key hospital financial metrics over time [14–17, 20]. While the number of admissions and the length of stay have both fallen, as demonstrated in Fig. 6.3, the cost of hospital care has risen dramatically, with inflation-adjusted hospital expenses increasing, on average, by 5% a year.

Staff wages and benefits always comprise the largest percentage of hospital costs, and as shown in Fig. 6.3, from 1965 to the present, there has been as a substantial increase in the ratio of staff to patients. As discussed in greater detail in Chap. 5, additional factors are responsible for driving up the costs of hospital care in the United States especially as compared with other developed countries. Among these are the routine utilization of costly technology, expendables such as pharmaceuticals, and commodities such as surgical implants and devices [21–23]. Thus, in sum over the last decade, as outpatient services have increased, the number of admissions to hospitals has fallen, the acuity of hospitalized patients has increased, and the need for highly trained, technically proficient, and more costly staff and more costly technology has concomitantly significantly increased.

Pressures on Hospitals and Forces for Change

The last decade has seen enormous disruption in the US healthcare industry creating new and amplified pressures on all classes of hospitals. The requirements for teaching hospitals, both Academic Medical Centers and other hospitals engaged in resident training, have expanded: there are more work-hour restrictions, more educational imperatives demanding greater training and outpatient care, and new educational requirements calling for protected time for research. All these changes have reduced the number of hours that residents and fellows (house staff) are engaged in direct inpatient medical care and necessitated the addition of mid-level practitioner such as nurse practitioners and physician assistants to the hospital workforce. These individuals are typically costlier than house staff and work fewer hours per week. It is sometimes stated that house staff "makes money for hospitals," but the data demonstrate that hospitals contribute substantial resources to the training of the next generation of physicians. Graduate medical education in the United States costs about $16 billion annually [9]. Medicare contributes about $3 billion each year toward training house staff. Smaller amounts of support are derived from Medicaid, the Veterans Administration, the Department of Defense, and the Public Health Service. The rest of the cost of training is subsumed by the hospitals themselves [9].

Additional economic pressures are faced by Academic Medical Centers and teaching hospitals. Academic Medical Centers care for the patients with the most critical levels of injury and often help to provide these highly technical services for at-risk patients who lack healthcare coverage and other resources. For example, 80% of all burn care is provided by Academic Medical Centers [9], as is a high proportion of trauma care, psychiatric emergency care, pediatric intensive care, and complex pediatric services such as pediatric neurosurgery, cardiothoracic surgery, and vascular surgery. These highly specialized services require extensive resources and specified levels of advanced certification and accreditation and are often inadequately reimbursed.

Top-level certifications, such as those required for level I trauma services, complex neonatal services, and oncology services, require that hospitals engage in clinical and/or basic bench science research to achieve and sustain certification. Grant support does not fully underwrite the cost of this research, and it is estimated that, overall, about 30–40% of the cost of research at academic health facilities is borne by the facilities themselves [24].

Thus, hospitals have been grappling with fewer inpatient admissions, in the face of increased use of expensive technology and an overall increase in hospital-related expenses. Meanwhile, overall healthcare expenditures were increasing, and in 2016, US healthcare spending reached $3.3 trillion or $10,348 per person. Hospital care accounted for approximately 32% of this overall healthcare expense [25].

Patient-Centered, Evidence-Driven, Value-Based Care

As healthcare costs continued to increase, the focus of healthcare reimbursement moved toward a value-based proposition, characterized as the Triple Aim [26] providing better, higher-quality outcomes to more patients at a lower cost. The hospital value-based program, signed into law as part of the Medicare Prescription Drug, Improvement, and Modernization Act of 2003, was designed to promote better clinical outcomes for hospital patients and to improve their in-hospital experience of care while simultaneously lowering costs [27].

Importantly, one of the value-based domains focuses on enhanced efficiency and cost reduction. This performance metric holds hospitals accountable for the patient's health status for the 30-day period following discharge. Thus, hospitals are now being required to participate in care across the entire healthcare continuum and are being held directly responsible for the care that occurs after discharge.

Not surprisingly, private insurance companies, such as Anthem Health, CIGNA, the UnitedHealth Group, and Aetna, have followed the footsteps of the Centers for Medicare and Medicaid Services (CMS) and have added to the financial stress of hospitals by also linking hospital reimbursement to outcome metrics and patient satisfaction scores [28].

While the intention of these programs is to incentivize hospitals to provide efficient, cost-effective, high-quality care, the approach places hospital reimbursement at risk. The value-based purchasing structure has a "revenue-neutral construct," so that some "at -risk" revenue is moved from poorly performing hospitals to higher-performing hospitals, which, counterintuitively, in turn, can limit the ability of a "poorly performing" hospital to afford ongoing clinical improvement initiatives. In addition to these challenges, healthcare disparities and the socioeconomic determinants of health are not factored into the current value-based scoring hospital metrics. Studies have demonstrated almost half of the variation in 30-day readmission rates following an admission for heart failure, a heart attack, or pneumonia was linked to community and social factors, such as access to care, rather than to the quality of care rendered within the hospital walls [29]. With these considerations in mind, it should not be surprising to learn that in 2016 academic teaching hospitals made up 17.9% of the 1235 hospitals that were penalized for inferior performance and comprised only 6.9% of the 1806 hospitals that received a bonus for performance on value-based metrics [30]. Similar findings have been reported for safety net hospitals which were shown to be disproportionately more likely to be assessed a reimbursement penalty based on a value-based payment system. For example, in 2014, the readmission penalty for safety net hospitals approached $500 per bed versus $314 for non-safety net hospitals [31]. In addition to a direct reduction in reimbursement, poor outcomes on quality metric determinants can tarnish a hospital reputation and status, which in turn can influence its role as a "provider of choice" for both patients and private insurance payers.

Overall, the net impact of the changes in hospital expenses and reimbursements has created a new set of challenges for many Academic Medical Centers, large teaching hospitals, and safety net institutions. These pressures are especially significant within Academic Medical Centers. Historically, these costly institutions sit at the top of the healthcare pyramid. Identified as delivering high-quality, advanced care, fueled by innovation and cutting-edge technology, Academic Medical Centers attract excellent clinicians, basic scientists, and affiliated staff. They were typically viewed as the provider of choice within their healthcare community and had several avenues of monetary support including philanthropy, public support for indigent care, commercial insurance payments, and research grant dollars. In the past clinical "excess revenue," over expenses could be used by these centers to underwrite uncompensated clinical care, as well as to cross subsidize the missions of research and teaching. Changing regulations, reduced public and research support, and the market forces which have moved less complex care from the hospital to the outpatient setting, coupled with rapidly changing and uncertain models of hospital reimbursement, have led to the prediction that over the next 2–3 years, the expenses of many Academic Medical Centers will outpace the growth of clinical revenues. As will be discussed later, these pressures and those being felt by other parts of the healthcare system have led academic centers to reassess their business approach to their mission and focus [32].

Financial pressures are also being experienced by small community, rural hospitals, and critical access hospitals. More than half of the hospitals in the country are rural hospitals, and in many regions they are the sole provider of inpatient, outpatient, emergency services and preventative services. Moreover in many regions these hospitals are separated from one another by long distances, and emergency access to care is compromised by inefficient or nonexistent modes of public transportation. The North Carolina Rural Health Research Program, funded by the Federal Office of Rural Health Policy, helps to track the health of these hospitals. Their data demonstrate that between 2010 and the present, 83 rural hospitals have closed, of which 29 were "critical access" hospitals, defined as those with under 25 beds and more than 35 miles from another healthcare facility. The majority of these closures were in the South and Southwest with 14 closures in Texas, 8 in Tennessee, and 6 in Georgia. Overall, half of all states experienced at least one rural hospital closure from 2010 to present [33]. These hospitals struggle for staff, resources, technology, and financial stability. The loss of these hospitals poses an enormous threat to the communities they serve, especially as the nation strives to improve the health of the population and overall access to patient-centered, efficient, and equitable care.

New Opportunities and Visions for Traditional Hospitals

Clearly, traditional hospitals, which have been a mainstay of our healthcare system, are experiencing disruptive pressures and must change and evolve to survive and continue to meet patient needs in an ever-changing healthcare system. The in-hospital environment is technically complex, and it is not easy for these brick-and-mortar buildings to flex to the changing healthcare needs of the country. For many hospitals, inpatient admissions and profitability have decreased, and simultaneously, the capabilities of ambulatory centers, which are often privately held and compete financially with hospitals, have expanded. Moreover, advances in tele-health and related technology have made it possible to quickly link healthcare providers and patients together, and with this it is likely that more types of advanced services will be safely provided outside of a hospital setting. These pressures are occurring against a backdrop of a shift toward value-based reimbursement, which demands that hospitals reengineer processes and create patient-centered care which focuses both on the patient's "experience" and the quality and safety of the clinical care during, and after, the hospital stay. The World Health Organization has questioned the role of the hospital in the changing healthcare environment and asked:

> If hospitals are to be integral parts of the healthcare system what should they look like? What size should they be? How should they be distributed within a geographical area? How can hospitals … enhance their performance both in terms of health outcomes and economic performance? [34]

To succeed, hospitals must "get beyond their walls." Academic centers and teaching hospitals must develop alliances with smaller community and rural hospitals and providers to ensure a flow of patients through their doors and at the same time must respect the individuality of their new partners. Conversely, the smaller allied hospitals and provider organizations must be willing to cede some local control and, in turn, gain resources and stability from their larger partner.

Predicated on the background information above, the sections that follow will outline new pathways that hospitals are forging within their changing, and challenging, environment.

Hospital Mergers and Acquisitions

In much of the world, "district" hospitals that provide high-technology intensive care operate within an organized system and are linked to local hospitals, which provide more basic inpatient, diagnostic, and surgical services, and to clinics and other providers of ambulatory community care [35].

Within most of the United States rather than a carefully planned healthcare system, competitive market forces have played the predominant role in determining linkages between hospitals and other providers. In the past many independent practicing physicians worked alone or in small groups and participated on the voluntary medical staff of a local community hospital. The pressures described, including reduced reliance on inpatient services, increased demand for advanced technology, integrated patient information systems, and the movement toward value-based reimbursement, which demands that care by coordinated across all sites, have driven previously independent organizations to affiliate or consolidate into more integrated delivery systems.

The structure of hospital mergers and consolidations can range from loose affiliations to a full acquisition [36]. The structures can include vertical integration, bringing together affiliated organizations providing different kinds of services such as hospital, ambulatory, ancillary care and social services, and/or horizontal integration, bringing together multiple organizations providing the same kind of services, such as hospitals or clinics [37].

Over the last few decades, the sprint to integrate has gathered speed. In 2013, HealthLeaders Media asked 159 healthcare leaders, primarily from academic health systems, teaching hospitals, and group practices, their plans regarding mergers or acquisition. Only 13% of hospital executives expected to remain fully independent from other healthcare systems [38]. Between 2012 and 2017, on average 103 mergers took place each year, and 115 hospital merges were announced in 2017 alone, an increase of almost 13% from the prior year. The planned mergers involve for-profit, non-profit, secular, and non-secular hospitals. Ten of the planned mergers involved hospitals with revenues of over $1 billion, and if approved by the courts and regulatory agencies, the planned merger between Dignity Health and Catholic Healthcare Initiatives, with revenues of over $27 billion, will create the largest not-for-profit health system in the country [39].

At the same time that hospitals have been consolidating, they have also been acquiring and directly employing physicians [38–40]. Twenty-seven percent of the Health Leaders Survey noted above responded that they had engaged in physician acquisitions in the last year and almost 60% said they plan to acquire physician groups going forward [38]. These employment arrangements represent a frame shift for practicing physicians. In 2012 only about 25% of physicians were employed by hospitals. This has increased almost 63% from 95,000 to 155,000 between 2012 and 2016 [41], and by mid-year of 2016, about 42% of practicing physicians were employed by hospitals [41]. These acquisitions have occurred in all states and in both urban and rural settings [38]. For physicians, mounting financial pressures including reduced reimbursement by almost all payer groups, the demands and risks of value-based reimbursement; the cost of acquiring and maintaining technology, including electronic medical record systems; and the costs establishing and maintaining an office practices have led physicians to trade professional independence for hospital employment [38–41]. Hospitals anticipate that by employing physicians, it will be easier to standardize care and improve quality and efficiency, while ensuring ongoing access to patient referrals for clinical care and research.

Hospitals and Their Communities

Many of these mergers and consolidations have been led by major Academic Medical Centers and were strategically designed to help reengineer their role in, and the structure of, the local and regional healthcare delivery systems. These consolidations share many common key goals. These include improving the overall quality of care by integrating best practices and processes throughout the healthcare system; implementing population-based, evidence-driven data analytics to improve disease management for patients with chronic illnesses thereby allowing them to stay healthy at home longer; coordinating care through the care continuum; improving access to all levels and sites of care by directly linking the Academic Medical Center, community providers, and patients through tele-health technology; and improving patient access to research initiatives and innovative medical care.

Hospital systems anticipated that hospital consolidation and physician employment would improve care, through the strategies noted, and reduce costs. The data regarding the success of this strategy are mixed. In fact, some experts have argued that these initiatives have increased the costs [41–43], without necessarily improving care. It is clear that mega-consolidations could lead to a consolidation of market share and increased bargaining leverage, which together could increase costs to the payers and patients, and reduce care options. The courts, providers, and consumers need to be keenly aware of these potential unintended consequences and monitor actual outcomes as the landscape of care delivery changes.

Though there is no set formula for all hospital mergers, it is clear that for mergers to successfully achieve the aims outlined above, hospitals must be able to have a meaningful impact on the health of the community. To accomplish this the Academic Medical Center must understand the socioeconomics and the social determinants of health affecting the population they serve. It has been suggested that less than 30% of a patient's health is related to their clinical medical care. Instead, the data suggest that about 30% of a patient's health is related to personal health habits such as exercise, diet, tobacco, and alcohol use; 40% is related to socioeconomic determinants such as education, the quality of one's social support network, healthcare literacy, income, and education; and 10% of a patient's health is related to environmental factors such as housing, access to transportation, and related issues that are well beyond direct clinical care [44, 45].

For the academic health centers to help improve the health of the population, they need data regarding the social determinants of health, population health, and local health [46]. These types of data must be used to inform decisions regarding sites of service, service consolidations, discontinuations, and additions. Successful consolidations add needed resources to underserved areas and reengineer current facilities to best fit the needs of the communities. These consolidations should include seamless systems of data transfer, such as integrated electronic records, to allow all providers to share key clinical data.

To better understand the social determinants of health and the needs of the community, a formal community needs assessment should be part of every well-planned hospital merger, and the road map and timeline for addressing those needs should be completed at the time of the acquisition.

In many cases, this planning process identifies the need for hospitals to enhance their access to primary care. Recently, direct physician employment has been a tactic used to quickly integrate hospitals with established primary care providers.

Patient-Centered Medical Homes and Medical Neighborhoods

An appreciation of the central role of primary care has in many cases led primary care providers, and their hospital partner, toward the model of a "patient-centered medical home" (PCMH) where practices use a team-based approach to provide consistent high-quality, coordinate, patient-centered care [47].

The local community hospital and the more distant, but technologically linked, academic center serve as critical members of this care team. To better coordinate and appropriately guide their patients care, PCMH use patient-level and population-level registry data to assess a given patient's risk factors and then appropriately arrange their care needs. In a fully integrated system, the PCMH serves as the linchpin between the patient and their "medical neighborhood" which in turn is comprised of all the separate independent entities providing healthcare services for patients within the local area, such as nonaffiliated hospitals, community and social service organizations, and state and local public health agencies [48]. In a well-functioning medical neighborhood, regular communication, collaboration, and shared decision-making across various sectors ensure the delivery of coordinated care.

Sustaining Healthy Communities

As part of the move toward value-based reimbursement and efficient, integrated, cost-effective care, hospitals and health systems are increasingly recognizing that creating and sustaining healthy communities are critical to the long-term sustainability of the hospital itself. Based on the present trends in care reviewed above, large Academic Medical Centers of the future will likely focus on the most highly specialized, evidence- and value-based care, grounded in technology and innovation, and will participate in focused clinical research that is carefully matched to the strengths of the hospital and its academic faculty and staff. In addition, the academic center will continue to engage in the education and training of the healthcare workforce but may participate more directly in the career planning of the residents and fellows especially with regard to their choice of specialties and practice sites.

The future role of the local or community hospital in the healthcare delivery system is less certain. Community hospitals are often economic drivers or "anchors" (as both consumers and employers) of their local economy [49]. The Academic Medical Centers with their affiliates often play a similarly important economic and civic role in larger metropolitan areas. In both settings hospitals can facilitate the coming together of other key stakeholders to positively influence health outcomes for the populations they serve [49]. Given the importance of the local hospital to the well-being of the community, and the importance of the vitality of the community to the sustainability of the hospital, appropriate new strategies will require a much broader reach into communities than hospitals have had historically [50].

Reaching beyond the traditional scope of healthcare to facilitate collaboration with educational institutions and local and regional economic development organizations to address workforce needs, housing and transportation issues will be a potent strategic market differentiator for the successful hospital of the future and will solidify its position as a region's preeminent employer and healthcare provider. Opportunities exist to partner with other anchor-like institutions such as universities and colleges, municipal governments, and faith-based organizations, among others. Often there will be a need, such as housing, that will necessitate collaboration with local community-based organizations, banks, and developers. Absent other anchor institutions' leadership, it may fall to the local hospital to spearhead these initiatives and engage all the relevant stakeholders in order to address issues around social and economic determinants of health.

Adopting an "anchor institution" mission aligns healthcare transformation with economic development strategies that will result in substantial benefits to hospitals and the communities they serve. Capitalizing on existing assets, hospitals can help communities that are challenged by multiple social and economic disparities to improve the health and quality of life for their residents and, thus, in turn, help to establish sustainable environments for the community.

Conclusion

The roadmap ahead for hospitals is not yet fully charted and is likely to be variably and perhaps simultaneously both rocky and rewarding. Some believe that only very complex care will be done in hospitals and that technology will enable most other levels of care to be accomplished in a completely outpatient realm. In this construct, following an ambulatory procedure, care will be completed in an outpatient or a home setting [51]. However, asking casually trained family members or other caregivers to provide care in the home setting may have unintended consequences for both the patient and the provider. The ability of home tele-monitoring to mitigate these risks has not, as yet, been fully tested through broad implementation. It is conceivable that financial or political motivations may hasten the move of traditional hospital services to other domains. These forces should be tempered by thorough analysis of carefully structured pilot projects, which includes outcome evaluations for patients from a diverse demographic and socio-economic makeup.

Hospitals can bring together highly trained, experienced staff equipped with advanced technology, available every hour of every day. This concentration of resources will remain an essential element of care for some patients ensuring that at least some hospitals will remain a critical component of the future healthcare delivery system. The challenge will be to integrate these highly concentrated and expensive resources into a healthcare delivery system that can also conveniently and efficiently deliver routine care close to home. A successful healthcare delivery system must also be both evidence-based and patient-/consumer-centric. This integration will require effective communication, sharing of information, and respectful relationships among the various types of providers making up the "medical neighborhood." It is also essential that hospitals coexist harmoniously with the communities they serve, respecting that health is more than healthcare.

References

1. Askitopoulou H, Konsolaki E, Ramoutsaki I, Anastassaki E. Surgical cures by sleep induction as the Asclepieion of Epidaurus. The history of anesthesia: proceedings of the fifth international symposium, by José Carlos Diz, Avelino Franco, Douglas R. Bacon, J. Rupreht, Julián Alvarez. Elsevier Science B.V, International Congress Series 1242(2002), pp. 11–17.
2. Online etymology dictionary. www.etymonline.com. Accessed 4 May 2018.
3. Morton TG, Woodbury F. The History of Pennsylvania Hospital, 1751–1895. Philadelphia: Times Printing House; 1897. p. 32.
4. Trueman CN, Semmelweis I. The history learning site, 2015. [cited 2018 May 18]; Available from: https://www.historylearningsite.co.uk/a-history-of-medicine.
5. Robinson DH, Toledo AH. Historical development of monitored anesthesia. J Investig Surg. 2012;25(3):141–9.
6. Richardson R. Joseph Lister's domestic science. Lancet. 2013;382:e8–e9, 28.
7. Beck AH. The flexner report and the standardization of American medical education. JAMA. 2004;291(17):2139–40.
8. Guterman S. Specialty hospitals: a problem or a symptom. Health Aff. 2006;25(1):95–105.
9. Grove A, Slavin PL, Willson MP. The economics of academic medical centers. N Engl J Med. 2014;370:2360–2.
10. Dobson A, DaVanzo J, Haught R. The financial impact of the american health care act's medicaid provisions on safety-net hospitals, The commonwealth fund. 2017. [cited 2018 May 23]; Available from: http://www.commonwealthfund.org/publications/fund-reports/2017/jun/financial-impact-ahca-on-safety-net-hospitals.
11. 2018 Edition AHA Hospital Statistics, Publisher: Health Forum LLC, Chicago, Ill, 2018, pp 8, 9.
12. CMS Fast facts for US hospitals 2018 [cited 2018 May 15]; Available from: https://www.aha.org/statistics/2018-01-09-fast-facts-us-hospitals.
13. CMS Fast Facts Archives. 2013 [cited 2018 May 15]; Available from: https://www.cms.gov/fastfacts.
14. American Hospital Association. 2018 edition AHA Hospital statistics, publisher. Chicago: Health Forum LLC; 2018. pp 2,3.
15. US Census Data: Cited June 5, 2018: Population estimates program, population division, US Census Bureau: Historical National Population Estimates: July 1, 1900 to July 1, 1999; Release Date: April 11, 2000, Revised date: June 28, 2000 [cited 2018 June 5]; Available from: https://www2.census.gov/programs-surveys/popest/tables/1900-1980/national/totals/popclockest.txt.
16. US Census [cited 2018 June 5]; Available from: https://factfinder.census.gov/faces/tableservices/jsf/pages/productview.xhtml?pid=DEC_00_SF2_PCT001&prodType=table.
17. 2017 (NST-EST2017-01) Source: US Census Bureau, population division; Release Date: 2017 December [cited, 2108 June 5]; Available from: https://www.census.gov/data/tables/2017/demo/popest/nation-total.html.
18. Weiss AJ (Truven Health Analytics), Elixhauser A (AHRQ). Overview of Hospital Stays in the United States, 2012. HCUP Statistical Brief #180. October 2014 Agency for Healthcare Research and Quality, Rockville, MD. [cited 2018 May 29]; Available from: http://www.hcup-us.ahrq.gov/reports/statbriefs/sb180-Hospitalizations-United-States-2012.pdf.
19. 2018 Edition American Hospital Association: Hospital statistics. Health Forum LLC, Chicago. 2018, P 13.
20. Bureau of Labor Statistics CPI Inflation Calculator: [cited 2018 May 27]; Available from: https://www.bls.gov/data/inflation_calculator.htm.
21. Papanicolas I, Woskie LR, Jha AK. Health care spending in the United States and other high-income countries. JAMA. 2018;319(10):1024–39.
22. Dieleman JL, Squires E, Bul AL, Campbel LM, Chapin A, Hamavid H, et al. Factors associated with increases in US health care spending, 1996–2013. JAMA. 2017;318(17):1668–78.
23. Fay B, Hospital and surgery costs. Debt.org. [cited 2018 May 31]; Available from: https://www.debt.org/medica. Available from: l/hospital-surgery-costs.
24. Dzau VJ, Cho A, Ellaissi W, et al. Transforming academic health centers for an uncertain future. N Engl J Med. 2013;369:991–3.

25. CMS Statistics National Health Expenditure Data, 2016 Highlights. [cited 2018 May 24]; Available from: https://www.cms.gov/research-statistics-data-and-systems/statistics-trends-and-reports/nationalhealthexpenddata/nationalhealthaccountshistorical.html.
26. Berwick DM, Nolan TW, Whittington J. The triple aim: care, health, and cost. Health Aff. 2008;27(3):759–69.
27. Hospital Value-based Purchasing a MLN booklet. [cited 2018 June1]; Available from: https://www.cms.gov/Outreach-and-Education/Medicare-Learning-Network-MLN/MLNProducts/downloads/Hospital_VBPurchasing_Fact_Sheet_ICN907664.pdf.
28. Japsen B. Medicare, commercial insurers agree on uniform health quality measures. 2016 [cited 2018 May 14]; Available from: https://www.forbes.com/sites/brucejapsen/2016/02/16/white-house-says-medicare-commercial-insurers-agree-on-health-quality-measures/#416a23711d9e.
29. Herrin J, St. Andre J, Kenward K, Joshi MS, Audet AJ, Hines SC. Community factors and hospital readmission rates. Health Serv Res. 2015;50:20–39.
30. Muhlestein D. Assessment-of-the-hospital-value-based-purchasing-program. [cited 2018 April 29]; Available from: https://www.accountablecarelc.org/sites/default/files/VBP-whitepaper-11.13.2015-FINAL1.pdf.
31. Matlin Gilman M, Hockenberry JM, Adams C, Milstein AS, Wilson IB, Becker ER. The financial effect of value-based purchasing and the hospital readmissions reduction program on safety-net hospitals in 2014: a cohort study. Ann Intern Med. 2015;163(6):427–36.
32. Guadagnolo G. Margin pressures for academic medical centers -Expert Perspective. 2018 March 30 [cited 2018 April 30]; Available from: https://www.eab.com/research-and-insights/business-affairs-forum/expert-insights/2018/segment-spotlight-academic-medical-centers.
33. 85 rural hospital closures NC Rural Health Research Program [cited 2018 June 15]; Available from: http://www.shepscenter.unc.edu/programs-projects/rural-health/rural-hospital-closures/.
34. McKee M, Healy J. The role of the hospital in a changing environment. Bull World Health Organ. 2000;78(6):803–8.
35. van Lerberghe W, Lafort Y, World Health Organi zation. Division of Strengthening of Health Services. In: Van Lerberghe W, Lafort Y, editors. The role of the hospital in the district: delivering or supporting primary health care? Geneva: World Health Organization; 1990. [cited 2018 May 27]; Available from: http://www.who.int/iris/handle/10665/59744.
36. Yanci J, Wolford M, Young P. What hospital executives should be considering in hospital mergers and acquisitions; [cited 2018 June 1]; Available from: https://www.dhgllp.com/industries/healthcare. Winter 2013.
37. Moore N. Difference between a vertically integrated company & a horizontally integrated production company [Updated, 2018 May 07; cited 2018 May 23]; Available from: http://smallbusiness.chron.com/difference-between-vertically-integrated-company-horizontally-integrated-production-company-32196.html.
38. Cheney C. Healthcare's consolidation landscape. 2017; [cited 2018 June 1]; Available from: https://www.healthleadersmedia.com/strategy/healthcare's-consolidation-landscape.
39. 2017-in-Review-The-Year-M & A -Shook- the Healthcare Landscape.pdf [cited 2018 June 1]; Available from: https://www.kaufmanhall.com/sites/default/files/2017-in-Review_The-Year-that-Shook-Healthcare.pdf.
40. Darves B. Understanding the physician employment "Movement". N EngJ Med Career Center. 2014 [cited 2018 June 1]; Available from: http://www.nejmcareercenter.org/article/understanding-the-physician-employment-movement.
41. Kacik A. Hospital-employed physicians drain Medicare. Modern Healthcare. 2017 [cited 2018 May 23]; Available from: http://www.modernhealthcare.com/article/20171114/NEWS/171119942.
42. Gamble M, Sachs B. l60 statistics and thoughts on healthcare, hospital and physician practice M&A. Becker Hospital Review. 2015 [cited 2018 May 23]; Available from: https://www.beckershospitalreview.com/hospital-transactions-and-valuation/60-statistics-and-thoughts-on-healthcare-hospital-and-physician-practice-m-a.html.
43. Livingston S, Bannow T. Hospital megamergers may lower overhead, but at what cost. Modern Healthcare. 2017 December 11[cited 2018 May 11]; Available from: http://www.modernhealthcare.com/article/20171211/NEWS/171219977.
44. Machledt D. Addressing the social determinants of health through medicaid managed care, 2017 [cited 2018 May 23]; Available from: Social Determinants of Health https://www.healthypeople.gov/2020/topics-objectives/topic/social-determinants-of-health.
45. Robert Wood Johnson foundation program what and why we rank. [cited 2018 June 1]; Available from: http://www.countyhealthrankings.org/. County health rankings and roadmap for Robert Wood Johnson foundation program what and why we rank.
46. Knettel A. The business case for academic health centers addressing environmental, social, and behavioral determinants of health. Washington, DC: Association of Academic Health Centers; 2011. [cited 2018 May 23]; Available from: www.aahcdc.org/portal.
47. Agency for Healthcare Research and Quality (AHRQ). PCMH: patient centered medical home resource center. AHRQ Website. [cited 2018 May30]; Available from: https://pcmh.ahrq.gov/page/defining-pcmh.
48. Taylor, E.F, Lake, T, Nysenbaum, J, Meyers, D. Coordinating care in the medical neighborhood: critical components and available Mechanisms White Paper (Prepared by Mathematica Policy Research under Contract No HHSA290200900019I TO2). Maryland: AHRQ Publication No 11–0064; 2011. [cited 2018

June 1]; Available from: https://pcmh.ahrq.gov/sites/default/files/attachments/Coordinating%20Care%20in%20the%20Medical%20Neighborhood.pdf.
49. Dubb S, McKinley S, Howard T. The anchor dashboard-aligning institutional practice to meet low-income community needs. The Democracy Collaborative at the University of Maryland. 2013 [cited 2018 June 1]; Available From: https://community-wealth.org/sites/clone.community-wealth.org/files/downloads/AnchorDashboardCompositeFinal.pdf.
50. Norris T, Howard T. Can hospitals heal America's communities? The Democracy Collaborative; [cited 2018 June 1]; Available from: https://democracycollaborative.org/content/can-hospitals-heal-americas-communities-0.
51. Emanuel E. Opinion – are hospitals becoming obsolete? – The New York Times 2018 [cited 2018 May 3]; Available from: https://www.nytimes.com/.../opinion/hospitals-becoming-obsolete.html.

Can Hospitals Advance Health Equity in the United States? The Influence of Technology, Economics, and Policy

7

Deborah Viola and Peter S. Arno

Introduction

Never, far from any social, political, or intellectual discourse are concerns about unequal health outcomes and inequalities in accessing care which stem from socioeconomic disparities in the United States, has been more prevalent. Despite the large evidence base supporting the depth and scope of these inequalities, there is little fundamental agreement among policy makers that these can be reduced in any meaningful way without burdening one group of constituents to support another, e.g., those who can afford insurance versus those who cannot.

This fundamental disagreement lags behind advances in care and the shift from acute to chronic disease management. Chronic care management transcends access to health insurance; as Elisabeth Rosenthal has noted, even the ACA has left individuals "insured but not covered" [1]. This is underscored by the Commonwealth Fund's latest Biennial Survey which reports that 28% of adults (aged 18–64) who were insured all year were "underinsured," i.e., their out-of-pocket expenditures or deductibles are so high that they are unable to adequately access needed healthcare [2]. This means that tens of millions of Americans are experiencing challenges in meeting the financial demands of caring for themselves and their families. The dual barriers presented by public policy and economic constraints are further exacerbated by and in turn handicap advances in medical and information technology that have the potential to reduce disparities in healthcare and outcomes.

We propose that hospitals are in a unique position to advance health equity in the United States. Although often portrayed as a big part of the healthcare cost equation, reimbursement pressures and the shift from acute care to the treatment of chronic illnesses are forcing hospitals to reconsider not only how and where to treat their patients but at lower costs. Since the most vulnerable, e.g., uninsured, low-income, racial/ethnic minority groups, are still more likely to visit a hospital emergency department for unnecessary care, there is opportunity for hospitals to leverage their investments in technology to shift costly, inappropriate utilization and reduce the detrimental impacts on health of socioeconomic disparities.

First, we provide an overview of the rise in health disparities and the impact of education and income inequality on health. Next we consider the evolution of hospitals and how the changing competitor landscape is forcing hospitals to reconsider the business of healthcare, including the impact of technology and big data on managing care. Finally we consider the impact of policy

D. Viola (✉)
Data Management and Analytics, Westchester Medical Center Health Network, Valhalla, NY, USA
e-mail: deborah.viola@wmchealth.org

P. S. Arno
Political Economy Research Institute, University of Massachusetts, Amherst, Amherst, MA, USA

R. Latifi (ed.), *The Modern Hospital*, https://doi.org/10.1007/978-3-030-01394-3_7

and payment reform and whether the economics and financing of hospitals support or undermine their ability to advance health equity.

Overview of Health Disparities and Inequalities in the United States

Although it is beyond the scope of this chapter to detail differences in disease prevalence or access to care by socioeconomic status (SES) or race/ethnicity, there is a wealth of evidence that these factors are major determinants of health outcomes. The widening wage gap since the 1970s has further intensified these links and contributed to a growing field of study on the relationship between income inequality and health. In a review of the literature exploring income inequality and health in 2006, Richard Wilkinson and Kate Pickett identified 168 studies, "the overwhelming majority of which showed a positive correlation" [3]. A 2015 study by the National Academies of Sciences, Engineering, and Medicine on mortality inequality stated "In summary, an abundance of research over the past two decades finds that SES differentials in mortality are widening, whether SES is measured by educational attainment or income quantile" [4]. The authors note that this trend is likely to continue and is further compounded by inequality in access to new health technologies, which occurs first among higher-income groups. Regardless of whether a particular health technology improves health or not, our point is that the adoption and diffusion of new health technologies are influenced by the same socioeconomic factors that determine disparities to begin with.

As dramatic as these differences are, nothing has grabbed the public's attention as much as the link between geography and health outcomes. As expressed by the catchy Robert Wood Johnson Foundation sound bite, "A ZIP code is 5 numbers meant to give mail to people—not indicate how long they live" [5]. The determination that our ZIP code is a stronger predictor of our health than our genetic profile has even contributed to a proliferation of ZIP health websites. Consider the impact of the following visualization, depicting a section of Delmar Boulevard in St. Louis, Missouri [6]. This stretch of the 9-mile boulevard literally reflects the classic "other side of the tracks" divide between a poor, black neighborhood in the north and a more affluent and "whiter" neighborhood in the south. As the map illustrates, residents in the north are less likely to have a bachelor's degree; their incomes reflect this as does their health status. Folks in the north are more likely to suffer from chronic diseases. These differences exist along a few miles of divide on a boulevard where the change from the City of St. Louis into University City in St. Louis County is marked by pillars depicting "Gates of Opportunity" (Fig. 7.1).

These relationships are consistent with hospital utilization more generally. Even among the employed, people with lower education levels and incomes are more likely to use the emergency department (ED) for nonemergency care. Blacks and Latinos are also more likely to visit an emergency room for nonemergency care than are their white coworkers. Medicaid beneficiaries use the ED at a twofold higher rate than the privately insured; higher use is often a result of unmet health needs or lack of access to "appropriate settings."

The relationships are complex. ZIP code level inequalities are "affected by the degree of residential segregation of rich and poor, and the health of people in deprived neighborhoods is likely to be poor, not because of the inequality within each of those small areas, but because they are deprived in relation to the wider society" [3]. Deprivation is defined as more than just inadequate access to healthcare and services; it includes inadequate access to transportation, employment, food sources, clean air, and safe parks—all of which are being more widely recognized as social determinants of health [7]. And deprived neighborhoods are generally comprised of racial/ethnic minorities, contributing to racial/ethnic disparities in health outcomes.

Hospitals also reside within ZIPs and their service areas span multiple ZIP codes. Not only do hospitals provide care, but they are often the major employer in their service areas and contribute to the local economies. Hospitals are community anchors and have an opportunity, an

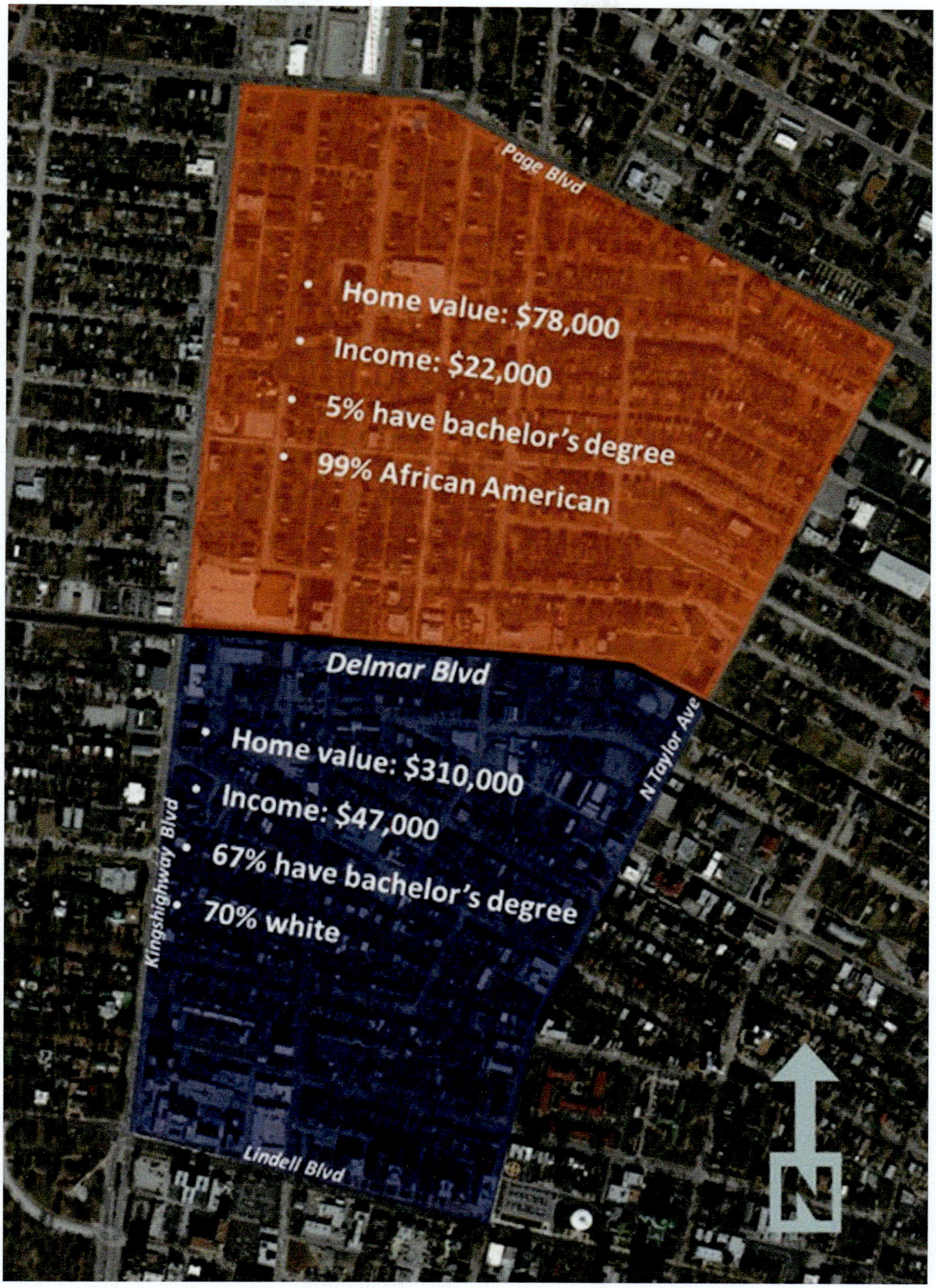

Fig. 7.1 Delmar divide. (Source: For the Sake of All, 2015. Used with permission)

obligation we would suggest, to participate in community health business partnerships, a model advanced by David Kindig at the University of Wisconsin and George Isham of HealthPartners. They note that "Most healthcare leaders are fully occupied with the more familiar goals of improving the experience of healthcare and reducing per capita cost of healthcare…the reality is that even major progress in these two areas over the next decade will not help us achieve our goals related to robust life expectancy and disparity reduction without explicit attention to improving health" [8]. Hospitals are beginning to invest in population health- and value-based initiatives that include not only primary care-based practices but care management teams and local community-based organizations. Hospitals routinely provide health education and improve the health literacy of the communities they serve. Hospitals are also moving toward improving care delivery (e.g., reducing preventable ED visits and readmissions) and reducing costs. These efforts in and of themselves could reduce unnecessary healthcare spending and provide resources that could be allocated into other deprived areas within communities, like improved access to healthy foods. It is estimated that as much as $500 billion of waste, and perhaps considerably more, accrue to the US healthcare system due to failures in care delivery, coordination, and overtreatment [9, 10].

As neighborhood anchors, hospitals can influence and support programs outside of their immediate delivery system while improving care delivery at the clinical level. Leveraging data allows them to understand the ecosystems within their neighborhoods and the impact of inequalities on health. Hospitals know how to identify their most vulnerable communities and can leverage data and technology that will not only improve outcomes but do so at lower costs.

Changing Care Continuums, Technology, and Big Data

Hospitals traditionally have provided acute and emergency care. As our colleagues in the preceding chapter have highlighted, hospitals are embracing new and emerging services and are undertaking new roles as participants in clinically integrated delivery systems. Advances in technology and changes in reimbursement, especially as a result of the Patient Protection and Affordable Care Act (2010), are challenging hospitals to focus on the "continuum of care," e.g., providing and coordinating patient care across all care settings. Further, EDs are experiencing increased visit volumes also as a result of technological advances. Primary care physicians are sending ill patients to the ED in lieu of admitting, and walk-ins have increased due to shortages in primary care and access issues. As a result, there is a growing use of EDs as diagnostic centers and as an important site for outpatient care, making EDs the main source of inpatient hospital admissions. If managed appropriately, the ED provides one opportunity for hospitals to advance health equity. And it may even be cost saving. "ED-based observation units prevent costly hospital admissions; the average cost of an ED visit is about $900. The average cost of a hospital stay is ten times that amount" [11] (Fig. 7.2).

If we are as healthy as our ZIP code, then local area health "hot spotting" is the logical first step. Health outcomes, socioeconomic indicators, crime data, transportation routes, availability of fresh fruit and vegetables, and number of clinics, i.e., the entire ecosystems of neighborhoods, can be captured and mapped to determine areas experiencing local health disparities and to help identify causes for those disparities. The Camden Coalition of Healthcare Providers shares information on patients through a locally developed health information exchange that enables care teams to extend their reach beyond hospitals or affiliated providers. The exchange enables data sharing among different hospital systems, primary care providers, community-based organizations, and even correctional facilities so that care teams are able to address the entire health ecosystem surrounding a patient. As a result they are able to direct resources where needed, whether it is assistance with medical care or housing [12].

Hospitals can also leverage their electronic health record, or EHR, data. Electronic health records track patient data, and current systems

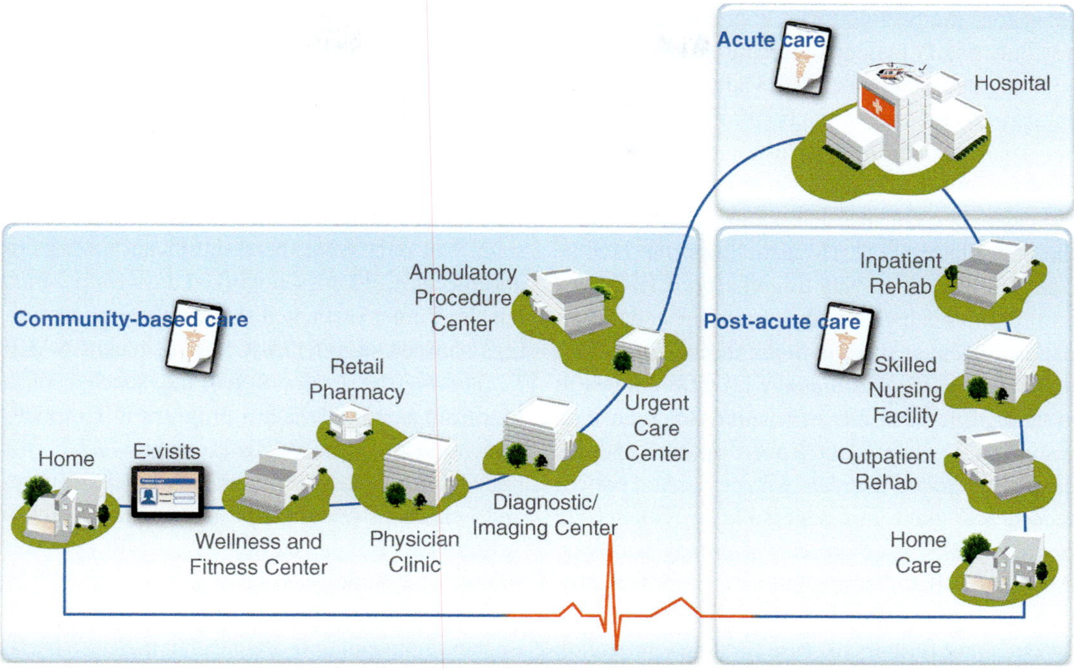

Fig. 7.2 Care continuum. (Source: Sg2, 2017. Used with permission)

can capture more than clinical information and allow sharing of patient information among all providers. In a commentary by Juliet Rumball-Smith and David Bates, they suggest that given the widespread adoption of EHRs, implementation and operational efforts should be directed at creating a "true EHR-equity marriage" [13]. This marriage can be achieved by capturing and integrating patient-generated data that enables analyses of disparities within care processes. Hospitals are also able to integrate social and economic determinants of health into clinical findings. The Area Deprivation Index (ADI), provided by the University of Wisconsin, represents the level of socioeconomic deprivation in geographic areas using 17 census markers; it is freely accessible and available for the entire United States [14]. Using a geographic information science (GIS) framework, more local or relative deprivation indices can be developed around hospital service areas by correlating these ADI values with hospitalization rate data [15]. Flags associated with patient ZIPs can be used as signals within EHRs or care plans to providers and care teams that a patient may be at risk due to socioeconomic challenges. This in turn could trigger a social determinants screening to accompany the medical exam. Patient care plans can include information on local resources, e.g., food pantries, in addition to where to go for a follow-up blood pressure screen. Technology vendors provide resource directories that are updated monthly and identify not only community services but assist health systems in tracking and coordinating referrals across the care continuum to assure that patient needs are met. When the University of Arkansas Medical Center launched prompts within their EHR to clinicians to query patients in areas related to these social determinants, they were able to reduce readmission rates by nearly 4% [16].

As neighborhood anchors, hospitals influence and support programs outside of their immediate delivery system while improving care delivery at the clinical level. Not only do they know how to identify their most vulnerable communities, but care management teams can identify barriers to achieving health equity and intervene to reduce or eliminate these barriers. The diffusion of technology and availability of digital infrastructures, as well as the proliferation of smart phones, has not only made patient outreach easier, but it is enabling a more democratized approach to medical care. At the end of his book, *The Patient Will See You Now*, Eric Topol notes that "Once the digitization of medicine got legs, it became increasingly clear that democratization would be the next phase" [17]. He also states that healthcare still has a long way to go before EHRs contain comprehensive and longitudinal data on patients because most patients receive care from different providers affiliated with different health systems. But the ability of hospitals to create data warehouses where data from disparate sources can be integrated to create a more holistic patient record and make this accessible to patients via portals on their smart phones is already available. And as we shall discuss, payment reform is providing a big incentive for hospitals to do this.

Dr. Topol furthers his case for democratization by suggesting that as healthcare providers increasingly become more data savvy, the increased use of predictive models to prevent chronic disease or anticipate a hospitalization will provide more opportunity to provide the right care to individuals. For populations at greater risk who have escaped early diagnosis in part because of access issues, the use of "Facebook" technology means we can learn not only about someone's shopping preferences but whether they are predisposed to a readmission, heart failure, or a missed appointment.

Hospitals have the ability to capture and analyze large amounts of data and wrap other technologies around the information to improve not only clinical outcomes but the patient experience. The use of telehealth can provide an opportunity for hospitals to leverage technology to advance health equity. Telehealth can lower the overall cost of care and improve access to the insured and the underinsured, as well as other potentially high utilizing and vulnerable patient populations, like the elderly and disabled. Telehealth is defined as "the use of technology to deliver health care, health information or health education at a distance" [18]. Telehealth consults between providers, or between provider and patient, also save time and travel expenses, in addition to the lags inherent in scheduling follow-up or additional appointments with specialists. For special populations, this could be significant. At the Marcus Autism Center in Georgia, pediatric patients with developmental disabilities and other psychiatric disorders were provided access to clinical specialties at over 35 satellite facilities across the state. Not only were there significant savings in absenteeism and missed worked days for parents, but the Center estimated that transportation savings were close to $175 K [19]. A recent AARP *Insight on the Issues* noted the success of a Medicaid home telehealth program in Colorado that reduced rehospitalizations by 62% for patients with diabetes, congestive heart failure, and chronic obstructive pulmonary failure. Additional savings accrued as a result of lower ED use and home visits [20].

Telehealth capabilities help remediate the impact of physician shortages, but there are barriers to the adoption of telehealth applications, including reimbursement and legislation. "Less than 1 percent of Medicare beneficiaries take advantage of telehealth technologies," in part due to CMS reimbursement favoring rural areas [18]. Current "originating site restrictions" limit billing for telehealth services to patients seen at traditional sites of care including provider offices, hospitals, clinics, and skilled nursing facilities. The inability to bill for services offered in a patient's home negates some of the biggest potential impacts telehealth could have on improving health outcomes and achieving health equity. Extending care management and monitoring into the home should be as ubiquitous as video streaming services. State variation in Medicaid coverage makes a summary challenging. However, almost all states provide some coverage for telehealth, and state programs have demonstrated far more flexibility than Medicare. Commercial insurers are increasingly making use of telehealth, and close to 30 states have parity laws requiring comparable reimbursement rates for telemedicine and office visits (Fig. 7.3).

Although the forecasted increase in telehealth visits over the next several years is rather robust, there are barriers to its widespread adoption by providers and patients that include "patient

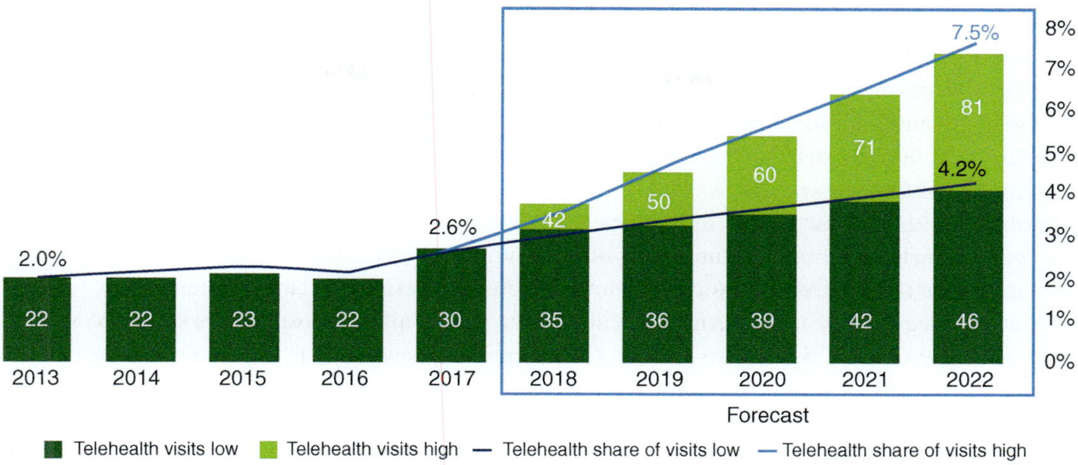

Fig. 7.3 US telehealth visits 2013–2022. (Source: IQVIA National Disease and Therapeutic Index, Jan 2018; IQVIA Institute, Feb 2018. Used with permission)

concerns about being treated by a random doctor, and providers' concerns about being paid for their time" [21]. Despite these barriers, there is some evidence that the number of telehealth visits may represent new utilization. In a study of commercial claims data over a 3-year period for acute respiratory illnesses, J. Scott Ashwood and colleagues discovered that almost 90% of telehealth visits were for new utilization, possibly explained by a "dose response with respect to convenience and utilization," and for conditions where treatment has been underutilized, e.g., diabetes and mental health, and for underserved populations, increased use of telehealth services may lead to increases in the value of care [22].

The use of telehealth could play an integral role in the success of value-based programs, suggesting a need for policy and payment reform designed to achieve health equity. These should include incentives to encourage patients and providers to seek and provide care at all appropriate sites.

Policy and Payment Reform

There is little question that expanding telehealth throughout the healthcare sector can be speeded up by easing restrictions and increasing provider reimbursement for these services. The degree to which telehealth can reduce racial/ethnic and geographic health disparities is likely to be positive but modest, yet its potential impact remains unknown.

Much of the discussion in the literature on achieving health equity focuses too little attention on the resources needed or where they could be found. Hospitals are by far the largest segment of the healthcare sector, accounting for one out of every three healthcare dollars. In 2016, expenditures in the hospital industry amounted to $1.1 trillion and are projected to increase by 5.5% per year to reach $1.8 trillion by 2026 [23]. If major changes in healthcare are to be made to improve health equity, it seems obvious that some of these resources must be reallocated either from or within the hospital sector.

There will always be a need for hospitals, but the hospital market is changing dramatically in a number of ways. It is clear that overall the number and rate of hospitalizations have been declining for more than a decade [24]. And we also know that utilization and costs vary significantly by payer, demographic group, and geographic region. Unfortunately, there is no comprehensive national database for outpatient utilization or costs, yet many analysts believe that changes in reimbursement have in recent years led to a shift from inpatient to outpatient services that is expected to continue for years to come [25].

Recent data on those under 65 with employer-sponsored health insurance tell a slightly different story. Analyzing a dataset of about 4 billion claims for 39 million insured per year, the Health Care Cost Institute reported that in 2016 increased spending on outpatient services was the biggest contributor to the annual growth in total spending, yet the increase in expenditures for outpatient (and inpatient) spending was driven almost entirely by price increases, not changes in utilization as displayed in the figure below [26] (Fig. 7.4).

Another significant change affecting the entire healthcare landscape has been the growing concentration in hospital markets across the country since at least the 1990s, but the pace appears to have picked up since the passage of the Affordable Care Act in 2010 [27]. Martin Gaynor, one of the nation's leading experts on concentration in healthcare markets, recently testified before Congress that in the last 20 years, there have been 1519 hospital mergers, with 680 since 2010 [28]. There is no doubt that in addition to gaining market share and negotiating leverage, the long-term reduction in the number of hospitalizations has led to an oversupply of beds and financial pressures that have forced many hospitals to either close or merge with larger systems.

These shifts in hospital markets have significant implications for the future of healthcare financing, how services are delivered and the ability to promote health equity. Extensive research demonstrates that increased market power has enabled hospitals to exert increased price-setting power, thus imposing higher prices resulting in increased healthcare expenditures. For example, Schulman and Richman find that "Monopoly hospitals, those that dominate a local market with no

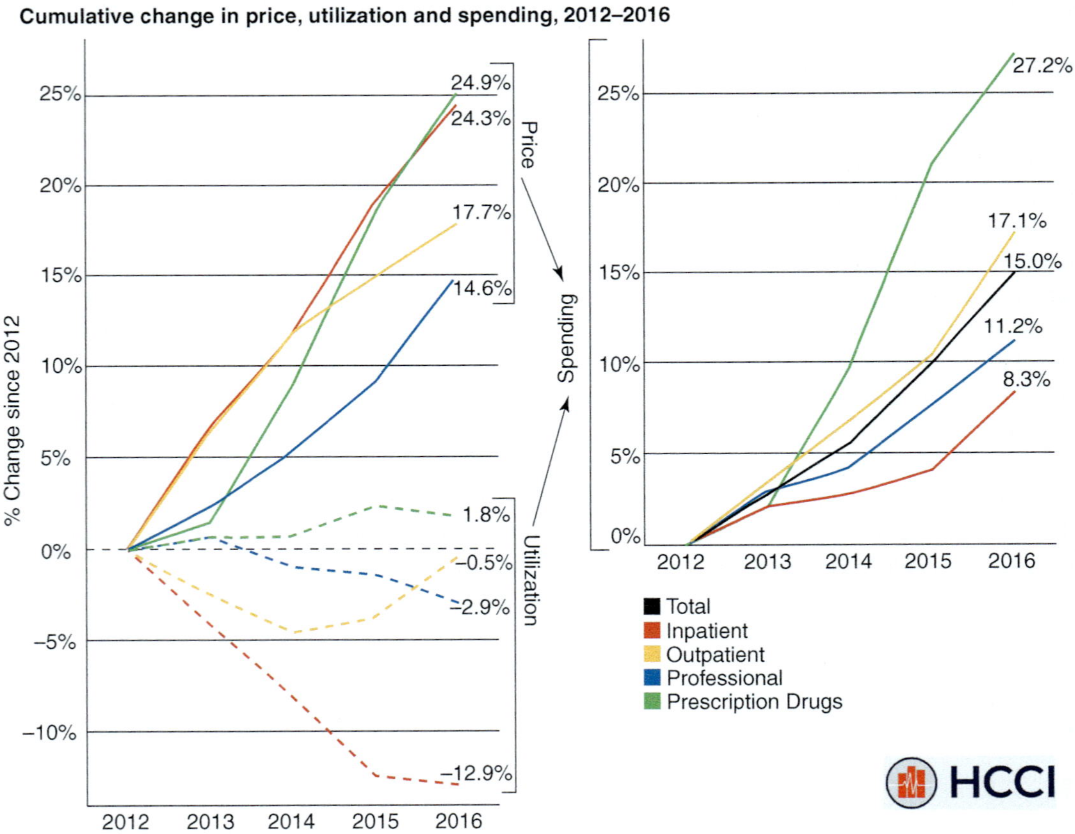

Fig. 7.4 Cumulative change in price, utilization, and spending, 2012–2016. (Source: Health Care Cost Institute. 2016 Health Care Costs and Utilization Report. 2018 Jan Used with permission)

other competing hospital, have 15.3 percent higher prices than hospitals in more competitive markets, and hospital consolidation is responsible for sharp price increases across markets within states" [29]. In a recent comprehensive study of the California healthcare market, researchers found that 76% of the state's counties had highly concentrated hospital markets [30].

In addition to higher hospital prices and expenditures, hospital concentration also bleeds into other segments of healthcare. For example, there has been an increasing trend of hospitals buying physician practices. The California study reports that the percentage of physicians working for foundations owned by hospitals increased from 24% to 39% between 2010 and 2016. Clearly, growing consolidation in healthcare markets affects not only hospitals but physician practices, commercial insurance markets, pharmaceutical manufacturers and distributers, etc. All of which lead to increased healthcare prices and expenditures, not less. The California study provides spectacular evidence of these trends: in highly concentrated markets, average inpatient procedures and outpatient physician prices were 79% and 35–63% higher (depending on physician specialty), respectively, when compared to less concentrated markets. Moreover, hospital consolidation which leads to reduced competition allows hospitals to negotiate higher prices on an ongoing basis, making this a long-term problem leading to rising prices over time. Finally, hospital concentration raises another concern, although here the data is not conclusive. A small but growing body of evidence suggests that patient health outcomes are significantly worse in hospitals in more concentrated markets [31–33].

The accelerating trend toward hospital market concentration must be slowed or reversed carefully to avoid creating new barriers to access in underserved markets. This can be done with regulatory oversight and through antitrust enforcement at the state and federal levels, heightened data transparency and consumer engagement, and more fundamentally, through the political will of policy makers to address this issue. If this trend can be stopped or reversed, it could lead to lowering healthcare costs, improving the quality of care and potentially freeing up resources allocated to promoting community health initiatives.

In a major effort to promote population health, the Affordable Care Act (ACA) enacted provisions to require that tax-exempt hospitals (the vast majority in the United States) expand the definition of charity care (part of the requirement for nonprofit status) to include direct spending on community health improvement and contributions to community groups for health improvement initiatives [34]. Yet data from 2010 through 2014 indicates that less than 1% of operating expenses have been allocated each year toward community health benefits. As in the past, prior to the ACA, the main portion of "community benefits" has gone toward unreimbursed patient care such as charity care. Rosenbaum and colleagues estimated that the value of the nonprofit hospital tax exemption was $24.6 billion in 2011, an amount that has surely risen in the last few years [35]. It is possible that hospitals have increased their contributions to community health benefits since 2014, but given the magnitude of the value of their tax exemption, hospitals should be required to contribute more funds to promote these benefits which could be used in a variety of ways to help hospitals integrate their clinical services with community-based initiatives and promote prevention and their local community's health status.

The underlying rationale behind the shift toward value-based care and payment—improving the quality of care at lower costs—is hard to fault. Yet the efficacy of this approach has not been demonstrated. The development and promotion of Accountable Care Organizations (ACOs) have been the mainstay of the federal government's strategy to accomplish this transformation. The ACO framework encourages hospitals and physicians to collaborate effectively by offering financial incentives if they improve both the quality and efficiency of care. There are now approximately 1000 ACOs serving more than 32 million people [36].

Despite the rapid growth of ACOs over the past few years, evidence of their impact on quality and costs has been decidedly mixed. For example, Song and Fisher writing in 2016 argue that cost savings from ACOs have been modest to date but that further savings are still achievable [37]. At the same time, they argue, quality improvements have been significant. Hsu et al. (2017) are also cautiously optimistic in their assessment of cost savings to date through the ACO framework [38]. They find, for example, that rates of emergency department visits and hospitalizations have fallen by an average of 6% and 8%, respectively, through implementing ACO operating systems.

Alternatively, Schulman and Richman write that "based on 3 published evaluations of the ACO program, the experiment so far has failed to produce needed efficiencies" [29]. Another large national study by Ryan and colleagues concluded that hospital-based value payment "was not associated with improvements in measures of clinical process or patient experience and was not associated with significant reductions in two of three mortality measures" [39]. More recently in a study examining hospital data from 2008 to 2014, Papanicolas et al. noted "We found no evidence to suggest that implementing Medicare's Hospital Value-Based Purchasing program accelerated the improvement of patient experience beyond secular trends, even among the hospitals with the poorest performance at baseline. Instead, we found that the rate of improvements in patient experience has slowed since the program was implemented" [40]. The future of ACOs remains in question. According to a 2018 survey conducted by the National Association of ACOs of its members, it found that more than 70% of ACO respondents indicated they are likely to leave the Medicare Shared Savings Program, Medicare's largest alternative payment model, as a result of having to assume increased risk [41].

Thus the record remains mixed at best, but it may just be a matter of time for ACOs and value-based payment schemes to establish a more successful record, or perhaps the incentives are far too weak and the risks too high. The opportunities for hospitals and physicians to avoid cost controls and even expand their profit opportunities within an ACO framework remain largely intact. Elizabeth Rosenthal's extensive reporting in her book *An American Sickness* (2017) describes this clearly:

> Providers—up and down the health care supply chain—rapidly devised ways to stay within the letter of the new law while often flagrantly flaunting its quality-promoting cost-saving intentions…The small incentives to encourage good behavior and coordinated medical care often paled compared to the profit that could be garnered by creative or aggressive billing that tested the boundaries of the law...[42]

We must ask the question whether the imposition of greater financial risk placed on providers is the most efficient or even the appropriate approach to improving the quality of care or reducing costs, particularly if it does not address the fundamental drivers of increasing costs—administrative waste and high prices in our fragmented healthcare system. It may also be wise to take an historical perspective on the changing financial reimbursement mechanisms that have been tried unsuccessfully to control costs over the years. Marmor and Oberlander raised serious concerns about the long-term viability of ACOs and value-based payment back in 2012:

> During the past four decades, American policymakers and analysts have embraced an ever changing array of panaceas to control costs, including managed care, consumer-directed health care, and more recently, delivery system reform and value-based purchasing. Past panaceas have gone through a cycle of excessive hope followed by disappointment at their failure to rein in medical care spending. We argue that accountable care organizations, medical homes, and similar ideas in vogue today could repeat this pattern… We believe that the U.S. needs less innovation and more emulation. That is, in order to control costs effectively, Americans should focus less on (re)inventing the latest delivery system or payment method, and instead pay more attention to what other countries do to slow health care spending. Global budgets, fee schedules, systemwide payment rules, and concentrated purchasing power may not be modern, exciting, or "transformational." But they have the advantage of working [43].

The ACO framework, or some iteration, may yet evolve into a system that some have called "place-based," which means instead of large providers assuming responsibility for individual patients they enroll, they become responsible for geographically based populations. This would foster greater collaboration and integration across local healthcare providers. It has the advantage of more holistically addressing the health of local populations by taking into account the larger scope of the social determinants of health ranging from enhancing employment opportunities to housing, safer neighborhoods, healthier food choices, etc. as well as promoting the diffusion of technologies such as telehealth. This is most likely to occur only if funding comes along with the increased responsibilities. This in turn would undoubtedly be linked with other and possibly more manageable tools for curbing healthcare expenditures such as global budgets and greater accountability for population-based health improvements. Changing incentives from financial risk to funding and rewarding changes in population health improvements may not be as far-fetched as it sounds. There are ACOs already experimenting with similar approaches in Maryland and Vermont, which if proven successful, could be replicated across the country. In a commentary by Louis Sullivan and Augustus White, they note that:

> Hospitals would be encouraged to join the fight if equality were included as a metric in the U.S. News and World Report rankings. These rankings are popular and closely watched. They bestow bragging rights on hospitals, but most important, provide guidance for people deeply interested in where they might go to receive the best care in the specialties that concern them most...Where do hospitals rank in their understanding of the problem of unequal care? What measures do they take to counteract the effects of prejudice in the treatment they provide? .... It would help U.S. health professionals understand health disparities and more effectively treat underserved and minority populations. Most important, it would help all patients and their families, not just those who need not worry about disparities in care, to know better where to go for the care they need [44].

Conclusion

The notion of truly advancing health equity requires facing some inconvenient truths. The single largest driver of health policy for the past few decades has been altering financial reimbursement mechanisms used to pay for healthcare in a dynamic economic environment. The latest iteration is unfolding as the transformation from "volume to value," through ACOs, bundled payments, clinically integrated networks, and other value-based payment schemes, but these latest efforts are still handicapped by public policy and existing economic incentives that discourage efforts to reduce disparities in healthcare access and outcomes.

The barriers to a more progressive role for hospitals are of our own doing. Hospitals can and should be economically incentivized to achieve more than reducing the per capita cost of healthcare. Hospitals can be important partners to recovering accrued and wasted dollars due to failures in care delivery and coordination that are in part responsible for current disparities in outcomes. Reallocating these dollars to and within hospital systems to improve data systems and technologies is essential. They should be required to support local surveillance to identify and care for the most disadvantaged patients and, further, to manage patients' care in alignment with local providers with clear service agreements. *This should not be an unrealistic challenge.* Hospitals already run command centers to manage patient transfers, transports, and flows within their own systems. They have demonstrated their ability to manage, evaluate, and report on patient care and adapt how they do so in accordance with the latest reimbursement schemas.

Hospitals serve as important community anchors and have already begun to encourage patients and position providers appropriately along the changing care continuum, despite and in some cases because of current reimbursement mechanisms. Knowledge of their local and regional markets allows for place-based care and an opportunity to leverage not just their local knowledge but their ability to scale and scope data and technology to improve population health. As the largest single component of our healthcare system, hospitals and their networks of physicians and clinics are well positioned to be the repositories of large analytic datasets that can identify, treat, and prevent community-wide health issues. To do so, however, will require a more holistic integration of clinical and community-based services on a regional level and an investment in the technology and resources that would be required. Today, it is rare to find interoperable data systems across clinical providers, let alone community-based service providers, that can share the kind of information that would be required in a truly integrated system.

The changes we do see occurring like the shift toward value-based payment and increased industry concentration are not occurring in a vacuum. They are in response to changes in financial reimbursement, a changing economic and demographic landscape, and to changes in technology. Individual stakeholders, such as hospitals, physicians, and even community-based providers, are not properly incented and cannot be expected to bring about these changes on their own. But as the largest stakeholder, hospitals can assume a leadership position in forging the working coalitions and demanding the necessary resources from our policy makers to facilitate a more equitable and integrated healthcare system. Improving health equity in our society is a goal we should all embrace. We believe that hospitals as an institution can and should play a leadership role in this endeavor. To the extent they fulfill this moral and public health imperative remains to be seen.

References

1. Rosenthal E. Insured but not covered. The New York Times. 2015. Available from: https://nyti.ms/2rD7qwS.
2. Collins SR, Gunja MZ, Doty MM. How well does insurance coverage protect consumers from health care costs? Kaiser Family Foundation. 2017. Available from: http://bit.ly/2zkg7yj.
3. Pickett KE, Wilkinson RG. Income inequality and health: a causal review AHRQ. 2015. Available from: http://bit.ly/2oBUbMg.
4. National Academies of Sciences, Engineering, and Medicine. The growing gap in life expectancy by income: implications for federal programs and policy responses. Washington, DC: The National Academies Press; 2015.
5. How does where you live affect how long you live? [Internet]. RWJF. Robert Wood Johnson; 2018 [cited 2018 Apr 16]. Available from: https://rwjf.ws/2IvRCDr.
6. For the Sake of All: A report on the health and well-being of African Americans in St. Louis and why it matters for everyone. This report was revised in July 2015. Available from: https://forthesakeofall.org/learn-more/publications/#book_close.
7. Artiga S, Hinton E. Beyond health care: the role of social determinants in promoting health and health equity. Kaiser Family Foundation. 2018 May. Available from: https://kaiserf.am/2IbpM3v.
8. Kindig DA, Isham G. Population health improvement: a community health business model that engages partners in all Sectors. Front Health Serv Manag. 30(4):3–20.
9. Cafarella Lallemand N. Reducing Waste in Health Care [Internet]. Health affairs health policy briefs. Robert Wood Johnson Foundation; 2016 [cited 2018 Apr 23]. Available from: https://rwjf.ws/2rV4oEB.
10. O'Neill DP, Scheinker D. Wasted health spending: who's picking up the tab? Health affairs blog. 2018. Available from: http://bit.ly/2kCsa4V.
11. Gonzalez M, Kristy SB, Blanchard JC, Abir M, Iyer N, Smith A, Vesely J, Okeke EN, Kellermann AL. The evolving role of emergency departments in the United States. Santa Monica: RAND Corporation; 2013. Available from: http://bit.ly/2rXCgl9.
12. Camden Coalition of Healthcare Providers; 2018. Available from: https://www.camdenhealth.org/.
13. Rumball-Smith J, Bates D. The electronic health record and health IT to decrease racial/ethnic disparities in care. J Health Care Poor Underserved. 2018;29(1):58–62.
14. University of Wisconsin Health Innovation Program. HIPxChange: sharing to transform healthcare. Area Deprivation Index. Available from: https://www.hipxchange.org/ADI.
15. Maroko AR, Doan TM, Arno PS, Hubel M, Yi S, Viola D. Integrating social determinants of health with treatment and prevention: a new tool to assess local area deprivation. Prev Chronic Dis. 2016;13(E128):1–5.
16. Dickson V. Mapping the impact of social determinants of health. Modern Healthcare. 2018. Available from: http://www.modernhealthcare.com/article/20180209/NEWS/180209899/.
17. Topol E. The patient will see you now: the future of medicine is in your hands. New York: Basic Books; 2015.
18. National Conference of State Legislatures. State coverage for telehealth services. Available from: http://bit.ly/2GvsT0h.
19. Virtual health aligning solutions with Enterprise-wide priorities. Sg2 Center for Clinical Technology. 2014.
20. Quinn WV, O'Brien EO, Springan G, Niehoff M. Using telehealth to improve home-based care for older adults and family caregivers. AARP Public Policy Institute. 2018. Available from: http://bit.ly/2KYwcAo.
21. IQVIA. 2018 and Beyond: outlook and turning points. 2018 March. Available from: http://bit.ly/2xcXMar.
22. Ashwood JS, Mehrotra A, Cowling D, Uscher-Pines L. Direct-to-consumer telehealth may increase access to care but does not decrease spending. Health Aff. 2017;36(3):485–91.
23. Cuckler GA, Sisko AM, Poisal JA, Keehan SP, Smith SD, Madison AJ, Wolfe CJ, Hardesty JC. National

health expenditure projections, 2017–26: despite uncertainty, fundamentals primarily drive spending growth. Health Aff. 2018;37(3):482–92.
24. Healthcare Cost and Utilization Project (HCUP). HCUP fast stats. Rockville: Agency for Healthcare Research and Quality; 2017. http://bit.ly/2qSuxnP.
25. McDowell M. Sg2 2017 impact of change forecast: finding growth. Sg2 analytics. 2017. Available from: http://bit.ly/2qUXzCu.
26. Health Care Cost Institute. 2016 Health care costs and utilization report. 2018. Available from: http://bit.ly/2HGcP0f.
27. Fulton BD. Health care market concentration trends in the United States: evidence and policy responses. Health Aff. 2017;36(9):1530–8.
28. Gaynor M. Hospital and Health Insurance Markets Concentration and Inpatient Hospital Transaction Prices in the U.S. Health Care Market. Statement before the Committee on Energy and Commerce Oversight and Investigations Subcommittee U.S. House of Representatives. 2018. Available from: http://bit.ly/2qQQGmh.
29. Schulman KA, Richman BD. Reassessing ACOs and health care reform. JAMA. 2016;316(7):707–8.
30. Scheffler RM, Fulton BD, Hoang BD, Shortell SM. Consolidation in California's health care market 2010–2016: impact on prices and ACA premiums. Berkeley: School of Public Health, University of California; 2018. http://bit.ly/2HerKMo.
31. Gaynor M, Moreno-Serra R, Propper C. Death by market power: reform, competition, and patient outcomes in the National Health Service. Am Econ J Econ Pol. 2013;5(4):134–66.
32. Romano PS, Balan DJ. A retrospective analysis of the clinical quality effects of the acquisition of Highland Park hospital by Evanston Northwestern healthcare. Int J Econ Bus. 2011;18(1):45–64.
33. Kessler DP, McClellan MB. Is hospital competition socially wasteful? Q J Econ. 2000;115(2):577–615.
34. Young GJ, Flaherty S, Zepeda ED, Singh SR, Rosen Cramer G. Community benefit spending by tax-exempt hospitals changed little after ACA. Health Aff. 2018;37(1):121–4.
35. Rosenbaum S, Kindig DA, Bao J, Byrnes MK, O'Laughlin C. The value of the nonprofit hospital tax exemption was $24.6 billion in 2011. Health Aff. 2015;34(7):1225–33.
36. Muhlestein D, Saunders R, McClellan M. Growth of ACOs and alternative payment models, in 2017. Health Affairs Blog. 2017. Available from: http://bit.ly/2L9SkY4.
37. Song Z, Fisher ES. The ACO experiment in infancy—looking back and looking forward. JAMA. 2016;316(7):705–6.
38. Hsu J, Price M, Vogeli C, Brand R, Chernew ME, Chaguturu SK, Weil E, Ferris TG. Bending the spending curve by altering care delivery patterns: the role of care management within a pioneer ACO. Health Aff. 2017;36(5):876–84.
39. Ryan AM, Krinsky S, Maurer KA, Dimick JB. Changes in hospital quality associated with hospital value-based purchasing. N Engl J Med. 2017;376(24):2358–66.
40. Papanicolas I, Figueroa JF, Orav EJ, Jha AK. Patient hospital experience improved modestly, but no evidence Medicare incentives promoted meaningful gains. Health Aff. 2017;36:133–40.
41. National Association of ACOs. Press Release, 2018. Available from: http://bit.ly/2JYIpEc.
42. Rosenthal E. An American sickness: how healthcare became big business and how you can take it back. New York: Penguin; 2017.
43. Marmor T, Oberlander J. From HMOs to ACOs: the quest for the Holy Grail in US health policy. J Gen Intern Med. 2012;27(9):1215–8. Available from: http://bit.ly/2fmelbU.
44. Sullivan LW, White AA. Inequality persists in health care. CNN Opinion. 2014. Available from: https://cnn.it/2rP6iYc.

8 The Tall Order of the Modern Hospital: Balancing Patient Care with Economics and Academic Missions – Administrators' Perspective

Ronald C. Merrell

Definitions

All hospitals in the USA today are perforce modern. There is no possibility for an anachronism to survive or certainly succeed in the demanding brew of technology, soaring expectation, regulation, and economics of health care in this century. There is no more demanding a situation than that of the Academic Health Center. There are now 5534 hospitals in the USA, and 4840 are community hospitals. Of these 2849 are nongovernmental not-for-profit hospitals [1]. Therefore the vast majority of acute care hospitals are in the private sector and subject to the forces of the marketplace. There are 1825 rural community hospitals and 3231 community hospitals are in a system. An Academic Health Center embraces all the elements of university life with a deep engagement with regulators, health payers, public attention, and the inevitable bottom line.

Balancing Missions

In order to prevail and succeed, administration of an Academic Health Center (AHC) must balance the many facets of interaction. Balance is an interesting term. It implies that there will be a fulcrum somewhere and no particular pull or draw or press can be allowed to displace the other elements. Balance also suggests that at the level of administrators, there will be decisions that cannot meet every expectation for support, funding, space, or time. Balance implies compromise and very tough choices. In order to make those decisions wisely and effectively, the administrators of an AHC must have broad experience in management, regulation, contracting, etc. to be sure that the balance does not slip into an ineffective tumble or slide into failure. No component can displace another and at the base of all decisions must be missions and practicality. All the component missions and interface organizations must have the conviction that they represent the sine qua non of the blended institution that it is an AHC. Administration pulls it together.

Players and Payers

The interface organizations which decide the fate of an AHC are numerous and not always without conflict. At the interface of academic and educational expectations, there is of course the Association of American Medical Colleges (AAMC). This organization has pressed for improvement and standards in academic health since its organization in 1876. Its mission is to serve and lead the academic medical community to better health care for all. There are four mission areas: medical education, patient care,

R. C. Merrell (✉)
Department of Surgery, Virginia Commonwealth University, Richmond, VA, USA
e-mail: ronald.merrell@vcuhealth.org

R. Latifi (ed.), *The Modern Hospital*, https://doi.org/10.1007/978-3-030-01394-3_8

medical research, and striving for diversity and inclusion [2]. AAMC reflects the interests of 151 US medical schools and 17 Canadian schools. The AAMC components convene 400 teaching hospitals including 51 Veterans Affairs hospitals. The AAMC represents the interests of 173, 000 full-time faculty members, 89,000 medical students, 129,000 residents, and 60,000 graduate students/postdoctoral fellows. The AAMC is a not-for-profit entity that is at the apex of a series of regulatory and advocacy groups. The AAMC is in alliance with the American Medical Association to name the Liaison Committee on Medical Education which is recognized by the Department of Education for setting standards and accrediting medical schools. Last year the US schools graduated 19,254 newly minted physicians. The AAMC delegates graduate matters to the Accreditation Council on Graduate Medical Education to certify and regulate residency programs. The Council accredits 29 primary board specialties and a total of 153 certificate programs. AHCs generally strive to train a comprehensive cadre of medical specialties, and the task is obviously onerous. The Council of Teaching Hospitals includes about 400 entities that all could recognize as full-service Academic Health Centers. Please note that of the over 5000 hospitals in the USA, there are only 400 AHCs. The AHCs are not only committed to medical students and residents. Their responsibilities include dentistry, graduate studies, nursing, pharmacy, public health, allied health, and veterinary medicine. That puts them at the very crux of all medical education and providing the public with competent, compassionate, and accredited health-care personnel in every aspect of patient care and research.

The education mission is separate somewhat from patient care accreditation. The Joint Commission is an independent not-for-profit organization that accredits some 21,000 health enterprises in the USA [3]. No AHC gets very far without complete and even exemplary accreditation from the Joint Commission. The regulatory requirements are broad and deep. In addition AHCs like all health units must meet the accreditation of all local, state, and federal regulators for patient care and safety. That regulation would include nuclear, hazardous waste, local disaster preparedness, street signage, parking, fire codes, etc. This litany is not intended to defend the AHC. On the contrary we all expect the accreditation requirements to be faithfully met and exceeded as part of the core mission. The AHC is expected to maintain the highest of internal credentials, quality assurance, patient safety, and workplace safety for the enormous number of workers which typically runs to the many thousands in an AHC.

Now this enterprise must be paid for by numerous, generally reluctant, sources. Expenditure for health care in the USA is the highest per capita in the world and growing. In 2016 spending rose 4.3% to 3.3 trillion dollars or 17.9% of the gross domestic product. Medicare accounts for 20% of the payments, while Medicaid covers 17%. Private insurance covers 34%, and 11% comes from out-of-pocket expenses. Put another way the federal government pays 28.3%, employer insurance covers 19.9%, while state and local governments pay 16.9% [4]. Of these payments 32% go to hospitals, 20% to physician and clinical services, and 10% for prescription drugs. Hospitals may be responsible for administration of some of the payments to physicians and for drugs.

All the payers have a keen interest in protecting stockholders, taxpayers, and subscribers. They make large demands on hospitals, records, standards, documentation, and accountability. Current payment systems are dynamic and unlikely to persist past the publication of this book. Payment will be based on performance, compliance, and medical record documentation. It is generally agreed that the current expenditures are not sustainable. Therefore things must change. Also it is unclear that the USA is ready for a single-payer system. It is not even clear that the USA is ready for a system! Perhaps the public is increasingly assigning to government that responsibility to assure health care. That has huge but only vaguely seen implications. The AHCs have a special role in the economics of health care in the USA. Even though they only represent 5% of all hospitals, AHCs provide 37% of all charity care in the USA and 26% of all Medicaid hospitalizations [5]. AHCs are the usual sites for burn units, and Level I trauma designation is customary. Over half of the National Institutes of Health extramural funding went to faculty at AHCs in 2011. However indirect cost reimbursement does not completely cover the cost of research at AHCs which absorbs 30% of the support. The cost of teaching is also a defining feature of AHC financing with direct costs of training residents and fellows, faculty supervision, equipment, and staff reaching some $16 billion annually. Medicare covers $3 billion, and the Department of Veterans Affairs, Department of Defense, Medicaid, and the Public Health Service provide more modest support. Medicare is the biggest source of Graduate Medical Education (GME) support and is the only entity that has a formula for ongoing support. However, the number of graduate slots has been essentially frozen since 1997, and there is no enthusiasm for any further government funding. In fact the energy is to draw down graduate training and perhaps charge tuition. Clearly most of the direct cost of GME is embraced by the AHCs.

There is an increase in the number of medical graduates who seek funded resident positions. There were 16 new allopathic schools opened in the early part of the century and 15 new osteopathic schools. Medical schools added about 30% new student slots. This adds up to a 49% increase in first year enrollment in the USA. With the cap on GME slots from Medicare, the states, VA, and various other entities have risen to the occasion, and there is no current shortage of resident positions. The accommodation reflects tremendous community and academic effort. To teach the new medical students, much of the expenses has fallen to the AHCs of course [6]. The AAMC called for a great expansion of medical students in 2006. The cost of each new student is in excess of $62,000 per year in variable costs. Obviously tuition will not cover this. There are several scenarios to anticipate the impact of these costs. New sources of revenue could be sought and certainly will be. Medical education could move to less expensive sites and become more efficient through innovation. This is an essential element for moving forward [7].

The costs of education, research, and extraordinary clinical care for the vulnerable make the AHCs a special challenge for administrators. The vagaries of funding and patient care income are certainly no better than any community hospital. Therefore the AHCs are in a constant state of study and evolution as health-care practice and funding bend and stretch for a new configuration.

Triumph of Excellence

Despite enormous pressures on the budgets and human resources, the AHC's leadership has continued to lead the nation in innovation and advances in health care. Last year the US news rankings of American hospitals declared that the top 20 hospitals in the USA were all AHCs. The criteria for ranking did not emphasize academic hallmarks of superiority. Instead the criteria included such hard facts as survival rates and staffing and low rates of medical error. The lead AHC on the list was the Mayo Clinic, and number two was the Cleveland Clinic. It should be noted that the top administrators at each are physicians. Dr. John Noseworthy, a noted neurologist, leads the Mayo Clinic, and Dr. Toby Cosgrove, a world-renowned cardiac surgeon, leads the Cleveland Clinic. Even as the challenges to AHCs are enumerated, the centers are carrying a disproportionate burden of burn care, trauma care, indigent care medical education, and resident education and a stunning role in medical research. They are a pride to their communities and nation [8].

Issues

It must be clear that the AHCs are not on some sort of privileged autopilot. Their issues are huge and only carefully coordinated responses can allow them to succeed. Anticipation of issues is a hallmark of the centers as they ride with the times and often determine the future of health care. Some of the emerging issues deserve mention.

Technology

The practice of medicine will continue to get better in the future as new technology changes practices and outcomes. The new technology must include advances in health informatics. The current electronic medical record is not mature. It is really an electronic version of legacy paper records merged with requirements for charge capture, materials management, and compliance with the myriad regulations of payers and credentialing activities. The electronic record is time-consuming, and that time could be applied to more personal contact with patients. Improvements are coming for sure, but the wait is excruciating. Great enhancements and challenges will come from the notion of artificial intelligence (AI). This computer wizardry will allow very fast integration of patient data, global experience, and probability to generate patient management schemes of unparalleled accuracy and effectiveness. All should be aware of the pitfalls, and the clinicians of the next few decades must be always vigilant for computer error that will come almost certainly from erroneous computer entry. AI will seamlessly guide respirator management and fluid therapy. Personalized medicine and genomics will allow highly specific patient-centered therapy with the expectation of great improvements in outcomes. We should expect great improvements in diagnostics including imaging, tissue analysis, invasive monitoring, and programmed interventions for surgery. The evolving technology must certainly be guided by wise decisions and careful incorporation into the generalities of medical practice. Some of the technology will certainly be disruptive and press medicine into unforeseen direction. Wise leadership and highly informed practitioners will keep the patient safe.

Venue

The hospital has been the crux of advanced health care and medical education since the time of Flexner over a century ago. Health care moved to the hospitals because that was the locus of the expensive and complicated technology that supported the highest objectives in radiology, surgery, diagnostics, and skill of the practitioners. Medical students and residents studied there because the new treatments predicted the likely future of their practices and the concentration of patients allowed concentrated experiences for rapid training. However, the technology has gotten smaller, cheaper, and easily distributed. Therefore, much of health care is moving to homes, the workplace, and wherever the patient might go. Through monitoring, data management, distant interaction, and patient education, the hospital could become a much less important player. The rare specialist can be dispatched into very remote sites as part of a virtual medical staff such that no practitioner need be isolated. Systems of transfer and pre-hospital care grow more sophisticated and effective. This could be a great challenge to the imminence of AHCs. However, the likelihood is great that the large medical centers will lead through networking and remain just as important as ever but through the mediation of telecommunications and information management. The large centers simply must abandon the notion of hospital as the sole physical venue and continue to support practitioners and patients through electronic and virtual means. Education would logically follow the patients to their source of care. Students and residents will obviously be spending more and more time in virtual environments evaluating patients and participating in their care. This is of course revolutionary. One would expect great resistance and a shortage of workable plans. However, in the long term the direction seems inevitable.

Conflicting Missions

The core missions of the AHCs must be under constant review and subject to modifications. If education eclipses patient care or if technology outstrips the professionalism of the practitioners, the system will of course fail. If efforts to become more efficient marginalize the creativity of the practitioners, the future is grim. If leadership moves to bureaucrats without attention to professionals and patients, there is no purpose. The missions all have their inherent strengths in the ultimate success of the AHC and those strengths are precious. Balancing those missions for the greater purpose is imperative of course.

Competition

The pull of the private sector has been an active element in faculty and staff retention for most of the last century and continues. Patients may find the amenities of private suburban settings with excellent advertising programs and convenient parking much more attractive than long drives into the urban domain of most AHCs. Payers are little interested in the special aspects of the AHC if they can buy the same service for less money elsewhere.

Leadership

The people who have led our AHCs in the last century did not follow career tracks that were designed for such a task. They often came from the ranks of academic practitioners who rose to the task from prominence in research, clinical practice, or a variety of power bases in the AHC community. Some were carefully groomed as academic nurses and administrators from premier graduate programs. One characteristic that has been true is that they almost grew up in the culture of the AHC with almost no one coming from industry or business outside. Whatever the source of leadership, the AHC has been very fortunate in the main in the cadre of committed insightful and energetic leaders. This has not always been the case of course, and one of the greater risks to the success of an AHC has been the poor choice of leaders. A successful clinician, investigator, or administrator does not guarantee the ability or skill set required to integrate the many missions and find the balance for success.

Requirements

Success of the AHC may take many approaches. However there are three essential components. First and foremost no matter the idealism of the enterprise, the budget must balance and prevail. Period. There can be no way forward if budgets fail, programs are cut for survival only, and the business plan of the entity is regularly compromised by competition. Second, the AHC through its administration must balance successfully its manifold missions with loss to none. Surely the missions will evolve and should be examined for their relative impact one upon the other, but in the end balance must prevail. Finally, the AHC cannot go forward with the precondition that tradition is its best guide. It is difficult to say what health-care reform will eventually look like in America, and speculation is probably not worthwhile. However, a paramount feature will involve compromise and a careful attention to the times, patient expectations, staff expectations, government expectation, and business realities. By astute listening and starting from a position of compromise, success is much more likely.

Emerging Solutions

Several strains of innovation and synergy can be identified that likely will have a major impact on the future success of the AHC. First it is important to recognize that success is not a certainty and that the AHC is not so important to health care in the USA that its perpetuation will always be assured by even artificial means. The whole enterprise could collapse in financial ruin, and education, research, advanced patient care, and community service could fragment into any configuration of components. That is not a desirable outcome and can be avoided. The greatest assurance in this regard will involve competent and insightful administration and leadership.

Leadership

Current practices to advance leaders in AHCs are not very orderly. The academic and health community will benefit from well-designed structures to bring along members of the community to positions of ever greater authority and responsibility toward the objective of leading the highly complex and interactive function of the AHC. These efforts should of course include graduate programs, business education, and health administration curricula as well as experiences outside the AHC in business, government, and industry. Through such career paths, the maturing future leader can nurture skills for integration and bring back to the AHC valuable skills from other sectors. The leader need not be any particular member of the AHC community. There is every reason to nurture the administrator, clinician, pharmacist, nurse, allied health individual, and others who by their particular abilities as leaders and their preparation could prove the requisite force for success. Every discipline in the AHC should be active in developing such individuals.

Contracting. Contracting for payers, suppliers, services, and patients cannot be causal. This is the lifeblood of business success. Worker contracts for staff must be clear, fair, and allow for individual development of employees. Sincere concern for the workers will not be new to all AHCs but might be refreshing in some and its enhancement a benefit to all. The staff can have the satisfaction of successful performance reports, fair evaluation, and a sense of personal growth. Staff development and retention cannot proceed in a workplace that does not recognize the dignity and worth of the employees. Training those individuals in the allied health area on site is certainly desirable, and contracts for long-term education relationships are most desirable. Contracts for other sites where education might be better served should not be of course ignored. This might imply system building, networking, or affiliation. The coming time in the history of health care and the AHC is not a good one for being insular or elitist.

Simulation and Team Building

Most AHCs have recognized that simulation training for medical students leads to greater confidence and safety. Simulation training for residents is a requirement for credentials in many settings. Simulation centers are expensive. They require space and personnel. This can be mollified if the center is not for a single purpose. Use the center to update current practitioners and to build team behaviors for patient safety and incorporation of new technology. Market the simulation center to the region. Every imaginable cognitive, mechanical, and team skill can be developed in a simulated environment away from the press of urgent patient care. Patients can be reassured that no trainee is confronting their needs without full credentialing in the procedure they are about to perform. The faculty can be reassured that they are not teaching someone this procedure for the first time as a complete novice but they are working with a trainee who has been fully credentialed in this endeavor in a simulated, safe, controlled environment. Simulation can be shared between medical schools, hospitals, and distant sites through distant teaching. Standardized curricula are well developed; outcomes have been vetted and are highly reproducible.

Discovery

In the rush of inpatient care, it is difficult to reflect on the outlier, the case that is not quite fitting the algorithm or the possibility of a unique observation. Carving out a way to catch these precious events should be a priority. It is hard to imagine today the discoveries at the Hotel Dieu in Paris with leisurely rounds led by imminent clinicians who gave their names to so many conditions: Laennec, Dupuytren, Charcot, etc. A recent proposal from the Massachusetts General puts just such opportunities into focus in the AHC and should be considered more broadly. The medical teaching service can be called when a case seems more complex and unusual or maybe just interesting [9].

Patient Education and Communication

Successful AHCs right now are heavily engaged in patient empowerment through website education, interactive groups, and specific instructions for a disease or regimen. It should be remembered that patients have not been particularly passive for a long time. The patients are computer savvy and well versed in the prudent use of social media. The more patients are involved, the more likely they will participate and assure their best outcome. Patient care can be made far more efficient by interactive telemedicine for instruction prior to coming to the hospital and for post-hospital surveillance. Early recognition of complications may avoid readmission, and recognition of troublesome problems prior to admission may avoid a scrubbed admission. The use of media by AHCs for caregivers, family, general public education, and community outreach is at its very infancy. Of course there will be mistakes and there will be some misinformation. The use of media for disease prevention is just at its beginning. AHCs should be in the vanguard to make these mechanisms of patient communication and involvement seamless and effective.

Telemedicine and e-health. These terms are simply a continuation of the communication themes outlined above. However, the terms have some connotation of their own. A successful AHC will be required to lead in these areas. Direct-to-consumer telemedicine will certainly be a stretch for highly organized AHCs. However, to ignore the demand, would be to invite unwanted competition from outside the AHC community. That may not be desirable if the AHC is to continue to essay for comprehensive health care and training. One should consider that a draw for the AHC has been the availability of rare specialists for consultation. However, in a telemedicine system, the superspecialist is only a click away. AHCs in order to maintain their competitiveness should consider joining and leading the telemedicine effort by making their specialists available through electronic consultation.

Efficiency: This Is at Once Hard and Easy

Hanging on to outdated programs, outdated leaders, old concepts, and low-demand service is really not workable. Every aspect of the AHC will be under scrutiny for effectiveness, quality, and economic viability. Certainly there are programs of less than obvious contribution to the bottom line. However, a better system of analyzing programs in terms of downstream profit will surely be developed. There is no room for waste in material management, housekeeping, parking or operating room times, supply consumption for a given procedure, or operating room start times. Time in the ER, length of stay, and waiting time for an outpatient appointment all go to the calculation of efficiency in the center. The opportunities for innovation and improvement in this regard are legion.

Conclusion

The Academic Health Center is a powerful contributor to medical innovation, education, and patient care in the USA. The role of the administration in this success is not to be underestimated. The administrator is responsible for the balance of potentially conflicting missions. It might be better said that the administrator is responsible to allow those missions to function in harmony. Balance may be a good term to indicate the tensions that are inevitable for such an enterprise. However, harmony invites a pleasant image of compatibility and synergy. The administration must be attuned to the present conditions and accurately anticipate the future to some degree. No administrator should be expected to be a savant or visionary. The leader will succeed by preparation and by listening acutely to the various constituents of their enormous organizations. The administrator is not the apex of a successful AHC. Neither is a conductor the uniquely gifted performer in an orchestra. Let us all strive for harmony and hope for a conductor with a good ear and a well-understood baton.

References

1. American Hospital Association (AHA). Home page. Retrieved from: www.AHA.org. Last accessed 15 May 2018.
2. Association of American Medical Colleges (AAMC). Home page. Retrieved from: www.aamc.org. Last accessed 15 May 2018.
3. The Joint Commission. Home page. Retrieved from: www.jointcommission.org. Last accessed 15 May 2018.

4. Centers for Medicare & Medicaid Services. Home page. Retrieved from: www.CMS.gov. Last accessed 15 May 2018.
5. Grover A, Slavin PL, Willson P. Perspective: the economics of academic medical centers. New England J of Medicine. 2014;370:2360–2.
6. Mullan F, Salsberg E, Weider K. Why a GME squeeze is unlikely. N Engl J Med. 2015;373:2397–9.
7. Schieffer D, Azevedo B, Culbertson R, Kahn M. Financial implications of increasing medical school size: does tuition cover cost? Permanente J. 2012;16:10–4.
8. Advisory Board. Daily briefing. August 2, 2016. Retrieved from: www.advisory.com/daily-briefing/2016/08/02. Last accessed 15 May 2018.
9. Armstrong K, Ranganathan R, Fishman M. Toward a culture of scientific inquiry-the role of medical teaching services. N Engl J Med. 2018;378:1–5.

Part II

Advanced Technologies and the New Mission of Modern Hospital

9 The Modern Hospital: Patient-Centered and Science-Based

Rifat Latifi and Colene Yvonne Daniel

Introduction

Today's modern hospital incorporates genomics, nanotechnology tools, robots, artificial intelligence, telemedicine, and other technologies to provide care. Clinicians now have a much greater knowledge of these mechanisms and the biology of disease. They understand where one can effectively disrupt transformation from normal to malignant tissue and how to influence the body's response to disease. This has resulted in a substantial metamorphosis of the hospital overall, as well as a particular metamorphosis of physicians and surgeons as part of the hospital revolution. For example, while the surgical foundation is fundamentally the same, the modus operandi of the practice of surgery has changed substantially [1]. While today's hospitals are heavily influenced by the financial bottom line, multiple layers of bureaucracy and administration, insurance companies, and continuing changing public policies and perceptions pertaining to health, hospitals continue to function in a collaborative environment. Clinicians and administrators strive to maintain the basic principles of caring, teaching, mentoring, and advancing the art and science of the surgical and medical discipline above everything else. The transformation in healthcare and surgical and medical practice has not changed the basic tenets: hospitals and physicians care for the sick and injured, are healers, strive for perfection, while respecting the rich surgical past and making teaching and scientific contributions. However, in order to be prepared for the future, the new modern hospital must constantly strive to understand and master the magnitude and complexities of the new body of knowledge, technology, and teamwork essential to optimal healthcare today. For the new generations of surgeons and physicians, training must be modified to abide by new requirements from government agencies and other regulatory bodies. Above all, the modern hospital must be adaptable, flexible, and prepared to incorporate technology that will come in successive waves to challenge our prejudice and demand the best in critical understanding of the changing options for patient care.

In this chapter, we discuss some of the elements that we believe are paramount in changing *the new hospital* while balancing the skills of comforting a patient while they heal or take their last breath and working effectively under exceptionally stressful situations such as war. In other words, the patient has been, remains, and will continue to be the epicenter of everything that we do in the hospital. Everything that we do, from

R. Latifi (✉)
New York Medical College, School of Medicine, Department of Surgery and Westchester Medical Center, Valhalla, NY, USA
e-mail: rifat_latifi@nymc.edu; rifat.latifi@wmchealth.org

C. Y. Daniel
The Bonne Sante Group, LLC, Washington, DC, USA

R. Latifi (ed.), *The Modern Hospital*, https://doi.org/10.1007/978-3-030-01394-3_9

the parking lot to the board room, in small hospitals or corporations, has to be patient-focused. This has been the norm for centuries. So, while the invention of new buzzwords like "patient-centered" has helped guide day-to-day activities, the fact remains that hospitals were always patient-centered. Surgeons, physicians, nurses, administrators, and all other healthcare workers are patient-centered in their work.

To discover what has occurred in the continuum of transition and transformation of surgery and what has changed during the last century or so, we do not really need to go very far. One only has to look back within our own practices and recognize the changes in surgery within our own lifetimes in order to realize how much surgery has been reinvented and how much surgeons have been transformed. If we do this, perhaps we may begin to understand the complexity of the process and the magnitude of adaptation required to stay current with surgical science. This chapter does not address whether we are better or worse, but merely acknowledges that we have become different surgeons and physicians and that the stage on which we practice surgery has been utterly transformed.

Hospital and Institution of Patient-Centered Care and Research

Today's healthcare provider, as never before, has to respond to and incorporate the ever-evolving changes of *the new hospital* including nanotechnology and surgical science yet maintains the skills of comforting a patient while they heal or take their last breath, as well as working effectively under exceptionally stressful situations such as war, other disasters, and a myriad variety of other emergencies. In all of this, the patient has been, remains, and will be the epicenter of everything that we do and will do in the hospital. Everything that we do, from the parking lot to the boardroom small or mega corporates that manage hospitals, has to do with the patient. It has been like this for centuries. So, while the new invention of jargons like "patient-centered" and others similar to that has taken more prominent places in the day-to-day discussions and perhaps activities, the fact remains that hospitals were always patient-centered and surgeons and physicians, nurses, and all others who work and are involved in the hospital being were and are patient-centered. What is new, is the fact that patients have become more educated about their medical problems and more active participants in the decision maing process.

In order to strive for emphasis on patient-centered practices, the US government established the *Patient-Centered Outcomes Research Institute* (PCORI). PCORI provides funding to researchers and institutions to conduct clinical effectiveness research (CER). CER is assisting patients, clinicians, purchasers, and policy-makers in making informed health decisions [1–10]. PCORI began funding research in 2012 and through 2017 has supported 466 projects for a total of $1.7 billion. During that first year, total funding was $72 million. In 2013, funding rose to $204 million. Between 2014 and 2018, per year funding has ranged from $295 million to $382 million.

While the patient-centered care concept has been adopted by clinicians, hospital administrators, the public, and the media, almost as new concept, we feel that we have been practicing patient centeredness all along. Nonetheless, this is an important transition of care where the central principle in PCORI's activities is the idea of engagement of all stakeholders. Stakeholders can come from various communities including caregivers, clinicians, healthcare institutions, researchers, policy-makers, professional societies, insurers, and industry, but patients lead this process first and foremost. The key objective of engagement is conducting research that is truly patient-centered and aims to answer questions or examine outcomes that matter to patients and their families or caregivers within the context of patient preferences. Engagement with stakeholders can occur at various stages of the research life cycle: developing research questions, prioritizing research questions, study design, participants recruitment and study conduct, review of the study report, and dissemination of findings. During study design and conduct, patients may be particularly helpful in identification of relevant outcomes, suggesting participant eligibility criteria and assisting in participant recruitment. Additional recommendations for researchers conducting PCORI-funded research can be found in

PCORI Methodology Standards. PCORI has established five research priorities that include (1) assessment of prevention, diagnosis, and treatment options, (2) research improving healthcare systems, (3) communication and dissemination of research findings, (4) disparities in healthcare, and, finally, (5) priority of enhancing research infrastructure and conducting research on CER.

While the concern has always been for the welfare and outcomes of the patient, patient-centered care refers to the shift in focus on who determines what is necessary and who can provide input on outcomes. In other words, in patient-centered models of medical and surgical practice, the patient is the real partner in managing his/her disease, and the patient-centered approach incorporates the perceptions and needs of the patient [10]. A quick look in PubMed on May 25, 2018, we identified 25,979 articles of which 12,008 are published in the last 5 years under "patient-centered care." The surge of all these original articles, review articles, case reports, and other reports in PubMed is a powerful illustration of the new trend that the clinicians, researchers, and academic hospitals are taking note of patient-centered care. A systematic review of 14 studies (seven of which were randomized clinical trials) on laparoscopic repair of ventral hernia (LVHR) [11] found that LVHR improved the overall health-related quality of life of patients (HRQoL) in 6 of the 8 studies. These authors found that LVHR demonstrated improved pain scores and improved functionality (in 12 studies). Patients returned to work within a ranged from 6 to 18 days postoperatively in 50% of studies, while the physical function scores were improved in the remaining 50% of the studies. Overall patient satisfaction improved after LVHR in all studies assessing patient satisfaction, including improving mental and emotional well-being (in six of the seven studies). *Patient-centered* concept is a specific metric that has now been incorporated into how surgeons and physicians and hospitals in general assess the outcomes and interact with patients. Using a patient-centered focus has broadly changed the environment in which we all work. To this end, patients' satisfaction with an operation has become a common theme and a focus in many important scientific deliberations and peer-reviewed journals [12].

Providing Patient-Centered Care: Involving the Patient in Surgical Decisions of a Difficult Problem

Involving the patient as a real partner in surgical decisions is of utmost importance, particularly in difficult situations, such as transplant, joint replacement, or any major surgical decisions.

For example, in our practice in patients in need of reconstruction of abdominal for complex defects, we explain to each patient and family, with the utmost clarity, that three main outcomes are possible with surgery:

1. We will complete the task, that is, perform lyses of adhesions, take down stomas or fistulas (when present), restore the continuity of the GI tract and reconstruct the abdominal wall, and then oversee a postoperative course that leads to recovery, without major incident.
2. We may not be able to accomplish any of the intended goals as specified in the first outcome (#1) and in fact make the patient worse.
3. We may successfully complete the initial operation, but the fistulas may recur, the anastomoses may leak, and a serious wound infection may develop that requires reoperation and possible mesh explantation essentially returning to square one, or even worse, the complications may prove fatal.

These outcomes are reviewed, not only with the patient but also with the family, as well as the preoperative, operative, and postoperative teams. Proper mental preparation is essential for the surgeon and surgical team as well as for the patient and family. So, in our mind and practice, the surgical team consists of the patient, surgeon, and the surgical personnel including anesthesiologist, nurses, scrub team, referring doctors, family, and friends. The more each and every one is involved, and they understand the process, the better the communications will be. Yet, the question that remains to be answered, however, despite all the research, is does this makes a major difference in real outcomes?

In a recent paper [13], the investigators conducted a stepped-wedge, cluster-randomized trial involving patients with a high risk of death and their surrogates in five intensive care units (ICUs) to compare a multicomponent family-support intervention delivered by the interprofessional ICU team with usual care in 1420 critically ill patients. The primary outcome of their study was the surrogates' mean score on the hospital anxiety and depression scale (HADS) at 6 months. Secondary outcomes were the surrogates' mean scores on the impact of event scale (IES), the quality of communication (QOC) scale, and a modified patient perception of patient centeredness (PPPC) scale, as well as the mean length of ICU stay. There was no significant difference between the intervention group and the control group in the surrogates' mean HADS score at 6 months or mean IES score. The surrogates' mean QOC score was better in the intervention group than in the control group, as was the mean modified PPPC score. The authors concluded that among critically ill patients and their surrogates, a family-support intervention delivered by the interprofessional ICU team did not significantly affect the surrogates' burden of psychological symptoms, but the surrogates' ratings of the quality of communication and the patient and family centeredness of care were better, and the length of stay in the ICU was shorter with the intervention than with usual care. Moreover, there was a shorter ICU LOS in the control group, but this was attributed to shorter mean length of stay of patients who died.

The take-home message from this major study is that while patient-centered care does not change the clinical outcome substantially, the family is better off with new communication efforts made by all of us, and that is something that we need to concentrate significantly. The educated patient about his/her disease is the best patient.

The Scientific Revolution and Impact on Clinical Practice

Science and scientists have led the hospital revolution. Integrating new innovative solutions in hospital routine practices is a challenging task, albeit less now than in the past. How does an innovation or individual idea or change in clinical practice that is a potential breakthrough makes it to mainstream clinical practice? In recent years researchers have been preoccupied with integration of these new scientific methods into hospital practice and why some of the innovation fail and other make it [14]. These authors conducted a qualitative study using a purposive sample of hospitals that participated in the State Action on Avoidable Rehospitalizations (STAAR) initiative, a collaborative to reduce hospital readmissions that encouraged members to adopt new practices. They reported that the key to full implementation of new practices at the initial state of implementation process is to select few key staff members that held the innovation in place for as long as a year while more permanent integrating mechanisms began to work. However, innovations that proved intrinsically rewarding to the staff, by making their jobs easier or more gratifying, became integrated through shifts in attitudes and norms over time.

The process of implementation of scientific breakthroughs, in clinical practice, however, is complex and often difficult and may take decades if not longer before they become a mainstream. But the scientist and clinicians cannot stop and have not stopped just because the initial results were not as good as expected or frankly were catastrophic in some cases. In this process often there was a disagreement between traditional practice and technological or simply common scientific discoveries. Those scientist or clinicians who have question the status quo often and mandated the changes were not treated always with respect or kindness, most often by their own peers. Below we will remind our readers about few examples.

Liver Transplant: From Disastrous Results to Standard of Care

One of the most dramatic changes in one procedure that was truly catastrophic initially and then transitioned to superb results is the development of orthotopic liver transplantation, which was only possible with persistence, and dedication, by Dr. Thomas Starzl [15].

Dr. Starzl on his paper in 1968 in the Annals of Surgery began the report with this:

> "Until last year, the kidney was the only organ which had been transplanted with subsequent significant prolongation of life. There had been nine reported attempts at orthotopic liver transplantation; seven in Denver and one each in Boston and Paris. Two of these patients had succumbed within a few hours after operation, and none had lived for longer than 23 days. This dismal picture has changed within the last 9 months, inasmuch as seven consecutive patients treated with orthotopic liver transplantation from July 23, 1967 to March 17, 1968 all passed through this previously lethal operative and postoperative period. Three of the recipients are still alive after 9, $2^{1/3}$, and 1 months; the others died after 2, $3^{1/2}$, $4^{1/3}$, and 6 months" [15].

Today, liver transplant is standard of care for liver failure and many other indications. Heart and lung transplant and pancreas transplant are also standard of care with excellent results and long-term outcomes and survival. This was made possible only with scientific persistence, development, and learning from mistakes and from one another.

Total Parenteral Nutrition (TPN)

Although the concept of feeding patients entirely parenterally by injecting nutrient substances or fluids intravenously was advocated and attempted long before the successful practical development of total parenteral nutrition (TPN) in the 1960s by Dr. Dudrick, as late as 1959, there were serious doubts that total parenteral nutrition (TPN) would actually be able to sustain life [16]. Yet, since 1968, TPN has become the standard of care for all patients who cannot or should not be able to maintain their nutritional status by oral or enteral means [17]. "Realization of this 400 year old seemingly fanciful dream initially required centuries of fundamental investigation coupled with basic technological advances and judicious clinical applications. Most clinicians in the 1950's were aware of the negative impact of starvation on morbidity, mortality, and outcomes, but only few understood the necessity for providing adequate nutritional support to malnourished patients if optimal clinical results were to be achieved. The prevailing dogma in the 1960's was that, 'Feeding entirely by vein is impossible; even if it were possible, it would be impractical; and even if it were practical, it would be unaffordable'" (thought and wrote by few prominent scientists) writes Dr. Stanley Dudrick in the history of parenteral nutrition [18]. Major challenges to the development of TPN were seen as detrimental to developing a safe formulation, biochemically compatible and able to sustain life. Today, TPN is a standard of care that has saved and continued to save millions of people around the world.

Mastectomy and Laparoscopic Cholecystectomy

When Dr. "Barney" Crile Jr. of Cleveland Clinic suggested that "we do not need to perform radical Halstedian mastectomy," he was expelled from the Cleveland Academy of Surgeons [19, 20]. Not only that radical mastectomy is never performed nowadays but has not been performed for decades.

He was not the only one rejected by his peers for innovative thinking. Prof. Dr. Med Erich Mühe of Böblingen, Germany, performed the first laparoscopic cholecystectomy (LC) on September 12, 1985 [21]. When he reported this accomplishment in 1986 to the German Surgical Society, he was rejected from the group. Yet, in 1992, he received their highest award, the German Surgical Society Anniversary Award, and, in 1999, he was recognized by SAGES for having performed the first laparoscopic cholecystectomy. Now LC is a standard of care throughout the world.

Another major development in implementation of scientific advances in surgery that was a result of laparoscopic surgery is robotic-assisted surgeries that have now become routine even in some of the smallest hospitals in this country and many tertiary hospitals around the world. In just about every clinical surgical discipline, and every part of the anatomy from the brain, neck, chest, abdomen, bones, and ligaments, robotic-assisted surgical applications are considered routine. The idea of performing robotic-assisted surgery is relatively new (couple of decades), but in most recent quick glance at PubMed, when using the phrase robotic surgery, there were 14,892 articles, of which 8781 were published in the last 5 years [22].

Not many discoveries have changed the life of patients as did the stent in vascular surgery that has gained more from the scientific development almost more than any other field in surgery. In 1990 Juan C. Parodi performed the first endovascular abdominal aortic aneurysm (AAA) repair in Buenos Aires. Two years later, in 1992, Parodi and Claudio Schonholz visited Montefiore Medical Center in New York to perform with us the first endovascular AAA repair to be done in the United States [23]. Since then 10,918 papers have been published on PubMed, of which 4595 articles were published in the last 5 years on endovascular stent for aortic aneurism on PubMed (as of May 25, 2018), and today endovascular surgery is a standard of care, sought after, both by patients and vascular surgeons worldwide.

The More You Do, the Better the Outcomes

As a result of many scientific and technological advances, many hospitals around the world, and with this great number of clinicians, have become highly specialized in a particular field. Patients undergoing complex surgical procedures at high-volume centers have better outcomes. This has been demonstrated in just about every procedure. A relevant example is aortic procedures [24]. In-hospital mortality correlates to center volume ($p = 0.014$) with low, intermediate, and high-volume centers having mortality rates of 23.4% ($n = 187$), 20.1% ($n = 62$), and 12.1% ($n = 15$), respectively. This relationship persisted when controlling for severity of comorbid illness ($p = 0.007$). The number of complications per patient varied significantly by center volume ($p = 0.044$), as well. Other examples of surgical excellence in high-volume centers that perform pancreatectomy have been clearly documented [25]. In a study performed at Johns Hopkins, all 1000 pancreaticoduodenectomies performed between March 1969 and May 2003 by a single surgeon reported an unprecedented mortality rate of 1% [25]. In addition, the median operative time decreased significantly over the five decades, with 8.8 h reported in the 1970s and 5.5 h during the 2000s. Postoperative length of stay dropped from a median of 17 days in the 1980s to 9 days in the 2000s. Overall 5-year survival was 18%; for the lymph node-negative patients, it was 32%; and for node-negative, margin-negative patients, it was 41%. Another report from the same institution [26] has demonstrated that patients who have cancers with favorable pathological features have statistically significant improved long-term survival.

As a result of scientific developments and innovative approaches to clinical practice, a team-based approach has become the new model for delivering hospital care. There has been a shift in the focus on how, for example, the surgical group works as a team, how they communicate, how they collaboratively make decisions, and how they manage tasks. While the surgeon has always worked with a team, the need for communication and group decision-making has recently been emphasized. In essence, every clinician is required to master the competency to work in a team. All members of the surgical team are required to focus on working together toward better proficiency. Maximizing the potential of how a team works together has been assessed as well. Recently an opinion piece in JAMA Surgery described "Evolution of Surgery: The Story of Two Poems" that summarizes wonderfully the transformation of surgery and the surgeon [27]. The message is clear; it is not all about the surgeon and his or her kingdom. Rather, it is about the patient, the team, the quality, the outcomes, and seeking new ways of providing the best possible care. Standards have changed, and some standards are changing rapidly, so that there is a need for all clinicians to be well informed at all times. While the need to be informed is imperative to the success and for optimum results, acquiring and retaining this new information can be overwhelming.

Intensive care units are now so complex that one needs a week of orientation to learn the environment, and often you cannot see the patient among all the computer hardware and technology. This is not always an easy milieu in which to work, but it is an improvement in many aspects. An intensive care unit (ICU) room can be transformed into a dialyzing unit or into an operating room within minutes. These are "All In One" ICU models where virtually anything can be done. You can see intubated patients walking through the corridors of hospitals hooked to cardiac devices while waiting for new hearts. The trauma room has an angio suite, an operating room, CT scan, MRI, and everything needed to care effectively for the patient.

One group of patients who have benefited greatly from advances in technology are those involved as military casualties [28, 29]. Now, a critically ill and severely injured military patient can get care from three different continents, all while flying above 10 thousand meters, attached to, and supported by, some of the most sophisticated machines that man has ever conceived and invented [29]. A retrospective review of Critical Care Air Transport Team (CCATT) of 975 of injured individuals from Iraq and Afghanistan transferred to Germany demonstrated a mortality of 2.1% and inflight mortality of 0.02%. The evacuation of the injured patients from the war zone is part of the damage control [30, 31]. All this occurs while the patient is being continuously monitored from the ground somewhere in North America. New civilian hospitals have video conferencing equipment and basic telemedicine ability in their patient's room, while the operating room looks more like the cockpit of the Airbus 380 than anything else. All of this is ergonomically and functionally friendly.

Summary

The modern hospital has become a place where patient-centered care and scientific and technological advances converge and work together for the betterment of humankind. The public, insurance companies, and multiple state and federal agencies look upon hospitals and expect them to provide the highest quality of care and best outcomes, and these outcomes are published both for individual practitioners and for institutions. On the surgery side, nationally, American College of Surgeons (ACS) and other groups have created a number of programs that measure quality (NSQIP, NTDB) and that have become models for the rest of the world.

Today's hospital has multiple challenges that are encountered while using exciting technology that has changed the quality of care and allowed clinicians to enhance their patient-centered practices. These challenges include rapidly changing technology, increasing bureaucratic logistics, and revisions in hospital design that enhance the quality of care, while incorporating more complexities. Because of these changes, the modern hospital and those who work in it are required to be informed, alert, up to date, and ready for change, incorporating new knowledge of disease and technology, all the while jumping over the multiple hurdles that have always been present and always keeping the patient foremost in mind. The human toll and the cost of working in the modern hospital are high, and we need to make sure we understand the intricacies of working in this new institution, known as *the modern hospital*, so we can ensure better care for our patients and ourselves.

References

1. Latifi R, Rhee P, Gruessner R, editors. Technological advances in surgery, trauma, and critical care, Springer. New York; 2015.
2. Anonymous. Methodological standards and patient-centeredness in comparative effectiveness research: the PCORI perspective. JAMA. 2012;307(15):1636–40.
3. Ellis LE, Kass NE. How are PCORI-funded researchers engaging patients in research and what are the ethical implications? AJOB Empir Bioeth. 2017;8(1):1–10.
4. Frank L, Basch E, Selby JV. The PCORI perspective on patient-centered outcomes research. JAMA. 2014;312(15):1513–4.
5. Selby JV. Patient-Centered Outcomes Research Institute seeks to find out what works best by involving 'end-users' from the beginning. J Comp Eff Res. 2014;3(2):125–9.
6. Selby JV, Forsythe L, Sox HC. Stakeholder-driven comparative effectiveness research: an update from PCORI. JAMA. 2015;314(21):2235–6.
7. Selby JV, Lipstein SH. PCORI at 3 years--progress, lessons, and plans. N Engl J Med. 2014;370(7):592–5.

8. Sheridan S, Schrandt S, Forsythe L, Hilliard TS, Paez KA. The PCORI engagement rubric: promising practices for partnering in research. Ann Fam Med. 2017;15(2):165–70.
9. Patient-Centered Outcomes Research Institute (PCORI). Getting to know PCORI. Arlington, VA. September 10–12, 2017.
10. Rickert J. Health Affairs Blog. Patient centered care: what it means and how to get there. Accessed from http://healthaffairs.org/blog/2012/01/24/patient-centered-care-what-it-means-and-how-to-get-there/. Accessed on 19 Nov 2014.
11. Sosin M, Patel KM, Nahabedian MY, Bhanot P. Patient-centered outcomes following laparoscopic ventral hernia repair: a systematic review of the current literature. Am J Surg. 2014;208:677–84.
12. Liang MK, Clapp M, Li LT, Berger RL, Hicks SC, Awad S. Patient satisfaction, chronic pain, and functional status following laparoscopic ventral hernia repair. World J Surg. 2013;37(3):530–7. https://doi.org/10.1007/s00268-012-1873-9.
13. White DB, Angus DC, Shields AM, et al. A randomized trial of a family-support intervention in intensive care. N Engl J Med. 2018;378:2365. https://doi.org/10.1056/NEJMoa1802637.
14. Brewster AL, Curry AL, Cherlin JE, et al. Integrating new practices: a qualitative study of how hospital innovations become routine. Implement Sci. 2015; 10:168.
15. Starzl TE, Groth CG, Brettschneider L, Penn I, Fulginiti VA, Moon JB, Blanchard H, Martin AJ Jr, Porter KA. Orthotopic homotransplantation of the human liver. Ann Surg. 1968;168(3):392–415.
16. Moore FD. Metabolic care of the surgical patient. Philadelphia and London: WB Saunders Co; 1959.
17. Dudrick SJ, Wilmore DW, Vars HM, Rhoads JE. Long-term total parenteral nutrition with growth, development, and positive nitrogen balance. Surgery. 1968;64:134.
18. Dudrick SJ. History of parenteral nutrition. J Am Coll Nutr. 2009;28(3):243–51.
19. Lerner BH. The breast cancer wars. Fear, hope, and pursuit of a cure in 20th century America. New York: Oxford University Press; 2001.
20. Saxon W. New York Times. Dr. George Crile Jr, 84, Foe of unneeded surgery dies. Found online at http://www.nytimes.com/1992/09/12/us/dr-george-crile-jr-84-foe-of-unneeded-surgery-dies.html. Accessed on 19 Nov 2014.
21. Reynolds W Jr. The first laparoscopic cholecystectomy. JSLS. 2001;5(1):89–94.
22. PubMed. https://www.ncbi.nlm.nih.gov/pubmed/. Accessed 25 May 2018.
23. Veith FJ, Marin ML, Cynamon J, Schonholz C, Parodi J. 1992: Parodi, Montefiore, and the first abdominal aortic aneurysm stent graft in the United States. Ann Vasc Surg. 2005;19(5):749–51.
24. Iribarne A, Milner R, Merlo AE, Singh A, Saunders CR, Russo MJ. Outcomes following emergent open repair for thoracic aortic dissection are improved at higher volume centers. J Card Surg. 2014. https://doi.org/10.1111/jocs.12470. [Epub ahead of print].
25. Cameron JL, Riall TS, Coleman J, Belcher KA. One thousand consecutive pancreaticoduodenectomies. Ann Surg. 2006;244(1):10–5.
26. Winter JM, Cameron JL, Campbell KA, Arnold MA, Chang DC, Coleman J, Hodgin MB, Sauter PK, Hruban RH, Riall TS, Schulick RD, Choti MA, Lillemoe KD, Yeo CJ. 1423 pancreaticoduodenectomies for pancreatic cancer: a single-institution experience. J Gastrointest Surg. 2006;10(9):1199–210; discussion 1210–1.
27. Freischlag JA, Kibbe MR. The evolution of surgery: the story of "two poems". JAMA. 2014;312(17):1737–8. https://doi.org/10.1001/jama.2014.14448.
28. Pruitt BA Jr. Combat casualty care and surgical progress. Ann Surg. 2006;243(6):715–29.
29. Blackbourne LH, Baer DG, Eastridge BJ, Kheirabadi B, Bagley S, Kragh JF Jr, Cap AP, Dubick MA, Morrison JJ, Midwinter MJ, Butler FK, Kotwal RS, Holcomb JB. Military medical revolution: prehospital combat casualty care. J Trauma Acute Care Surg. 2012;73(6 Suppl 5):S372–7. https://doi.org/10.1097/TA.0b013e3182755662.
30. Ingalls N, Zonies D, Bailey JA, Martin KD, Iddins BO, Carlton PK, Hanseman D, Branson R, Dorlac W, Johannigman J. A review of the first 10 years of critical care aeromedical transport during operation Iraqi freedom and operation enduring freedom: the importance of evacuation timing. JAMA Surg. 2014;149(8):807–13. https://doi.org/10.1001/jamasurg.2014.621.
31. Palm K, Apodaca A, Spencer D, Costanzo G, Bailey J, Blackbourne LH, Spott MA, Eastridge BJ. Evaluation of military trauma system practices related to damage-control resuscitation. J Trauma Acute Care Surg. 2012;73(6 Suppl 5):S459–64. https://doi.org/10.1097/TA.0b013e3182754887.

Modern Hospitals, Airports, Surgeons, and Pilots: What Do They Have in Common?

10

Rifat Latifi, Shekhar Gogna, and Elizabeth H. Tilley

Introduction

To explain the relationship and commonalities between the modern hospital and airport, we will analyze two most known representatives of hospitals (surgeons) and airports (i.e., airline industry) (pilots). We are fully aware that neither surgeons nor pilots are the most important people in hospitals or airline industry. Other physicians and nurses, as well as all levels of support staff, are critical to the function of the hospital; without them, there would be no hospital. The airline industry functions much the same. While without pilots, there will be no airline industry (although recent developments on drones may question this), without so many other professionals (air traffic controllers and others), there would not be an airport. Surgeons undergo extensive and prolonged training before they can work in a hospital and make decisions that affect the lives of patients. Similarly, pilots undergo intensive training as well in order to fly commercially, militarily, or privately. While pilot training is not as intense as a surgeon's training, the ultimate gravity of how their performance and decisions affect the lives of people is the same. Both of these highly sophisticated professions require extensive training, but this training cannot always predict who will commit errors and who will handle emergency situations effectively. Numerous factors play a part in how these situations are handled. In addition to their particular technical and professional preparedness, the most important factors of success include communication with other personnel, the technical skill and mental state of the pilot or surgeon, and environmental factors. For example, noise and a lack of cohesion among the team can affect the focus of the pilot or surgeon.

A critical predictor of effectiveness for both surgeons and pilots is extensive training, so that when an emergency occurs, he/she does not have to think about the basic procedures for their job. This allows the surgeon or pilot to focus solely on the current emergency and how to handle it. Both, however, rely extensively on team support.

Performing complex surgery or being a successful and safe clinician is much like flying a plane. Both take an enormous amount of training, which at times can be grueling. Surgery itself can be dangerous and time-pressured, and while much of it depends on surgical decision-making and the technical skills of the surgeon, other factors and nontechnical elements contribute to the success of an operation. Both of these high-pressure, high-demand professions share numerous

R. Latifi (✉)
New York Medical College, School of Medicine, Department of Surgery and Westchester Medical Center, Valhalla, NY, USA
e-mail: rifat_latifi@nymc.edu; rifat.latifi@wmchealth.org

S. Gogna · E. H. Tilley
Department of Surgery, Westchester Medical Center, Valhalla, NY, USA

R. Latifi (ed.), *The Modern Hospital*, https://doi.org/10.1007/978-3-030-01394-3_10

commonalities. First and foremost is the institution. These institutions, both hospital and airport, are not to be underestimated. Their functionality is critical to the success of the surgeon and the pilot. This chapter reviews commonalities and differences between the decision-making among pilots and surgeons as well as the institutions in which they operate, by incorporating the concepts of situational awareness, sensemaking, and concise communication, and how these phenomena can be applied to understanding the process of dynamic decision-making and efficient functioning which will lead to customer satisfaction in both realms. Ultimately, both institutions can learn from one another, but airport institutions have made great strides in providing communication that enhances efficient customer flow.

The Safety of Airline Industry

Flying a plane (or occasionally riding in a plane, for that matter) can be dangerous business but still much safer than everyday activities such as driving a car. In fact, it is one of the safest activities we do. There were approximately 9,709,000 scheduled passenger flights. Given the low number of fatal crashes that year (7), you would statistically have to fly 5,342,857 times for every accident. The average for 2010–2014 is lower but still better than any previous 5-year period, one fatal crash per 2,925,000 flights. That means a 0.72% risk. You have never been less likely to fly on a plane that will crash and experience fatalities [1]. Still the list of fatalities is extensive and often high-profile [1]. Recent fatalities include the AF Andrade Empreendimentos e Participações Cessna 560XLS+ Citation Excel in Guarujá, Brazil, where five passengers and a pilot were killed after crashing into a residential area on 13 August 2014. On 10 August 2014, Sepahan Airlines HESA IrAn 140, flight 217 near Nardaran, Azerbaijan, 5 crew members and 18 passengers were killed when the aircraft crashed shortly after takeoff. On 24 July 2014, Air Algerie MD83, EC-LTV, flight AH5017, near Gossi, Mali, crashed after the pilot contacted the control tower to request a different route due to weather conditions, killing 6 crew members and 119 passengers. Despite all of these, the airline industry is one of the safest industries today.

The Hospital

Throughout the recorded history of the institution of the hospital, there is a constant evolution of practices, technology, and systems, beginning with the first recorded hospital in the East Roman Empire in the fifth and sixth centuries AD to the modern twenty-first century technology-driven hospitals [2]. The dynamic institution known as the hospital is extremely complex and involves a large mix of interrelated services such as intensive care units, outpatient clinics, clinical laboratories, imaging, emergency rooms, operating rooms, and other procedure suites. While the previously listed units are service-related, there are also hospitality-based functions, such as front desk reception, technical and engineering services, food services and housekeeping, and the fundamental inpatient care or bed-related functions [3]. In other words, the hospital is much like a small city, where there is a continuous influx and outflux of short-term residents (patients). The hospital is a community of healthcare providers (doctors, nurses, healthcare allies, administrative personnel, security, engineers, media personnel, and many others). Quality of patient care has become a forefront of national media and educational discussion. This has intensified the call for more effective and efficient use of scarce resources through integrated service design model [4]. Integrated service design is a team-based, client focused approach to provide health and social services under one roof. Because the hospital is a complex system required to provide exceptional patient care, much can be learned from other industries [5]. Many airports serve millions of people every year. Each year the five busiest airports in the world serve between 75 million to 101 million. The Hartsfield–Jackson Atlanta International Airport serves 101.5 million per year; Beijing Capital International Airport, 90.1; Dubai International Airport, 83.6; O'Hare International Airport, 76.9 (2015); and

London Heathrow Airport, 75.7 [6]. These are highly complex and fast-paced environments that are able to manage multiple airlines, industries, and people.

Training and Complex Decision-Making

The safety of airlines is clearly multifactorial, but pilots play a major role, and becoming a pilot takes intensive training. For example, to get a private pilot's license, you must hold an aviation medical certificate, have a minimum of 40 flight training hours, and pass several written and oral exams. However, to become a commercial pilot, the rules differ based on the aircraft you will be flying. According to the Federal Aviation Administration (FAA), there are several certifications and exams that must be passed. A commercial pilot is responsible for the lives of many people, so intensive flight simulation scenarios are a major part of the training process.

Performing surgery is also a dangerous and extremely complex process. The training that goes into becoming a medical doctor is even more intensive than becoming a pilot. Medical doctors typically have between 11 and 16 years of training, including residency. The training is very complex and it is not an easy process. Such training is necessary in order for the medical doctor to become a surgeon, an expert who is ready to deal with the unexpected. Much like the scenario of a pilot who does not have to think about the basics when an emergency occurs, a surgeon and medical doctor cannot waste time on thinking through basics of operating during a procedure.

There is a difference between how surgical residents and pilots are selected. Potential aviators are currently selected using the Aviation Selection Test Battery (ASTB). The ASTB is a written test designed to evaluate math and verbal skills, mechanical comprehension, aviation and nautical information, and spatial apperception (https://militaryflighttests.com/astb-test). The ASTB has a strong predictive validity through primary flight training. While the ASTB evaluates many skills necessary to aviation, it is correlated with performance; it does not account for the natural genetic variation in physiological stress response. Once selected by the ASTB, all naval pilot trainees undergo water survival training in the Modular Egress Training Simulator (METS) device, which is a highly demanding and stressful test. In contrast, potential surgical residents are interviewed, have to demonstrate that they have done well in the past education, and show dedication, but there is no physical test. Actually, the senior author (RL) observed few years ago chief resident of surgery (last year of training) struggling while removing a gallbladder. When asked if he needs an optometrist for new glasses, he admitted that he had a depth perception problem that could not be fixed. He was a fine surgeon by all means; however, clearly this important element of surgical skills was missing. We should test our future surgeons just like we test pilots before they are selected for the residency and flying schools.

While there are a number of similarities among pilots and surgeons, still there are some other significant differences between surgeons and pilots with respect to public involvement. Every pilot error is recorded, scrutinized, analyzed, and made public; rarely are the errors of surgeons made public. There is no recording of the procedures, and thus it is impossible or very difficult to replay them and make them public. Furthermore, because of privacy issues, only a few major mistakes by surgeons ever make it to the news. Both pilots and surgeons have dangerous jobs; these types of careers take the lives of other people in their hands while engaging in tasks that are played out in dynamic, ever-changing contexts. Paying attention to all available cues is of the utmost importance. After all, people's lives depend on it!

Like pilots, surgeons work in dynamic environments while taking responsibility for the lives of individuals and managing to complete difficult tasks such as a pancreaticoduodenectomy, liver or lung resection, or takedown of complex multiple fistulas. While these and the countless other surgical procedures may seem very difficult for nonsurgeons or novice and inexperienced surgeons, the well-trained surgeon can complete these procedures safely, but when a crisis arrives, things change dramatically. Perhaps, surgeons have a bit "more time" to address crises, as the operating room is not flying at 1000 km/h. Still, the environments of surgeons and pilots are considered dynamic, meaning there is continual change occurring within the environment.

When broken down by steps, work within dynamic environments can be fit into three major categories. First, the pilot or surgeon must continually monitor and assess the situation. While this is the first step in the process, it is also continual. The pilot or surgeon has to assess the situation with each development in order to process how to respond and which step to take next. He or she must then make appropriate reactions based on assessment. Once appropriate action is taken, evaluation of results must be made. The cycle then repeats itself [7].

Both jobs are intensely stressful, not only because people's lives are dependent upon decisions that are made, but there is no "downtime" while performing these jobs. A surgeon can't go take a break during a long and intense surgery. A pilot can't stop flying a plane if he doesn't feel well. Additionally, a key aspect to functioning successfully in complex dynamic environments is the ability not only to observe and seek information but to understand what that information means in the larger context of a task goal [8]. Moreover, an ability to then anticipate events in that environment leads to better prediction and understanding of future events. The cognitive components of these processes are of interest to researchers and will briefly be discussed in this chapter. While these cognitive components are of interest, a major goal of this chapter is to establish what may be occurring when a surgeon or pilot seemingly makes a "gut-level" decision. There are a whole host of other factors that the operator is not aware of, such as the integration of the information they have learned through training and experience. This phenomenon can be called situational awareness, sensemaking, or unconscious processing of environmental cues. Regardless of the term used, the concept has been reviewed in a number of ways, particularly in the literature on the abilities of pilots [9–11].

Both pilots and surgeons, and often other clinicians, have to make serious decisions that are time dependent and may have serious consequences. While the pilot is supported by the most sophisticated technologies of the flying machine, the surgeon has to make decisions that are dependent on his or her experience, knowledge, and this seemingly surreal gut-level decision-making. Overall, these decisions are made in dynamic environments. Awareness of the individual state of the surgeon and pilot is crucial and accompanies the awareness of the operating environment, such as communication dynamics among the teams. Not being aware of certain subtleties in communication may be detrimental to both surgical and piloting outcomes. In situations that are fluid and dynamic, checklists, while possibly viewed as something to be used by novices only, have been shown to be helpful. Checklists can allow the surgeon or pilot to focus on the multiple acting parts of an operation and clear the mind of clutter [12–14].

Finally, there is much to learn regarding how and why individuals make decisions, particularly decisions that appear to be gut level or unconscious. The research in this field is valuable and informative for professions that make decisions in dynamic environments that will affect the lives of other individuals.

What Can Hospitals Learn from Airports?

The authors assume that every reader of this chapter has traveled through a busy airport, and moreover, every reader has worked, has been, or will go to the hospital. Having spent most of our adult lives at various hospitals and airports around the world, we thought that the future hospitals should, in fact, mimic the efficiency of the airport. It took the senior author of this chapter less than 12 min to get a boarding pass, check his luggage, go through the security line, put his boots back on, and collect the computer bag on the other line before he was ready to get a cup of coffee at one of the busiest airports.

Could the modern hospitals learn from airports in meeting the needs of patients? We believe the efficiency of airports and airline industry can be delivered at a hospital just as it is at an airport. What will make this compatibility even better would be high technological advancements that are used by both institutions. Of course, it is clear that while hospitals have made great strides, the airline industry has made greater advances in communication.

The American Hospital Association conducts an annual survey of hospitals in the United States. According to the report published in 2018, the total number of registered hospitals in the United States is 5,534 of which 4,840 are community hospitals and 209 are federal government hospitals. The total number of nonfederal psychiatric hospitals is 397. Community hospitals mentioned in the report include academic medical centers or other teaching hospitals if they are nonfederal short-term hospitals [15]. On the other hand, there are about 5,136 public airports and 14,112 private airports is in the United States [16]. Hospitals are divided into academic and nonacademic types. For purposes of trauma classification, hospitals can also be classified as level I, II, and III based on their acuity level to manage and handle emergencies. Similarly, airports are divided into large, medium, and small hub airports or non-hub types depending on number of passengers traveling through them and the level of commercial activity. While there are several things that we have pointed out that hospitals can learn from airports, these two entities do have more things in common than expected. Table 10.1 summarizes how airport compares with hospitals.

Importance of Functional Designs at Hospitals

Recent attention in healthcare has been focused on patient safety as an outcome of better architectural design of a hospital facility, including its technology, equipment, and efficient staff. Research psychologists have proved beyond doubt that physical environment bears a significant impact on safety

Table 10.1 Comparison of hospitals and airports

	Hospitals	Airports
Pre-visit formalities	Patients make prior appointment for office visits by telephone. Dial 911 in case of emergencies	Passengers book online tickets and online check-in and get boarding pass, more emergently rush to the airport, and buy ticket at the counter
Entry	Front desk for patients and their relatives, which guide them to front desk where all necessary paperwork regarding identity, appointment details, and type of service, i.e., inpatient versus outpatient status and valid insurance papers, are reviewed	Airport reservation desk provides various services like check-in, review of valid passport and visa, and baggage drop and then proceeds security checks, frisking zones after passing through immigration
Waiting time	Patients and their relatives can rest quietly in waiting area, read magazine, watch TV, and talk to the fellow patients	Passengers can go shopping, dine multi-optional cuisine, can use luxurious facilities like spa, or can hang out in lounge
Service delivery	Service is provided. Hopefully there will be no complications	Service is provided. Hopefully you will arrive at the destination without any major issues
Post visit experience	Hospital may send you a long survey to complete… You may need post op visit. Hopefully you will see the same surgeon or surgeon who looked after you. You will never see the nurses or others who looked after you while in the hospital	You fill a survey, mostly sent to you by agency that booked your ticket. You will most likely never see the same airport or airline personnel ever again
Safety	100–300 thousand patients die each year in the United States alone from medical errors	No data on people dying at airport; however, average of seven fatal flights per year for last few years

and human performance [16]. "Latent conditions" are organizational/system factors that can potentially create the conditions conducive for errors. Latent conditions behave like "resident pathogens" that are usually dormant within a system and become apparent only when a disaster strikes. These conditions are not usually visible to the naked eye; however, close scrutiny often identifies them before adverse effect strikes [17]. Clinicians and healthcare policy makers can improve patient and staff outcomes by targeting latent conditions by using evidence-based designs to make a patient's hospital visit efficient and more meaningful than imagined. The Institute of Medicine published a report, Crossing the Quality Chasm: A New Health System for the 21st Century which described six key elements critical for ensuring patient safety and quality care [18]. Table 10.2 lists these points which are important in conceptualizing the functionality-based designs.

Effective functional design of the hospital in simpler terms is an affordable, approachable, and efficient healthcare system which provides patients and the accompanying visitors with a stress-free environment and gives them a sense of satisfaction. High-quality hospitals have better performance measures in terms of providing patient care and generating revenues at the same time. The importance of patient experience as a key quality metric has been underscored by the inclusion of the Hospital Consumer Assessment of Healthcare Providers and Systems (HCAHPS) scores into the Centers for Medicare and Medicaid Services (CMS) Value-Based Purchasing Program (VBP). In 2013, the VBP program put at risk 1% of total [19].

Medicare payments will rise to 2% by 2017; thus, poor performance on patient satisfaction metrics may represent a substantial financial risk for hospitals [18]. The Quality Payment Program (QPP) was implemented in 2015 and rewards providers who provide quality care and high value. The program is able to reduce costs because providers who do not meet the performance standards receive reduced Medicare payments [20]. Patient satisfaction is a proxy but a very effective indicator to measure the success of doctors and hospitals [21]. There is cumulating evidence that better patient experience is associated with improved adherence to medications and treatments, improved clinical and other health outcomes, and greater safety and reduced adverse events [22, 23].

Table 10.2 Six key elements critical for ensuring patient safety and quality care

Patient centered	Safety centered	Effectiveness	Efficiency	Timeliness	Equity
Using variable acuity rooms and single bedrooms	Improving the availability of assistive devices to avert patient falls	Use of lighting to enable visual performance	Standardizing room layout, location of supplies, and medical equipment	Ensure rapid response to patient needs	Ensuring the size of structure
Posting clearly marked signs to navigate the hospital	Better interdependencies of care, at work spaces and work processes	Controlling the effects of noise	Minimize potential safety threats	Eliminate inefficiencies in the processes of care delivery	Layout of the structure
Better access to healthcare information	Ventilation and filtration systems to control and prevent the spread of infections	Use of natural lighting	Improving patient satisfaction by minimizing patient transfers with variable-acuity rooms	Facilitate the clinical work of nurses	Functions of the structure
Ensuring sufficient space to accommodate family members	Facilitating handwashing with the availability of sinks and alcohol hand rubs				
	Using surfaces that can be easily decontaminated				

When Things Do Not Go the Way We Want, What Can We Learn from Airline Industry Root Cause Analysis?

In medicine and surgery as well as other fields, when things do not go well, we have a number of ways that we analyze and try to improve the system. There are however, a wide range of discrepancies as to how things are handled when things do not go the way we want, and the main factors include the type of the hospital, private, community, academic, government, etc. Most academic hospitals, however, have a morbidity and mortality (M&M) conference, and some call it improvement conference for each of the clinical disciplines that are part of the quality department. The M&M usually occurs on a daily basis and allows for all levels of attending to review cases. For example, if a patient has an anastomotic leak, although a very known complication after colonic resection, there will be an open departmental presentation, usually by the most senior residents or the residents that assisted in the surgery. During this presentation, the patient data and hospital course are reviewed. Most pertinent literature is also reviewed, and then the conclusion may be one of the several options: (1) patient disease and standard of care were met; (2) there was a technical error or error in judgment; and (3) there was a communication error or in case of trauma can be individual provider or system error with or without opportunity for improvement. In more severe cases, errors or deviation from the standard of care, than the surgeon or other individual surgeon or nurse, can be reeducated, can be re-trained, or can simply be dismissed. Every significant complication is reviewed in a well-established peer-review process, which ultimately provides recommendation for the final action to the departmental leadership. This process reviews the outcomes (no adverse outcome, minor adverse outcome, major adverse outcome of death) and establishes the degree that the patient's care was affected (care not affected; added additional treatment/interventions; increased monitoring/observation; or life sustaining treatment/intervention) as the result of the intervention. Medical records are reviewed and the reviewers established if there was an issue with the documentation (no issue with documentation; documentation does not substantiate clinical course of treatment; documentation is missing or not present; or documentation is illegible). At this point, the reviewer needs to assess issues or no issues. If issues are related to the surgeon, he/she can say that there are issues with diagnosis, judgment, and technique/skill; communication or implementation of the treatment plan; policy/compliance; supervision of allied health professionals; or supervision of house staff. The final action proposed to the leadership of the department is based on any of these: no action warranted or variance from standard of care but care appropriate or care inappropriate. Ultimately, there is a clear and delineated process to be followed when reviewing difficult cases where something may have gone wrong.

What the leadership of the department decides to do with the information is based on these findings and can be anything from surgeon self-acknowledged plan sufficient; educational letter sent to surgeon sufficient; and initiation of informal improvement plan with surgeon or develop a formal improvement plan with the surgeon. In most outrageous and disastrous complications, the privileges of the surgeon may be terminated immediately and reviewed by peers and the hospital or, for the worst cases, reported to state and national agencies where the surgeon or the physician can potentially lose the license to practice medicine or surgery. In either surgery or aviation a thorough examination of complication needs to be reviewed. Below, you can find a recent route-cause analysis of a plane crash as recorded at on the public website [24].

Uncontained Engine Failure and Subsequent Fire American Airlines Flight 383 Boeing 767-323, N345AN

Executive Summary

On October 28, 2016, about 1432 central daylight time, American Airlines flight 383, a Boeing 767-323, N345AN, had started its takeoff ground roll at the Chicago O'Hare International Airport, Chicago, Illinois, when an uncontained engine failure in the right engine and subsequent fire occurred. The flight crew aborted the takeoff and stopped the airplane on the runway, and the flight attendants initiated an emergency evacuation. Of the 2 flight crewmembers, 7 flight attendants, and 161 passengers on board, 1 passenger received a serious injury and 1 flight attendant and 19 passengers received minor injuries during the evacuation. The airplane was substantially damaged from the fire. The airplane was operating under the provisions of 14 Code of Federal Regulations Part 121. Visual meteorological conditions prevailed at the time of the accident.

Probable Cause

The National Transportation Safety Board determines that the probable cause of this accident was the failure of the high-pressure turbine (HPT) stage 2 disk, which severed the main engine fuel feed line and breached the right main wing fuel tank, releasing fuel that resulted in a fire on the right side of the airplane during the takeoff roll. The HPT stage 2 disk failed because of low-cycle fatigue cracks that initiated from an internal subsurface manufacturing anomaly that was most likely not detectable during production inspections and subsequent in-service inspections using the procedures in place. Contributing to the serious passenger injury was (1) the delay in shutting down the left engine and (2) a flight attendant's deviation from company procedures, which resulted in passengers evacuating from the left over wing exit while the left engine was still operating. Contributing to the delay in shutting down the left engine was (1) the lack of a separate checklist procedure for Boeing 767 airplanes that specifically addressed engine fires on the ground and (2) the lack of communication between the flight and cabin crews after the airplane came to a stop.

This is a report of an accident and provides a detailed description of what went wrong and how it could have been avoided. At the same time, concrete measures were taken to avoid similar events. The M&M conference is the comparison activity to the root cause analysis done by the FAA when there was a technical issue that caused a flight crew to abort a takeoff. However, unless there is major catastrophe from medication use or similar event, the improvement processes from one hospital do not become "law of the land" as they do for the FFA.

Leadership of Pilots and Surgeons

There are few people who do not know the story of flight 1549. At 3:25 p.m. on 15 January 2009, US Airways Flight 1549 took off on what was supposed to be a routine flight from New York's LaGuardia Airport en route to Charlotte, North Carolina, with 5 crew members and 150 passengers on board. One hundred seconds later, the aircraft, commanded by Captain Chesley "Sully" Sullenberger, crossed paths with a flock of migrating Canada geese. The aircraft collided with several of the large birds, which pelted both engines. As the giant turbines, spinning at over 10,000 revolutions per minute, began to disintegrate, the engines were irreparably damaged and shut down. In the next 3 min and 28 s, Sullenberger and his copilot Skiles had to act quickly to save every soul on that flight. They landed the jetliner in the middle of a frozen river, and then they and the crew proceeded to get every person safely out of the aircraft and onto rafts or the wings of the crippled plane. From there, NY Waterway ferries, coast guard, and New York fire and police department vessels, well-trained in emergency rescues, along with passing sightseeing cruise boats, quickly retrieved them all. Later, the reality of what happened on that cold January day began to emerge, and it had nothing to do with miracles or solo heroic action. The successful landing, evacuation, and rescue of Flight 1549 was the direct result of a concerted effort to make flying safer by refining communication and teamwork, as well as workload and threat and error management—a program commonly known in the aviation industry as crew resource management (CRM) [25]. This incident and overall evaluation of functionality of airports provides invaluable ideas that can be implemented for facilitating effective and valuable patient care at hospitals.

Good leadership is a central aspect of quality and safety in healthcare organizations. As a leader, the surgeon sets the direction for the team, teaches, and ensures the safety and desired outcomes of patients. A good leader communicates openly in timely manner; these attributes are common in good pilots and better surgeons. Leaders should be accessible and approachable and ensure that team members are not isolated. Maintaining "cordial" and healthy relations with administrative and nonclinical staff is very important for the surgical/medical departments as it ensues the ease of workflow within the unit. Importantly, leadership skills can be taught and learned. The myth that leaders are born and not made is not really true; it is the hard work and honesty that matters!

Summary

Hospitals of the future will become an integral part of the continuum of care aimed at restoring health for the patients they serve with the goal to provide an environment promoting the well-being of patients, surgeons, nurses, and support staff. An "airport"-like model of healthcare will be the next-generation hospital model. Airports teach us to set up contingency plans, safety checks, and effective backup to ensure patient safety and avoid future mistakes. The focus on efficiently communicating to airport visitors and streamlining their pass through the airport, with kiosk setups at appropriate places, eases the stress of navigating through airports, and it saves lot of time and energy. This model can be used to inform hospital design. Better communication with the patients beginning prior to coming to the hospital regarding their time and place of appointment and timely information about changes, if any, in the plans definitely goes a long way in establishing a good rapport with the patient and community. Improved communication and integration among various services and departments ensures that the demands and needs of patients are met in a timely manner, under one roof. Most importantly, courteous hospitality with effective healthcare and satisfied patients and their relatives is the ultimate goal of any hospitals, healthcare providers, and policy makers. While surgeons and pilots undergo very similar rigorous training and have to constantly engage situational awareness, the hospital systems have much to learn from the communications used to facilitate efficient airport visitor flow through at airports.

References

1. Federal Aviation Administration. Aviation data and statistics. Found at https://www.faa.gov/data_research/aviation_data_statistics/. Retrieved on June 8 2018.
2. Miller TS. The birth of the hospital in the Byzantine Empire. Baltimore: Johns Hopkins University Press; 1997.
3. Readying for takeoff: An 'airport model' would help a hospital struggling to secure a future to fly. Mod Healthc. 1999: 40. Health Reference Center Academic.
4. Fleury MJ. Integrated service networks: the Quebec case. Health Serv Manag Res. 2006;19:153–65.
5. Shaw J, Calder K. Aviation is not the only industry: healthcare could look wider for lessons on patient safety. Qual Saf Health Care. 2008;17:314.
6. Gifford E, Galante J, Kaji AH, et al. Factors associated with general surgery residents' desire to leave residency programs: a multi-institutional study. JAMA Surg. 2014;149(9):948–53. https://doi.org/10.1001/jamasurg.2014.935.
7. Endsley MR. A survey of situation awareness requirements in air-to-air combat fighters. Int J Aviat Psychol. 1993;3:157–68.
8. Endsley MR. Measurement of situation awareness in dynamic systems. Hum Factors. 1995;37:65–84.
9. Endsley MR. The application of human factors to the development of expert systems for advanced cockpits. In: Proceedings of the 7th International Symposium on Aviation Psychology. Columbus: Ohio State University; 1987. p. 167–171.
10. Durso FT, Sethumadhavan A. Situation awareness: understanding dynamic environments. Hum Factors: J Hum Factors Ergon Soc. 2008;50:442–50. https://doi.org/10.1518/001872008X288448.
11. Mehtsun WT, et al. Surgical never events in the United States. Surgery. 2013;153(4):465–72.
12. Smith D. Introduction to aeronautical decision making. 2002. Retrieved 08 October 2009 from the World Wide Web: ADM.
13. Aircare. An aviators guide to good decision making. Welligton: Aircare; 2006.
14. Gawande A. The checklist manifesto: how to get things right. New York: Metropolitan Books, Henry Holt and Company, LLC; 2009.
15. American Hospital Association. Fast facts on US hospitals. 2018. Retreived from http://www.aha.org/products-services/aha-hospital-statistics.html
16. Leape LL. Error in medicine. JAMA. 1994;272:1851–7.
17. Reason J. Making the risks of organizational accidents. Aldershot: Ashgate Publishing; 1997.
18. Institute of Medicine. Crossing the quality chasm: a new health system for the 21st century. Washington, DC: National Academy Press; 2001.
19. CMS issues final rule for first year of hospital value-based purchasing program. 2011. Available at: http://www.cms.gov/apps/media/press/factsheet.asp?Counter=3947
20. Quality Payment Program. Found at https://qpp.cms.gov/about/qpp-overview. Retrieved on 8 June 2018.
21. Prakash B. Patient satisfaction. J Cutan Aesthet Surg. 2010;3(3):151–5.
22. Doyle C, Lennox L, Bell D. A systematic review of evidence on the links between patient experience and clinical safety and effectiveness. BMJ Open. 2013;3(1):e001570.
23. Price RA, Elliott MN, Zaslavsky AM, Hays RD, Lehrman WG, Rybowski L, et al. Examining the role of patient experience surveys in measuring health care quality. Med Care Res Rev. 2014;71(5):522–54.
24. National Transportation Safety Board. Found at https://www.ntsb.gov/investigations/AccidentReports/Pages/AAR1801.aspx. Accessed 1 June 2018.
25. Sullenberger C, Chesley B. 'Sully' Sullenberger: making safety a core business function. Healthc Financ Manage. 2013;67:50–4.

Disease-Oriented Regionalization Approach: Quality of Care and Volume Above All

11

Nabil Wasif

Introduction

Modern healthcare has evolved into a multifaceted enterprise that requires coordination and efficient allocation of resources to function efficiently. This is particularly true for delivery of complex, tertiary level healthcare. In particular, ideal delivery of healthcare should be of consistently high quality and delivered with minimal variation. In reality this is a standard that is rarely achieved even in highly evolved systems. Often the quality of care delivered is highly variable for different patients presenting with the same disease process, which in turn leads to variation in outcomes following treatment.

Why does this variation exist? A combination of patient, provider, and system factors leads to this phenomenon. For one, patients have variable disease courses and inherent differences in comorbidity that may correlate to differential responses to treatment. Second, providers may have different approaches to treatment when dealing with a patient presenting with a similar problem. Finally, the system itself may channel patients to a provider who may not be best equipped to deal with that particular problem. As an example let us consider two patients with rectal cancer. Patient A is a relatively healthy 65-year-old male with stage III rectal cancer, whereas patient B has the same problem but in addition is uninsured and has diabetes with early-stage kidney disease. Patient A is seen at a tertiary care facility and undergoes preoperative chemoradiation followed by surgical removal of his rectum with negative margins. His final pathology shows the tumor has been downstaged and he has an uncomplicated recovery and survives long term without any recurrence of his cancer. Patient B however is seen at his local hospital and taken straight to surgery by the surgeon on call. The patient's rectum is removed and he is given a colostomy. However he has positive margins and also goes into renal failure after the surgery. His recovery is complicated and 6 months later his cancer recurs in the pelvis. Could this have been prevented if patient B had been treated the same way as Patient A?

The implementation of a national policy of regionalization has been proposed to help prevent precisely this kind of variation in patient outcomes following complex surgery. The empirical basis for this policy is the volume-outcome relationship. In this chapter I discuss some of the evidence behind the volume-outcome relationship, define the phenomenon of regionalization, and then discuss the pros and cons of enacting such a policy nationally.

N. Wasif (✉)
Department of Surgery, Mayo Clinic Arizona, Phoenix, AZ, USA
e-mail: wasif.nabil@mayo.edu

R. Latifi (ed.), *The Modern Hospital*, https://doi.org/10.1007/978-3-030-01394-3_11

Volume-Outcome Association

The volume-outcome relationship was first described by Luft et al. in 1979 [1]. They showed that mortality following open-heart surgery, vascular surgery, transurethral resection of the prostate, and coronary bypass was 25–41% lower in hospitals that had a higher annual volume of these procedures. Birkmeyer et al. built on this work to establish a clear correlation between operative mortality (outcome) and the number of cases of a particular surgery performed (volume) for 14 types of procedures related to cardiovascular diseases and cancer [2]. Absolute differences in adjusted mortality rates between very low-volume and very high-volume hospitals ranged from 0.2 to 12%. While noting these differences in complex surgery, both studies also noted that for simpler surgeries such as cholecystectomy variation in outcomes was not seen. Hence, the volume-outcome relationship was seen only for complex surgery with relatively high postoperative mortality and not for low-mortality operations. Although the magnitude of the association may vary, the overall trend is a clear correlation between lower mortality as the number of cases goes up. Or put otherwise, "practice makes perfect."

A multitude of studies were published over the next decade, mostly utilizing large administrative databases or cancer registries, examining this volume-outcome association across a variety of surgical procedures. In a systematic review of 135 studies looking at this topic, 70% found a statistically significant association between higher volume and lower postoperative mortality [3]. Furthermore, it has been estimated that hundreds of patient deaths could be avoided in the United States if elective high-risk surgeries were preferentially shifted away from low-volume to high-volume hospitals [4].

Regionalization

This shift of complex surgery from low-volume to high-volume hospitals has been dubbed regionalization or centralization. As the preponderance of evidence pointed toward the existence of a clear volume-outcome relationship, regionalization in the absence of any concerted policy was demonstrated by several authors. For example, Finks et al. demonstrated an increase in the median hospital volume of four cancer resections (lung, esophagus, pancreas, and bladder) as well as repair of abdominal aortic aneurysm from 1999 to 2008 [5]. At the patient level, the likelihood of surgery at a low-volume center decreased for esophageal, pancreatic, and colorectal resections from 1999 to 2007, with a corresponding increase in the proportion of patients undergoing surgery at a high-volume center [6]. Taken together, studies such as these suggested that a preferential shift to high-volume hospitals was seen in the first decade after dissemination of the volume-outcome studies (Fig. 11.1) [6]. Whether this was due to patient choice or awareness, change in referral practices or more restrictive insurance networks remains unclear, and it is likely that all of these factors played a part.

Mortality

As regionalization was being demonstrated across the United States, a simultaneous improvement in postoperative mortality following complex surgery was also seen. For example, risk-adjusted mortality following surgery decreased by 11–19% for major cancer operations and by 8–36% for cardiovascular operations [5]. As more reports accumulated, surgical thought leaders at three major hospital systems, Dartmouth-Hitchcock Medical Center, the Johns Hopkins Hospital, and the University of Michigan Health System, publically announced a "Take the Volume Pledge" campaign. The goal was to encourage hospitals and individual surgeons to voluntarily restrict performance of 10 high-risk surgical procedures if they did not meet certain minimum thresholds of annual number of cases. The debate following release of this pledge reflects both the pros and cons of regionalization.

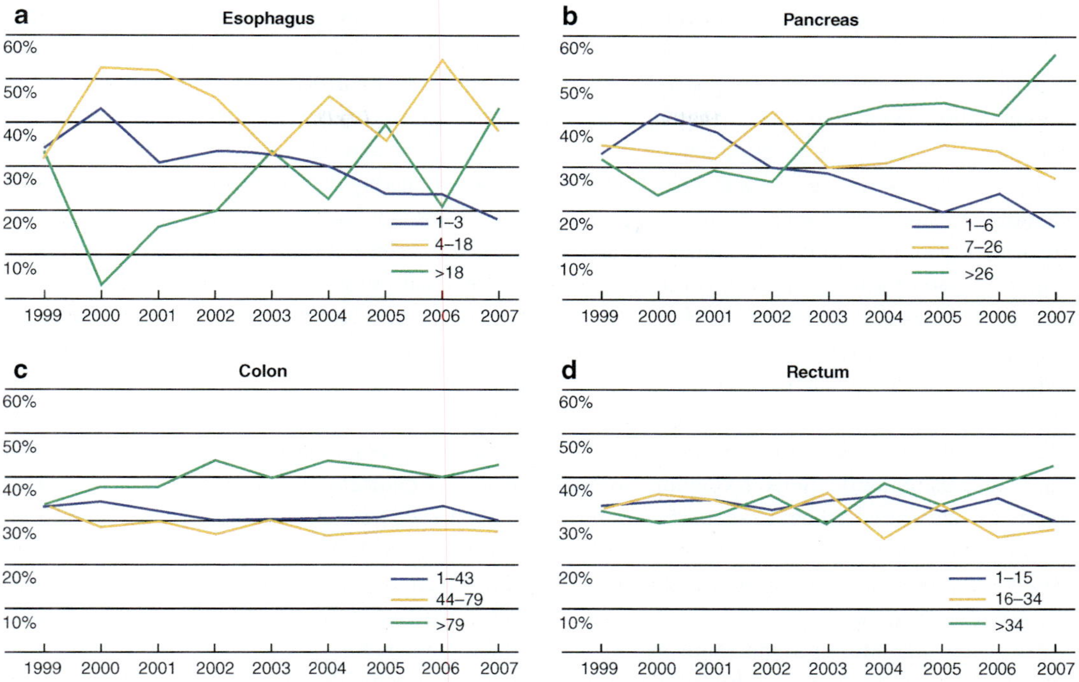

Fig. 11.1 Proportion of patients undergoing surgery from 1999 to 2007 stratified by annual volume of cases at the treating hospital. (**a**) Esophagus. (**b**) Pancreas. (**c**) Colon. (**d**) Rectum. (Reprinted from Stitzenberg and Meropol [6]. With permission from Springer Nature)

The Argument for Regionalization

The most compelling argument for regionalization remains the reduction in postoperative mortality for complex surgical resections when performed at a hospital that does a high number of such operations. As mentioned earlier, this has the potential to prevent a proportion of postoperative deaths that may result from these surgeries being performed at low-volume hospitals. Putting aside the binary variable of postoperative mortality, other differences are also seen in the care of these patients at high- and low-volume centers. For one, a reduction in the length of stay following surgery at a high-volume hospital compared to a low-volume hospital is often seen. Finley et al. demonstrated a 19% reduction in length of stay following pulmonary resection in Canada, and Gordon et al. had similar findings for patients undergoing complex gastrointestinal surgery in the United States at a high-volume hospital [7, 8].

For cancer surgeries in particular, highest-volume hospitals are associated with improved long-term survival in addition to better postoperative mortality [9]. There is some evidence to suggest that this improvement in long-term survival may in part be attributed to the fact that high-volume centers are often better at delivering guideline-compliant, standardized treatment and also at achieving oncologically important outcomes, such as a negative margin and adequate lymph node retrieval [10]. There may also be a “halo” effect in play at high-volume hospitals. Urbach et al. showed that hospitals that performed a high volume of lung resections were associated with a lower mortality for pancreatic resections as well [11]. This association was stronger than the direct correlation of mortality from pancreatic resections and hospital volume for the same. This suggests that the ability of a hospital to successfully perform complex surgery of one kind leads to advantages that translate into improvements in general postoperative care.

Some of the structural and process factors present at high-volume hospitals that are associated with improved postoperative outcomes have been identified. Improved patient selection, for example, by the more frequent use of cardiac stress tests prior to surgery, and higher frequency of invasive monitoring in the perioperative period have both shown to be higher at high-volume hospitals [12]. A higher proportion of skilled nonsurgical expertise, such as critical care intensivists and advanced endoscopy and interventional radiologists, can often "rescue" patients when serious complications following surgery occur. In fact this "failure to rescue" has been shown to be a prime determinant in the postoperative difference in mortality between high- and low-volume hospitals [13]. Finally, surgeons with subspecialty training and more experience are more likely to be present at high-volume hospitals. A meta-analysis of more than 54,000 articles found that higher surgeon volume and evidence of specialization were associated with improved outcomes across a multitude of procedures [14].

Disadvantages of Regionalization

Despite the evidence presented so far on the volume-outcome relationship and the potential benefits likely to accrue secondary to regionalization, the majority of complex cancer surgery in the United States is still performed outside of high-volume centers. Why this discrepancy? In the following paragraphs, I examine the flip side of the coin for regionalization.

In a classic paper, Finlayson et al. conducted a discrete choice experiment on patients with pancreatic cancer [15]. They were given the choice of having an operation locally or travelling to a regional facility. To help inform this choice, they were also given the respective mortality rates following surgery for each facility. Compared to a mortality rate of 6% for the local facility, when the patients were informed that the regional facility had a mortality rate of 3% for the same operation, 45 out of 100 patients still preferred surgery locally. Even when the local risk went up to 12%, 23 out of 100 patients preferred surgery locally. This suggests that a significant proportion of patients factor in other variables besides mortality when making decisions about undergoing surgery. These include family support, convenience, and familiarity with local healthcare networks.

Regionalization of complex surgery to high-volume centers has also been shown to impose a greater travel burden on patients. On average, the median distance travelled for surgery to a high-volume center compared to a low-volume center is higher for patients undergoing colon, esophageal, liver, and pancreas surgery (Fig. 11.2) [16]. This travel burden has not diminished over time and with further regionalization is also likely to increase and play a factor in patient decision-making process. When patients travel far for surgery, the likelihood of fragmentation of care also arises. If a patient who underwent complex surgery at an index hospital is readmitted in the postoperative period to a "non-index" hospital, a higher risk of morbidity and mortality is seen compared to patients who were readmitted back to the index hospital [17].

A further concern that has been raised is the issue of disparities in access to high-volume centers. Although regionalization improves postoperative mortality, these gains are not shared equally among patient subsets. In particular, African-American and socioeconomically disadvantaged patients are less likely to undergo surgery at high-volume hospitals [18]. Other than travel distance, problems with lack of insurance or underinsurance, rurality, and restrictive insurance networks may play a role in this discrepancy. Without addressing these issues, including universal access to healthcare, continued regionalization is likely to exacerbate existing disparities. Finally, this may also increase the average wait time for surgery for many patients with a corresponding delay in treatment that may be unacceptable for many patients, especially those with aggressive cancers [19].

Moving on from the perspective of the patient to that of the hospital system itself, there is a finite capacity to shift the burden of complex surgery from all low-volume hospitals to high-

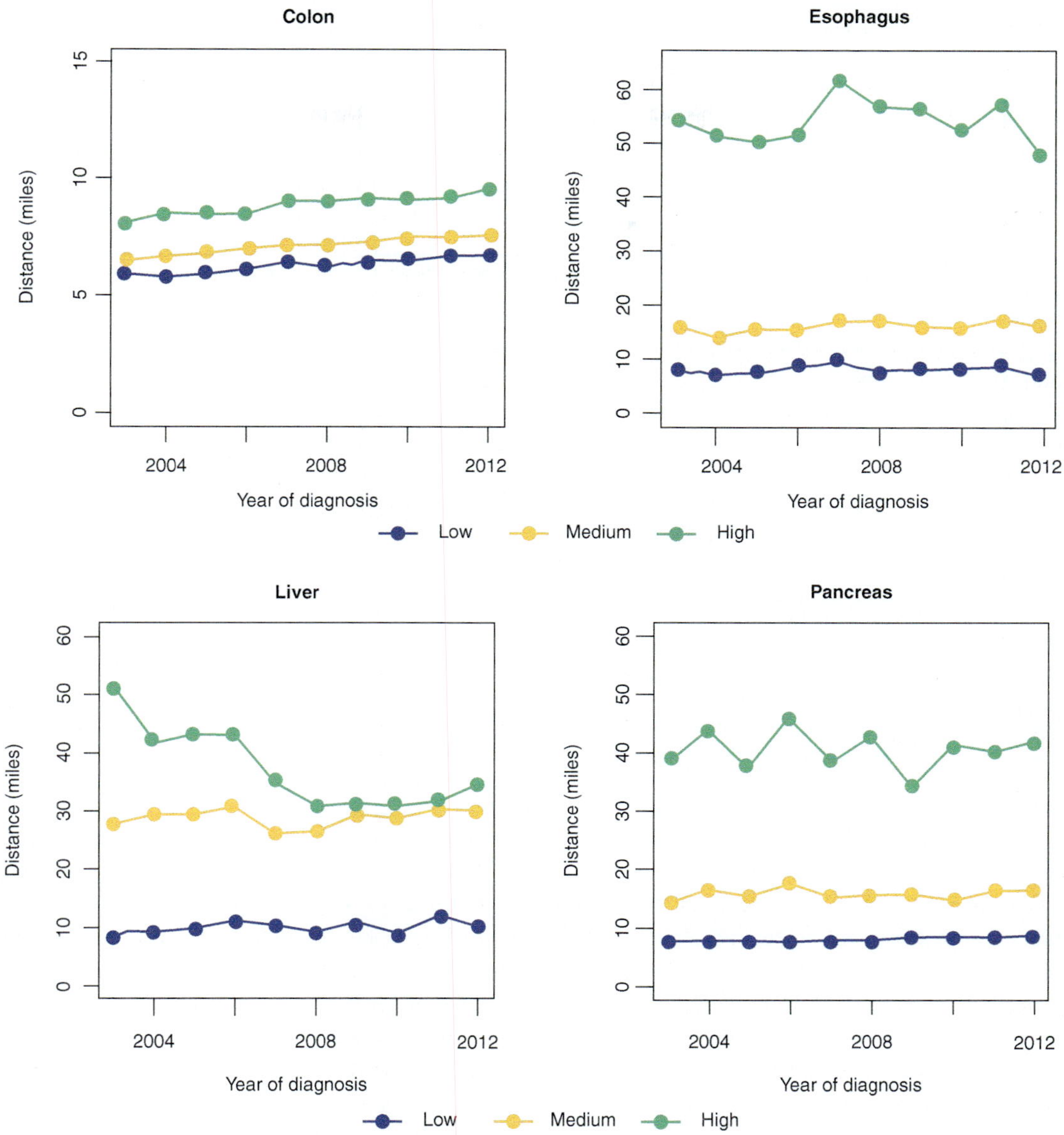

Fig. 11.2 Median distance travelled in miles by patients for surgery at low-, medium-, and high-volume hospitals. (Reprinted from Wasif et al. [16]. With permission from Springer Nature)

volume ones. Our group has demonstrated that the majority of complex surgery performed in the United States currently still occurs in low-volume hospitals [16]. A purely volume-based referral system would quickly inundate high-volume hospitals and make for an unsustainable system. For these hospitals, any such policy measure would necessitate an immediate need for expansion of resources such as hospital beds and nursing staff to accommodate these patients.

The very definition of a high-volume hospital itself has also been brought into question. Traditional analytic methods to divide hospitals into low, medium, and high volume have been criticized, especially the use of somewhat arbitrary cutoffs to designate a hospital as high volume. Such categorization tends to exaggerate the differences between volume groups as compared to when volume is treated as a continuous variable [20]. Even if volume is associated with improved

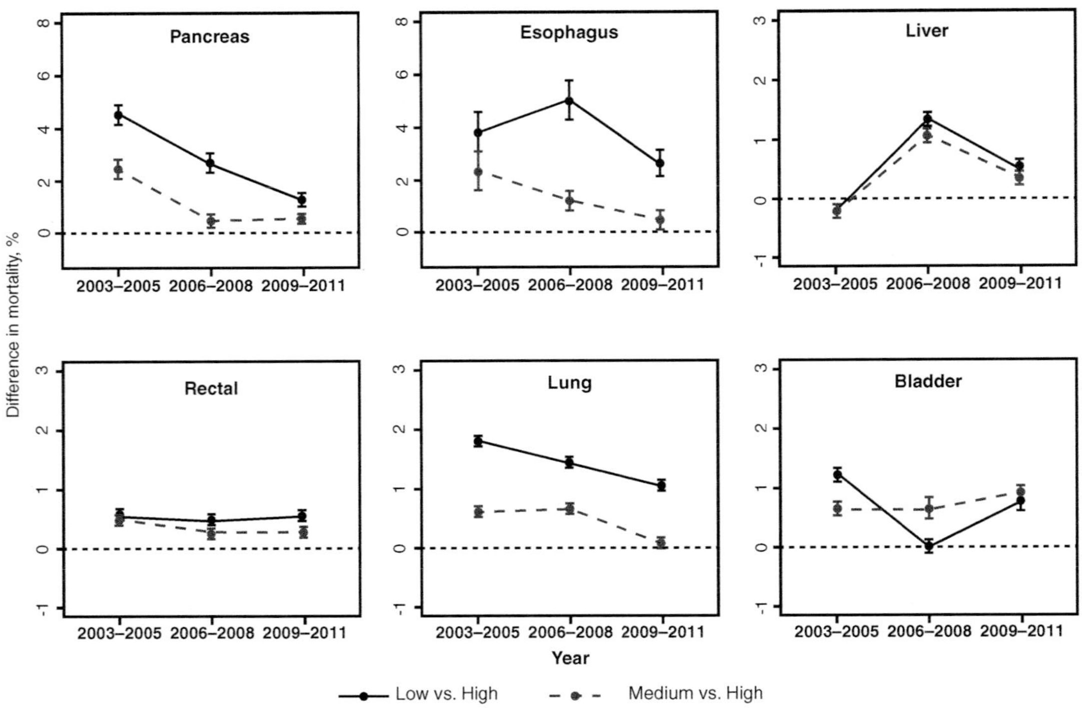

Fig. 11.3 Adjusted mean difference in mortality between low-, medium-, and high-volume hospitals over time. (Reprinted from Wasif et al. [22]. with permission from Elsevier)

outcomes, it may only account for a proportion of the variation seen in outcomes between hospitals. For example, Thabut et al. showed that annual procedure volume was associated with only 15% of the variation in mortality seen among US lung transplant centers [21]. Any volume threshold would also have to be procedure specific as the number of cases needed to achieve optimal outcomes increases as the complexity of the surgery increases. In fact, for relatively common surgeries such as colon resection or gallbladder removal, most studies do not show a volume-outcome association with mortality.

Another consideration is the mortality associated with the complex surgery itself. Work by our group has shown that postoperative mortality has decreased over the last decade. This is true for all hospitals irrespective of low-, medium-, or high-volume status and can be attributed to improvements in overall perioperative care. Consequently, this has led to the "attenuation" of the volume-outcome relationship that was initially described at the turn of the century. Furthermore, this improvement is seen to a greater extent in low- and medium-volume hospitals compared to high-volume hospitals so that outcomes between medium- and high-volume hospitals are now generally comparable (Fig. 11.3) [16, 22]. This time period coincides with the dawn of the "surgical quality movement." Following publication of the Institute of Medicine *To Err is Human: Building a Safer Health System* in 1999, hospital systems recognized the need to reduce medical errors and focus on quality improvement measures [23]. In the surgical world, this led to the implementation of several quality initiatives such as the National Surgical Quality Improvement Program (NSQIP), public reporting of operative outcomes, and surgical checklists, all of which have been shown to be associated with improved postoperative outcomes.

Future Directions

So where do we go from here? I believe the best strategy may be one of "regionalization-lite" where both medium- and high-volume centers are the ones designated for performing complex surgery. For the reasons delineated above, a complete transfer of all patients to high-volume hospitals is not feasible; however the very low-volume "hobbyist" centers and possibly surgeons should be discouraged from performing these operations. The likelihood of implementation and acceptance of regionalization is higher if expansion of access for patients and payers to both medium- and high-volume hospitals is pursued. Furthermore, for low- and medium-volume hospitals to achieve comparable outcomes to high-volume hospitals, strategies should be put in place that are evidence based. These include having subspecialty surgeons, in-house intensivists for postoperative monitoring, and advanced endoscopy or interventional radiology services to "rescue" patients when complications do occur. By implementing such measures, the variability in the outcomes following complex surgery will likely be reduced without restrictions to access or exacerbating current disparities.

References

1. Luft HS, Bunker JP, Enthoven AC. Should operations be regionalized? The empirical relation between surgical volume and mortality. N Engl J Med. 1979;301(25):1364–9.
2. Birkmeyer JD, Siewers AE, Finlayson EV, et al. Hospital volume and surgical mortality in the United States. N Engl J Med. 2002;346(15):1128–37.
3. Halm EA, Lee C, Chassin MR. Is volume related to outcome in health care? A systematic review and methodologic critique of the literature. Ann Intern Med. 2002;137(6):511–20.
4. Dudley RA, Johansen KL, Brand R, Rennie DJ, Milstein A. Selective referral to high-volume hospitals: estimating potentially avoidable deaths. JAMA. 2000;283(9):1159–66.
5. Finks JF, Osborne NH, Birkmeyer JD. Trends in hospital volume and operative mortality for high-risk surgery. N Engl J Med. 2011;364(22):2128–37.
6. Stitzenberg KB, Meropol NJ. Trends in centralization of cancer surgery. Ann Surg Oncol. 2010;17(11):2824–31.
7. Finley CJ, Bendzsak A, Tomlinson G, Keshavjee S, Urbach DR, Darling GE. The effect of regionalization on outcome in pulmonary lobectomy: a Canadian national study. J Thorac Cardiovasc Surg. 2010;140(4):757–63.
8. Gordon TA, Bowman HM, Bass EB, et al. Complex gastrointestinal surgery: impact of provider experience on clinical and economic outcomes. J Am Coll Surg. 1999;189(1):46–56.
9. Fong Y, Gonen M, Rubin D, Radzyner M, Brennan MF. Long-term survival is superior after resection for cancer in high-volume centers. Ann Surg. 2005;242(4):540–4; discussion 544–547.
10. Bilimoria KY, Bentrem DJ, Ko CY, et al. Multimodality therapy for pancreatic cancer in the U.S.: utilization, outcomes, and the effect of hospital volume. Cancer. 2007;110(6):1227–34.
11. Urbach DR, Baxter NN. Does it matter what a hospital is "high volume" for? Specificity of hospital volume-outcome associations for surgical procedures: analysis of administrative data. BMJ. 2004;328(7442):737–40.
12. Birkmeyer JD, Sun Y, Goldfaden A, Birkmeyer NJ, Stukel TA. Volume and process of care in high-risk cancer surgery. Cancer. 2006;106(11):2476–81.
13. Ghaferi AA, Birkmeyer JD, Dimick JB. Variation in hospital mortality associated with inpatient surgery. N Engl J Med. 2009;361(14):1368–75.
14. Chowdhury MM, Dagash H, Pierro A. A systematic review of the impact of volume of surgery and specialization on patient outcome. Br J Surg. 2007;94(2):145–61.
15. Finlayson SR, Birkmeyer JD, Tosteson AN, Nease RF Jr. Patient preferences for location of care: implications for regionalization. Med Care. 1999;37(2):204–9.
16. Wasif N, Etzioni D, Habermann EB, et al. Racial and socioeconomic differences in the use of high-volume commission on cancer-accredited hospitals for cancer surgery in the United States. Ann Surg Oncol. 2018;25(5):1116–25.
17. Zafar SN, Shah AA, Channa H, Raoof M, Wilson L, Wasif N. Comparison of rates and outcomes of readmission to index vs nonindex hospitals after major cancer surgery. JAMA Surg. 2018;153:719.
18. Stitzenberg KB, Sigurdson ER, Egleston BL, Starkey RB, Meropol NJ. Centralization of cancer surgery: implications for patient access to optimal care. J Clin Oncol. 2009;27(28):4671–8.
19. Bilimoria KY, Ko CY, Tomlinson JS, et al. Wait times for cancer surgery in the United States: trends and predictors of delays. Ann Surg. 2011;253(4):779–85.
20. Livingston EH, Cao J. Procedure volume as a predictor of surgical outcomes. JAMA. 2010;304(1):95–7.
21. Thabut G, Christie JD, Kremers WK, Fournier M, Halpern SD. Survival differences following lung transplantation among US transplant centers. JAMA. 2010;304(1):53–60.
22. Wasif N, Etzioni DA, Habermann EB, et al. Does improved mortality at low- and medium-volume hospitals lead to attenuation of the volume to outcomes relationship for major visceral surgery? J Am Coll Surg. 2018;227(1):85–93.e9.
23. PSNet. To err is human: building a safer health system. January 2000. Retrieved from: https://psnet.ahrq.gov/resources/resource/1579/to-err-is-human-building-a-safer-health-system

Volume, Quality, and Research of the Modern Hospital: The Survivable Strategy

12

Xiang Da (Eric) Dong and Rifat Latifi

Background

The majority of healthcare cost centers on in-hospital care in developed countries [1]. In the United States alone, a third of all healthcare spending is concentrated on hospital care, a sum exceeding $1082 billion alone in fiscal year 2016 [1]. The rapid and continued rise in hospital expenditures has led to increased scrutiny of how healthcare dollars are spent, as well as the return on investment in the form of patient outcome, patient satisfaction, availability of services, community outreach, and regional impact of services [2].

For a hospital to survive and flourish, the revenue based on services rendered must exceed the costs incurred providing care to patients. A profitable hospital needs to control the cost while maintaining the quality of care [3]. There is a correlation, although not always proportional, between the quality of care offered by a hospital and their bottom line [4, 5]. However, providing excellent care will frequently improve hospital profitability, likely through increased patient volume and better payor-mix population. A hospital can drive patient volume through expansion of services by increasing research investments into new technologies. The added volume of service is clearly important, although there is a limit due to the cost of adapting new technologies for the new hospital. For clinical programs to flourish, it would, therefore, need to marry three tenets of a successful hospital, namely, volume, quality, and research and development. Initial investment in research and development takes time to see the results, and one cannot expect immediate return on investment.

However, the most highly profitable hospital, based on federal data from 2013, on nearly 3000 hospitals are actually nonprofit hospitals [6, 7]. Although tax exempt status has been identified as a reason, research and reputation have traditionally gone a long way for these nonprofit institutions performing so well [6, 7]. Patient satisfaction is also closely linked to increase in patient volume [8]. Hospitals with high patient satisfactions will ultimately improve their volume and quality of care based on patient preferences [9].

In this chapter, we will review the history supporting the regionalization of complex surgeries and the positive correlation between volume and quality of care. We will also discuss the policies and initiatives that promoted regionalization of care, along with the barriers to implementation in the United States. Finally, the keys to surviving a marketplace healthcare system like the United States, where social media and published outcomes influence the consumer of healthcare

X. D. Dong (✉)
New York Medical College, School of Medicine, Department of Surgery, Surgical Oncology, Westchester, Medical Center, Valhalla, NY, USA
e-mail: xiang.dong@wmchealth.org

R. Latifi
New York Medical College, School of Medicine, Department of Surgery and Westchester Medical Center, Valhalla, NY, USA

R. Latifi (ed.), *The Modern Hospital*, https://doi.org/10.1007/978-3-030-01394-3_12

services, are highlighted. The need to focus on patient outcome, to invest in key drivers of technology, and to add research to strengthen the quality of care will be discussed as well.

Hospital Quality Reporting: History and Change

The association between quality of care with high-volume hospitals and surgeons is a well-observed phenomenon over the last four decades [10–13]. The reason for the improved outcome is a reflection of the high-volume surgeon versus the process improvements from a high-volume hospital has also been dissected in order to analyze the reason for the differences. Nowhere is the need for superior outcomes more evident nowadays with public reporting than high-risk procedures such as cardiac surgeries and complex oncologic surgeries [14–17]. The effect is measured in terms of patient outcome prominently denoted by in-hospital mortality rates [18]. Although early studies lacked sufficient case-mix adjustments, the creation of specialized databases have permitted improvements in analyses. Initial evaluations focused on statewide registries that listed several high-risk procedures which carried differences in 30-day mortalities [14, 19]. Other lower-risk procedures seem to result in similar outcomes between low-volume and high-volume hospitals based on various aspects of assessments [20].

Back in the 1970s and 1980s, crude data collection and analysis was already under way for cardiac surgeries to evaluate patient outcome [19]. The results were imperfect due to surgeon bias and disparities in patient selection. At the time, a firestorm was released when the state of New York decided to publish the first physician-specific mortality report, hailed by consumer advocates for the public release of data and vilainized by operating surgeons who viewed the data as inaccurate due to patient selection and sampling [19, 21]. Beginning in the 1970s, the state of New York first initiated the Cardiac Surgery Reporting System (CSRS) which was quite controversial at the time of inception, due to the fear of challenging the practice patterns of individual surgeons. The collection of statewide data was carried out with the results reported to the state's Department of Health. Included in the reporting system were demographics, risk factors, complications, discharge status, surgeon, and hospital. Following the collection of the data, CSRS developed risk adjustment tools to account for patient factors such as congestive heart failure and low ejection fraction which would complicate postoperative outcomes. Initial decision was to publish the results but keeping the identities of the hospitals and surgeons confidential [18]. However, the data was ultimately released to the public by Dr. Axelrod via an article in *New York Newsday* [21]. The article titled "Ranking Open-Heart Surgery: State Study Lists Best Hospitals" was published on December 4, 1990 [21]. As expected, it created an immediate media battle between operating surgeons and consumer advocates in terms of support and criticism for outcomes reporting [21]. Subsequently, a follow-up article was published on December 18, 1991, on the individual surgeon outcomes, much to the disappointment of many underperforming surgeons [22].

However, the publication of the data to the public set in motion of what would become an era of provider outcome reporting. The *New York Post* article reported the results of all cardiac surgeons who performed CABGs in 1989 and 1990 in New York State [22]. What was disturbing in the data was that surgeons who performed fewer than 50 cases a year had a mortality rate of 6.1% in comparison to surgeons averaging more than 50 operations per year which was around 3% [22]. The correlation of volume on outcome is soon discovered in other surgical specialties as well [20].

As a result of the findings, the Cardiac Advisory Committee took the initiative to improve the outcome of hospitals with higher than expected patient mortality. Site visits, process reviews, and recommendations were implemented. Low-volume surgeons were restricted or changes implemented to their practice patterns. A dramatic drop in mortality in cardiac surgery was soon observed in those low-volume hospitals which led others to tout the success of volume reporting [19].

It is likely that the release of patient outcome data prompted a rapid change in the way that data was reported. Under-coding was soon replaced with over-coding to minimize the risk of the consequences from poor outcomes [22]. From 1989 to 1992, there was a 21% decrease in actual cardiac surgery mortality and a 41% decrease in risk-adjusted mortality [22]. Parallel to this decrease in mortality is also the possibility of surgeons' cherry picking the best candidates suitable for surgery [19, 22]. Fortunately, this limitation to access did not appear to be borne out in real-life data as hospitals and surgeons learned to grade their patients in various categories of risk.

An unintended effect of the dissemination of data from New York hospitals is that data reporting soon became available in other states as well [19]. More interestingly, states also showed that risk-adjusted mortality decreased from 1990 to 1994 in states without previous statewide reporting of CABG results. Massachusetts showed a 42% decline in risk-adjusted mortality for CABG, likely a result of the perceived threat of public reporting going to Massachusetts and hospitals and surgeons preparing for the change to their practice from the publicly available data [19]. In the end, the changes to cardiac surgery data reporting set the stage for changes in other complex surgeries, notably higher-risk surgeries including vascular and cancer operations.

Surgical Volume and Outcome

The relationship between high volume and low mortality seen with cardiac surgery translated to major cancer surgeries as well [20]. Initially, regional and statewide databases on cancer patients demonstrated the discrepancy in the outcomes for patients treated at high-volume centers versus those treated in low-volume centers. Eventually, the statewide data would translate into nationwide data, which showed a similar pattern [20]. In 2002, Birkmeyer and colleagues published a landmark study showing that higher-volume hospitals had lower operative mortality rates for several high-risk operations [20]. Using information from the national Medicare claims database and the Nationwide Inpatient Sample, the authors examined the immediate postoperative mortality of patients for six types of cardiovascular procedures and eight types of major cancer resections. In order to address limitations to previous smaller statewide studies, the authors used data from the Medicare population, which accounts for the majority of patients undergoing high-risk procedures in the United States. In addition, the authors excluded those under 65 years of age or over 99 years of age to prevent discrepancies from extremes of age [20]. The absolute magnitude of the relation between volume and outcome differed between the types of procedures. However, the differences in survival based on volume data were striking and undeniable.

Similarly, using information from the all-payer Nationwide Inpatient Sample from 1995 to 1997, Finlayson and colleagues published in 2003 the operative mortality in cancer surgery only with relation to hospital volume [23]. As expected, mortality was higher for high-risk procedures including esophagectomy, pancreatic resections, and pulmonary lobectomy. Mortality reductions were not as prominent for gastrectomy, cystectomy, and pneumonectomy and insignificant for nephrectomy and colectomy [23]. This strengthened the argument that only high-risk procedures favored larger institutions for better outcomes.

In spite of the previous findings, volume data alone has been criticized for the lack of vigorous evaluation as the sole predictor of mortality [24]. There were differences on the outcome of the data from the statewide and nationwide samples. Studies that took into account clinical data instead of administrative data, which lacked case-mix index, tended to show greater differences in outcome or mortality. However, although patients at low-volume rural hospitals tended to be slightly older, comorbidity did not vary significantly by volume. Studies based on clinical data have not reported weaker volume–outcome relationships than those based on administrative data [13, 24].

Overall, the takeaway message is that certain high-risk procedures have marked differences in patient outcome depending on the location where the surgeries was performed. For instance, differences in mortality in procedures such as pancreatectomy and esophagectomy differed by well over 12% between the lowest-volume and the highest-volume hospitals. Relatively small differences were found for other more common procedures such as carotid endarterectomy or colectomy. The findings by Birkmeyer and colleagues were scrutinized and confirmed for a variety of diseases treated by physicians [20]. For 20 years prior to his landmark paper and 20 years since, many studies have described higher rates of operative mortality in certain high-risk procedures at low-volume surgical centers [25]. Through the use of Medicare claims data, patients undergoing several high-risk procedures continue to show significantly lower mortality rate in high-volume centers despite the recent improvements in surgical care [25]. The importance of surgical experience and hospital volume has disseminated to consumer-oriented outlets and websites (e.g., https://www.healthscope.org and www.leagfroggroup.org).

The number of potential avoidable deaths was also scrutinized with selective referral to high-volume hospitals [18]. Although early studies lacked sufficient case-mix adjustment, the creation of specialized databases has allowed more sophisticated analysis leading to more concrete evidence of benefits from referrals to high-volume centers [26–29]. Selective referral of high-risk disease processes known to receive better outcome in large-volume centers will likely generate better outcomes. A study on the initiative to facilitate referral to high-volume centers to reduce hospital mortality in California was done focusing on several known high-risk procedures [18]. Of the high-risk procedures or diseases identified in a California study, an estimated 602 deaths could potentially be avoided out of 58,306 patients admitted to low-volume hospitals [18]. With this kind of numbers touted by referral to high-volume centers, the time was ripe for development of referral centers to mitigate the impact of low-volume surgeries in low-volume hospitals [26–29].

Specialization and Regionalization of Care

The quality of care in the twenty-first century is increasingly trending toward specialization [11, 12]. Much of the care given for medical and surgical diseases saw a shift toward regionalization of care. Nowhere is the immediate benefit more prevalent than the surgical mortality of high-risk cardiovascular or major cancer resection procedures performed in high-volume hospitals [20]. However, this does bring into question the problems associated with the regionalization of care model, which is limiting access to patients with these major surgical problems as the treatment of certain diseases became more concentrated in urban areas [30–32]. Regionalizing of care leads to undue stress on patients and their families, because of the travel burden necessary to seek specialized care. The burden for patients is also pronounced when undergoing ongoing cancer treatments. The regionalization model also augments the loss of patient volume seen in smaller already-struggling hospitals which serve a critical need to patients in rural areas. The loss of patient volumes leads to a vicious cycle where emergency care, which still needs to be delivered, becomes even less frequent adding to an already poorly prepared rural hospital [33–36]. In addition, the recruitment and retention to smaller hospitals of experts in the field becomes ever more difficult. The intention of the regionalization model was to drive the patient population with complex disease problems toward the urban area to improve overall outcomes. However, this model became a direct assault on the rural, smaller hospitals which does serve a critical need for large swarms of the country [33–36].

With the regionalization of care comes the problem that is incumbent to rural facilities. The balance and trade-off between providing a wide range of services and maintaining excellence of care becomes ever more difficult. Drivers of change also included the shift of care from inpatient to outpatient settings, rapid advances in medical technology, inadequate supply and difficulty in attracting medical personnel to rural areas, and the increased need for substantial investment in managing specific conditions for which the return of investment may not justify the cost. All of these factors help explain why many rural hospitals are in economic decline with difficult choices to make to avoid closure all together. [33] Investments in technologies to increase volume to improve outcome is difficult to guarantee success.

Although outcome-based research has consistently showed that volume and outcome are intertwined, there is also no threshold to set as different diseases have variable numbers that are deemed high-volume hospital [37, 38]. The intricacies of transitioning to a high-volume referral pattern are more complicated than increasing the availability of services. For starters, high-volume hospitals produce better results because of the inference that experience produces better results or that referral of healthy patients able to travel distances intrinsically leads to better outcomes. Although the idea of selective referral is beneficial based on nationwide registry studies, it is inherently disruptive to the patients and their families. The continuity of care, the distance to obtain care, and limits in choice of care based on health plans are all constraints in expanding the volume–outcome relationship [37, 38].

The Leapfrog Project

The potential benefits from regionalization of care invited broader efforts to improve patient outcome. Specifically, performing coronary artery bypass graft, abdominal aortic aneurysm, coronary angioplasty, esophagectomy, and carotid endarterectomies at high-volume centers only could save over 2581 patient lives per year by requiring hospital volume standards for high-risk procedures [28]. A large group of hospitals was therefore organized in an attempt to manage and treat patients with needs for specialized surgeries at high-volume centers [28].

In 1998, a consortium of large US healthcare purchasers created the Leapfrog project to improve patient outcomes [39]. The initiative was supported by the Health Care Financing Administration and US Office of Business Group on Health by functioning as liaison purchasers. Hoping to improve quality of care, the project would focus on innovations in healthcare and education of the consumer patients.

Reports by the Institute of Medicine (IOM) have pointed to the failure of healthcare system to recognize and reward quality medical care [2]. This has led to a history of healthcare purchasers getting various levels of health products from suppliers without a clear picture of expectations.

With the shortcomings of traditional medical purchasing expectations and results, the Leapfrog project aimed to ensure that patients receive safer and higher-value healthcare through information dissemination and comparative performance measurements. The members of the Leapfrog group planned to use nationally recognized performance assessment sources, such as the National Committee for Quality Assurance, Joint Commission on Accreditation of Healthcare Organizations, and national medical specialty societies [2]. The initial planned incentives that were built into the Leapfrog initiative were patient volume, increased price compensation, and public recognition which ultimately translated into patient volume as well [2].

Since the adoption of the Leapfrog project, retrospective analysis of the implementation of the project showed that there is decreased incidence of complications [40, 41]. The impact of the Leapfrog project shows promise, although its effects may not be as profound as initially hoped for [40, 41]. The three goals of the Leapfrog project aimed for public release of the performance measurements, increased use of information systems in healthcare, and tie-in of reimbursement to quality of care [2]. The goals of the Leapfrog project have led to variable success rates. The public release of health measures has seen an increase in the United States since the early years of public reporting of information. Following the cardiac surgery data releases, this has expanded to neonatal units, cancer treatment outcomes, and ICU care [40]. The number of hospitals that have adopted computerized order entry as well as electronic medical records were at first slow to catch up in the early 2000s due to resistance from the industry. However, implementation is now in full swing with widespread adoption in the industry, although years after the initial enthusiasm to support its use. Finally, the tie-in of reimbursement to quality of care has been met with variable results.

Survival of the Rural Hospitals and Quality Metrics

In general, quality of care varied by the state, region of the state (rural versus urban), and the time period. There is a trend or perception that teaching, larger, and more urban hospitals have better quality of care than nonteaching, smaller, and rural hospitals [36]. With pay-for-performance becoming an integral part of care, there is now a pressing need for hospitals to achieve higher standards of quality in attracting new patients [42, 43].

Moreover, the adoption of new health plans and switching based on quality metrics may be more difficult than initially thought. Most of the econometric data finds that consumers tend to favor plans with expanded choices and favorable quality metrics [15]. However, focus groups also suggest that consumers are not sufficiently aware of the plan specifics to make informed choices [44, 45]. A survey of Medicare beneficiaries found that over 30% of patients knew the differences between Medicare HMO and standard coverage, while only 11% had enough information to make informed choices [44–46].

Compared with high-volume centers, critical access hospitals, which face greater challenges in delivering high-quality care due to the limited resources, showed a lower score on measured process of care and higher mortality rates for patients with acute myocardial infarction, congestive heart failure, or pneumonia [34]. Interestingly, however, they do receive higher patient satisfaction scores in providing access to inpatient care [35].

The challenges faced by rural hospitals include decreasing patient volume, capital expenditures, and understanding the cost of care. In a time when patients are migrating to the urban areas along with programs designed to shift the complicated patients toward larger tertiary centers, the loss of patient volume remains the most pressing issues for rural hospitals, which starts the cascade of many other issues that will follow. These issues include lack of research and high-quality outcome data. In addition, the demands of new technology, electronic medical records, and keeping pace with changes in medical care put unsustainable pressure on the rural hospitals to keep pace. Finally, the cost of care is not necessarily related to the benefits it brings to a hospital bottom line as well as the community it serves. For instance, the cost of bringing pancreatic cancer specialists into community practice is not sustainable in the long term, due to the lack of volume [47].

Research and Technology of the New Hospital

In this difficult financial environment, one of the best strategies not only for the survival of an existing clinical programs but also initiating new programs or new hospitals is to embrace technological advances and invest in the research and outcome data reporting. Only programs that keep strict data and analyze and report the data to national agencies and organizations such as NSQIP, NTDB, and others will be able to objectively assess their results and find ways to improve outcomes. While this requires advanced technologies and human capacities, it is one of the best ways to ensure progress.

At times, aging hospitals are faced with serious dilemma on how to proceed with changes required. Should one continue to struggle with replacement of parts of technologies or should there simply be a decision to change dramatically the entire hospital from the ground up?

This dilemma has been faced by many hospitals in challenging, competitive environments. As an example, the average operating margin for hospitals in New Jersey was just 1.7%, well short of the national average of 4.4% [48, 49]. However, in the midst of this competitive state, several aging hospitals such as Capital Health elected to relocate to a new multimillion-dollar campus by ditching aging technology and replacing their nineteenth-century medical center in Mercer, New Jersey, with another spa-like hospital located a few miles further down the road. Similarly, Princeton Healthcare, with the backing of generous donors, moved their 92-year-old campus to a large 630,000-square-foot building several miles away. Both strategic moves have proved successful in the long run following the initial outlay in expenditures [50].

Patient Choice as Driver of Change

The choice of hospitals and the competition among hospitals will guide the survivability of the new hospitals. With the implementation of changes related to centralization of care, centralized systems such as the UK National Health Service have seen the benefits and difficulties associated with changes guided by competition and well-informed patients [51–54]. Between 2010 and 2014, there was a rise in robotic prostatectomies worldwide. During this time, a number of centers in England transitioned from performing open radical prostatectomies to robotic prostatectomies. The system that the British utilizes is partly a quality based service where the patients can choose to travel to any hospital [51–54]. During the abovementioned time period, centralization of care for cancer surgery such as esophageal surgery and prostate surgery was promoted due to the previous findings that high-volume hospitals tend to deliver care with lower operative 30-day mortality. Although the expected patient referral pattern would centralize the patients in urban centers, the rapid and widespread adoption of robotic surgery rendered commissioned guidelines obsolete, despite being published as recent as 2015 for prostate surgery in England [52]. In the end, rather than a policy of centralization, patient choice and hospital competition became the drivers of change with patients choosing the providers and hospitals as well as hospitals offering competitive and well-publicized cancer care [55]. During the years studied, patients with prostate cancer gravitated toward centers that offered robotic approaches to radical prostatectomy, regardless of the outcomes or date supporting its use [52]. The lesson learned from this sweeping change in management of prostate cancer was that centers that were slow to adopt new technologies were forced to close their programs [53]. Competition will continue to drive those changes. Unfortunately, performance indicators are problematic due to a long lag time. This lag time allows clinical practice to change substantially, similar to what has come to pass with the adoption of robotic surgery worldwide. In conclusion, patient choice and hospital competition will have an outsized influence on the type of services provided by a hospital. Surrogate markers of quality performance will only have a limited role in the patient choices in this age of rapid technological adoption.

Summary

The modern hospital is a dynamic institution where it has to adapt to the changing needs of the patient population. Information dissemination is making comparisons for the level of care a key to selecting the hospital of choice. Patients are armed with the information following research into the availability of services in their region prior to making educated decisions. For the modern hospital to flourish, they need to focus on the needs of their resident patient population and select several services capable of matching the outcomes seen in the best hospitals as reported by multiple news and media outlets.

References

1. NHE Fact Sheet. Historical NHE 2016. CMS.gov website. https://www.cms.gov/research-statistics-data-and-systems/statistics-trends-and-reports/nationalhealthexpenddata/nhe-fact-sheet.html
2. Milstein A, Galvn RS, Delbanco SF, Salber P, Buck CR. Improving the safety of health care: the leapfrog initiative. Eff Clin Pract. 2000;6:313–6.
3. Dong GN. Performing well in financial management and quality of care: evidence from hospital process management for treatment of cardiovascular disease. BMC Health Serv Res. 2015;15:45. https://doi.org/10.1186/s12913-015-0690-x.

4. Jha AK, Li Z, Orav J, Epstein AM. Care in U.S. hospitals – the hospital quality alliance program. NEJM. 2005;353:265–74. https://doi.org/10.1056/NEJMsa051249.
5. Harkey J, Vraciu R. Quality of health care and financial performance: is there a link? Health Care Manag Rev. 1992;17:55–63. PMID: 1428860.
6. Bai G, Anderson GF. A more detailed understanding of factors associated with hospital profitability. Health Aff. 2016;35:5. https://doi.org/10.1377/hlthaff.2015.1193.
7. Horwitz JR. Making profits and providing care: comparing nonprofit, for-profit, and government hospitals. Health Aff. 2005;24:3. https://doi.org/10.1377/hlthaff.24.3.790.
8. Hall MF. Looking to improve financial results? Start by listening to patients: improving patient satisfaction can have a direct impact on your hospitals reputation--and financial results. Healthc Financ Manage. 2008:76+. Academic OneFile, Accessed 17 Apr 2018.
9. Jha AK, Orav EJ, Zheng J, Epstein AM. Patients' perception of hospital care in United States. N Engl J Med. 2008;359:1921–31. https://doi.org/10.1056/NEJMsa0804116.
10. Hughes RG, Hunt SS, Luft HS. Effects of surgeon volume and hospital volume on quality of care in hospitals. Med Care. 1987;25:489–503.
11. Luft HS, Bunker JP, Enthoven AC. Should operations be regionalized? The empirical relation between surgical volume and mortality. N Engl J Med. 1979;301:1364–9.
12. Begg CB, Cramer LD, Hoskins WJ, Brennan MF. Impact of hospital volume on operative mortality for major cancer surgery. JAMA. 1998;280:1747–51.
13. Halm EA, Lee C, Chassin MR. Is volume related to outcome in health care? A systematic review and methodologic critique of the literature. Ann Intern Med. 2002;137:511–20. https://doi.org/10.7326/0003-4819-137-6-200209170-00012.
14. Hannan EL, Kilburn H Jr, O'Donnell JF, Lukacik G, Shields EP. Adult open heart surgery in New York state: an analysis of risk factors and hospital mortality rates. JAMA. 1990;264:2768–74.
15. Dranove D, Stekas A. Start spreading the news: a structural estimate of the effects of New York hospital report cards. J Health Econ. 2008;27:1201–7. https://doi.org/10.1016/j.healeco.2008.03.001.
16. Birkmeyer JD. Should we regionalize major surgery? Potential benefits and policy considerations. J Am Coll Surg. 2000;190:341–9.
17. Birkmeyer JD. High risk surgery – follow the crowd. JAMA. 2000;283:1191–3.
18. Dudley RA, Johansen KL, Brand R, Rennie DJ, Milstein A. Selective referral to high-volume hospitals: estimating potentially avoidable deaths. JAMA. 2000;283:1159–66.
19. Harlan BJ. Presidential address: statewide reporting of coronary artery surgery results: a view from California. J Thorac Cardiovasc Surg. 2001;121:409–16.
20. Birkmeyer JD, Siewers AE, Finlayson EVA, Stukel TA, Lucas FL, Batista I, Welch G, Wennberg DE. Hospital volume and surgical mortality in the Unites States. N Engl J Med. 2002;346:1128–37. https://doi.org/10.1056/NEJMsa012337.
21. Zinman D. Ranking open-heart surgery: state study lists best hospitals. New York Newsday. 1990 Dec 4; Sec. A:4.
22. Hannan EL, Kumar D, Racz M, Siu AL, Chassin MR. New York State's cardiac surgery reporting system: four years later. Ann Thorac Surg. 1994;58:1852–7.
23. Finlayson EVA, Goodney PP, Birkmeyer JD. Hospital volume and operative mortality in cancer surgery. Arch Surg. 2003;138:721–5.
24. LaPar DJ, Kron IL, Jones DR, Stukenborg GJ, Kozower BD. Hospital procedure volume should not be used as a measure of surgical quality. Ann Surg. 2012;256:606–15. https://doi.org/10.1097/SLA.0b012e31826b4be6.
25. Reames BN, Ghaferi AA, Birkmeyer JD, Dimick JB. Hospital volume and operative mortality in the modern era. Ann Surg. 2014;260:244–51. https://doi.org/10.1097/SLA.0000000000000375.
26. Daley J. Invited commentary: quality of care and the volume-outcome relationship – what's next for surgery? Surgery. 2002;131:16–8.
27. Gordon TA, Bowman HM, Tielsch JM, Bass EB, Burleyson GP, Cameron JL. Statewide regionalization of pancreaticoduodenectomy and its effect on in-hospital mortality. Ann Surg. 1998;228:71–8.
28. Birkmeyer JD, Finlayson EVA, Birkmeyer CM. Volume standards for high-risk surgical procedures: potential benefits of the Leapfrog initiative. Surgery. 2001;130:415–22. https://doi.org/10.1067/msy.2001.117139.
29. Christian CK, Gustafson ML, Betensky RA, Daley J, Zinner MJ. The Leapfrog volume criteria may fall short in identifying high-quality surgical centers. Ann Surg. 2003;238:447–57. https://doi.org/10.1097/01.sla.0000089850.27592.eb.
30. Boudourakis L, Wang T, Roman S, Desai R, Sosa J. Evolution of the surgeon-volume, patient-outcome relationship. Ann Surg. 2009;250:159–65. https://doi.org/10.1097/SLA.0b013e318a77cb3.
31. Bruce H, Hamilton B, Richards K, Bilimoria K, Cohen M, Ko C. Does surgical quality improve in the American College of Surgeons National Surgical Quality Improvement Program: an evaluation of all participating hospitals. Ann Surg. 2009;250(3):363–76. https://doi.org/10.1097/SLA.0b013e3181b4148f.
32. Epstein AM. Volume and outcome – it is time to move ahead. N Engl J Med. 2002;346:1161–4.
33. Moscovice IS. Rural hospitals: a literature synthesis and health services research agenda. Health Serv Res. 1989;23:892–930.
34. Joynt KE, Harris Y, Orav EJ, Jha AK. Quality of care and patient outcome in critical access rural hospitals. JAMA. 2011;306:45–52.

35. Casey MM, Davidson G. Upper Midwest rural health research center final report #10: patient assessments and quality of care in rural hospitals. Minneapolis: Upper Midwest Rural Health Research Center, University of Minnesota; 2010.
36. Keeler EB, Rubenstein LV, Kahn KL. Hospital characteristics and quality of care. JAMA. 1992;268:1709–14. https://doi.org/10.1001/jama.1992.03490130097037.
37. Studnicki J, Craver C, Blanchette CM, Fisher JW, Shahbazi S. A cross-sectional retrospective analysis of the regionalization of complex surgery. BMC Surg. 2014;14:55. https://doi.org/10.1186/1471-2482-14-55.
38. Finks JF, Osborne NH, Birkmeyer J. Trend in hospital volume and operative mortality for high-risk surgery. NEJM. 2011;364:2128–37. https://doi.org/10.1056/NEJMsa1010705.
39. Birkmeyer JD, Dimick JB. Potential benefits of the new Leapfrog standards: effect of process and outcomes measures. Surgery. 2004;135:568–75. https://doi.org/10.1016/j.surg.2004.03.004.
40. Galvin RS, Delbanco S, Milstein A, Belden G. Has the Leapfrog group had an impact on the health care market. Health Aff. 2005;24:1. https://doi.org/10.1377/hlthaff.24.1.228.
41. Brooke BS, Perler BA, Dominici F, Makary MA, Pronovost PJ. Reduction of in-hospital mortality among California hospitals meeting Leapfrog evidence-based standards for abdominal aortic aneurysm repair. J Vasc Surg. 2008;47:1155–64.
42. Lindenauer PK, Remus D, Roman S, Rothberg M, Benjamin EM, Bratzler DW. Public reporting and pay for performance in hospital quality improvement. NEJM. 2007;356:486–96. https://doi.org/10.1056/NEJMsa064964.
43. Kolstad JT, Chernew ME. Quality and consumer decision making in the market for health insurance and health care services. Med Care Res Rev. 2009;66:28S–52S.
44. Hibbard JH, Peters E. Supporting informed consumer health care decisions: data presentation approaches that facilitate the use of information in choice. Annu Rev Public Health. 2003;24:413–33. https://doi.org/10.1146/annurev.publhealth.24.100901.141005. Epub 2001, Nov 6. PMID: 12428034.
45. Hibbard JH, Jewett JJ, Engelmann S, Tusler M. Can Medicare beneficiaries make informed choices? Health Aff. 1998;17:181–93.
46. Tunis SR, Messner DA. Medicare policy on bariatric surgery: decision making in the face of uncertainty. JAMA. 2013;310(13):1339–40. https://doi.org/10.1001/jama.2013.278849.
47. Allison A. The community hospital survival guide: strategies to keep the doors open. Becker Hospital CFO report. 2015.
48. Anderson GF. From 'soak the rich' to 'soak the poor': recent trends in hospital pricing. Health Aff. 2007;26:3. https://doi.org/10.1377/hlthaff.26.3.780.
49. AHA 2016 annual survey. AHA Hospital Statistics, 2018 edition. https://www.aha.org/statistics/fast-facts-us-hospitals
50. Kaysen R. To survive, medical companies in New Jersey are building new hospitals. The New York Times. 2011.
51. Ho V, Town RJ, Heslin MJ. Regionalization versus competition in complex cancer surgery. Health Econ Policy Law. 2007;2:51–71.
52. Aggarwal A, Lewis D, Mason M, Purushotham A, Sullivan R, van der Meulen J. Effect of patient choice and hospital competition on service configuration and technology adoption within cancer surgery: a national, population-based study. Lancet Oncol. 18:1453–45.
53. Nguyen PL, Gu X, Lipsitz SR. Cost implications of the rapid adoption of newer technologies for treating prostate cancer. J Clin Oncol. 2011;29:1517–24. [PubMed: 21402604].
54. Frencher SK, Ryoo JJ, Ko CL. Emerging importance of certification: volume, outcomes, and regionalization of care. J Surg Oncol. 2009;99:131–2.
55. Urbach DR, Baxter NN. Does it matter what a hospital is "high volume" for? Specificity of hospital volume-outcome associations for surgical procedures: analysis of administrative data. Qual Saf Health Care. 2004;13:379–83. https://doi.org/10.1136/bmj.38030.642963.AE.

Precision Medicine: Disruptive Technology in the Modern Hospital

13

Michael J. Demeure

Introduction

Physicians have long strived to deliver personalized medicine. They evaluate each patient's own unique health history and presentation before recommending a treatment plan. Precision medicine is the next iteration in truly personalized medicine. The term precision medicine has evolved to describe the use of genetics and genomics when they are applied to the care of a particular individual patient. This has become practical due to the development of genomic technologies such that the results of genetic analysis are available rapidly and at decreasing costs. The promise of delivering more effective treatments with reduced toxicity and at a lower cost has only begun to be realized and only in limited applications. Most healthcare providers and payers know that precision medicine is the future but are not certain what it is, how it will be applied, when it will be used, and for which circumstances will payment for testing and treatments be provided. Nonetheless, while the field of precision medicine faces hurdles toward widespread adoption, the modern hospital must be prepared to embrace these new technologies. Hospitals will increasingly be asked to take leadership roles in the healthcare system to shepherd the use of genomics to better the health of the populations they serve.

M. J. Demeure (✉)
Hoag Family Cancer Institute, Hoag Memorial Hospital Presbyterian, Newport Beach, CA, USA

Translational Genomics Research Institute, Phoenix, AZ, USA
e-mail: michael.demeure@hoag.org

Genetics and Genomics in Medicine

Genetics describes the study of the DNA code that each individual harbors in every cell of their body. Inherited diseases based on germline genetics such as hemophilia or cystic fibrosis can be assessed by the analysis of DNA from a patient's white blood cells obtained with a simple venipuncture or of the DNA obtained from a buccal swab. Genomics applies to the analysis of somatic disease-bearing tissue such as testing a lung cancer specimen for a gene fusion involving the ALK gene to inform potential treatment of the cancer [1]. Newer technologies now allow one to detect shed genetic material from tumors in peripheral blood as well, which may in many cases obviate the need for a more invasive biopsy. Most often, discussion of genetic tests involves testing of DNA sequences; however, it is also possible to analyze RNA, epigenetic modifications, or protein level changes such as phosphorylation status. The genetic code is carried in DNA in chromosomes. DNA encodes proteins by its sequence of nucleotide codons. DNA information is transcribed into RNA which is then translated to a protein sequence. Options for DNA testing include whole-genome analysis, sequencing of

R. Latifi (ed.), *The Modern Hospital*, https://doi.org/10.1007/978-3-030-01394-3_13

the coding genome called exome, sequencing of subsets of genes generally referred to as panel testing, or sequencing of individual genes or specific areas of genes. In general costs of sequencing are dependent on the expanse of the genome covered and the sequencing depth. Analysis and annotation also add cost. Overall, the ability to sequence DNA with next-generation sequencing has resulted in rapid results at a rapidly decreasing cost allowing tractability in patient care.

Genomic analysis of DNA has taken the lead in molecular medicine largely because the technology is most robust, DNA is easily obtained from paraffin blocks, and the analytic tools are more advanced than for other molecular assays. Sequence analysis of RNA for gene fusions and gene expression yields important information about the importance of particular gene mutations and may expose additional potential targets for therapy. Researchers are also able to sequence the methylome, proteome, and microbiome. Precise characterization of immune cell profiles will be important in the management of transplant recipients, patients with autoimmune diseases, and immunotherapy of cancer. These types of assays must undergo rigorous clinical development and the process of FDA approval but will eventually be brought into the clinic.

Applications in Clinical Medicine

The promise of precision medicine transcends all fields of medicine. While oncology is, perhaps, leading the adoption of genomics into clinical practice, it is relevant in virtually all specialties. In primary care fields, genomics can inform wellness and identification of disease for which patients are at increased risk prompting prevention strategies, screening, and early intervention. Pharmacogenomics may help doctors select and prescribe drugs with greater efficacy and safety because genomics can inform a physician about the metabolism of drugs, the potential for adverse events, or interactions with other drugs in a particular patient. Similarly cardiologists can identify patients at increased risk for aortic dissection or be guided in their selection of lipid-lowering pharmaceuticals. Much of precision medicine is used in a sporadic and ad hoc manner by individual physicians, particularly in nonacademic hospitals or academic hospitals that do not have their own clinical sequencing facilities on site. Some hospitals and medical centers are adopting preferred vendor relationships with favorable contracts for specific genomic testing services. The adoption of precision medicine is important for hospitals because it offers the promise of being able to deliver better healthcare outcomes at lower cost.

The purpose of this section is to illustrate examples where genomics is currently impacting patient care in order to illustrate the rationale to support the adoption of precision medicine initiatives by hospitals. Perhaps the initial widespread adoption of genetic testing has been in the field of prenatal diagnosis of genetic disease through amniocentesis, and now analysis of fetal DNA is maternal blood. Each state has a law that requires that newborns be tested for a panel of metabolic, endocrine, and other disorders. Most states test for the 32 conditions specified by the Health Resources and Services Administration (HRSA) in their Recommended Uniform Screening Panels, but additional disorders that may be included in each state's panels vary. In pediatrics, children with suspected anomalies may undergo genetic analysis, or pharmacogenetics may guide selection and dosage of drugs to treat a variety of disorders. Pharmacogenetics is the application of the knowledge of how germline variations or polymorphisms of genes may affect drug metabolism, efficacy, or toxicity. The FDA has associated over 120 drugs and 22 genes with drug-gene associations in prescription drug labels. The following are but two of many similar findings related to common genetic variants identified affecting drug safety. Genetic variants or polymorphisms of the genes VKORC1 and CYP2C9 have been associated with increased risk of bleeding complications and lower dosing recommendations for warfarin [2, 3]. Complications from inappropriate overdosing of warfarin are one of the most common causes of adverse medication reactions causing visits to hospital emergency rooms [4]. Rather than the empiric dosing commonly done, a better approach is recommended that incorporates a patient's genotype [5]. Another single nucleotide polymorphism in the SLCO1B1 gene is associated with a 4.5-fold increased risk of muscle toxicity and heart damage in patients treated with simvastatin, a common cholesterol-lowering medication [6]. For these patients, it may be possible to choose an alternative statin drug such as pravastatin [7]. Assessment by sequencing of the gut microbiome is another emerging area of importance with potential application in many fields, in particular the study of drug metabolism, immunology, and health maintenance [8]. The gut microbiome is generally stable in health but can be altered by diet, administration of antibiotics, and disease states [9]. The gut microbiome alters drug metabolism, and thus perturbations in the gut bacteria could potentially expose patients to toxicity from drugs with a narrow therapeutic window such as digoxin [10, 11]. Over 60 drugs have been identified as having microbiome-related interactions [12]. Recently, it has even been shown that the gut microbiome affects the efficacy of immune-modifying anticancer drugs in that the antitumor effects of CTL-4 blockade appear dependent on the presence of specific gut bacteria including *B. fragilis* or *B. thetaiotaomicron* [13]. Computers and machine learning of metadata can predict patient health and disease. Target stores can predict a pregnant woman's due date and customers' other major life events based on purchases of mundane items, such as unscented lotions, cleaning supplies, and cotton balls, and then use the information to send targeted mailings with coupons [14]. Similar application of machine learning and data science when combined with genomics can be used to predict suicide attempts from mood-focused smartphone apps and genetic blood tests, thereby offering an opportunity for intervention [15, 16].

In cancer, genetics may be used to identify patients who will undoubtedly develop cancer, as in the case of a germline RET mutation and medullary cancer of the thyroid. Patients who harbor an inherited pathogenic variant of the RET gene will develop medullary thyroid cancer. Prior to the availability of genetic testing for this variant, patients who had an affected parent had to undergo yearly screening blood tests because they had a 50% chance of inheriting the predisposition gene from their affected parent. Presently, a single genetic test can be done, and if negative, the individual is not at increased risk and can forego yearly screening. If affected, patients can then be counseled to undergo a prophylactic thyroidectomy. More commonly, genetics may indicate an increased risk but not a certainty of developing cancer as in the case of BRCA1 and BRCA2 mutations. Affected patients are at increased risk of developing breast, ovarian, pancreatic, or prostate cancer. These patients may elect to have increased screening for breast cancer or to have prophylactic mastectomies or oophorectomy. The risk profile of these operations makes them acceptable choices. The option of prophylactic pancreatectomy to avoid the possible development of pancreatic cancer does not seem warranted for most patients given the risks of the operation and the sequelae of exocrine and endocrine insufficiency, so our center and others are studying the possible benefit of high-risk screening clinics for patients at increased risk of pancreatic cancer due to their genetics or family history. Recently, a blood test for various cancers used a combination of a multiplex PCR panel of cancer-related genes and assay for protein biomarkers to identify early stage potentially resectable cancer with high sensitivities [17]. Particularly encouraging is the ability to detect early cancers of the ovary, liver, stomach, pancreas, and esophagus because there currently are no available screening tests. These types of tests are or will soon be commercially available.

New technologies and protocols are being adopted for screening of high-risk individuals for early cancers. An example of this is the use of surveillance with whole body MRI in patients with pathogenic germline TP53 mutations (Li-Fraumeni syndrome) to minimize the need for radiation exposure due to serial CT scans. These patients are at increased risk for a variety of cancers including soft tissue and bone sarcomas, breast cancer, adrenal cancers, and central nervous system cancers including gliomas, neuroblastomas, and choroid plexus carcinomas. Less commonly, these patients may develop lung cancers, leukemias, kidney cancers, thyroid cancers, melanomas, pancreatic or colon cancer, or germ cell cancers. At initial screening with whole body MRI, the prevalence of detected new primary cancers has been reported to be 7–13% [18, 19]. Our hospital initiated whole body MRI in a registry trial for patients identified as harboring pathogenic germline TP53 mutations. At present there are many other known genetic variants that may predispose one to an increased risk of cancer. The availability of genetic counselors and the medical directorship is key to identify the genetic testing needed for each patient and their kindred based on a thorough review of the patient's history and that of their family. Genetic testing labs offer a variety of single gene tests and tailored panels. Selection of appropriate testing must be cost-effective but sufficiently comprehensive. Our hospital has also initiated high-risk cancer screening programs in our institute for women's health for breast and gynecologic cancers and for prostate cancer, pancreatic cancer, gastrointestinal cancers, neurologic cancers, urologic cancer, neurologic cancers, and rare cancer syndromes including multiple endocrine neoplasia and Li-Fraumeni syndromes (germline TP53 mutations). There may be an overlap between these screening programs in that one pathogenic germline variant may predispose a patient to multiple cancers in different systems, so a coordinated approach is needed. Nurse navigators assist in assuring patients have appropriate screening and coordination between programs. These protocols have established a paradigm for future programs designed to allow for early detection of hereditary cancers.

Somatic testing of tumors to guide treatment of cancer is becoming increasingly relevant to treatment decisions [20]. In the case of early stage breast cancer, testing of tumor tissue can predict the likelihood of relapse and help guide decisions regarding adjuvant chemotherapy [21], including possibly sparing patients from the cost and morbidity of chemotherapy if their risk of recurrence is low [22]. In stage IV lung cancer, it is now standard of care to test lung tumor tissue for a panel of gene mutations, fusions, and amplifications including the epidermal growth factor receptor gene (EGFR), ALK, ROS1, BRAF, MET, and others. Treatments with targeted agents improve outcomes and are associated with less toxicity than cytotoxic chemotherapy [1, 23, 24]. The greatest current potential may be the application of sequencing in patients whose tumors have progressed despite standard chemotherapy or for patients with rare tumors for which there are no good options. The Bisgrove study [25] demonstrated for the first time in a prospective trial that patients with tumors refractory to prior chemotherapy could benefit from treatment based on a molecular analysis of their tumors including immunohistochemistry, fluorescent in situ hybridization, and gene expression microarray. These patients experienced an improved progression-free survival when compared to the results that were associated with their previous regimen. Later studies have shown benefit associated with tumor analysis using next-generation sequencing [26]. For patients with rare cancers, treatments based on solid prospective randomized phase III clinical trials showing efficacy may be lacking, so treatment is based on data from case reports or small single institutional series [27]. The additional guidance of the knowledge of potential driver mutations is useful for physicians to select potential off-label chemotherapies or to guide patients toward clinical trials from which he or she would most likely benefit [28].

The oncology field including doctors, testing labs, pharmaceutical firms, patient advocacy groups, and payers are still trying to resolve when genomic testing should be used and importantly when insurers should or will pay for testing and then the treatment recommended based on the genomic analysis. One consortium of these interested parties, the Center for Medical Technology Policy, attempts to offer some guidance recommending payment for comprehensive large panel (greater than 50 genes) testing for a patient who "is newly diagnosed with Stage IV adenocarcinoma of the lung, or is newly diagnosed with carcinoma of unknown primary site, or is newly diagnosed with Stage IV rare or uncommon solid tumors for whom no systemic treatment exists in clinical care guidelines and/or pathways, or is newly diagnosed with Stage IV solid tumors where the median overall survival is less than two years (e.g., pancreatic cancer), or has stage IV solid tumors and has exhausted established guideline-driven systemic therapy options and requisite molecular testing and maintains functional status (ECOG score 0-2), or has newly diagnosed hematologic malignancies with limited treatment options in defined clinical care guidelines" [29]. Alas, payers are not often on board with these types of recommendations yet. Only recently has the FDA approved a large next-generation sequencing panel test by a commercial lab, and CMS is following suit with a favorable coverage decision for next-generation sequencing tests for some advanced cancers for patients who have not had their tumors sequenced previously and who continue to seek treatment for their cancer [30].

The diagnosis of neurologic disorders has advanced through the application of genomic analysis. In hereditary neurologic diseases such as ataxia, Duchenne muscular dystrophy, Cowchock syndrome, or Charcot-Marie-Tooth disease, a genomic diagnosis provides helpful information regarding prognosis, possible treatments, and support for treatment needs [31]. Genetic counseling and prenatal testing for subsequent pregnancies for parents may be offered. For later onset neurologic diseases such as Huntington's disease, patients may or may not want to know, and genetic counseling is vitally important in their care. The genomics of Alzheimer's disease is polygenic and complex [32], beyond solely polymorphism of the APOE gene, but genetic testing identifying patients at risk may allow them to be closely monitored, and treatment started possibly even before the earliest sign of the disease in order to slow progression [33].

The genetic study of cardiovascular disease has identified an extensive list of monogenic disorders, but the phenotypic expression is variable indicating that much remains to be learned regarding other modifying factors in expression of the genetic variants [34]. The causal genetic basis of aortic aneurysms has been linked to mutations of the FBN1 gene in Marfan's syndrome and the COL3A1 gene in vascular Ehlers-Danlos syndrome [35]. For other vascular diseases, the cause and severity are more multifactorial with involvement of at least 19 genes identified as monogenic causes of very low or high levels of LDL cholesterol [34]. Other examples linking gene mutations to cardiovascular disease include mutations in KLHL3 as a cause of hypertension due to familial hyperkalemic hypertension or pseudohypoaldosteronism type II [36, 37] and BAG3 mutations in dilated cardiomyopathy [38].

An emerging area of interest, as the availability of genomic sequencing increases and costs decrease, is the application of genomic medicine into health maintenance [39]. Layering other technologies on to traditional wellness exams including electronic monitoring aids, assessment of metabolomics, and determination of an individual's gut microbiome is being used in pilot projects to tailor lifestyle modification and medical management [40]. Presently, these programs are not covered by insurance payers so are either by self-pay subscription as part of concierge medical practices or clinical research programs. If clinical utility is demonstrated and costs continue to decrease, genomic health will become widespread clinical practice. As hospital systems become increasingly at risk for population health outcomes rather than doing business in pay for service models, then it becomes imperative for hospitals to employ technologies that offer the opportunity to prevent diseases and improve overall health. Physicians are increasingly partnering with hospitals either through employment, joint venture, or accountable care organizations, so it behooves hospitals to provide resources for learning and increased adoption of genomic technologies to physicians in their community as well.

Hospital-Based Programs

Hospitals have a duty to provide value in high-quality healthcare to their patient population. The promise of precision medicine is that applied properly, genomics will allow for targeted screening, timely detection of disease, and more effective treatments with less toxicity, all of which will result in overall cost savings to the healthcare system. The promise has not yet been fulfilled, and the field needs outcome data to demonstrate clinical utility and value. Hospitals must decide how to develop, support, and measure the performance of programs related to precision medicine. Competition amongst demands for resources require that potential return on investment be calculated. As the field is evolving rapidly and outpacing coverage decisions by payers, there are added complexities in adoption of technologies. The investment of hospital resources must be devoted to developing precision medicine.

Staffing and education are essential. Genetic counselors, a medical director, and educational and support staff are required. Genetic counselors are specialists with professional training in medical genetics and in the communication of the selection, interpretation, and use of the results of genetic tests. They may be employed by hospitals or be independent practitioners. Genetic counselors generally will have a bachelor's degree in biology, social science, or a related field and then have received additional specialized training. Master's degrees in genetic counseling are offered by programs accredited by the Accreditation Council for Genetic Counseling (ACGC). Some states also require licensure of genetic counselors. There are currently an estimated 4000 genetic counselors in the United States. The workforce study commissioned by the National Society of Genetic Counselors showed their workforce had grown by 88% from 2006 to 2016, and they identified a need for an additional growth of 72% over the next decade. Therefore, training of additional genetic counselors and additional tools to assist counselors to be more efficient in their delivery of services are needed. Additionally, some hospitals may need to turn to other resources to provide necessary services such as web-based counseling or substitute providers. Genetic counselors often work in concert with a physician who serves as the medical director of the medical genetics program. Support staff to schedule appointments, obtain and collate records, and process insurance approval and billing are needed. Physical clinic space must be provided as well.

Other staff are needed as well. Navigators may be nurses, physician assistants, or other well-trained individuals to welcome and guide patients into programs and through appropriate appointments, tracking outcomes, and assuring compliance. Physicians who are knowledgeable in the field of genomic medicine need to assume leadership roles with resources available to bring necessary technologies. It is likely that physician leaders will be tasked with developing education programs to improve the knowledge and capabilities of existing staff. Staff knowledgeable in the insurance regulations related to genetic and genomic testing assists in securing insurance payment for services.

The integration of genomic data into the clinical information housed in the electronic health records of individual patients is essential in order for the full benefit of precision medicine to be realized [41]. Work flow for physicians and other healthcare providers is at times very inefficient in that clinical data is housed in different locations that do not communicate with each other. It is routine for an EHR to react to a physician order for a medication to which a patient has a known allergy by presenting an alert on the computer screen. Similarly, if a patient has pharmacogenetic data, in his or her EHR, which would suggest an alternative drug or dosing schedule or the increased possibility of an adverse event, then an alert could also come up on the computer screen. The ordering physician would have available links to additional information to further discern the choice of prescribed drug and dose. Furthermore, as germline genomic data such as pharmacogenomics is immutable for each patient, it makes sense for the EHR systems at different facilities to share this data in the interest of patient safety. Alternatively, there should exist a central repository of genomic data that each hospital's EHR could access, and then the relevant information could be downloaded into the EHR. In order for this to be possible, common widely accepted data standards must be adopted. Patients must also have the ability to restrict or grant access to their individual genomic data. Healthcare systems that are integrated with employed or a single contracted medical staff and relatively stable patient populations such as the Geisinger Clinic [42] or Kaiser Permanente may be a good platform to link genomic data to clinical data in their EHR, whereas hospitals that are not closed systems in that their medical staff are largely private practice physicians who are not employed by the hospital also have the challenge of effectively linking outpatient data with inpatient clinical data. The Health Information Technology for Economics and Clinical Health (HITECH) Act of 2009 was designed to promote the meaningful adoption of electronic health records and facilitate sharing of information across platforms [43, 44].

Challenges and Barriers

Precision medicine is a lofty goal but there remain significant barriers to widespread and full implementation. In a survey of physicians and healthcare professionals in North America and Europe, two-thirds of respondents had already seen an improvement in patient outcomes due to the implementation of precision medicine, and 92% believed that the role of precision medicine will continue to increase and eventually replace traditional approaches to care [45]. These same healthcare leaders note that there is a lot of work to be done in the governance, culture, and related information technology. Big data storage with related privacy policies augmented by security safeguards and better annotation by predictive analytics are key hurdles. Investments will be needed to educate healthcare providers in the use of new technologies. Additionally mechanisms for quality assessment and improvement mechanisms have not been developed to evaluate and improve how physicians may use or misuse genomic data. For example, a healthcare system may need to address data that demonstrates some breast surgeons are recommending prophylactic mastectomy based on variants of undermined significance (VUS) in the BRCA1/2 genes if it is happening in their patients [46]. One finding from the same study showed that many of the patients who underwent bilateral mastectomy and had BRCA1/2 VUS had not seen a genetic counselor. The reasons are not clear but may relate to surgeons having incorrect interpretation of the VUS or the lack of availability of a genetic counselor. There exists a shortage of genetic counselors at the same time that there will be a predicted need with the increased use of genetic testing [47]. Conversely, there are advocates for broad genetic testing without what is seen as the restriction of a requirement to see a genetic counselor. The rationales for this opinion include that doctors can be adequately knowledgeable with direct education. Vassy et al. showed that primary care physicians, if supported with access to genetic counselors or medical geneticists, could, after 6 h of training regarding testing whole-genome sequencing, provide pretest counseling, discuss results, and arrange management [48]. The requirement to see a genetic counselor before testing adds a barrier to testing that disproportionately disadvantages women, African Americans, and Latinos [49]. A mandate requiring pretesting genetic counseling by a major insurance payer resulted in a marked increased cancellation rates for genetic testing even for patients for whom testing was recommended per NCCN guidelines. The increased cancellation rates were greatest for patients that were members of a minority group [50, 51]. Additionally, there already exists direct patient access to genetic testing that is provided by commercial labs. Patients may receive results and then seek interpretation and advice for their physician or a genetic counselor. Ultimately, as genetic testing becomes more widely used, multiple points of access to genetic expertise will be needed, and hospitals will be the most likely provider.

Another major challenge revolves around payment and insurance coverage for genetic and genomic testing. Germline testing for BRCA1/2 in patients with breast cancers and insurance coverage for counseling and testing are fairly ubiquitous. Additionally due to mandated coverage by the Affordable Care Act signed into law by President Obama in 2010, women without cancer but who are concerned about their family history of breast or ovarian cancer can obtain counseling and testing. Coverage and payer indications for genetic counseling and testing in other tumor types are also generally available depending on indications. Notably, Medicare does not currently provide coverage for counseling provided by genetic counselors, but this may change if a proposal to include genetic counselors as Medicare providers is adopted.

Lawsuits of failure to obtain genetic testing in accordance with published guidelines have been reported [52]. Potential claims could result alleging that there had been a missed or delayed detection of cancer. A patient in Connecticut sued and was awarded $4 million after she developed ovarian cancer. Her physician failed to suggest genetic testing be done because she had a strong family history of breast cancer [53]. Other cases are being adjudicated related to inaccurate genetic tests, incomplete genetic testing that fails to consider all variants, inaccurate interpretation of the results of genetic testing, complications to drug treatment that could have been avoided with a priori pharmacogenetic testing, and other issues related to genetic testing.

Hospital Programmatic Development

The commitment to delve into and develop robust programs as early adopters of precision medicine requires significant investment. Certain costs can constrain and may indeed be the primary barrier to adoption of precision medicine, but the good news is that sequencing technology is decreasing rapidly [54]. Sources of funds largely include philanthropic sources, industry partnerships, and operational funds. A hospital system is fortunate if it enjoys significant financial and programmatic support from a healthy and committed donor base. The medical industry including informatics platform vendors, testing labs, and pharmaceutical firms all have a potential interest in collaborating with hospital systems that have well-developed clinical data on their patient population to demonstrate clinical utility of their offerings. The allocation of operational funds is subject to competition with other programmatic needs, and service lines within the hospital and decisions are influenced by an assessment of the potential return on the investment. In the case of at-risk care models, ROI may be realized over time and indirectly as manifest by fewer readmissions to the hospital and fewer emergency room visits due to drug adverse events following the implementation of pharmacogenetics [55]. A precision medicine approach resulted in prolonged survival and no increase in costs when compared to traditional chemotherapy or supportive care [56]. Hospitals can develop early detection of cancers based on screening programs targeted to patients at increased genetic risk. Outcomes will be improved but so will utilization of services including additional imaging and screening tests, biopsy procedures, and surgical services. Identification of germline genetic variant will result in cascade testing of family members that may avail themselves of care at the hospital facilities. Lastly, it is hard to quantify the intangible value of the hospital enhancing its reputation by being an early adopter of genomic technologies and precision medicine for the purpose of improved patient care.

Programmatic needs can be looked at in categories including physical space and resources, personnel, and informatics. Personnel decisions include deciding on leadership. Will there be a single leader to shepherd the program forward, and how will the leader be empowered and with what resources? There will need to be administrative support, genetic counselors, nurses and navigators, and a marketing team personnel. These people need to receive training with an ongoing continuous effort, so a senior PhD level educator is required. There need to be funds for membership in professional societies and to support attendance at meetings related to precision medicine. Data support means IRB and HIPPA compliance and information technology support for internal databases, linkage to multicenter system databases, and bioinformatics support. Data coordinators are needed for data entry. Strategic partnerships of nonacademic hospitals with university programs and industry can provide synergy. Hospitals have the patients that can accrue in trials at university hospitals or in industry-sponsored trials. Library and journal access are needed for research and ongoing patient care. Precision medicine programs are ideally linked to hospital clinical research programs so that patients not only have access to novel diagnostic modalities but can get novel therapeutic agents that may be more efficacious due to the genomic variants identified.

It's About the Patient

Ultimately, it is all about the patient receiving the best value in healthcare. Widespread adoption of new technologies does not occur unless one is able to discern how the technology can enhance one's life [57]. So, a focus on the patient means that hospitals need to facilitate enhancing the patients' knowledge regarding the hospital program in precision medicine and how the application of genetics and genomics can enhance the health of the patients and their families. Dedicated staff at the hospital are needed to provide education, along with additional education materials and informational online resources. Logistical support staff are needed to assure samples are properly submitted to testing labs and results are provided to the patients and their doctors and other healthcare providers. Financial counselors and coordinators are needed to help the patient assist in getting lab tests paid and also to assist in getting payment for the treatments recommended based on the results of the genetic tests. For those with financial hardship, knowledge of and guidance in securing existing patient assistance funds are important. Patients can use their own data to promote their own access to precision medicine. A knowledgeable patient can be empowered to be their own best advocate given the appropriate support and assistance.

Summary

The field of precision medicine is rapidly evolving, and there have been notable successes in many fields of medicine resulting in better outcomes for patients with potential cost savings. There remain numerous challenges including the need for healthcare providers to learn about the interpretation and proper use of genomic testing, integration of genomic data into electronic health records, and for payers to reimburse testing when it can help patients. Hospitals will be key entities in the evolving movement toward value-based care; therefore, the modern hospital will need to foster the proper use of genomics to improve the care of patients they serve. The potential rewards are healthier patients, earlier detection of disease, safer drug use, and better outcomes at a lower cost.

References

1. Solomon BJ, Mok T, Kim D-W, et al. First-line crizotinib versus chemotherapy in ALK-positive lung cancer. N Engl J Med. 2014;371:2167–77.
2. Higashi MK, Veenstra DL, Kondo LM, et al. Association between CYP2C9 genetic variants and anticoagulation-related outcomes during warfarin therapy. JAMA. 2002;287:1690–8.
3. Rieder MJ, Reiner AP, Gage BF, et al. Effect of VKORC1 haplotypes on transcriptional regulation and warfarin dose. N Engl J Med. 2005;352:2285–93.
4. Shehab N, Sperling LS, Kegler SR, Budnitz DS. National estimates of emergency department visits for hemorrhage-related adverse events from clopidogrel plus aspirin and from warfarin. Arch Intern Med. 2010;170:1926–33.
5. Klein TE, et al. International warfarin pharmacogenomics consortium. Estimation of warfarin dose with clinical and pharmacogenetic data. N Engl J Med. 2009;360:753–64.
6. Link E, Parish S, Armitage J, et al. SLCO1B1 variants and statin-induced myopathy – a genomewide study. N Engl J Med. 2008;359:789–99.
7. Voora D, Ginsburg GS. Clinical application of cardiovascular pharmacogenetics. J Am Coll Cardiol. 2012;60:9–20.
8. Kuntz TM, Gilbert JA. Introducing the microbiome into precision medicine. Trends Pharmacol Sci. 2017;38:81–91.
9. Shreiner AB, Kao JY, Young VB. The gut microbiome in health and in disease. Curr Opin Gastroenterol. 2015;31:69–75.
10. Haiser HJ, Turnbaugh PJ. Developing a metagenomic view of xenobiotic metabolism. Pharmacol Res. 2013;69:21–31.
11. Saad R, Rizkallah MR, Aziz RK. Gut pharmacomicrobiomics: the tip of an iceberg of complex interactions between drugs and gut-associated microbes. Gut Pathogens. 2012;4:16–29.
12. Rizkallah MR, Gamal-Eldin S, Saad R, Aziz RK. The pharmacomicrobiomics portal: a database for drug-microbiome interactions. Curr Pharmacogenomics Person Med. 2012;10:195–203.

13. Vétizou M, Pitt JM, Daillère R, et al. Anticancer immunotherapy by CTLA-4 blockade relies on the gut microbiota. Science. 2015;350:1079–84.
14. Duhigg C. How companies learn your secrets. New York Times magazine. Feb 16, 2012.
15. Levey DF, Niculescu EM, Le-Niculescu H, et al. Towards understanding and predicting suicidality in women: biomarkers and clinical risk assessment. Mol Psychiatry. 2016;21(6):768–85.
16. Niculescu AB, Levey DF, Phalen PL, et al. Understanding and predicting suicidality using a combined genomic and clinical risk assessment approach. Mol Psychiatry. 2015;20:1266–85.
17. Cohen JD, Li L, Wang Y, et al. Detection and localization of surgically resectable cancers with a multi-analyte blood test. Science. 2018;359:926–30.
18. Ballinger ML, Best A, Pai ML, et al. Baseline surveillance in li-Faumeni syndrome using whole-body magnetic resonance imaging: a meta-analysis. JAMA Oncol. 2017;3:1634.
19. Bojadzieva J, Amini B, Day SF, et al. Whole body magnetic resonance imaging (WB-MRI) and brain MRI baseline surveillance in TP53 germline mutation carriers: experience from the Li-Fraumeni syndrome education and early detection (LEAD) clinic. Familial Cancer. 2018;17:287. https://doi.org/10.1007/s10689-017-0034-6.
20. Dancey JE, Bedard PL, Onetto N, Hudson TJ. The genetic basis for cancer treatment decisions. Cell. 2012;148:409–20.
21. Kuijer A, Straver M, den Dekker B, et al. Impact of 70-gene signature use on adjuvant chemotherapy decisions in patients with estrogen receptor–positive early breast cancer: results of a prospective cohort study. J Clin Oncol. 2017;35:2814–9.
22. Loncaster J, Armstrong A, Howell S, et al. Impact of oncotype DX breast recurrence score testing on adjuvant chemotherapy use in early breast cancer: real world experience in greater Manchester, UK. Eur J Surg Oncol. 2017;43:931–7.
23. Kris MG, Johnson BE, Berry LD, et al. Using multiplexed assays of oncogenic drivers in lung cancers to select targeted drugs. JAMA. 2014;311:1998–2006.
24. Ramalingam SS, Yang JCH, Lee CK, et al. Osimertinib as first-line treatment of EGFR mutation–positive advanced non–small-cell lung cancer. J Clin Oncol. 2017;36(9):841–9. Epub ahead of print.
25. Von Hoff DD, Stephenson JJ Jr, Rosen P, Loesch DM, Borad MJ, Anthony S, et al. Pilot study using molecular profiling of patients' tumors to find potential targets and select treatments for their refractory cancers. J Clin Oncol. 2010;28(33):4877–83. https://doi.org/10.1200/JCO.2009.26.5983.
26. Kato S, Kurasaki K, Ikeda S, Kurzrock R. Rare tumor clinic: the University of san Diego Moores Cancer Center experience with a precision therapy approach. Oncologist. 2018;23:171–8.
27. Greenlee RT, Goodman MT, Lynch CF, et al. The occurrence of rare cancers in U.S. adults, 1995-2004. Public Health Rep. 2010;125:28–43.
28. Schwaederle M, Zhao M, Lee JJ, et al. Impact of precision medicine in diverse cancers: a meta-analysis of phase II clinical trials. J Clin Oncol. 2015;33:3817–25.
29. http://www.cmtpnet.org/docs/resources/Full_Release_Version_August_13__2015.pdf. Accessed Feb 1, 2018.
30. https://www.cms.gov/medicare-coverage-database/details/nca-proposed-decision-memo.aspx?NCAId=290&bc=AAAAAAAAAAQAAA%3D%3D. Accessed February 5, 2018.
31. Huang Y, Yu S, Wu Z, Tang B. Genetics of hereditary neurologic disorders in children. Transl Pediatr. 2014;3:108–19.
32. Escott-Price V, Shoai M, Pither R, Williams J. Polygenic score prediction captures nearly all common genetic risk for Alzheimer's disease. Neurobiol Aging. 2017;49:214.e7–11.
33. Crous-Bou M, Minguillon C, Gramunt N, Molinuevo JL. Alzheimer's disease prevention: from risk factors to early intervention. Alzheimers Res Ther. 2017;9:71–80.
34. Kathiresan S, Srivastava D. Genetics of human cardiovascular disease. Cell. 2012;148:1242–57.
35. Superti-Furga A, Gugler E, Gitzelmann R, Steinmann B. Ehlers-Danlos syndrome type IV: a multi-exon deletion in one of the two COL3A1 alleles affecting structure, stability, and processing of type III procollagen. J Biol Chem. 1988;263:6226–32.
36. Boyden LM, Choi M, Choate KA, et al. Mutations in kelch-like 3 and cullin 3 cause hypertension and electrolyte abnormalities. Nature. 2012;482:98–102.
37. Glover M, Ware JS, Henry A, et al. Detection of mutations in KLHL3 and CUL3 in families with FHHt (familial hyperkalaemic hypertension or Gordon's syndrome). Clin Sci (Lond). 2014;126:721–6.
38. Norton N, Li D, Rieder MJ, et al. Genome-wide studies of copy number variation and exome sequencing identify rare variants in BAG3 as a cause of dilated cardiomyopathy. Am J Hum Genet. 2011;88:273–82.
39. Patel CJ, Sivadas A, Tabassum R, et al. Whole genome sequencing in support of wellness and health maintenance. Genome Med. 2013;5:58–61.
40. Price ND, Magis AT, Earls JC, et al. A wellness study of 108 individuals using personal, dense, dynamic data clouds. Nat Biotech. 2017;35:747–56.
41. Sitapati A, Kim H, Berkovich B, et al. Integrated precision medicine: the role of electronic health records in delivering personalized treatment. WIREs Syst Biol Med. 2017;9:e1378. https://doi.org/10.1002/wsbm.1378.
42. Carey DJ, Fetterolf SN, Davis FD, et al. The Geisinger MyCode community health initiative: an electronic health record-linked biobank for precision medicine research. Genet Med. 2016;18:906–13. https://doi.org/10.1038/gim.2015.187.
43. Blumenthal D. Lauching HITECH. N Engl J Med. 2010;362:382–5.

44. Waldren S, Kibbe D, Mitchell J. "Will the feds really buy me an EHR?" and other commonly asked questions about the HITECH Act. Fam Pract Manag. 2009;16:19–23.
45. Davis J. Providers say they're ready to progress to precision medicine. Healthcare IT News. May 2016. Retrieved from: http://www.healthcareitnews.com/news/providers-say-theyre-ready-progress-precision-medicine.
46. Kurian AW, Li Y, Hamilton AS, et al. Gaps in incorporating germline genetic testing into treatment decision-making for early-stage breast cancer. J Clin Oncol. 2017;35:2232–9.
47. Hoskovec JM, Bennett RL, Carey ME, et al. Projecting the supply and demand for certified genetic counselors: a workforce study. J Genetic Couns. 2017;27:16. https://doi.org/10.1007/s10897-017-0158-8.
48. Vassy JL, Christensen KD, Schonman EF, et al. The impact of whole-genome sequencing on primary care and outcomes of healthy adult patients. Ann Intern Med. 2017;167:159–69.
49. Hughes KS. Genetic testing: what problem are we trying to solve? J Clin Oncol. 2017;35:3789–92.
50. Whitworth P, Beitsch P, Arnell C, et al. Impact of payer constraints on access to genetic counseling. J Oncol Pract. 2017;13:e47–56.
51. Childers CP, Childers KK, Maggard-Gibbons M, et al. National estimates of genetic testing in women with a history of breast cancer or ovarian cancer. J Clin Oncol. 2017;35:3800–6.
52. Merchant GE, Lindor RA. Personalized medicine and genetic malpractice. Genet Med. 2013;15:921–2. https://doi.org/10.1038/gim.2013.142.
53. Downs v Trias, 49 A.3d 180 (Conn. 2012).
54. Real-world precision medicine: challenges and opportunities in hospitals across the US *in* Becker's Hospital review. June 12, 2017.
55. Elliott LS, Henderson JC, Neradilek MB, et al. Clinical impact of pharmacogenomics profiling with a clinical decision support tool in polypharmacy home health patients: a prospective pilot randomized controlled trial. PLoS One. 2017;12:1–16. https://doi.org/10.1371/journal.pone.0170905.
56. Haslem DS, Van Norman SB, Fulde G, et al. A retrospective analysis of precision medicine outcomes in patients with advanced cancer reveals improved progression free survival without increased health care costs. J Oncol Pract. 2017;13:e108–19.
57. Moore GA. Crossing the chasm: marketing and selling disruptive products to mainstream customers. 3rd ed. New York: Harper Collins; 2014.

Nanotechnology: Managing Molecules for Modern Medicine

14

Russell J. Andrews

Introduction

Medicine has been using nanotechnology for millennia – any process involving molecular interactions is in essence a nanotechnique. More recently nano-sized particles have been employed in more technically advanced medical applications, e.g., the MRI contrast agent gadolinium is a particle of nanometer dimensions.

The term nanotechnology comes from the Greek *nanos* – dwarf. One nanometer is 10^{-9} meter (m); one micron (μ) equals 1000 nanometers (nm) or 10^{-6} m (Fig. 14.1) [1]. However, more important than the small size of the nanorealm (1–100 nm) is the concept of constructing or manipulating materials molecule by molecule or atom by atom – as opposed to cutting materials smaller (the traditional key to precision surgery and precision manufacturing alike). Top-down molecular etching (nanolithography) and bottom-up particle deposition or self-assembly are the keys to nanotechnology – for both medical and industrial applications.

A brief introduction to the advantages of working at the nanoscale for sensing – from bacteria and toxin detection to DNA and troponin monitoring – is appropriate. In a 2016 article entitled "Toward the Responsible Development and Commercialization of Sensor Nanotechnologies" (whose authors were from the National Nanotechnology Coordination Office, the National Cancer Institute, the National Institute for Occupational Safety and Health, and the Center for Nanotechnology, NASA Ames Research Center), the following definition of a sensor is provided:

> A sensor produces a measurable signal as a result of physical, chemical, biological or any combination of the aforementioned stimuli. [2]

Several sensing transduction methods and the relevant nanomaterials employed are provided in Fig. 14.2 [2]. Additionally, three unique physiochemical characteristics of engineered nanomaterials (ENMs) advantageous for sensing are described:

> First, the high surface-to-volume ratio of materials at the nanoscale allows for enhanced chemical reactivity, a feature that can be modulated by particle type, shape, and surface topography. Second, the ability to precisely craft nanomaterials with functional ligands can confer single-molecule sensitivity and specificity. Third, an important attribute of ENMs is the possibility to engineer them as highly integrated systems that can offer more rapid and multiplexed detection of analytes using advanced transduction mechanisms. [2]

The field of nanoparticles for applications such as selective targeting of cancer cells – to enhance both diagnosis and therapy – is well known and will not be repeated here. This

R. J. Andrews (✉)
Department of Nanotechnology & Smart Systems, NASA Ames Research Center, Moffett Field, CA, USA
e-mail: rja@russelljandrews.org

R. Latifi (ed.), *The Modern Hospital*, https://doi.org/10.1007/978-3-030-01394-3_14

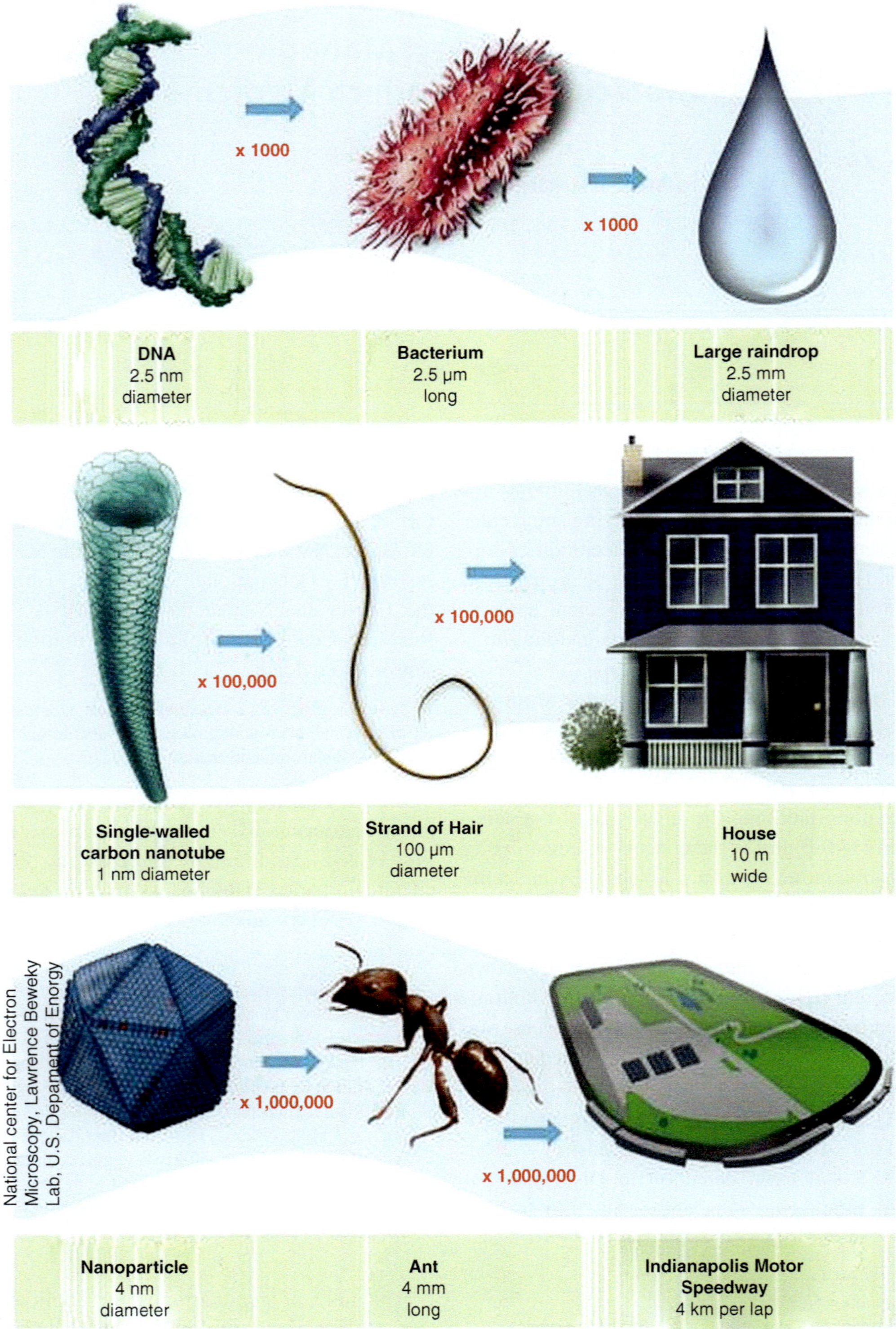

Fig. 14.1 Examples of the nanoscale. (Reprinted from National Nanotechnology Coordination Office [1]. https://www.nano.gov/nanotech-101/what/nano-size. Used with permission from the Creative Commons License 3.0: https://creativecommons.org/licenses/by/3.0/us/?utm_source=www.domtail.com)

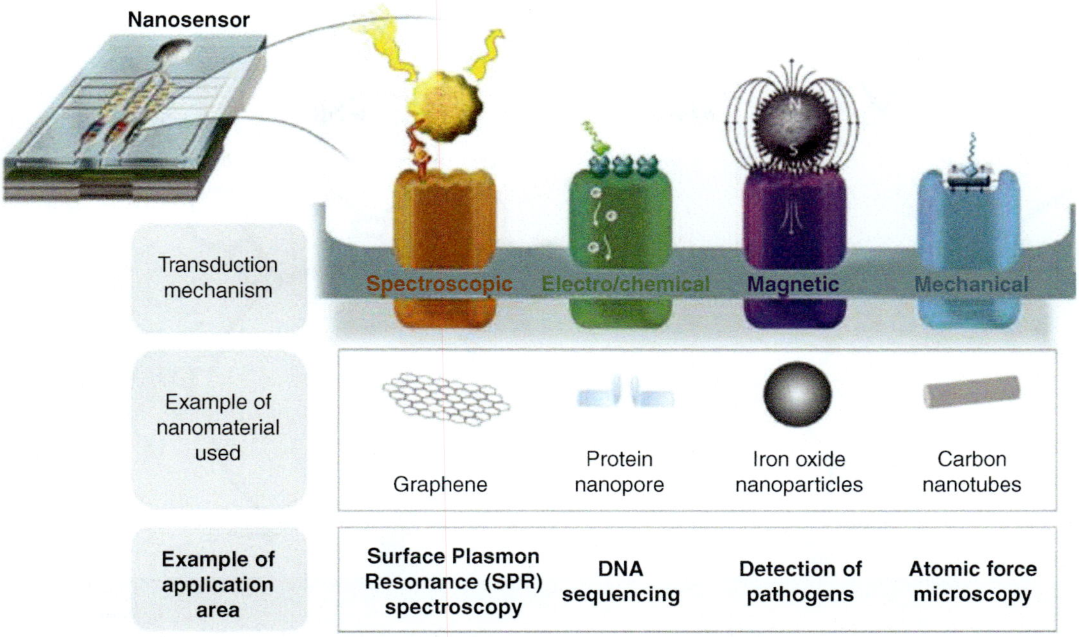

Fig. 14.2 Types of nanosensors. (Reprinted with permission from Fadel et al. [2]. © (2016) American Chemical Society)

chapter provides an overview of nanotechnology for modern medicine by presenting several other examples:

1. Nanotechnologies for inexpensive point-of-care (POC) testing
2. Wearable devices for real-time continuous diagnosis and therapy, as well as energy harvesting
3. Nanoparticles to enhance the effectiveness of radiation therapy (RT)
4. Nanotechnology to enhance the brain-machine interface (BMI) for precision monitoring and modulating of brain electrochemical activity

Nanotechnologies for Inexpensive Point-of-Care (POC) Testing

The past decade has seen dramatic advances in nanotechniques for inexpensive POC testing – progress essential for increasing the scope of health care into more universal settings beyond traditional (typically quite expensive) laboratory instruments. Examples include detection of (1) C-reactive protein (CRP) using a carbon nanofiber-based sensor [3] and (2) cardiac troponin 1 (for acute myocardial infarction) using silicon nanowire field-effect transistors [4]. Perhaps even more impressive is a recent report on the fabrication of disposable paper-based sensors for DNA detection [5]. This approach uses room-temperature, solvent-less plasma-enhanced chemical vapor deposition to produce a DNA sensor that is rapid, highly sensitive, and low cost.

Another application of sensors is for detection of pathogens (e.g., bacteria) and toxins (from noxious gases to nerve agents). Regarding the former, a recent article documents a graphene biosensor in which binding of the *Escherichia coli* bacteria results in a measurable electrical signal [6]. Graphene is a two-dimensional form of carbon atoms in a hexagonal lattice (i.e., resembling chicken wire) that has several remarkable properties, perhaps the most relevant for this application being its high electronic conductivity. To selectively detect *E. coli*, a sensing probe consisting of a pyrene-tagged DNA aptamer (PTDA) attached to the graphene undergoes a

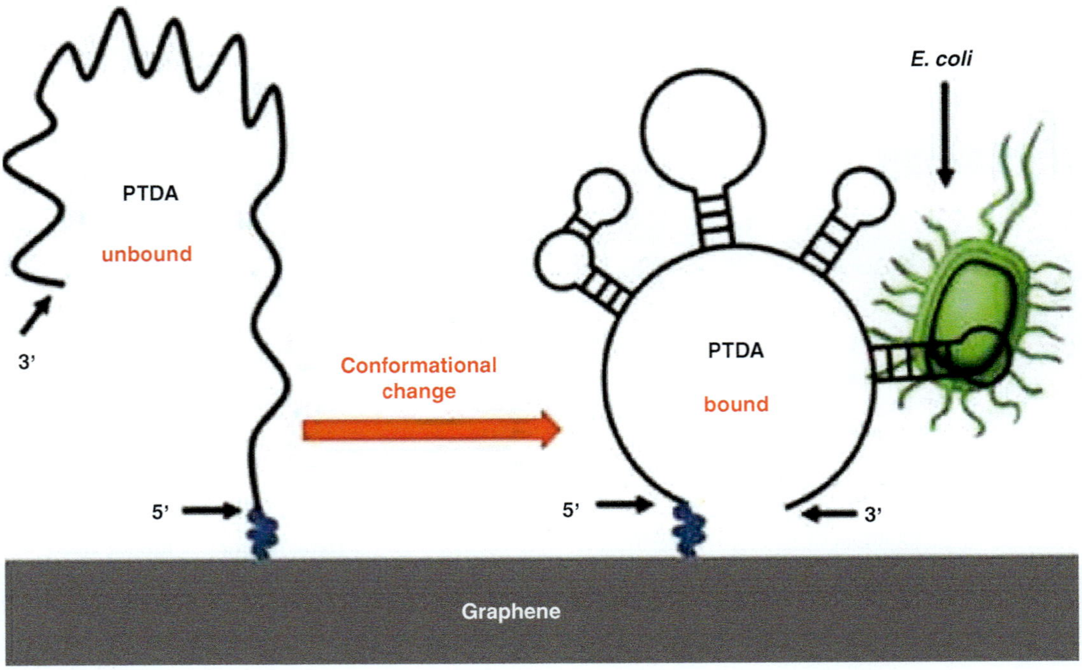

Fig. 14.3 Graphene biosensor for *E. coli* (see text for abbreviations). (Reprinted from Wu et al. [6]. With permission from John Wiley & Sons)

conformational change that results in a detectable current (Fig. 14.3) [6].

Regarding the detection of toxins, the gas methane is one of the several environmental pollutants of concern – methane being an order of magnitude more detrimental than carbon dioxide as a greenhouse gas, explosive when its concentration exceeds 10% in air, and a major component of natural gas. Specially functionalized carbon nanotubes have been used to fabricate a sensor that can distinguish between methane, sulfur dioxide, and ammonia, with the advantages over conventional sensing methods of being smaller, less expensive, and more efficient with regard to power consumption [7]. Nano-multisensor devices promise to fill the need for an "E-nose"; integration of the sensor with a smartphone has been demonstrated (Fig. 14.4) [7].

Flexible and Wearable Nanodevices

Flexible nanodevices have many applications in future medicine – from incorporating into the fabric of clothing (e.g., to monitor toxic gases in the wearer's environment), to monitoring parameters ranging from heart rate to body chemistries (e.g., blood glucose) both easily and continuously, to improving wound healing (e.g., in burn patients). Figure 14.5 illustrates how flexible graphene gas nanosensors are incorporated into fabric [8]. Figure 14.6 shows a nanofabricated "Band-Aid" for continuous pulse monitoring [8].

Patches or Band-Aids with microneedles are being fabricated for continuous and minimally invasive monitoring of body fluids (e.g., blood glucose) [9]. The polymer gel microneedles are so small the sensation when the patch is applied is similar to touching Velcro. Moreover, the microneedles swell and become soft with use – so when they are removed, there is no danger of a needle-stick injury and potential infection.

Three-dimensional printed cellulose nanofibrils will likely have numerous medical applications. They possess desirable properties such as flexibility, liquid (e.g., tissue fluid) absorption, ability to act as a carrier of proteins, and biodegradability [10]. One application is wound care, especially in burn patients, where the properties of fluid absorption and protein delivery are desirable;

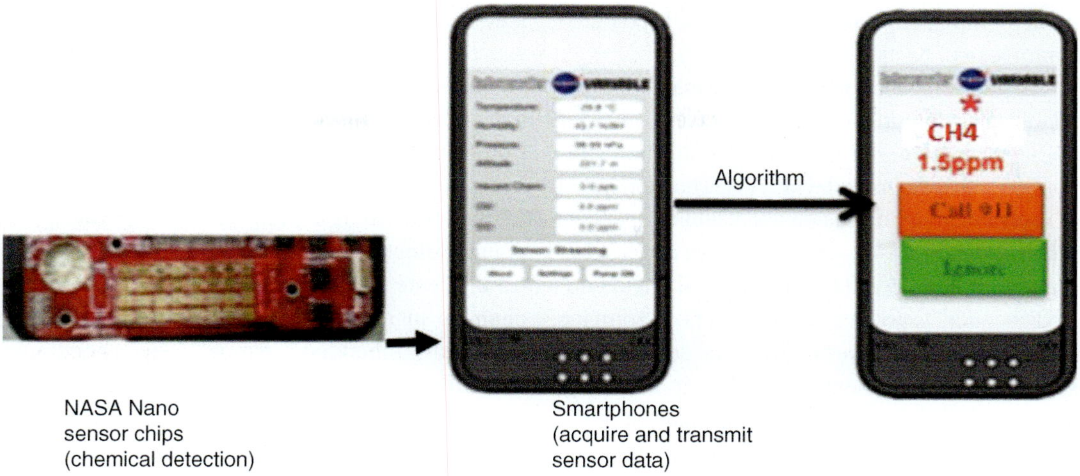

Fig. 14.4 "E-nose" toxic chemical nanosensor + smartphone. (Reprinted from Hannon et al. [7]. With permission from the Creative Commons License 4.0: https://creativecommons.org/licenses/by/4.0/)

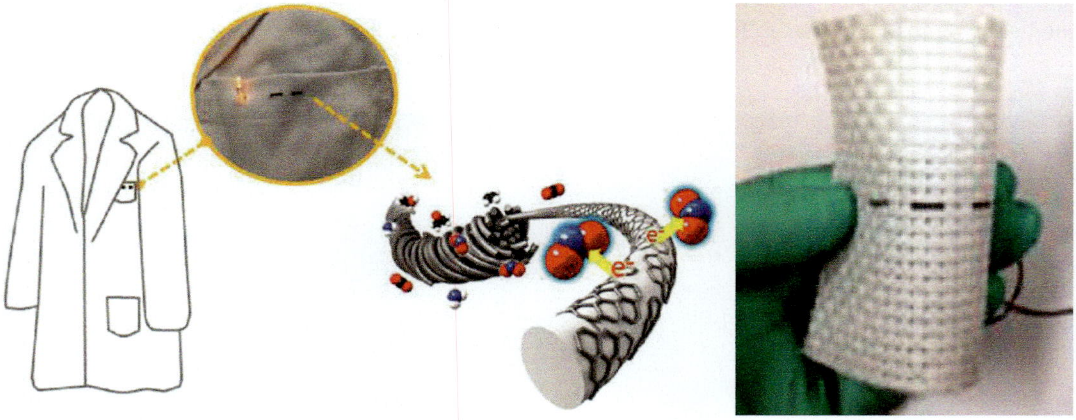

Fig. 14.5 Left: schematic of nanosensor in fabric yarn. Right: resulting "nanosensor" cloth. (Reprinted with permission from Singh et al. [8]. © (2017) American Chemical Society)

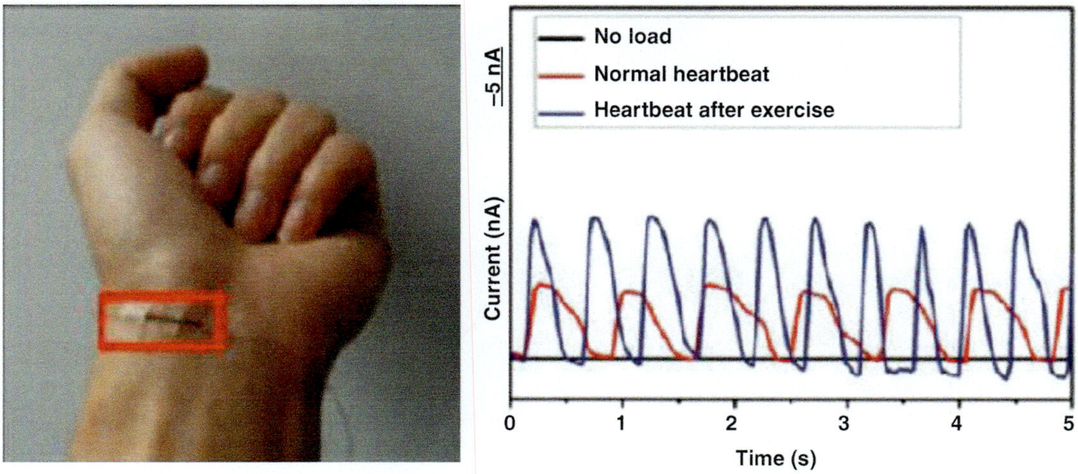

Fig. 14.6 Nanofabricated "Band-Aid" for continuous pulse monitoring. (Reprinted with permission from Singh et al. [8]. © (2017) American Chemical Society)

tissue temperature and pH are other potential parameters to be monitored (Fig. 14.7).

Another application using flexible cellulose nanofibrils – important for wearable electronics for both information storage and identification purposes – is as a memory device [11]. The fabrication of such a memory device on nanocellulose paper is illustrated in Fig. 14.8 [11]. It involves inkjet printing to form the top and bottom electrodes and initiated chemical vapor deposition (iCVD) to form the resistive switching layer (RSL). One advantage of such paper-based memory is that it is readily destroyed by simple burning – important in medical applications where privacy and security are major concerns. Examples of the conformable nature of these nanocellulose paper-based memory devices are provided in Fig. 14.9 [11].

For remote POC testing, a self-powered medical diagnostic device is clearly more desirable than a device requiring an outside energy source (e.g., conventional electric current or a battery). Various methods of energy harvesting have been proposed, from piezoelectric generation (where changes in pressure are converted into electricity) to triboelectric generation (TEG – in which a nanostructured surface and contact electrification plus electrostatic induction create electricity when subjected to changes in mechanical force) [12]. A floating oscillator-embedded triboelectric generator (FO-TEG) has been described which can power an LED array solely by the motion of a human runner (Fig. 14.10) [12]. Such techniques make self-contained wearable diagnostic and therapeutic medical devices feasible. A prototype self-powered, paper-based diagnostic device for POC blood testing utilizing TEG has been described [13].

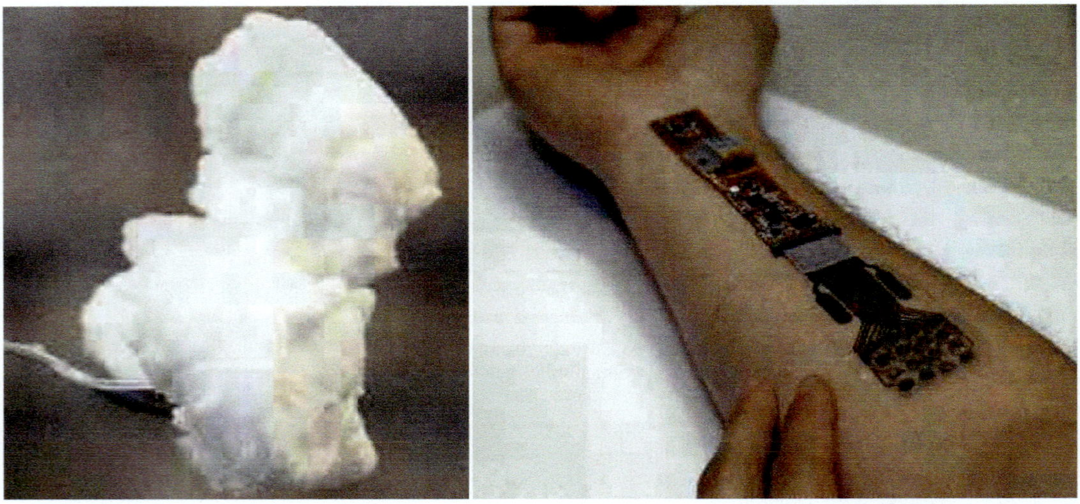

Fig. 14.7 Left: nanocellulose. Right: prototype nanocellulose wound care monitor. (Courtesy of VTT)

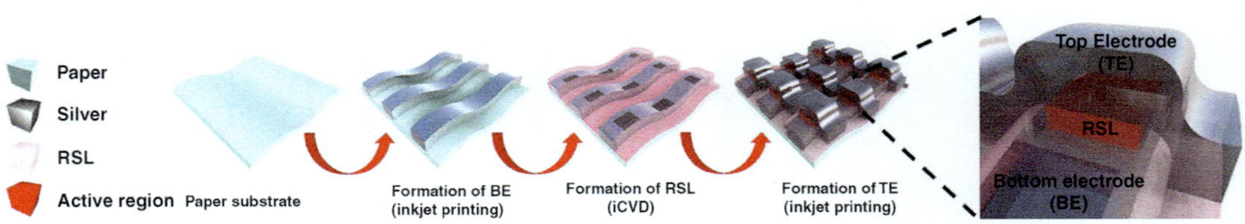

Fig. 14.8 Fabrication of nanocellulose paper memory device for wearable electronics. (Reprinted from Lee et al. [11]. With permission from the Creative Commons License 4.0: https://creativecommons.org/licenses/by/4.0/)

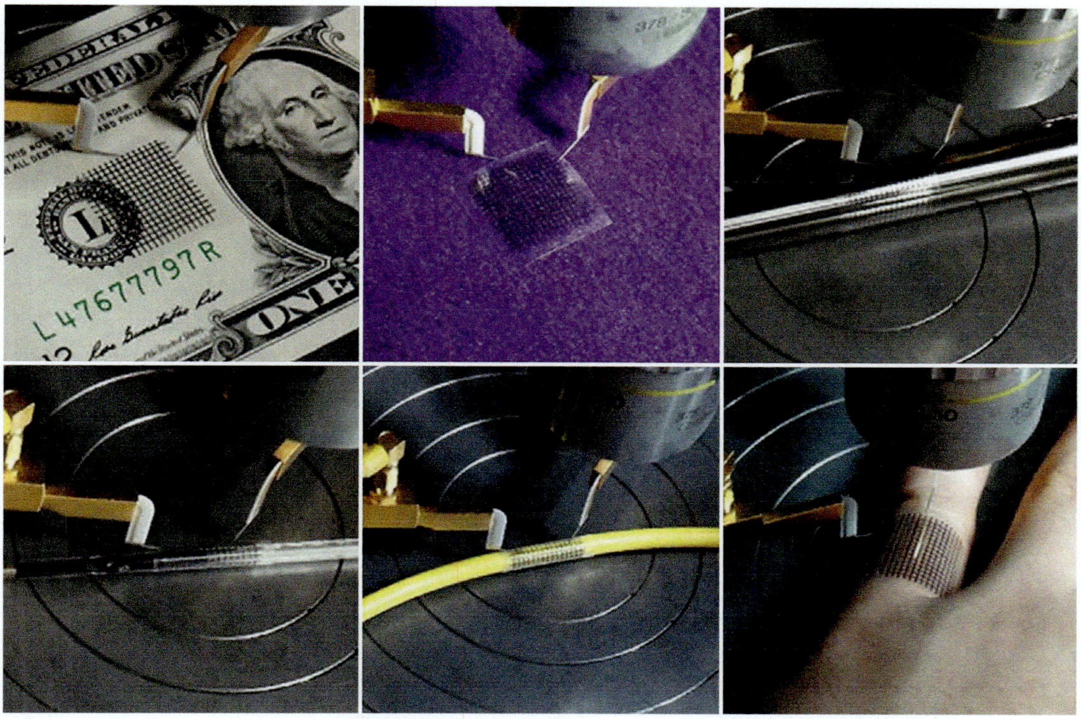

Fig. 14.9 Conformability and potential applications of nanocellulose paper-based memory. (Reprinted from Lee et al. [11]. With permission from the Creative Commons License 4.0: https://creativecommons.org/licenses/by/4.0/)

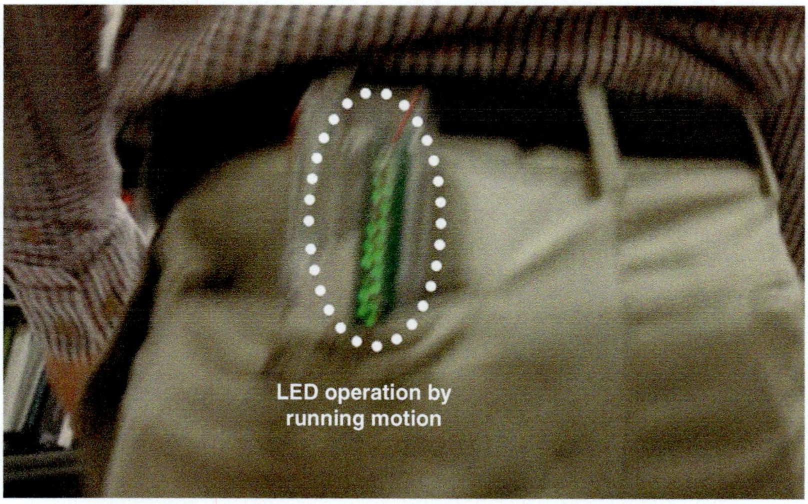

Fig. 14.10 LED array powered by a runner using a triboelectric generator (TEG). (Reprinted from Seol et al. [12]. With permission from the Creative Commons License 4.0: https://creativecommons.org/licenses/by/4.0/)

Nanoparticles for Radiation Therapy

There are numerous examples where interactions of nanoparticles (NPs) with molecules or cells are used for therapeutic purposes. One such area is the use of NPs to enhance the biological effect of radiation therapy (RT) on tumor cells [14, 15]. As an example – because of its progress into extensive clinical trials – the use of hafnium oxide NPs activated by radiotherapy for cancer treatment is considered here.

Hafnium oxide NPs belong to the class of transition metals that possess a high electron density. These NPs are characterized by one single intratumoral administration and designed for cancer cell uptake. Once injected, they can be activated solely by ionizing radiations such as RT yielding a tumor-localized high-energy deposit and increased cell death compared to the same dose of radiation (Fig. 14.11). Hafnium oxide NPs were successfully evaluated in a phase II/III trial in patients with locally advanced soft tissue sarcoma [NCT01433068] and are currently evaluated in phase I/II for head and neck squamous cell carcinoma [NCT01946867; NCT02901483] and prostate [NCT02805894], liver [NCT02721056], rectum [NCT02465593], and recurrent/metastatic head and neck squamous cell carcinoma or metastatic non-small cell lung cancer [NCT03589339] [16, 17]. Interestingly, hafnium oxide NPs for cancer treatment are considered to be a drug by the Food and Drug Administration (FDA) in the USA but a device in the EU.

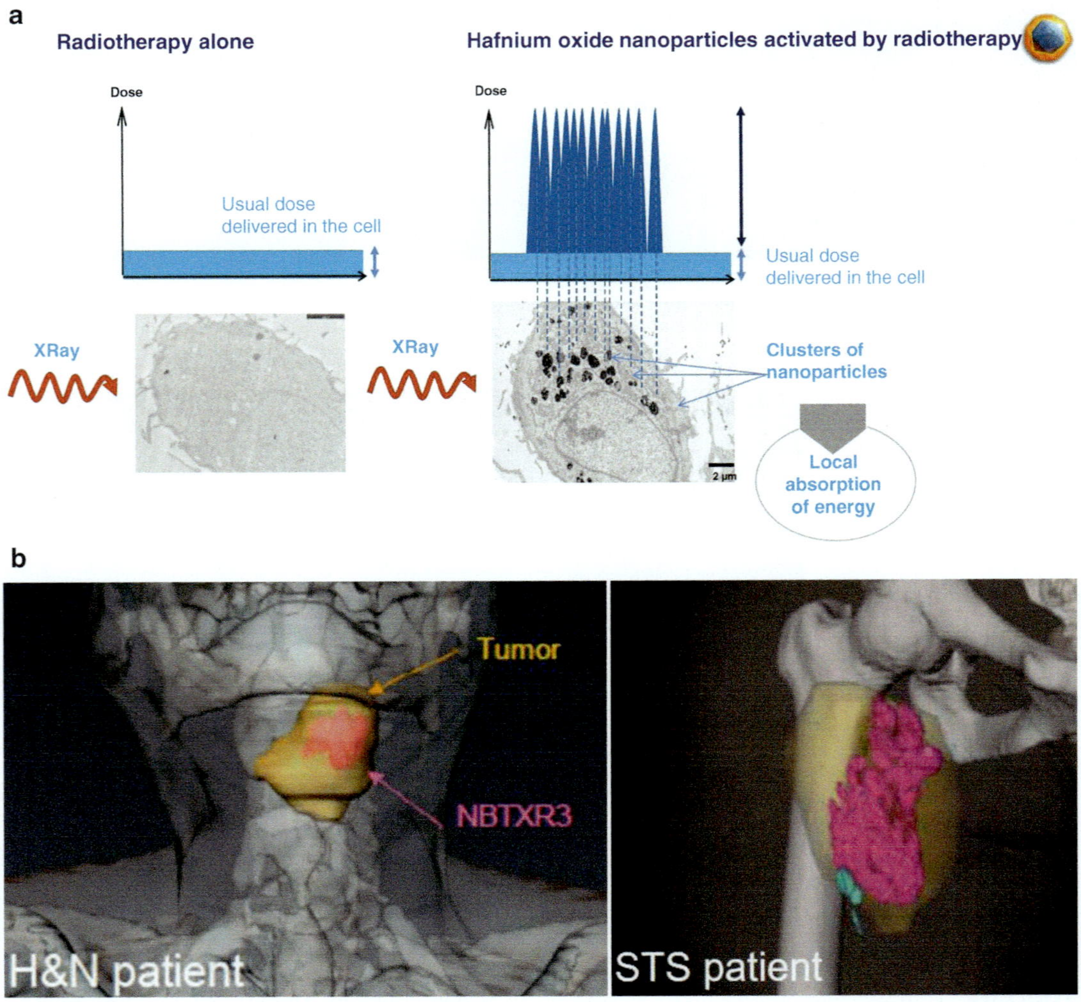

Fig. 14.11 (**a**) Schematic of increased intratumoral electron generation due to hafnium oxide nanoparticles (NBTXR3). (**b**) Intratumoral administration of hafnium oxide nanoparticles in patients with head and neck squamous cell carcinoma (H&N) and locally advanced soft tissue sarcoma (STS). (Courtesy of Nanobiotix)

Nanotechnology to Enhance the Brain-Machine Interface (BMI)

Traditional methods of monitoring brain electrical function include, most commonly, the electroencephalogram (EEG). The EEG has the advantage of being noninvasive but has the disadvantage of each electrode recording electrical activity from a large volume of brain tissue. This can be acceptable for detecting gross events such as seizure activity but is of little use in understanding brain function at a more precise (e.g., neuronal) level. Similarly, traditional therapeutic brain stimulation methods such as (1) transcranial magnetic stimulation (TMS) and (2) deep brain stimulation (DBS) also lack precision – and in the case of DBS – have the disadvantage of requiring a surgical procedure to implant the electrode(s).

Thus considerable effort is being spent to develop more precise methods of monitoring brain electrical activity. The most advanced device to date is Neuropixels – a microelectrode 1 cm in length, 20 × 70 microns in cross section, and containing 960 recording sites (each approximately 20 microns across) which can be individually addressed (up to 384 sites at a time) (Fig. 14.12) [18]. Each site is composed of titanium nitride and is complementary metal-oxide-semiconductor (CMOS) compatible. Although tens of microns are not quite within the strict definition of the nanorealm, when multiple such electrodes are implanted, in vivo recording in rodents allows resolution of single neuron electrical activity.

Brain function depends on both electrical and chemical (i.e., neurotransmitter (NT)) activities. Until recently less progress had been made regarding precise localization of brain chemical activity due to a lack of appropriate monitoring equipment. Standard techniques such as fast-scan cyclic voltammetry and differential pulse voltammetry (DPV) using traditional (glassy carbon) microelectrodes are reasonably successful at detecting and monitoring a single NT (e.g., dopamine or serotonin – two NTs involved in severe depression and other mood disorders) – but when

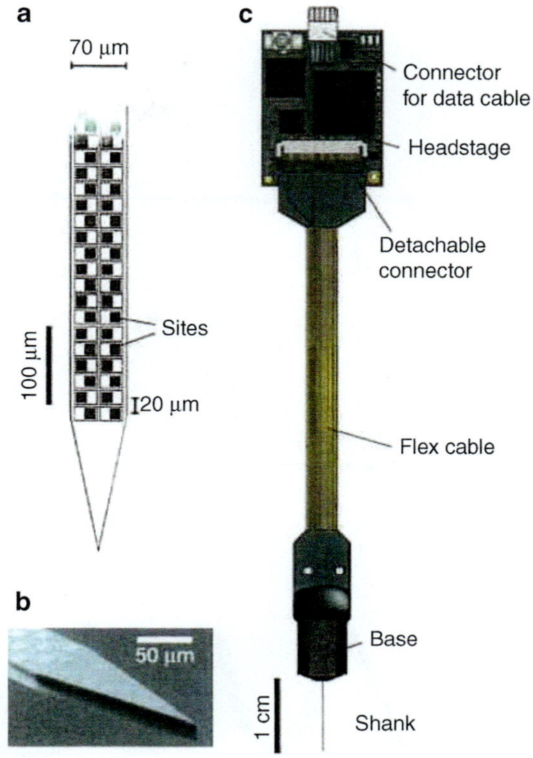

Fig. 14.12 (**a**) Illustration of sensing portion, showing checkerboard site layout (dark squares). (**b**) Scanning electron microscope image of probe tip. (**c**) Probe packaging, including flex cable and headstage for bidirectional data transmission. (Reprinted from Jun et al. [18]. With permission from Springer Nature)

in an environment similar to that in brain tissue (in which ascorbic acid is ubiquitous), traditional microelectrodes suffer from substantial cross talk that precludes monitoring multiple NTs in close proximity. However, appropriately characterized nanoelectrodes are capable of distinguishing dopamine and serotonin in the presence of ascorbic acid (Fig. 14.13) [19].

Another major advantage of nanoelectrodes is the improved charge transfer over metal electrodes – resulting in orders of magnitude decrease in impedance and increase in capacitance [20, 21]. The improvement is likely due in part to the greatly increased surface area of nanoelectrodes as well as the coating of the electrodes with conductive polymers [21]. These advances not only improve the sensitivity of

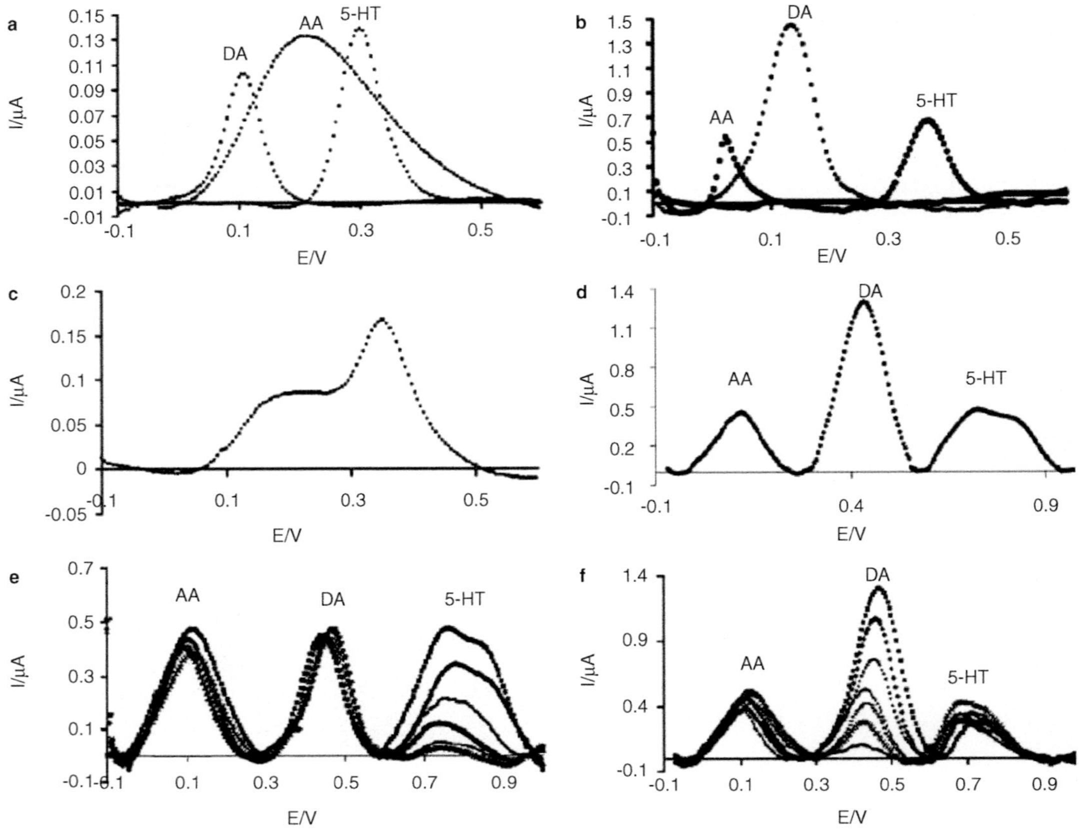

Fig. 14.13 (**a**) Baseline-corrected DPV plots of individual detection of 10 mM DA (dopamine), 1 mM AA (ascorbic), and 10 mM 5-HT (5-hydroxytriptamine – serotonin) with a glassy carbon electrode; (**b**) baseline-corrected DPV plots of individual detection of 10 mM DA, 1 mM AA, and 10 mM 5-HT with a carbon nanofiber electrode; (**c**) baseline-corrected DPV plots of a ternary mixture of 10 mM DA, 1 mM AA, and 10 mM 5-HT with a glassy carbon electrode; (**d**) baseline-corrected DPV plots of a ternary mixture of 10 mM DA, 1 mM AA, and 10 mM 5-HT with a carbon nanofiber electrode; (**e**) baseline-corrected DPV plots of a ternary mixture of 1 mM AA, 10 mM DA, and 5-HT (10 mM, 5 mM, 2.5 mM, 1 mM, 0.5 mM, and 0.25 mM) with a carbon nanofiber electrode; (**f**) baseline-corrected DPV plots of a ternary mixture of 1 mM AA, 10 mM 5-HT, and DA (10 mM, 5 mM, 2.5 mM,1 mM, 0.5 mM, 0.25 mM, and 0.1 mM) with a carbon nanofiber electrode. (Reprinted from Rand et al. [19]. With permission from Elsevier)

electrical activity monitoring but also allow equivalent stimulation of brain tissue with much less risk of electrolysis (i.e., permanent brain injury due to excessive charge).

The greatest advance in the treatment of movement disorders (notably Parkinson's disease) over the past half century has been DBS, as initially discovered serendipitously by Benabid and colleagues in France in the late 1980s. However, DBS has been much less successful in treating epilepsy and disabling mood disorders (e.g., depression, schizophrenia) – which afflict many more people worldwide than Parkinson's disease and other movement disorders. The possibility of understanding the electrical and chemical changes underlying these nervous system disorders – because we have the tools to understand brain electrical and chemical activity in both health and disease – makes the application of nanotechnology to the BMI one of the most exciting aspects of nanotechnology for modern medicine.

References

1. National Nanotechnology Coordination Office. Nanotechnology: big things from a tiny world. Downloaded from website www.nano.gov. Feb 11, 2018.
2. Fadel TR, Farrell DF, Friederesdorf LE, et al. Toward the responsible development and commercialization of sensor nanotechnologies. ACS Sens. 2016;1:207–16.
3. Gupta RK, Periyakaruppan A, Meyyappan M, Koehne JE. Label-free detection of C-reactive protein using a carbon nanofiber based biosensor. Biosens Bioelectron. 2014;59:112–9.
4. Kim K, Park C, Kwon D, et al. Silicon nanowire biosensors for detection of cardiac troponin 1 (cTn1) with high sensitivity. Biosens Bioelectron. 2016;77:695–701.
5. Gandhiraman RP, Nordlund D, Jayan V, Meyyappan M, Koehne JE. Scalable low-cost fabrication of disposable paper sensors for DNA detection. ACS Appl Mater Interfaces. 2014;6:22751–60.
6. Wu G, Dai Z, Tang X, et al. Biosensing: graphene field-effect transistors for the sensitive and selective detection of *Escherichia coli* using pyrene-tagged DNA aptamer. Adv Healthc Mater. 2017;6(19):1700736 (9pp). https://doi.org/10.1002/adhm.201700736.
7. Hannon A, Lu Y, Li J, Meyyappan M. A sensor array for the detection and discrimination of methane and other environmental pollutant gases. Sensors. 2016;16(8):1163. (11pp).
8. Singh E, Meyyappan M, Nalwa HS. Flexible grapheme-based wearable gas and chemical sensors. Appl Mater Interfaces. 2017;9:34544–86.
9. Donnelly R. Microneedle patch for body fluid testing. BioOpticsWorld. 2014.
10. Lahtinen P. 3D nanocellulose for wound care. Med Design Briefs. 2017:52.
11. Lee BH, Lee DI, Bae H, et al. Foldable and disposable memory on paper. Sci Rep. 2016;6:38389. (11pp).
12. Seol ML, Han JW, Jeon SB, Meyyappan M, Choi YK. Floating oscillator-embedded triboelectric generator for versatile mechanical energy harvesting. Sci Rep. 2015;5:16409. (10pp).
13. Martinez RV. Self-powered, paper-based devices for medical diagnostics. Technol Briefs. 2018.
14. Mi Y, Shao Z, Vang J, Kaidar-Person O, Wang AZ. Application of nanotechnology to cancer radiotherapy. Cancer Nano. 2016;7:11. (11pp).
15. Levy L. Nanoparticle technology enhances effectiveness of radiotherapy. Med Design Briefs. 2017:36–7.
16. Bonvalot S, Le Pechoux C, De Baere T, et al. First-in-human study testing a new radioenhancer using nanoparticles (NBTXR3) activated by radiation therapy in patients with locally advanced soft tissue sarcomas. Clin Cancer Res. 2017;23:908–17.
17. Nanobiotix website (www.nanobiotix.com). Accessed 16 Feb 2018.
18. Jun JJ, Steinmetz NA, Siegle JH, et al. Fully integrated silicon probes for high-density recording of neuronal activity. Nature. 2017;551:232–6.
19. Rand E, Periyakaruppan A, Tanaka Z, et al. A carbon nanofiber based biosensor for simultaneous detection of dopamine and serotonin in the presence of ascorbic acid. Biosens Bioelectron. 2013;42:434–8.
20. Keefer EW, Botterman BR, Romero MI, Rossi AF, Gross GW. Carbon nanotube coating improves neuronal recordings. Nat Nanotechnol. 2008;3:434–9.
21. de Asis ED Jr, Nguyen-Vu TDB, Arumugan PU, et al. High efficient electrical stimulation of hippocampal slices with vertically aligned carbon nanofiber microbrush array. Biomed Microdevices. 2009;11:801–8.

15 Advanced Technologies: Paperless Hospital, the Cost and the Benefits

Charles R. Doarn

Introduction

In antiquity, communications were conducted in many different forms. Smoke signals, cave paintings (petroglyphs), pictograms, ideograms, oral discourse, and eventually writing. Sumerians and Egyptians were the first to begin cuneiform script, which continued to evolve across the entire world in many forms. The Rosetta Stone is one example of how societies communicated. Pheidippides, a hemerodrome, was one way of medical information that was sent from village to village in antiquity [1]. Scrolls and parchment eventually led to paper, and once Gutenberg's printing press was invented in 1439, books were printed, and literacy became relevant to almost anyone. His invention fueled the Renaissance and the Reformation in Europe, which led the development of science and discovery and eventually the modern world. Concurrent to this was the Islamic Golden Age, where science, culture, engineering, and medicine flourished [2]. Writing and paper provided a foundation for everything to move forward. Advances in civilization, culture, language, communications, and most importantly medicine.

This paradigm remained as the foundation of all of humanity until the early twenty-first century, where today we communicate in vastly different ways, often without paper at all. Libraries, once the hallowed halls of academia, are no longer teaming with intellectual curiosity. We just google it [3]. We communicate at the speed of light. We transfer patient information from one location to another instantaneously. We store terabytes of data in small devices. A generation ago, storage would consume significant floor space in a clinic or hospital setting. What humankind took thousands of years to perfect has literally and fundamentally changed in one generation!

You might ask, what does this have to do with the future of healthcare? Let me opine. With the integration of computers, telecommunications, and intelligent software, paper is slowly disappearing. You can transfer money or deposit a paper check without going to the bank. You can board a plane without a paper ticket – your smartphone is your boarding pass. Your physician can give you a prescription without a paper copy – you just go to your local pharmacy and pick it up. This innovation, which we have at our fingertips, has fundamentally changed our society. The way we live, the way we think, the way we survive as a species. Certainly, medicine has evolved. Although some may disagree with that tenant [4], Le Fanu posits that "…with alternative medicine in the ascendancy and unaccounted for explosion in health-service costs."

C. R. Doarn (✉)
Family and Community Medicine,
University of Cincinnati, College of Medicine,
Cincinnati, OH, USA
e-mail: Charles.doarn@uc.edu

R. Latifi (ed.), *The Modern Hospital*, https://doi.org/10.1007/978-3-030-01394-3_15

With any new technological innovation, there are those who are naysayers. When Laennec invented the stethoscope in 1816, his colleagues quipped that he was going against the grain – the standard of care in this period was for the physician to place his head on the patient's chest in order to hear heart and lung sounds [5]. Analogous to this affront to the nineteenth century, medical establishment was the concept of "gentlemen do not have dirty hands." Puerperal fever was rampant in Europe in the 1840s, and Ignaz Semmelweis observed high mortality in birthing mothers in the obstetrical clinics. The midwives of the day were not experiencing this same mortality. The inquisitive Semmelweis asked the midwives why this was the case. It basically came down to handwashing. Semmelweis began to institute this concept between patient encounters, and this resulted in much consternation from his peers and their scientific and medical opinions [6]. It took many decades before the stethoscope and handwashing became standard medical practice.

Healthcare and paperless hospitals are areas that have seen significant adoption of technology. However, these fields remain far behind other industries. The technical revolution or age of computing in the mid-twentieth century is a key contributor to these changes. Even before television had been invented, Radio News published its monthly issue in April 1924 of a young patient being examined by this physician via a television – very futuristic at that time (Fig. 15.1).

While physicians like Osler and others were at the forefront of this medical evolution in the early twentieth century, I doubt they had in mind the kinds of technology and intelligence built into the inanimate physician – the computer [7]. Christakis writes about the development of modern medical thought during the first part of the twentieth century and the text used in training medical students about internal medicine [8]. Many medical students and, for that matter, most students do not really need to buy textbooks or even physically go to class or the library. They can get what they need on their personal device wherever they are. Furthermore, distance learning, around since the late 1950s, provides a "virtual" presence, where students and faculty may not physically need to meet on campus very often or ever. That as both cost and benefits – positively and negatively.

What is the scope and the impact of the integration of various technologies in moving healthcare in a truly new paradigm? Furthermore, what are the costs and benefits of this integration – not only financial but also quality of service and perhaps even equity?

The integration of new technology and the change it brings can often cause significant challenges and often result in unintended consequences. This will be discussed later in the area of data integrity and cybersecurity.

Innovation

Technological innovation often comes about to meet a need – warfare, space exploration, lifestyle, and better ways of doing things are just few examples. While each of these has traditionally been the purview of governments or large corporations, people today are much more intimately involved in change. It still requires money, often lots of it; just look at Elon Musk or Jeff Bezos. They are going into space in partnership with NASA as a customer – the government is buying services not developing them! They would not be able to do what they do without their own financial backing. Moreover, with communication tools now available to us, we see the concept of crowdsourcing as a tool. To illustrate, GE Aircraft Engines required a new part for a jet engine. Rather than design it in-house, they announced a competition through crowdsourcing, and a young Serbian student designed it, printed it on a 3D printer, and submitted it. He won the prize, and GE began testing and manufacturing it. What used to take 2–3 years now took less than 6 months.

It is often those of us who think outside the box, like Uber, Lyft, Amazon, and Tesla, that move things forward. They found a profitable way. Health faces the same opportunities but can be constrained by personalities, barriers, and

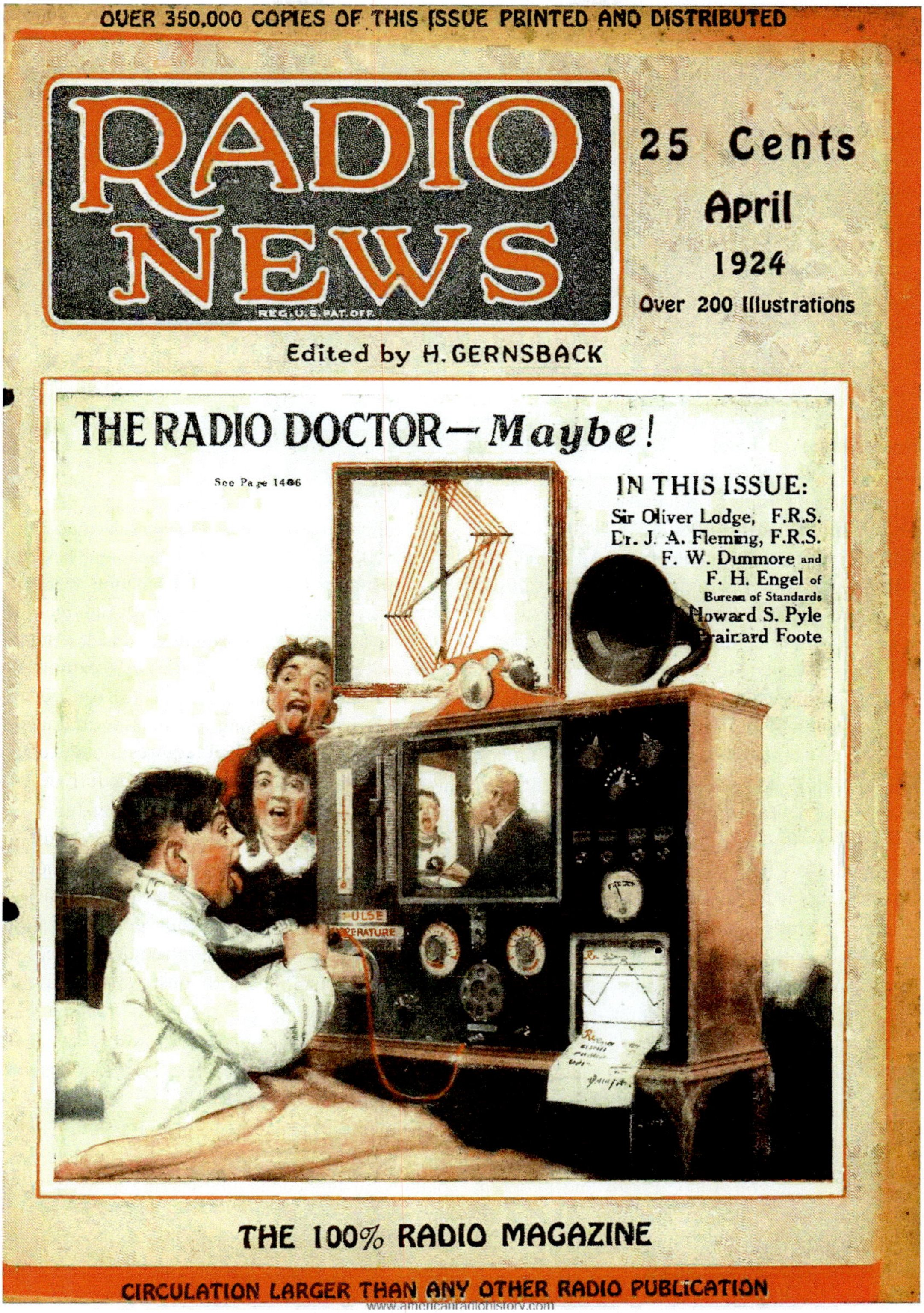

Fig. 15.1 Future of healthcare as seen in 1924. (Used with permission from AmericanHistory.com. Retrieved from https://www.americanradiohistory.com/Archive-Radio-News/20s/Radio-News-1924-04-R.pdf)

often unsurmountable challenges. Nevertheless, there are early adopters who are disrupters, and they challenge the status quo.

Innovation specific to healthcare includes a wide variety of areas. For the purpose of this narrative, we will limit these to computing power, telecommunications, imaging, sensors, artificial intelligence, and human capabilities. Each has great potential and of course there are risks. Continuous innovation in these areas has led us to new disciplines like telemedicine, e-health, robotic surgery, electronic health records, home healthcare, and global health.

One example of how this need and the change that was brought about is the development of the electronic health record (EHR) of Epic. In the late 1970s, Judith Faulkner founded the Human Services Computing as a database management system for medical systems. Each patient's longitudinal health is a chronicle of life. An "epic" tale if you will. While Epic is just one platform used today, the question going forward is "is this the right platform or approach for moving forward?" [9]. This is especially important in the era of cloud computing and initiatives like Web 2.0.

Is a paperless and filmless health record safe, secure, and saving the healthcare industry money and providing high-quality care? Depends on whom you ask. There is a plethora of observations and data that is quite illustrative of the success and impact of this EHR. Just imagine what workflow would be like without it. Clarke et al. conducted a qualitative study on the impact of electronic records on patient safety in the UK's National Health System. This study was conducted at the beginning of the implementation and identified perceived risk to patient safety [10]. The economic and organizational models in the USA are different than in the UK, and conclusions of the Clarke et al. study only have a tangential impact on the US marketplace. Yoldi-Negrete et al. recently reported on Adobe Forms and Dropbox as low-cost data collection systems [11]. Perhaps this is a future direction that could fundamentally change the healthcare industry.

Hanoon reports positive feedback from operating room staff regarding a paperless patient tracking system [12]. Computer-based systems, while costly in capital expense and in maintenance, have many positive impacts, including improvements in scheduling, reduction in cancellation, tracking of patients, reduction in supplies (e.g., paper), productivity, etc. Even the introduction of robotic-assisted surgery has shown cost savings [13].

The calculation of cost and benefit often ignores or minimizes the opportunity costs in healthcare. Its inclusion is key to understand the true impact of technology adoption in healthcare [14–16]. The analysis must include other intrinsic costs such as the cost of doing nothing at all. Inaction will have a huge downstream impact.

Computing Power

The computers we have access to today are incredibly fast, effective, and highly capable. They can be programmed to access information from all kinds of sources, run algorithms, and provide answers in the blink of eye. Just consider IBM's Watson. Computers linked to one another, embedded with sensors, and extremely fast processors, allow users the opportunity to do things that were once done by a significant workforce. Yes, technology and innovation have eliminated jobs, but they have also created new jobs. Inventory systems in retail, industry, and healthcare institutions are becoming fully automated, requiring little human interaction and of course no paper. Several institutions are exploring radio-frequency identification (RFID) systems for tracking supplies and equipment and managing patient flow [17]. This has social dimensions that must be understood prior to wide-scale adoption and integration [18]. Ker et al. examine the impact of health information systems on improving healthcare [19].

Much has changed in the use of computers over the last few decades. Today, of course, computers are embedded in everything from cars, appliances, toys, and even in our bodies. The human condition has forever been altered as a result of this integration of computers. Fairchild Semiconductor founder Gordon Moore observed in 1965 that the semiconductor, which powers the computer, doubles in capacity every year or two.

This became known as Moore's law. The faster it is, the more it can do. In medicine today, we have computing power in nearly every facet of our work. Much of which no longer needs paper. Even the operating manuals are in the cloud.

Storage

Medicine and healthcare are data-rich disciplines. The practice of medicine today requires significant storage of images (photography and various scans/films), video, lab results, notes, and longitudinal studies of individuals, and the list goes on. Until computers were integrated into medicine, storage was all paper-based. All of this data can now be stored on computer-based storage systems, which makes the data easily accessible via dashboards and business analytics tools. Artificial intelligence is slowing being integrated into medicine. Informatics and data mining become highly relevant tools [20–22]. The integration of data systems and analytic tools has ushered in a new era of big data. Hurlen et al. discuss big data and how it can minimize the need for paper [23].

With new technology in storage capacity and capability also comes challenges. Who manages the data? Who owns the data? How is it kept secure? How is data and information integrity supported? These are but a few of the questions facing the healthcare sector and data. Data is protected in each country by laws, policies, and regulations. In the USA, there is the Privacy Act and the Health Insurance Portability and Accountability Act. Data systems have several layers of encryption and user authentication. This limits and controls access to data to only those who have a need. A significant amount of data is in the "cloud" and is not physically maintained where the patient-physician encounter occurs [24].

Large data repositories are ideal for research initiatives, population health, and epidemiology. The success of informatics is dependent in part on data and immediate access and security of the data. Cai et al. discuss the Internet of Things using big data storage systems and cloud computing [25].

It is worth noting at this juncture that in the 1970s it was generally thought that personal computers would eliminate or at least minimize the need for paper to print documents. UNESCO reported in 1999 that the world would need 756,000,000 trees to produce 1 year of paper [26]. Conversely, many publications such as newspapers, magazines, textbooks, and yes even peer-reviewed journals are going paperless [27].

Storage of information electronically must be secure and must be quickly accessible. Large data sets cannot be maintained and utilized effectively without such storage systems.

Telecommunications

In 1885, Alexander Graham Bell founded the American Telephone and Telegraph (AT&T) Company to promote a new way of communication, the telephone, which he developed in 1874. In an early twentieth-century radio interview with Thomas Watson, Watson explained how the very first words transmitted on the telephone were "Mr. Watson come here! I want you!" Watson and Bell were in different rooms of the laboratory, and when Bell spilled battery acid on his pants, he uttered those words, and Watson heard them on the phone [28]. The introduction of the telephone permitted much more efficient communication in real time. In 1888, Heinrich Rudolf Hertz proved the existence of electromagnetic waves, which he quipped "It's of no use whatsoever…." We of course use his discovery everyday of our lives in nearly everything we do [29].

Mobile telephony has been around since Martin Cooper invented the cellular phone at Motorola in 1973. It was not until the 1990s that cellular communications became more widespread. At this same time, personal digital assistants (PDAs) were being used. In the mid-1990s, these became integrated into what was termed the "smartphone." QWERTY keyboards and resistive touchscreens were incorporated, and in 2007, Apple introduced the iPhone. Today, there has been more smartphones manufactured and sold in the past 18 months than there have been televisions manufactured and sold in the entire world since it was commercially available in the 1930s.

The proliferation of these devices puts enormous resources in the hands of healthcare personnel anywhere they may in the world. Ernsting et al. report on smartphones and health apps for managing health behaviors [30]. There are hundreds of thousands of apps on Google Play and Apple for consumers to manage every aspect of their lives and for healthcare professionals. Physicians today can have many medical resources on their phone. The current smartphones and tablet computers have significantly reduced the need for paper in the health setting. Tablet computers can actually serve as the interface with the patient [31–34]. Paper charts may be a thing of the past, but there is still some reticence to change and challenges in implementation [35–38].

The Internet is the information superhighway that literally links everyone the plane to one another. If you have mobile phone, you can reach anyone anywhere they are located or gain access to information at your fingertips.

Imaging and Sensors

Imaging and sensors have become key tools in medicine and healthcare. Small devices embedded on the body, in the patient's home or location, can provide a wide variety of data, including a patient's location, their vital signs, whether a person is supine or standing, medicine adherence, and other important attributes [39]. There are even handheld ultrasound systems that are commercially available. Small sensors, linked wirelessly to a system, enable home health and remote monitoring [40, 41].

When Wilhelm Röntgen discovered X-rays in 1895, the nascent technology was crude and cumbersome. Over the next 100 years or so, X-ray images transition from film to digital, such that radiologists can look at the films in the comfort of their home [42]. Computed tomography (CT) scans, magnetic resonance imaging (MRI) scan, and positron emission tomography (PET) as well as pathology slides can all be digitally acquired, stored, and transmitted worldwide at the speed of light [43, 44].

In addition to the ability to obtain all of this information digitally, it can be stored and retrieved very quickly and efficiently. Image comparison can be made using algorithms and decision support systems [45]. Images obtained in a hospital in the USA can be sent to a radiologist in India and receive a response with diagnosis back very rapidly [44].

While there are still films used, this technology will slowly be phased out as digital technology is ubiquitous across all of healthcare. The next step will be the integration of artificial intelligence (AI). This step will provide assistance to the radiologists in ways not previously imagined.

Artificial Intelligence

In Stanley Kubrick's 2001: A Space Odyssey, a computer system, named Heuristically programmed ALgorithmic computer (HAL), is a sentient computer that controls the spacecraft. HAL in the 1968 film adaption is an artificial intelligent system that challenges authority and actually emulates human emotion. Fictitious as this may be, conceptually computer systems, like IBM's Watson, are becoming much more versatile in their capability. Harnessing this power will enable healthcare to achieve a much higher level of fidelity.

A computer that mimics cognitive functions can bring data in from sensors and make decisions with little or no human interaction. While we may be a few years away from robust systems, there are those who rail against this. Some big names in the information technology world may even be alarmists.

A PubMed search on the term "artificial intelligence in medicine" yields 1329 items. Three selections convey where this field is moving. da Costa et al. discuss vital sign monitoring in hospital wards [46], Valmarska et al. review how symptoms and medication change patterns in Parkinson's patient using different algorithms [47], and Hamet discusses two branches in AI, virtual and physical, with the use of robotics in monitoring treatment [48].

While AI in medicine may be in an early development stage, it is not beyond the realm of possibilities that AI capabilities may double every 2 years or less. Recall Moore's law. The acceleration can only enable better-quality healthcare.

Human Capabilities

Education has been at the cornerstone of extending human life. Our understanding of medicine and life's processes is based on the knowledge gained and passed down to the next generation. Plumbers and electricians train as apprentices – "the watch how I do it concept." Medical training can also be similar. However, today in the early part of the twenty-first century, there is a need to get physicians and nurses into practice soon. The demand is high and the supply is low [49]. High-fidelity medical simulators have been developed and deployed. Surgical simulators can provide a high degree of accuracy in training new surgeons. Such systems mimic anatomical structures and incorporate imaging and other data sets so that the trainee can perform the task over and over without harm [50]. With any new technology, it takes a while for wide adoption [51]. Surgical simulators can be analogous to actual surgical care, and haptics may play a role [52].

Medical education as well as education in the health sciences continues to evolve. Students utilize a wide variety of tools, including simulators, virtual reality, and even social medical that has changed dramatically from the past [53]. Even microscopy and pathology can be taught virtually [54].

Using tablet computer and high-speed telecommunications, students of all kinds can literally get an education without ever leaving the comfort of their home or favorite coffee shop.

Cybersecurity

The more advanced technology becomes and the more valuable data becomes, the risk continues to increase on vulnerability and security. Before the age of computers and vast data repositories, patient files were kept under lock and key. Often visible to each and every patient that entered the clinic, they obviously could not access it. But it was visible nonetheless. With the integration of mobile devices, computer systems, off-site data storage facilities, and new healthcare entrants like Google, Microsoft, and Amazon, the IT budget and vigilance of the IT staff are a significant portion of any healthcare enterprise.

Business processes and data collection, transfer, and storage are done virtual private networks (VPNs), but there are always nefarious acts that can impact everyone. There have been cyberattacks on individuals and organizations [55, 56]. Recent intrusions into healthcare settings by nefarious actors demand a ransom be paid in order to turn computers back on or somehow release them from attack. There have also been vulnerabilities in monitoring of patients. Slotwine et al. report on cybersecurity vulnerabilities of implanted cardiac devices [57].

While data is much more secure than it has ever been, there are constant threats and ongoing development of new authentication and security processes for gaining access. The more computers are integrated and capable of decision-making, the more we must remain vigilant as individuals and as organizations.

The Paperless Hospital

Integration of these disciplines discussed above is literally the only way healthcare can meet the growing demand. We know there is a shortage of physician and allied health workers worldwide to not only teach but to educate as well [58, 59]. We also know that we, as a species, are living longer, and with longevity come increases in disease [60]. Finally, we know that our environment is changing and that is where advanced technologies can help humanity.

In the modern healthcare setting, the patient is a customer of service. Patients will shop around, and if they see a medical center that has marketed themselves as high tech – they have a surgical robot, or they are affiliated to a university – the patient will choose that cite.

The advanced technologies that enable EHRs, robotic telesurgery, remote monitoring, home healthcare, and telemedicine and e-health are at the forefront of the evolution in healthcare.

Robotic Surgery

In the late 1990s, telemanipulation systems were being deployed to medical centers for a variety of surgical procedures. With research and development from NASA research (Computer Motion's Zeus platform) and DARPA research (SRI and eventually Intuitive Surgical's da Vinci platform), robotic surgery was set to become a new tool in surgical intervention worldwide. After a lengthy legal battle, Intuitive Surgical acquired Computer Motion. Much has been written about robotic surgery [61]. In 2005, researchers at the University of Cincinnati demonstrated remote wireless surgery in an underwater habitat [62] and in the high desert using a drone for wireless communications [63, 64] and conducted a total porcine nephrectomy over a 2500-mile distance [65].

In 2018, robotic surgical systems are more common than at any other time. They have been shown to be challenging and cost-effective. According to a most recent publication on cost-effectiveness of robotic vs open partial nephrectomy, the robotic approach was nominally lower, but there were few perioperative complications [66].

Remote Monitoring

The innovation discussed above, regarding personal devices, sensor, and telecommunications, has permitted the further development, acceptance, and utility of home healthcare and telemedicine. Patients can be seen by their care provider wherever they are located. It is not necessary to travel to the clinic, the physician's office, or the hospital for routine care. Weinstein et al. report the clinical components of telemedicine [67]. Bashshur et al. have compiled several studies on the empirical evidence of telemedicine in chronic disease management [68], primary care [69], telepathology [43], teleradiology [44], telemental health [70], teledermatology [71], and diabetes management [72].

Telemedicine has been used in space [73], battlefield [74], disasters [75], and many other clinical applications. In addition, Latifi et al. have used telemedicine in training and for trauma support [76, 77].

Conclusion

Over the course of human history, technology and innovation have helped shape what we do, how we do it, and how we interact with one another. This took thousands of years to perfect. There has been more innovation in the past 120 years or so than the 10,000 years preceding the beginning of the twentieth century. We are naïve to think that this unbridled growth we are witnessing now will fundamentally change humanity. There are costs and benefits of integrating technology in our lives. In medicine, diagnosis and treatment have been greatly enhanced, yet if we are not vigilant, there may be someone in the shadows trying to steal data and change data or with some the nefarious intent.

References

1. Doarn CR, Merrell RC. Hemerodrome: a messenger and medicine. Telemed J E Health. 2018;24(3):171–2.
2. Falagas ME, Zarkadoulia EA, Samonis G. Arab science in the golden age (750–1258 CE) and today. FASEB J. 2006;20(10):1581–6.
3. Carr N. Is Google making us stupid? Yearbook Nat Soc Study Educat. 2008;107(2):89–94.
4. Le Fanu J. Rise and fall of modern medicine. Lancet. 1999;354(9177):518.
5. Roguin A. Rene Theophile Hyacinthe Laënnec (1781–1826): the man behind the Stethoscope. Clin Med Res. 2006;4(3):230–5.
6. Ataman AD, Vatanoğlu-Lutz EE, Yıldırım G. Medicine in stamps-Ignaz Semmelweis and Puerperal Fever. J Turkish German Gynecol Assoc. 2013;14(1):35–9.
7. Osler W. Evolution of modern medicine. New Haven: Yale University Press; 1943.
8. Christakis NA. The ellipsis of prognosis in modern medical thought. Social Sci Med. 1997;44(3): 301–15.
9. Congdon K. Is epic future proof. Health IT outcomes. 2014. https://www.healthitoutcomes.com/doc/is-epic-future-proof-0001. Last accessed 24 May 2018.
10. Clarke A, Adamson J, Watt I, Sheard L, Cairns P, Wright J. The impact of electronic records on patient safety: a qualitative study. BMC Med Inform Decis Mak. 2016;16:62.
11. Yoldi-Negrete M, Morales-Cedillo IP, Navarro-Castellanos I, Fresán-Orellana A, Panduro-Flores R, Becerra-Palars C. Combining adobe forms and dropbox to obtain a low-cost electronic data collection system. Telemed J E Health. e-Pub Jun 22, 2018.

12. Hanoon M. OR staff reap rewards of paperless patient tracking system. OR Manager. 2015;31(6):22–3.
13. Ho C, Tsakonas E, Tran K, Cimon K, Severn M, Mierzwinski-Urban M, Corcos J, Pautler S. Robot-assisted surgery compared with open surgery and laparoscopic surgery: clinical effectiveness and economic analyses [Internet]. Ottawa: Canadian Agency for Drugs and Technologies in Health; 2011 (Technology report no. 137). [cited 2011-09-20]. Available from: http://www.cadth.ca/en/products/health-technology-assessment/publication/2682. Last accessed 24 May 2018.
14. Russell LB. Opportunity costs in modern medicine. Health Aff. 1992;11(2):162–9.
15. Lomas J, Claxton K, Martin S, Soares M. Resolving the "cost-effective but unaffordable" paradox: estimating the health opportunity costs of nonmarginal budget impacts. Value Health. 2018;21(3):266–75.
16. Sandmann FG, Robotham JV, Deeny SR, Edmunds WJ, Jit M. Estimating the opportunity costs of bed-days. Health Econ. 2018;27(3):592–605.
17. Abugabah A. Integrating RFID with healthcare information systems: toward smart hospitals. Asian J Inform Technol. 2017;16(9):734–7.
18. Fisher JA, Monahan T. Tracking the social dimensions of RFID systems in hospitals. Int J Med Inform. 2008;77(3):176–83.
19. Ker J-I, Wang Y, Hajli N. Examining the impact of health information systems on healthcare service improvement: the case of reducing in patient-flow delays in a US hospital. Technol Forecast Social Change. 2018;127:188–98.
20. Cios KJ, Moore GW. Uniqueness of medical data mining. Artif Intell Med. 2002;26(1–2):1–24.
21. Shortliffe EH, Barnett GO. Medical data: their acquisition, storage, and use. In: Medical informatics. New York: Springer; 2001. p. 41–75.
22. Chang V, Wills G. A model to compare cloud and non-cloud storage of Big Data. Future Gener Comput Sys. 2016;57:56–76.
23. Hurlen P, Pedersen J. Can big data solve small problems? Paper use in a paperless hospital. Stud Health Technol Inform. 2016;228:542–6.
24. Devadass L, Sekaran SS, Thinakaran R. Cloud computing in healthcare. Int J Stud Res Technol Manage. 2017;5(1):25–31.
25. Cai H, Xu B, Jiang L, Vasilakos AV. IoT-based big data storage systems in cloud computing: perspectives and challenges. IEEE Internet Things J. 2017;4(1):75–87.
26. Norman J. Computes have not caused a reduction in paper usage or printing. http://www.historyofinformation.com/expanded.php?id=1394. Last accessed 24 May 2018.
27. Williams TL, Lindsay MJ, Burnham JF. Online vs. Print Journals. J Electron Resour Med Libr. 2008;3(1):1–8.
28. CBC Broadcast of an Interview of Thomas Watson. http://www.cbc.ca/archives/entry/alexander-graham-bell-and-thomas-watson. Last accessed 5 Jun 2018.
29. Mulligan JF. The influence of Hermann von Helmholtz on Heinrich Hertz's contributions to physics. Am J Phys. 1987;55(8):711–9.
30. Ernsting C, Dombrowski ST, Oedekoven M, O'Sullivan JL, Kanzler M, Kuhlmey A, Gellert P. Using smartphones and health apps to change and manage health behaviors: a population-based survey. J Med Internet Res. 2017;19(4):e101.
31. Li J, Yazdany J, Trupin L, Izadi Z, Gianfrancesco M, Goglin S, Schmajuk G. Capturing a patient-reported measure of physical function through an online electronic health record **patient** portal in an ambulatory clinic: implementation study. JMIR Med Inform. 2018;6(2):e31.
32. Kauppinen H, Ahonen R, Mäntyselkä P, Timonen J. Medication safety and the usability of electronic prescribing as perceived by physicians-a semistructured interview among primary health care physicians in Finland. J Eval Clin Pract; 23(6):1187–94. Epub 2017 May 4.
33. Ong AP, Devcich DA, Hannam J, Lee T, Merry AF, Mitchell SJ. A 'paperless' wall-mounted surgical safety checklist with migrated leadership can improve compliance and team engagement. BMJ Qual Saf. 2016;25(12):971–6. Epub 2015 Dec 30.
34. Dudek NL, Papp S, Gofton WT. Going paperless? Issues in converting a surgical assessment tool to an electronic version. Teach Learn Med. 2015;27(3):274–9.
35. Boonstra A, Broekhuis M. Barriers to the acceptance of electronic medical records by physicians from systematic review to taxonomy and interventions. BMC Health Serv Res. 2010;10(1):231.
36. Hatton JD, Schmidt TM, Jelen J. Adoption of electronic health care records: Physician heuristics and hesitancy. Procedia Technol. 2012;5:706–15.
37. Landman AB, Rokos IC, Burns K, Van Gelder CM, Fisher RM, Dunford JV, Cone DC, Bogucki S. An open, interoperable, and scalable prehospital information technology network architecture. Prehosp Emerg Care. 2011;15(2):149–57.
38. Singh VK, Lillrank P, editors. Planning and designing healthcare facilities: a lean, innovative, and evidence-based approach. Boca raton: CRC Press; 2017. p. 95–130.
39. Potter P, Allen K, Costantinou E, Klinkenberg WD, Malen J, Norris T, O'Connor E, et al. Evaluation of sensor technology to detect fall risk and prevent falls in acute care. Jt Comm J Qual Patient Saf. 2017;43(8):414–21.
40. Majumder S, Mondal T, Deen MJ. Wearable sensors for remote health monitoring. Sensors. 2017;17(1):130.
41. Casselman J, Onopa N, Khansa L. Wearable healthcare: lessons from the past and a peek into the future. Telematics Inform. 2017;34(7):1011–23.
42. Morozov S, Guseva E, Ledikhova N, Vladzymyrskyy A, Safronov D. Telemedicine-based system for quality management and peer review in radiology. Insights Imaging. 2018;9(3):337–41.

43. Bashshur RL, Krupinski EA, Weinstein RS, Dunn MR, Bashshur N. The empirical foundations of telepathology: evidence of feasibility and intermediate effects. Telemed J E Health. 2017;23(3):155–91.
44. Bashshur RL, Krupinski EA, Thrall JH, Bashshur N. The empirical foundations of teleradiology and related applications: a review of the evidence. Telemed J E Health. 2016;22(11):868–98.
45. Jaffray DA, Das S, Jacobs PM, Jeraj R, Lambin P. How advances in imaging will affect precision radiation oncology. Int J Radiat Oncol Biol Phys. 2018;101(2):29.
46. da Costa CA, Pasluosta CF, Eskofier B, da Silva DB, da Rosa Righi R. Internet of health things: toward intelligent vital signs monitoring in hospital wards. Artif Intell Med. 2018;89:61–9. pii: S0933-3657(17)30136-7.
47. Valmarska A, Miljkovic D, Konitsiotis S, Gatsios D, Lavrač N, Robnik-Šikonja M. Symptoms and medications change patterns for Parkinson's disease patients stratification. Artif Intell Med. 2018. pii: S0933-3657(17)30587-0.
48. Hamet P, Tremblay J. Artificial intelligence in medicine. Metabolism. 2017 Apr;69S:S36–40.
49. Salsberg ES. Is the physician shortage real? Implications for the recommendations of the institute of medicine committee on the governance and financing of graduate medical education. Acad Med. 2015;90(9):1210–4.
50. Dawe SR, Pena GN, Windsor JA, Broeders JA, Cregan PC, Hewett PJ, Maddern GJ. Systematic review of skills transfer after surgical simulation-based training. Br J Surg. 2014;101(9):1063–76.
51. Zevin B, Aggarwal R, Grantcharov TP. Surgical simulation in 2013: why is it still not the standard in surgical training? J Am Coll Surg. 2014;218(2):294–301.
52. Salkini MW, Doarn CR, Kiehl N, Broderick TJ, Donovan JF, Gaitonde K. The role of haptic feedback in laparoscopic training using the LapMentor II. J Endourol. 2010;24(1):99–102.
53. Richardson A, Hazzard M, Challman SD, Morgenstein AM, Brueckner JK. A "Second Life" for gross anatomy: applications for multiuser virtual environments in teaching the anatomical sciences. Anat Sci Educ. 2011;4(1):39–43.
54. Lee LMJ, Goldman HM, Hortsch M. The virtual microscopy database-sharing digital microscope images for research and education. Anat Sci Educ. 2018;11:510–5.
55. Armstrong DG, Kleidermacher DN, Klonoff DC, Slepian MJ. Cybersecurity regulation of wireless devices for performance and assurance in the age of "medjacking". J Diabetes Sci Technol. 2015;10(2):435–8.
56. Arora S, Yttri J, Nilse W. Privacy and security in mobile health (mHealth) research. Alcohol Res. 2014;36(1):143–51.
57. Slotwiner DJ, Deering TF, Fu K, Russo AM, Walsh MN, Van Hare GF. Cybersecurity vulnerabilities of cardiac implantable electronic devices: communication strategies for clinicians-proceedings of the heart rhythm society's leadership summit: endorsed by the Heart Rhythm Society Board of Trustees. Heart Rhythm. 2018. pii: S1547-5271(18)30467-3.
58. Hoyler M, Finlayson SR, McClain CD, Meara JG, Hagander L. Shortage of doctors, shortage of data: a review of the global surgery, obstetrics, and anesthesia workforce literature. World J Surg. 2014;38(2):269–80.
59. Mercer C. Family medicine faces shortage of doctors willing to teach. CMAJ. 2018;190(21):E666.
60. Pandya A, Gaziano TA, Weinstein MC, Cutler D. More Americans living longer with cardiovascular disease will increase costs while lowering quality of life. Health Aff (Millwood). 2013;32(10):1706–14.
61. Moses GR, Doarn CR. Barriers to wider adoption of mobile telerobotic surgery: engineering, clinical and business challenges. Stud Health Technol Inform. 2008;132:309–12.
62. Doarn CR, Anvari M, Low T, Broderick TJ. Evaluation of teleoperated surgical robots in an enclosed undersea environment. Telemed J E Health. 2009;15(4):325–35.
63. Harnett BM, Doarn CR, Rosen J, Hannaford B, Broderick TJ. Evaluation of unmanned airborne vehicles and mobile robotic telesurgery in an extreme environment. Telemed J E Health. 2008;14(6):539–44.
64. Lum MJH, Rosen J, King H, Friedman DCW, Donlin G, Sankaranarayanan G, Harnett B, Huffman L, Doarn C, Broderick TJ, Hannaford B. Telesurgery via unmanned aerial vehicle (UAV) with a field deployable surgical robot. Stud Health Technol Inform. 2007;125:313–5.
65. Sterbis JR, Hanly RJ, Herman BC, Marohn MR, Broderick TJ, Shih SP, Harnett B, Doarn CR, Schenkman NS. Transcontinental telesurgical nephrectomy using the da Vinci robot in a porcine model. Urology. 2008;71(5):971–3.
66. Buse S, Hach CE, Klumpen P, Schmitz K, Mager R, Mottrie A, Haferkamp A. Cost-effectiveness analysis of robot-assisted vs open partial nephrectomy. Int J Med Robot. 2018;28:e1920.
67. Weinstein RS, Krupinski EA, Doarn CR. Clinical examination component of telemedicine, telehealth, m-health, and connected health practices. Med Clinics North Am. 2018;102(3):533–44.
68. Bashshur RL, Shannon GW, Smith BR, Alverson D, Antoniotti N, Barsan W, Bashshur N, Brown EM, Coye MJ, Doarn CR, Ferguson S, Grigsby J, Krupinski EA, Kvedar JC, Linkous J, Merrell RC, Nesbitt T, Poropatich R, Rheuban K, Sanders J, Watson A, Weinstein RS, Yellowlees P. The empirical foundations of telemedicine interventions for chronic disease management. Telemed J E Health. 2014;20(9):769–800. ePub June 26.
69. Bashshur RL, Howell JD, Krupinski EA, Harms KM, Bashshur N, Doarn CR. The empirical foundations of telemedicine intervention in primary care. Telemed J E Health. 2016;22(5):342–75.

70. Bashshur RL, Shannon GW, Bashshur N, Yellowlees PM. The empirical evidence for telemedicine interventions in mental disorders. Telemed J E Health. 2016;22(2):81–113.
71. Bashshur RL, Shannon GW, Tejasvi T, Kvedar JC, Gates M. The empirical foundations of teledermatology: a review of the research evidence. Telemed J E Health. 2015;21(12):953–79.
72. Bashshur RL, Shannon GW, Smith BR, Woodward MA. The empirical evidence for the telemedicine intervention in diabetes management. Telemed J E Health. 2015 May;21(5):321–54.
73. Doarn CR, Nicogossian AE, Merrell RC. Application of telemedicine in the United States Space Program. Telemed J. 1998;4(1):19–30.
74. Poropatich R, Lai E, McVeigh F, Bashshur R, The US. Army telemedicine and m-health program: making a difference at home and abroad. Telemed J E Health. 2013;19(5):380–6.
75. Doarn CR, Latifi R, Poropatich RK, Sokolovich N, Kosiak D, Hostiuc F, Zoicas C, Arafat R. Development and validation of telemedicine for disaster response: the NATO Multinational System. Telemed J E Health. 2018. ePub January 4, 2018.
76. Latifi R, Dasho E, Shatri Z, Tilley E, Osmani KL, Doarn CR, Dogjani A, Olldashi F, Koçiraj A, Merrell RC. Telemedicine as an innovative model for rebuilding medical systems in developing countries through multipartnership collaboration: the case of Albania. Telemed J E Health. 2015;21(6):503–9.
77. Latifi R, Tilley EH. Telemedicine for disaster management: can it transform chaos into an organized, structured care from the distance? Am J Disaster Med. 2014;9(1):25–37.

16 Newer Does Not Necessarily Mean Better

David J. Samson and Rifat Latifi

One of the most important reasons for hospital transformation and modernization has been research and technological advances. However, in research on policy diffusion, the belief that new ideas should always be adopted has been referred to as pro-innovation bias [1]. This belief is widespread in health care [2, 3] and certainly applies to medical technologies introduced into practice in hospitals. Given that medical technology is the main driver of health-care costs [4], hospital administrators and clinicians would be prudent to challenge this belief when making decisions about whether to acquire new technology or to encourage use of new interventions.

Only thorough and careful critical appraisal of evidence can ultimately provide a basis for concluding whether a new technology is better or not. The evidence-based medicine (EBM) movement [5] has been a major force in molding beliefs about the need for good quality evidence to support decisions at many levels within health care. Thus, EBM could be viewed as the main defense against potentially unwise decisions based on pro-innovation bias. The systematic review (SR) has been a vital tool in the EBM movement. Methods and standards for SRs have evolved over the years, in large part due to the activities of the Cochrane Collaboration [6], founded in 1993. Cochrane Reviews are considered being among the most rigorous of SRs and are excellent sources on which to base health-care decisions. The use of such SR methods leads to more reliable findings to base conclusions than use of less systematic methods.

Frameworks have been developed to systematically synthesize the findings of SRs into conclusions. One prominent framework is the Grading of Recommendation, Assessment, Development, and Evaluation (GRADE) system [7]. For a specific research question, application of GRADE can result in one of the four strengths or qualities of evidence levels: high, moderate, low, or very low [8]. The balance of beneficial outcomes against any intervention-related harms would be described as the net outcome. Comparison of the net outcome of an intervention and comparator can entail making judgments about the relative importance or trade-offs between the benefits and harms of the intervention and comparator.

Several potential conclusions can be reached about a body of evidence comparing a newer intervention with an older, established intervention. Below are descriptions of multiple reasons to conclude that newer is not necessarily better than older.

- *Insufficient evidence*. When evidence is insufficient to permit conclusions about the comparative effectiveness of the newer and older

D. J. Samson (✉)
Department of Surgery, Westchester Medical Center, Valhalla, NY, USA
e-mail: david.samson@wmchealth.org

R. Latifi
New York Medical College, School of Medicine, Department of Surgery and Westchester Medical Center, Valhalla, NY, USA
e-mail: rifat.latifi@wmchealth.org

R. Latifi (ed.), *The Modern Hospital*, https://doi.org/10.1007/978-3-030-01394-3_16

interventions, the key element is uncertainty. Uncertainty may be due to the low quantity of evidence, high risk of bias among included studies, inconsistency of results, lack of direct evidence, and imprecision of findings. Rephrased, we could state that we are uncertain whether newer is better than older. While this is not exactly the same as knowing the comparative effectiveness of newer versus older, the practical implications would be similar. Adoption of a new technology should wait until evidence allows for clear conclusions of comparative effectiveness.

- *Equivalence/noninferiority*. In this instance, evidence is sufficient to conclude that the newer intervention is either equivalent or at least noninferior to an older intervention. Ideally, studies addressed by SRs reaching this conclusion should be specifically designed to assess equivalence or noninferiority.
- *No net health outcome improvement*. This conclusion connotes that studies comparing a newer intervention to placebo or no active intervention control show that the intervention is ineffective. In some cases, a transient short-term benefit may be evident, but it is outweighed by risks of harms.
- *Similar net health outcome balance*. Here the newer and older interventions each have different benefits and harms. However, when the net outcome of newer and older is compared, the balance of benefits and harms for newer and older is concluded to be similar.
- *Inferiority*. We are surprised whenever SRs conclude that an older intervention is superior and the newer intervention is inferior. Inferiority may occur because the beneficial outcome favors the older intervention. Also, the newer intervention may be associated with more serious harms, leading to a poorer net health outcome than the older intervention.

Finding SR Examples Concluding Newer Is Not Better

This chapter will describe examples of SRs that concluded that newer interventions are not necessarily better than older interventions. To find these examples, I performed a PubMed search of SRs (using text words for SRs in titles and abstracted), limited to English language citations. The search was limited to the following sources (see Table 16.1):

Table 16.1 Sources of systematic reviews

Evidence report/technology assessment, full report or summary (Agency for Healthcare Research and Quality)
Cochrane Database of Systematic Reviews
Health technology assessment (UK National Health Service Programme)
Systematic Review
Journal of Comparative Effectiveness Research
The New England Journal of Medicine
Journal of the American Medical Association
Annals of Internal Medicine
Journal of the American College of Surgeons
Annals of Surgery
Journal of the American College of Cardiology
Circulation
Journal of Clinical Oncology
Cancer
British Medical Journal
The Lancet

I screened titles and abstracts of citations published between 2013 and 2018. I sought SRs that concluded that a newer intervention was not significantly superior to an older intervention. Content areas were limited to inpatient procedures that could be conducted by these services: medicine, surgery, cardiology, oncology, and hematology/oncology. Of 3638 citations screened, I selected 25 SRs selecting RCTs to serve as examples. *A* *M*easurement Tool to Assess *S*y*T*em*A*tic *R*eviews (AMSTAR) was applied to all SRs, and they were generally rated very favorably, particularly the Cochrane Reviews. Examples of 25 SRs (27 specific key questions) are summarized in Tables 16.1, 16.2, 16.3, 16.4, and 16.5 in order of reason for concluding the newer intervention was not necessarily better than the older intervention.

Insufficient Evidence

Table 16.2 summarizes information for 16 specific key questions, showing that insufficient evidence (statistically nonsignificant results) was the most frequent reason for concluding that newer

Table 16.2 Systematic reviews concluding newer is not better due to insufficient evidence

Author year	Key question(s)	Population	Intervention	Comparator	Outcomes	Conclusion
Jagannath 2016 [25]	Evaluate the effectiveness and safety of different types of allogeneic HSCT, in patients with severe transfusion-dependent ß-thalassemia major, ß-thalassemia intermedia, or ß0/+−thalassemia variants requiring chronic blood transfusion	Diagnosis of (transfusion-dependent) homozygous ß0/+−thalassemia, severe variants requiring chronic blood transfusion and iron chelation therapies	Any type of HSCT (bone marrow transplantation, peripheral blood cell transplantation, umbilical cord blood transplantation)	Each other or standard therapy	Event-free survival, overall response, quality of life, time to donor hematological reconstitution, stable mixed chimerism, acute/chronic GVHD, graft rejection with recurrence or persistence of β-thalassemia	Limited evidence to either support or refute the effectiveness and safety of different types of stem cell transplantation in people with severe transfusion-dependent ß-thalassemia major or ß0/+−thalassemia variants requiring chronic blood transfusion
Oringanje 2016 [26]	Examine the cure rate and risks of HSCT for people with sickle cell disease	Children and adults with sickle cell disease of all phenotypes, either gender and in all settings	Methods of HSCT	Different methods of HSCT, supportive care	Event-free survival, mortality, transplant-related mortality, acute GVHD, chronic GVHD, neurological complications, late SCD complications, quality of life, graft rejection with sickle cell disease recurrence/ persistence, other transplant-related morbidities	Evidence limited to observational, other less robust studies; no RCTs found; need for a multicenter RCT assessing the benefits and possible risks of HSCT comparing sickle status and severity of disease in people with sickle cell disease
Zhao 2014 [27]	Assess the comparative effectiveness and safety of different intermittent pneumatic compression (IPC) devices with respect to the prevention of venous thromboembolism in patients after THR	18+ years, undergone total hip replacement THR and with or without concomitant use of other types of thromboprophylactic measures together with IPC devices	IPC systems by different technical aspects	Different IPC methods	Symptomatic VTE, symptomatic proximal/distal DVT (fatal and nonfatal), symptomatic nonfatal PE, fatal PE, asymptomatic VTE	Lack of RCT evidence to make an informed choice of IPC device for preventing venous thromboembolism (VTE) following THR

(continued)

Table 16.2 (continued)

Author year	Key question(s)	Population	Intervention	Comparator	Outcomes	Conclusion
Fisher 2015 [28]	Determine the safety and efficacy of autologous adult bone marrow stem cells as a treatment for AMI, focusing on clinical outcomes	Any participants with a clinical diagnosis of AMI with no restriction on age	Stem cells following successful revascularization by angioplasty or CABG	No intervention or placebo	All-cause mortality, cardiovascular mortality, composite measures of MACE, periprocedural AEs, morbidity including reinfarction, incidence of arrhythmias, incidence of restenosis, target vessel revascularization and rehospitalization for HF, quality of life, LVEF	Insufficient evidence for a beneficial effect of cell therapy for AMI patients; however, most of the evidence comes from small trials that showed no difference in clinically relevant outcomes; further adequately powered trials are needed
Noelck 2016 [29]	Assess benefits and harms of surgical or percutaneous left atrial appendage (LAA) occlusion or removal	AF patients who are eligible for percutaneous LAA exclusion	6 LAA exclusion devices	Usual care without LAA exclusion	Stroke, mortality, cardiovascular morbidity, other reported health outcomes, HLOS, ICU LOS, bleeding infection, need for surgical intervention	Limited evidence; the Watchman device may be noninferior to long-term OAC in selected patients; percutaneous LAA devices associated with high rates of procedure-related harms; although surgical LAA exclusion during heart surgery does not seem to add incremental harm, there is insufficient evidence of benefit
Raman 2016 [30]	Compare benefits and harms of percutaneous transluminal renal angioplasty with stent placement (PTRAS) versus medical therapy alone in adults with ARAS	Atherosclerotic renal artery stenosis (ARAS)	Percutaneous transluminal renal angioplasty with stent placement (PTRAS)	Medical therapy alone	All-cause mortality, kidney function, BP control, CVD (including CHD), AEs (including medication-related and procedural complications)	Strength of evidence is low; studies have generally focused on patients with less severe ARAS; 7 RCTs and 8 other studies failed to support a beneficial effect of PTRAS on clinical outcomes for most patients with ARAS

Riemsma 2013 [14]	Assess beneficial and harmful effects of transarterial (chemo) embolization compared with no intervention or placebo intervention in patients with liver metastases	Patients with liver metastases no matter the location of the primary tumor	Transarterial (chemo) embolization	No intervention or placebo	Mortality, time to mortality, all AEs, and complications (serious AEs, non-serious AEs)	One small RCT showed no significant survival benefit or benefit on extrahepatic recurrence was found in the embolization group in comparison with the palliation group; high probability for selective outcome reporting bias
Khan 2016 [15]	Assess the effects of postoperative external beam radiation dose escalation in adults with high-grade glioma (HGG)	Adults 18+ pathological diagnosis of HGG (glioblastoma, anaplastic astrocytoma, anaplastic oligodendroglioma, anaplastic mixed oligoastrocytoma)	Hypofractionated, hyperfractionated, accelerated radiotherapy (RT)	Conventional fractionated RT or no RT (supportive care alone)	Overall survival, AEs, progression-free survival, quality of life	Insufficient data regarding hyperfractionated vs conventional fractionation RT (without chemotherapy) and for accelerated RT vs conventional fractionated RT (without chemotherapy)
Kucukmetin 2013 [16]	Compare the effectiveness and safety of laparoscopically assisted radical vaginal hysterectomy (LARVH) and radical abdominal hysterectomy (RAH) in women with early-stage (1–2A) cervical cancer	Adult women requiring radical surgery for histologically confirmed early-stage (stage 1 to 2A) cervical cancer	Laparoscopically assisted radical vaginal hysterectomy (LARVH)	Radical abdominal hysterectomy (RAH)	Overall survival, progression-free survival, disease-free survival, blood loss, HLOS, quality of life, AEs: direct surgical morbidity, surgically related systemic morbidity, recovery, longer-term problems, others	1 underpowered RCT (mod RoB), small number of women in each group, low number of observed events. Absence of reliable evidence precludes any definitive conclusions; RCT did not report data on long-term outcomes
Dumville 2015 [17]	Assess the effects of NPWT for treating pressure ulcers in any care setting	Adults with a pressure ulcer (category II or above), managed in any care setting	NPWT	No NPWT, different brand of NPWT	Complete wound healing and AEs (serious, non-serious), pain, infection	Currently no rigorous RCT evidence available regarding the effects of NPWT compared with alternatives for treatment of pressure ulcers; high uncertainty remains about the potential benefits or harms of using this treatment for pressure ulcer management

(continued)

Table 16.2 (continued)

Author year	Key question(s)	Population	Intervention	Comparator	Outcomes	Conclusion
Dumville 2015 [18]	Assess the effects of NPWT on the healing of surgical wounds by secondary intention (SWHSI) in any care setting	Adults with surgical wound healing by secondary intention (SWHSI)	NPWT	No NPWT, different brand of NPWT	Complete wound healing and AEs (serious, non-serious), pain, infection	Currently no rigorous RCT evidence available regarding clinical effectiveness of NPWT in treatment of surgical wound healing by secondary intention; the potential benefits and harms of using this treatment for this wound type remain largely uncertain
Dumville 2015 [19]	Assess the effects of negative-pressure wound therapy (NPWT) for treating leg ulcers in any care setting	Having leg ulcers, managed in any care setting	NPWT	No NPWT, different brand of NPWT	Complete wound healing and AEs (serious, non-serious), pain, infection	Limited evidence regarding the use of negative-pressure wound therapy (NPWT) for the treatment of leg ulcers, with only one small trial available that compared the use of NPWT with standard care before and after skin grafting
Eskes 2013 [20]	Summarize the evidence for the effects of HBOT as a treatment for acute surgical and traumatic wounds	Acute wounds (e.g., surgical wounds, penetrating wounds, lacerations, skin transplantations (surgical procedure), animal bites, and traumatic wounds)	HBOT	Any other intervention, dressings, steroids, or sham HBOT, different HBOT regimens	Wound healing, measured objectively, e.g., time to complete healing (days), number of wounds completely healed at a time point (proportion). AEs (visual disturbance (reversible myopia)), barotrauma, oxygen toxicity, infection, reoperations	Lack of high-quality, valid research evidence regarding the effects of HBOT on wound healing; two small trials suggested that HBOT may improve the outcomes of skin grafting and trauma; these trials were at risk of bias; further evaluation by high-quality RCTs is needed

Chang 2016 [21]	Assess effectiveness of subintimal angioplasty vs other treatments for people w/lower limb arterial chronic total occlusions	Chronic lower limb ischemia (IC or CLI, or both) treated for an iliac, femoral, popliteal, or crural occlusion by subintimal angioplasty	Subintimal angioplasty	PTA, surgical bypass, other techniques	Clinical improvement (relief of rest pain, healing of ulcers, and improvement in walking distance); tech success, vessel patency, limb salvage, complications	Insufficient evidence to support SIA over other techniques; only two trials, both at overall low RoB, but small number of studies, small sample sizes, and the differences in treatment techniques and control groups between the studies resulted in evidence being less applicable
Ambler 2014 [12]	Analyze RCTs comparing atherectomy against any established tx for PAD to evaluate the effectiveness of atherectomy	Symptomatic PAD with either claudication or critical limb ischemia and evidence of lower limb arterial disease	Atherectomy	Any established treatment for PAD	Primary vessel patency at 6 months/1 year, ACM 6 months/1 year, fatal/nonfatal CVEs, immediate procedural angiographic outcomes, target vessel revascularization, complications, morbidity, quality of life	Poor-quality evidence to support atherectomy as alternative to balloon angioplasty in maintaining primary patency, any time interval; except for mortality, no evidence atherectomy is better on any outcome; distal embolization was not reported in all atherectomy RCTs

(continued)

Table 16.2 (continued)

Author year	Key question(s)	Population	Intervention	Comparator	Outcomes	Conclusion
Griffin 2014 [13]	Assess the effects of low-intensity pulsed ultrasound (LIPUS), high-intensity focused ultrasound (HIFUS), and extracorporeal shockwave therapies (ECSW) as part of the treatment of acute fractures in adults	Skeletally mature adults, age of 18+ years, with acute traumatic fractures	LIFUS, HIFUS, ECSW	No additional treatment or placebo (sham US)	Overall quantitative functional improvement; time to fracture union; confirmed non-union or secondary procedure, such as failure of fixation or for delayed or non-union; AEs, pain, costs, adherence	Potential benefit of US for treatment of acute fractures in adults cannot be ruled out; the currently available evidence from heterogeneous trials is insufficient; future trials should record functional outcomes and follow up all trial participants
Dong 2016 [31]	Inquire whether pancreatic stents are useful in preventing pancreatic fistula after pancreaticoduodenectomy	Underwent pancreaticoduodenectomy for benign or malignant pathologies of the pancreas or periampullary region	Stents, internal, replacement of pancreatic juice	No stent, external, no replacement	Incidence of pancreatic fistula, in-hospital mortality, reoperation, HLOS, overall complications	Unable to ascertain the effects of pancreatic duct stenting on the risk of pancreatic fistulas, in-hospital mortality, and length of hospital stay after pancreaticoduodenectomy

Table 16.3 Systematic reviews concluding newer is not better due to equivalence/noninferiority

Author year	Key question(s)	Population	Intervention	Comparator	Outcomes	Conclusion
Briceno 2015 [22]	Compare novel oral anticoagulants (NOACs) and Watchman device to therapy with warfarin for the prevention of stroke in pts w/ NVAF	Nonvalvular AF	Watchman device, NOACs	Warfarin	Stroke and systemic embolism (SSE), all-cause mortality, safety: adjudicated major bleeding during treatment or device-/procedure-related complications	NOAC is superior to warfarin for prevention of stroke and death in patients with nonvalvular AF; Watchman is a reasonable noninferior alternative to warfarin for stroke prevention, but cautious use is essential given safety concerns
Jenks 2014 [9]	Compare the effectiveness of balloon angioplasty (with and without stenting) with medical therapy for the treatment of atherosclerotic renal artery stenosis in patients with hypertension	Adults 18+ with hypertension (DBP 95+ mm Hg) and uni- or bilateral atherosclerotic renal artery stenosis (stenosis greater than 50%)	Primary balloon angioplasty (with or without insertion of a stent)	Medical therapy	SBP, DBP, renal function, number and defined daily doses of antihypertensives, restenosis of the renal artery (defined as a stenosis of greater than 50%), CV AEs, procedural complications, med AEs	Hypofractionated radiation therapy has similar efficacy for survival as compared to conventional radiotherapy, particularly for individuals aged 60 and older with glioblastoma
Khan 2016 [15]	Assess the effects of postoperative external beam radiation dose escalation in adults with high-grade glioma (HGG)	Adults 18+ pathologic diagnosis of HGG (glioblastoma, anaplastic astrocytoma, anaplastic oligodendroglioma, anaplastic mixed oligoastrocytoma)	Hypofractionated, hyperfractionated, accelerated radiotherapy (RT)	Conventional fractionated RT or no RT (supportive care alone)	Overall survival, AEs, progression-free survival, quality of life	Insufficient data regarding hyperfractionated vs conventional fractionated RT (without chemotherapy) and for accelerated RT vs conventional fractionated RT (without chemotherapy)

(continued)

Table 16.3 (continued)

Author year	Key question(s)	Population	Intervention	Comparator	Outcomes	Conclusion
Hamilton 2017 [10]	Assess the analgesic efficacy and AEs of liposomal bupivacaine (LB) infiltration at the surgical site for the management of postoperative pain	Aged 18 years and older undergoing elective surgery at any surgical site, without restriction on any comorbidities	Single dose of liposomal bupivacaine infiltrated at the surgical site	Placebo or other types of analgesia delivered systemically or locally	PROs of pain, use of supplemental opiate analgesia (incidence of supplemental analgesia, time to supplemental analgesia, mean and total opiate consumption, opiate or other analgesia-related AEs), measures of cost-effectiveness, withdrawals, and AEs	LB at the surgical site does appear to reduce postoperative pain compared to placebo; however, limited evidence does not demonstrate superiority to bupivacaine hydrochloride; no SAEs or withdrawals
Adam 2013 [11]	Assess the comparative effectiveness of NOACs and standard thromboprophylaxis regimens in total hip replacement (THR) and total knee replacement (TKR)	THR, TKR	NOACs: factor Xa inhibitor (FXaI), direct thrombin inhibitor (DTI)	Low molecular weight heparin (MWH)	Symptomatic DVT, other VTE events, death, bleeding outcomes	DTI vs LMWH: death/ symptomatic DVT/ symptomatic PE/major bleeding no important differences

Table 16.4 Systematic review concluding newer is not better due to no net health outcome improvement

Author year	Key question(s)	Population	Intervention	Comparator	Outcomes	Conclusion
Thorlund 2015 [23]	Assess benefits and harms of arthroscopic knee surgery involving partial meniscectomy, debridement, or both for middle-aged or older patients with knee pain and degenerative knee disease	Patients ranging from degenerative meniscal tears and no radiographic signs of osteoarthritis (OA) to degenerative meniscal tears and more severe signs of OA	Arthroscopic surgery involving partial meniscectomy, debridement, both	Non-surgical treatments: sham surgery (including lavage), exercise, medical treatment	Pain and physical function, radiographic OA, OA grade, AEs	Small inconsequential benefit from interventions that include arthroscopy for degenerative knee is limited in time and absent at 1–2 years; knee arthroscopy is associated with harms; taken together, evidence does not support the practice of arthroscopic surgery

interventions are not necessarily better than older interventions. The first three studies in Table 16.2 reach this conclusion because in each instance, zero studies meet study eligibility criteria. Jagannath et al. [25] stated that evidence was limited against either supporting or refuting the effectiveness and safety of hematopoietic stem cell transplantation (HSCT) in treating patients with β-thalassemia. Oringanje et al. [26] concluded that a robust, multicenter RCT was needed to overcome the limitations of observational study evidence to assess benefits and risks of HSCT for people with sickle cell disease. Zhao et al. [27] compared different intermittent pneumatic compression (IPC) devices for patients who have undergone total hip replacement (THR). Their assessment of the evidence was that there was a lack of RCT evidence to make an informed choice of IPC device for preventing venous thromboembolism (VTE) following THR.

Among SRs that identified at least one eligible study for analysis, Fisher et al. [28] compared autologous adult bone marrow stem cells with no intervention or placebo as a treatment for acute myocardial infarction (AMI). They concluded that there was insufficient evidence for a beneficial effect of cell therapy for AMI patients. They also mentioned that most of the evidence comes from small trials that showed no difference in clinically relevant outcomes. Noelck et al. [29] assessed the Watchman device, versus usual care, used for surgical or percutaneous left atrial appendage (LAA) occlusion or removal in patients with atrial fibrillation (AF). These reviewers found limited evidence that the Watchman device may be noninferior to long-term optimal anticoagulation in selected patients. However, percutaneous LAA devices may be associated with high rates of procedure-related harms. Although surgical LAA exclusion during heart surgery does not seem to add incremental harm, there is insufficient evidence of benefit. Raman et al. [30] found that evidence failed to support a beneficial effect of percutaneous transluminal renal angioplasty with stent placement (PTRAS) versus medical therapy alone for patients with atherosclerotic renal artery stenosis (ARAS).

Riemsma et al. [14] identified one small RCT showing no significant survival benefit or benefit on extrahepatic recurrence in comparing transarterial chemoembolization to palliative care for liver metastases. These authors suspected a high probability for selective outcome reporting bias. Khan et al. [15] judged that, in treatment of high-grade intracranial gliomas, data were insufficient on the comparative effectiveness of hyperfractionated versus conventional fractionation radiotherapy (without chemotherapy) and for

Table 16.5 Systematic review concluding newer is not better due to similar net health outcome balance

Author year	Key question(s)	Population	Intervention	Comparator	Outcomes	Conclusion
Honda 2013 [24]	Compare hand sewing and mechanical methods for esophagogastric anastomosis after esophagectomy, and examine the contribution of each method to the occurrence of anastomotic leakages and strictures	Any age/sex/ethnic group underwent esophagectomy + reconstruction using a gastric tube for any esophageal cancer, any histological type, or benign disease	Hand-sewn (HS)	Circular stapler (CS)	Primary outcomes were (1) anastomotic leakage and (2) strictures; secondary outcomes included (3) operative time and (4) postoperative mortality	Use of a CS contributed to reducing the length of the operation but was associated with an increased risk of anastomotic strictures; both the CS and the HS methods are viable alternatives in the reconstruction after esophagectomy
Adam 2013 [11]	Assess the comparative effectiveness of NOACs and standard thromboprophylaxis regimens in total hip replacement (THR) and total knee replacement (TKR)	THR, TKR	NOACs: factor Xa inhibitor (FXaI), direct thrombin inhibitor (DTI)	Low molecular weight heparin (MWH)	Symptomatic DVT, other VTE events, death, bleeding outcomes	FXaI vs LMWH: death/nonfatal PE no important difference, lower risk of symptomatic DVT; risk of major bleeding increased

accelerated radiotherapy vs conventional fractionated radiotherapy (without chemotherapy). In a SR on laparoscopically assisted radical vaginal hysterectomy (LARVH) versus radical abdominal hysterectomy (RAH) in women with early-stage (1–2A) cervical cancer, Kucukmetin et al. [16] found one small RCT with a low number of observed events. They concluded that the absence of reliable evidence precludes any definitive conclusions that RCT did not report data on long-term outcomes.

Dumville and associates performed three separate SRs on the use of negative-pressure (vacuum) wound therapy for pressure ulcers, surgical wounds, and leg ulcers [17–19]. For the first two indications, these reviewers concluded that no rigorous RCT evidence was available regarding the effects of NPWT compared with alternatives and that high uncertainty remains about the potential benefits or harms of using this treatment. Regarding treatment of leg ulcers, the authors described the evidence as limited, consisting of one small trial. Another SR on wound treatment was performed by Eskes et al. [20] who noted the lack of high-quality, valid evidence regarding the effects of hyperbaric oxygen therapy (HBOT) on healing of acute surgical and traumatic wounds. Specifically, two small trials suggested that while HBOT may improve the outcomes of skin grafting and trauma, these trials were at risk of bias; further evaluation by high-quality RCTs is needed.

Chang et al. [21] reported insufficient evidence to support subintimal angioplasty for symptomatic peripheral arterial disease (PAD) over other techniques. There were only two relevant trials, and the small number of studies, the small sample sizes, and the differences in treatment techniques and control groups between the studies resulted in evidence being difficult to interpret. Another SR on PAD was published by Ambler et al. [12], who mentioned that poor quality evidence was available to support atherectomy as an alternative to balloon angioplasty in maintaining primary patency at any time interval. Further, except for mortality, there was no evidence that atherectomy is better on any outcome; distal embolization, an important potential adverse outcome, was not reported in all atherectomy RCTs.

Griffin et al. [13] compared low-intensity pulsed ultrasound (LIPUS), high-intensity focused ultrasound (HIFUS), and extracorporeal shockwave therapies (ECSW) as part of the treatment of acute fractures in adults with no additional treatment or placebo. These investigators concluded that although potential benefit of US for treatment of acute fractures in adults cannot be ruled out, the evidence from heterogeneous trials is insufficient.

Dong et al. [31] were unable to ascertain the effects of pancreatic duct stenting on the risk of pancreatic fistulas, in-hospital mortality, and length of hospital stay after pancreaticoduodenectomy.

Equivalence/Noninferiority

In Table 16.3, asking a different key question than Noelck et al. [29] Briceno et al. [22] compared the Watchman device with warfarin in non-valvular AF, concluding that Watchman is a reasonable noninferior alternative to warfarin for stroke prevention, but cautious use is essential given safety concerns. Jenks et al. [9], like Raman et al. [30], compared balloon angioplasty (with and without stenting) with medical therapy for the treatment of atherosclerotic renal artery stenosis in patients with hypertension, reaching a somewhat different conclusion. These authors concluded that data are insufficient that balloon angioplasty, with or without stenting, is superior to medical therapy. However, given small improvement in diastolic blood pressure (DBP) and small reduction in antihypertensive drug requirements, it appears safe and results in similar numbers of cardiovascular and renal adverse events to medical therapy. Khan et al. [15], mentioned previously, found that hypofractionated radiation therapy has similar efficacy for survival as compared to conventional radiotherapy.

Hamilton et al. [10] assessed liposomal bupivacaine (LB) infiltration at the surgical site for the management of postoperative pain compared with placebo or other forms of analgesia. These investigators concluded that LB at the surgical site appears to reduce postoperative pain compared to placebo; however, evidence does not demonstrate superiority to bupivacaine hydrochloride. Adam et al. [11] found no important differences between direct thrombin inhibitors (DTI) and low molecular weight heparin (LMWH) regarding death, symptomatic DVT, symptomatic pulmonary embolism (PE), and major bleeding.

No Net Health Outcome Improvement

Thorlund et al. [23] (Table 16.4) reported that, compared to nonsurgical treatment, there is a small inconsequential benefit from interventions that include the following: arthroscopy for degenerative knee is limited in time and absent at 1–2 years; knee arthroscopy is associated with harms; and taken together, evidence does not support the practice of arthroscopic surgery for degenerative knee conditions.

Similar Net Health Outcome Balance

Honda et al. [24] (Table 16.5) concluded that use of a circular stapler (CS) contributed to a shorter length of the operation but was associated with an increased risk of anastomotic strictures and that both the CS and the HS methods are viable alternatives in the reconstruction after esophagectomy. The SR by Adam et al. mentioned earlier noted that regarding factor X inhibitors (FXaI) versus LMWH, there were no important difference in death and nonfatal PE, a lower risk of symptomatic DVT, and an increased risk of major bleeding increased.

Inferiority

Farquhar et al. [32] (Table 16.6) stated there was high-quality evidence of increased treatment-related mortality and little or no increase in survival by using high-dose chemotherapy with autograft for women with early poor prognosis breast cancer. Fu et al. [33] observed that use of recombinant human bone morphogenetic protein-2 (rhBMP-2) in spinal fusion has no proven clinical advantage over bone graft and may be associated with important harms, making it difficult to identify clear indications for rhBMP-2.

Discussion

Skepticism of whether newer technology is better has been expressed in many areas of medical practice in recent years. Authors have noted that newer is not necessarily superior regarding pharmaceuticals [34], critical care mechanical ventilation [35], medical therapy for benign prostatic hyperplasia [36], medical treatment of female urinary incontinence [37], surgery for urinary incontinence and pelvic organ prolapse [38], drug-eluting coronary stents [39], surgical management of esophageal cancer [40], cancer treatment [41], glaucoma surgery [42], shoulder surgery [43], treatment of renal calculi [44], urologic and gynecologic surgery [45], antihypertensive medications [46], and treatment of metastatic melanoma [47].

Several studies have attempted to quantify the frequency with which randomized controlled trials (RCTs) have shown innovative interventions to be superior or not to either standard active interventions or placebo/inactive interventions.

In 1997, Machin et al. [48] reviewed the results of trials completed across a 30-year period with support from the UK Medical Research Council Cancer Therapy Committee. The authors included 32 RCTs that made 36 comparisons between interventions. Only 8 of 36 (22%) comparisons resulted in a statistically significant difference favoring an innovative intervention over an older, standard intervention. Johnston and colleagues [49] reviewed all phase III randomized trials funded by the National Institute of Neurological Disorders and Stroke (NINDS) conducted before the year 2000. Of 28 RCTs, 6 yielded measureable improvements in health (21%). Thus, 78% and 79%, respectively, failed to show that the newer

Table 16.6 Systematic review concluding newer is not better due to inferiority

Author year	Key question(s)	Population	Intervention	Comparator	Outcomes	Conclusion
Farquhar 2016 [32]	Compare the effectiveness and safety of high-dose chemotherapy HD CHT and autograft (either autologous bone marrow or stem cell transplantation) with conventional chemotherapy for women with early poor prognosis breast cancer	Women any age with early poor prognosis breast cancer either at 1st dx or as a recurrence, whether or not previously treated with CHT	HD CHT with autologous bone marrow or stem cell transplantation	Conventional chemotherapy	Overall, event-free survival; treatment-related mortality; morbidity such as non-hematological toxicities, e.g., nausea and vomiting, white cell measures, new malignancies, quality of life	High-quality evidence of increased treatment-related mortality and little or no increase in survival by using high-dose chemotherapy with autograft for women with early poor prognosis breast cancer
Fu 2013 [33]	Assess the effectiveness and harms of recombinant human bone morphogenetic protein-2 (rhBMP-2) in spinal fusion	Spinal fusion	Spinal fusion with rhBMP	Any control, spinal fusion with rhBMP	"Overall success" (at 24 months); fusion was primary end point in the remainder; pain, disability, neurologic status, function, and return to work; AEs	In spinal fusion, rhBMP-2 has no proven clinical advantage over bone graft and may be associated with important harms, making it difficult to identify clear indications for rhBMP-2

intervention was significantly better than the older intervention.

A team based at the University of South Florida (USF) has published two landmark articles documenting the frequency of different result patterns among RCTs comparing newer and older interventions. A JAMA article from 2005 [50] focused on RCTs funded through the National Cancer Institute (NCI) by the Radiation Therapy Oncology Group (RTOG). Fifty-nine comparisons were made in 57 RCTs. Of these, only seven trials found a statistically significant between-group difference in outcome. Six trials (10%) found a significant advantage favoring an innovative intervention, while one study (2%) significantly favored a standard, older intervention. Of the 52 RCTs that did not find a statistically significant difference between innovative and standard treatments (88%), 34 trials were classified as true-negative findings (no treatment effect was determined to be present, analogous to equivalence or noninferiority). Among all RCTs, true negatives comprised 58%, and false-negative results occurred in 18 trials (31%).

In 2008, Djulbegovic and USF colleagues [51] expanded their work from one Cooperative Oncology Group (COG) to eight. They identified 624 trials that made 781 comparisons, while at least some data were available for 743. Statistically significant results were observed in 221 instances (30%), while results were nonsignificant in 70%. Results from 89 comparisons (12%) were not further classifiable due to missing data or non-relevant outcomes. Of the remaining 433 comparisons, 12 (3% of the entire total) were classified as truly negative. An additional 218 comparisons (29%) were described as truly inconclusive because there was an equal chance of innovative treatment being better than standard treatment or vice versa. Of 2 remaining categories, 119 comparisons (16%) were considered inconclusive because it was highly unlikely that innovative treatments are better, and 84 comparisons (11%) were called inconclusive because it was highly unlikely that standard treatments are better.

Using the same classification scheme as the Djulbegovic and USF team, in 2011, Dent and coauthors analyzed 51 RCTs (85 comparisons) published by the UK Health Technology Assessment Programme in May 2008. Statistically significant results occurred in 20 comparisons (24%), and results were nonsignificant in 76%. Sixteen comparisons significantly favored the new intervention (19% of the entire set), and four favored the control intervention (5%). Nineteen (22%) were classified as true negative, 24% as truly inconclusive, 18% as inconclusive favoring the new intervention, and 13% as inconclusive favoring the control intervention.

The previously discussed examples, along with studies of the low frequency of RCTs finding statistically significant superiority of newer interventions over older ones, support skepticism rather than assuming that newer technology is necessarily better than older technology.

References

1. Smith DW, Zhang JJ, Colwell B. Pro-innovation bias: the case of the Giant Texas SmokeScream. J Sch Health. 1996;66:210–3.
2. Greenhalgh T. Five biases of new technologies. Br J Gen Pract. 2013;63:425.
3. Chalmers I. What is the prior probability of a proposed new treatment being superior to established treatments? BMJ. 1997;314:74–5.
4. Callahan D. Health care costs and medical technology. In: From birth to death and bench to clinic: The Hastings Center bioethics briefing book for journalists, policymakers, and campaigns. Garrison: The Hastings Center; 2008. p. 79–82.
5. Eddy DM. The origins of evidence-based medicine – a personal perspective. Virtual Mentor. 2011;13:55–60.
6. Chandler J, Higgins JP, Deeks J, Davenport C. Chapter 1: Introduction. In: Clarke MJ, editor. Cochrane handbook for systematic reviews of interventions version 5.2.0. The Cochrane Collaboration; 2017. (updated February 2017). https://training.cochrane.org/handbook.
7. Guyatt GH, Oxman AD, Schünemann HJ, Tugwell P, Knottnerus A. GRADE guidelines: a new series of articles in the Journal of Clinical Epidemiology. J Clin Epidemiol. 2011;64:380–2.
8. Balshem H, et al. GRADE guidelines: 3. Rating the quality of evidence. J Clin Epidemiol. 2011;64:401–6.
9. Jenks S, Yeoh SE, Conway BR. Balloon angioplasty, with and without stenting, versus medical therapy for hypertensive patients with renal artery stenosis. Cochrane Database Syst Rev. 2014;CD002944. https://doi.org/10.1002/14651858.CD002944.pub2.
10. Hamilton TW, et al. Liposomal bupivacaine infiltration at the surgical site for the management of postoperative pain. Cochrane Database Syst Rev. 2017;(2):CD011419.
11. Adam SS, McDuffie JR, Lachiewicz PF, Ortel TL, Williams JW. Comparative effectiveness of new oral anticoagulants and standard thromboprophylaxis in patients having total hip or knee replacement: a systematic review. Ann Intern Med. 2013;159:275–84.
12. Ambler GK, Radwan R, Hayes PD, Twine CP. Atherectomy for peripheral arterial disease. Cochrane Database Syst Rev. 2014;CD006680. https://doi.org/10.1002/14651858.CD006680.pub2.
13. Griffin XL, Parsons N, Costa ML, Metcalfe D. Ultrasound and shockwave therapy for acute fractures in adults. Cochrane Database Syst Rev. 2014;CD008579. https://doi.org/10.1002/14651858.CD008579.pub3.
14. Riemsma RP, Bala MM, Wolff R, Kleijnen J Transarterial (chemo)embolisation versus no intervention or placebo intervention for liver metastases. Cochrane Database Syst Rev. 2013;CD009498. https://doi.org/10.1002/14651858.CD009498.pub3.
15. Khan L, et al. External beam radiation dose escalation for high grade glioma. Cochrane Database Syst Rev. 2016;CD011475. https://doi.org/10.1002/14651858.CD011475.pub2.
16. Kucukmetin A, Biliatis I, Naik R, Bryant A. Laparoscopically assisted radical vaginal hysterectomy versus radical abdominal hysterectomy for the treatment of early cervical cancer. Cochrane Database Syst Rev. 2013;CD006651. https://doi.org/10.1002/14651858.CD006651.pub3.
17. Dumville JC, Webster J, Evans D, Land L. Negative pressure wound therapy for treating pressure ulcers. Cochrane Database Syst Rev. 2015;CD011334. https://doi.org/10.1002/14651858.CD011334.pub2.
18. Dumville JC, Owens GL, Crosbie EJ, Peinemann F, Liu Z. Negative pressure wound therapy for treating surgical wounds healing by secondary intention. Cochrane Database Syst Rev. 2015;CD011278. https://doi.org/10.1002/14651858.CD011278.pub2.
19. Dumville JC, Land L, Evans D, Peinemann, F. Negative pressure wound therapy for treating leg

ulcers. Cochrane Database Syst Rev. 2015;CD011354. https://doi.org/10.1002/14651858.CD011354.pub2.
20. Eskes A, Vermeulen H, Lucas C, Ubbink DT. Hyperbaric oxygen therapy for treating acute surgical and traumatic wounds. Cochrane Database Syst Rev. 2013;CD008059. https://doi.org/10.1002/14651858.CD008059.pub3.
21. Chang Z, Zheng J, Liu Z. Subintimal angioplasty for lower limb arterial chronic total occlusions. Cochrane Database Syst Rev. 2016;(11):CD009418.
22. Briceno DF, et al. Left atrial appendage occlusion device and novel oral anticoagulants versus warfarin for stroke prevention in Nonvalvular atrial fibrillation: systematic review and meta-analysis of randomized controlled trials. Circ Arrhythm Electrophysiol. 2015;8:1057–64.
23. Thorlund JB, Juhl CB, Roos EM, Lohmander LS. Arthroscopic surgery for degenerative knee: systematic review and meta-analysis of benefits and harms. BMJ. 2015;350:h2747.
24. Honda M, Kuriyama A, Noma H, Nunobe S, Furukawa TA. Hand-sewn versus mechanical esophagogastric anastomosis after esophagectomy: a systematic review and meta-analysis. Ann Surg. 2013;257:238–48.
25. Jagannath VA, Fedorowicz Z, Al Hajeri A, Sharma A. Hematopoietic stem cell transplantation for people with ß-thalassaemia major. Cochrane Database Syst Rev. 2016;(11):CD008708.
26. Oringanje C, Nemecek E, Oniyangi O. Hematopoietic stem cell transplantation for people with sickle cell disease. Cochrane Database Syst Rev. 2016;CD007001. https://doi.org/10.1002/14651858.CD007001.pub4.
27. Zhao JM, et al. Different types of intermittent pneumatic compression devices for preventing venous thromboembolism in patients after total hip replacement. Cochrane Database Syst Rev. 2014;CD009543. https://doi.org/10.1002/14651858.CD009543.pub3.
28. Fisher SA, Zhang H, Doree C, Mathur A, Martin-Rendon E. Stem cell treatment for acute myocardial infarction. Cochrane Database Syst Rev. 2015;CD006536. https://doi.org/10.1002/14651858.CD006536.pub4.
29. Noelck N, et al. Effectiveness of left atrial appendage exclusion procedures to reduce the risk of stroke: a systematic review of the evidence. Circ Cardiovasc Qual Outcomes. 2016;9:395–405.
30. Raman G, et al. Comparative effectiveness of management strategies for renal artery stenosis: an updated systematic review. Ann Intern Med. 2016;165:635–49.
31. Dong Z, Xu J, Wang Z, Petrov MS. Stents for the prevention of pancreatic fistula following pancreaticoduodenectomy. Cochrane Database Syst Rev. 2016;CD008914. https://doi.org/10.1002/14651858.CD008914.pub3.
32. Farquhar C, Marjoribanks J, Lethaby A, Azhar M. High-dose chemotherapy and autologous bone marrow or stem cell transplantation versus conventional chemotherapy for women with early poor prognosis breast cancer. Cochrane Database Syst Rev. 2016;CD003139. https://doi.org/10.1002/14651858.CD003139.pub3.
33. Fu R, et al. Effectiveness and harms of recombinant human bone morphogenetic protein-2 in spine fusion: a systematic review and meta-analysis. Ann Intern Med. 2013;158:890–902.
34. Wertheimer AI. Not everything new is better. Int J Pharm Pract. 2009;17:197–8.
35. Vitacca M. New things are not always better: proportional assist ventilation vs. pressure support ventilation. Intensive Care Med. 2003;29:1038–40.
36. Roehrborn CG. Drug treatment for LUTS and BPH: new is not always better. Eur Urol. 2006;49:5–7.
37. Starkman JS, Scarpero H, Dmochowski RR. Emerging periurethral bulking agents for female stress urinary incontinence: is new necessarily better? Curr Urol Rep. 2006;7:405–13.
38. Norton P. New technology in gynecologic surgery: is new necessarily better? Obstet Gynecol. 2006;108:707–8.
39. Waksman R. Drug-eluting stents: is new necessarily better? Lancet. 2008;372:1126–8.
40. Gao S, Lee P. Prof. David Watson: new things are not always better. J Thorac Dis. 2017;9:E855–6.
41. Grann A, Grann VR. The case for randomized trials in cancer treatment: new is not always better. JAMA. 2005;293:1001–3.
42. Higginbotham EJ, Alexis D. Is newer necessarily better? The evolution of incisional glaucoma surgery over the last 100 years. Am J Ophthalmol. 2018;191:xxv–xxix. https://doi.org/10.1016/j.ajo.2018.04.009.
43. Dilisio MF. Editorial commentary: our mentors were right, new is not always better: the posterolateral shoulder trans-rotator cuff portal is safe for SLAP repairs. Arthroscopy. 2018;34:396–7.
44. Gerber R, Studer UE, Danuser H. Is newer always better? A comparative study of 3 lithotriptor generations. J Urol. 2005;173:2013–6.
45. Wilensky GR. Robotic surgery: an example of when newer is not always better but clearly more expensive. Milbank Q. 2016;94:43–6.
46. Smetana GW. Newer is not always better: all antihypertensive medications do not equally reduce cardiovascular risk. J Gen Intern Med. 2012;27:618–20.
47. Puzanov I, Skitzki J. New does not always mean better: isolated limb perfusion still has a role in the management of in-transit melanoma metastases. Oncology (Williston Park). 2016;30:1053–4.
48. Machin D, et al. Thirty years of Medical Research Council randomized trials in solid tumours. Clin Oncol (R Coll Radiol). 1997;9:100–14.
49. Johnston SC, Rootenberg JD, Katrak S, Smith WS, Elkins JS. Effect of a US National Institutes of Health programme of clinical trials on public health and costs. Lancet. 2006;367:1319–27.
50. Soares HP, et al. Evaluation of new treatments in radiation oncology: are they better than standard treatments? JAMA. 2005;293:970–8.
51. Djulbegovic B, et al. Treatment success in cancer: new cancer treatment successes identified in phase 3 randomized controlled trials conducted by the National Cancer Institute-sponsored cooperative oncology groups, 1955 to 2006. Arch Intern Med. 2008;168:632–42.

The Winning Team: Science, Knowledge, Industry, and Information

17

Gabriel Gruionu, Lucian Gheorghe Gruionu, and George C. Velmahos

Introduction: It Takes a Village – Creating a Winning Team for Medical Innovation

Translating basic or clinical research into novel medical products requires more than a clinician scientist and their laboratory or clinical team. Although innovation is on the mission statement of almost every university or teaching hospital such as the Massachusetts General Hospital [1], usually there is no infrastructure for innovation execution within a clinical division or department. Beyond information and education sessions, what busy clinicians and scientists need is a functional innovation social network (ISN) which can execute each step in the innovation process. In addition to the subject matter experts represented by medical doctors and scientists, the ISN must also contain business experts, engineers, intellectual property experts, manufacturing, sales, and customer support to ensure that the new solution is clinically and commercially viable.

We have recently introduced a new intrapreneurship model of medical academic innovation at our institution and described the process of turning a new idea into a product [2]. Other works describe the stages of innovation process in great detail [3, 4]. While knowledge about the process is crucial for knowing what work needs to be done, building the team who can actually perform the work is key to accelerating innovation. Here we will focus less on the process of innovation (advancing from an idea to a commercialized product) and more on the crucial process of building the innovation team, managing the information and knowledge necessary for advancing innovation, and building the bridge between academia and industry. We argue that the winning team, the "village" needed for successful innovation, should include inventors, scientists, engineers, business development experts, as well as capital investors and other funding agencies.

G. Gruionu (✉)
Division of Trauma, Emergency Surgery and Surgical Critical Care, Massachusetts General Hospital/ Harvard Medical School, Boston, MA, USA
e-mail: ggruionu@mgh.harvard.edu

L. G. Gruionu
Medical Engineering Laboratory, Faculty of Mechanics and the INCESA Institute, University of Craiova, Craiova, Doli, Romania

G. C. Velmahos
Division of Trauma, Emergency Surgery, and Surgical Critical Care, Massachusetts General Hospital, Boston, MA, USA

The Industry Research and Development Network (RDN)

To build an academic ISN, we were inspired by industry research and development networks (RDN). In industry, the RDN for a family of products is coordinated by a product specialist

R. Latifi (ed.), *The Modern Hospital*, https://doi.org/10.1007/978-3-030-01394-3_17

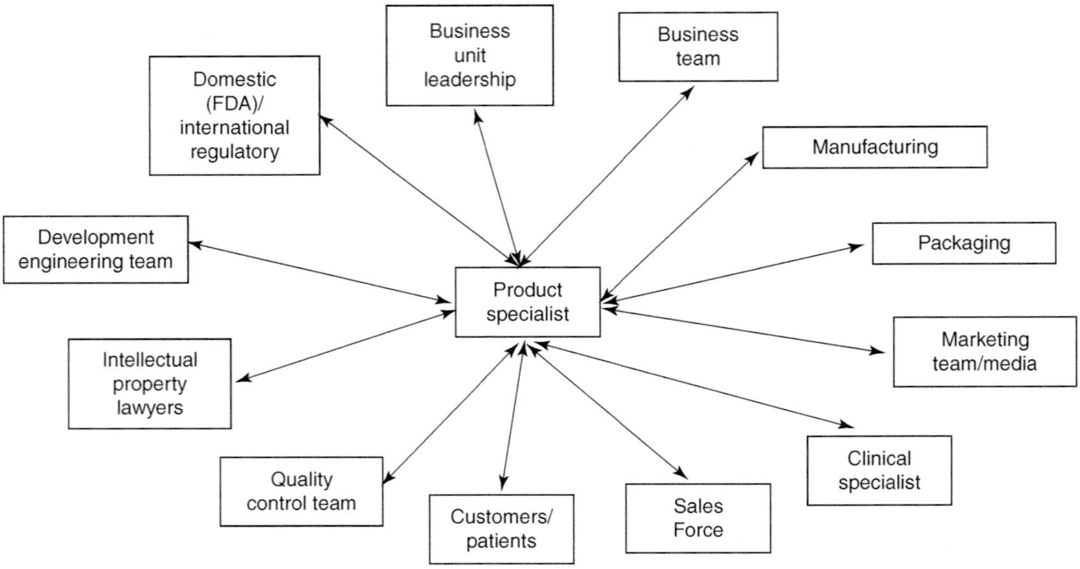

Fig. 17.1 The industrial research and development network (RDN) contains all functions necessary to support both new and commercialized products

(PS). His or her role is to insure fitness for use of the new product for the market from all different clinical, engineering, business, manufacturing, and sales perspectives (Fig. 17.1).

The main role of the PS, whose background can be a PhD or a MD, is to translate the clinical observations into a defined clinical need and functional requirements to be used by the engineering team to create a solution. The engineering prototyping team is usually a small team of engineers who are very versatile in combining many medical product technologies. They will usually try many different engineering solutions. The job of the project manager is to focus the exploration process so that the team creates a product that meets the product requirements and meets the development deadlines.

After a technically feasible solution was developed, it is the job of the PS to make sure that the proposed engineering solution meets the clinical and business requirements. The new product has to also be patentable; therefore the intellectual property (IP) lawyers are involved in the process throughout all stages of the development. They will review each element of the engineering solutions and determine if (1) it is novel and (2) it can be built by the company, meaning that it has freedom to operate (FTO). The IP consultations happen as often as a new engineering feature of the product is added or modified.

Regulatory specialists are needed along with IP lawyers, as there is a contradictory relationship between strong IP and the regulatory pathway that needs to be addressed. The more novel a product is, the stronger the IP, and the harder it is to pass regulatory standards. Sometimes novel academic inventions such as nanotechnology cannot even be evaluated by FDA before the agency develops its own understanding of the technology and designs the relevant regulatory testing. For novel approaches or applications, the FDA has to collaborate with the scientific community and the industry to develop these novel tests [5]. Academic innovation is by design novel, even ahead of its time; therefore the collaboration with regulatory experts is very important to ensure that the solutions can be implemented in clinical practice. Sometimes a less novel, intermediary solution should be pursued toward commercialization if the regulatory pathways are more clearly defined.

The rest of the RDN is part of the normal industry structure that exists in any medical technology company to support new and commercialized products. The manufacturing, packaging, sales, and customer support are as important for commercialized products as they are for new product development. For example, the sales and marketing experts can give feedback on whether a new product will be well received on the market or what price and sale volume can be expected.

While it offers a comprehensive support to a specific field of innovation, the RDN is company specific and specialized to the company's core technology. To accommodate the diversity of academic innovation within a hospital or a university, the RDN would have to be either very large or very versatile. We propose to use some elements of the RDN and build a new concept of an academic innovation support network.

The Academic ISN

A similar academic ISN (aISN) is necessary to support any new, brilliant idea in order for it to be successfully adopted by industry or financed by venture capital investors (Fig. 17.2). In the aISN, the role of the PS is played by the director of medical innovation (DMI). Like the PS in industry, the DMI does not always have to be the inventor of every new technology but will coordinate with several innovation projects for a clinical division or academic department (the innovation unit, IU). The advantage of having a MID is that the IU can develop a R&D process that can be repeated to many different ideas developed by the doctors or scientists instead of having every group developing their own model of innovation. However, the role of innovation director or innovation officer is a new function within the academia whose required skills are still under discussion [6]. One opinion is that, besides the professional training, the job requires intrapreneurial vision (entrepreneurship within a large organization), transdisciplinary thinking, and ability to thrive in the gray zone [6]. We cannot agree more. Such "soft" skills were necessary in our everyday work of spinning off three academic start-up companies, combining engineering and clinical knowledge to create new medical products from an idea, and dealing with multiple projects in the pre-feasibility stages at the same time.

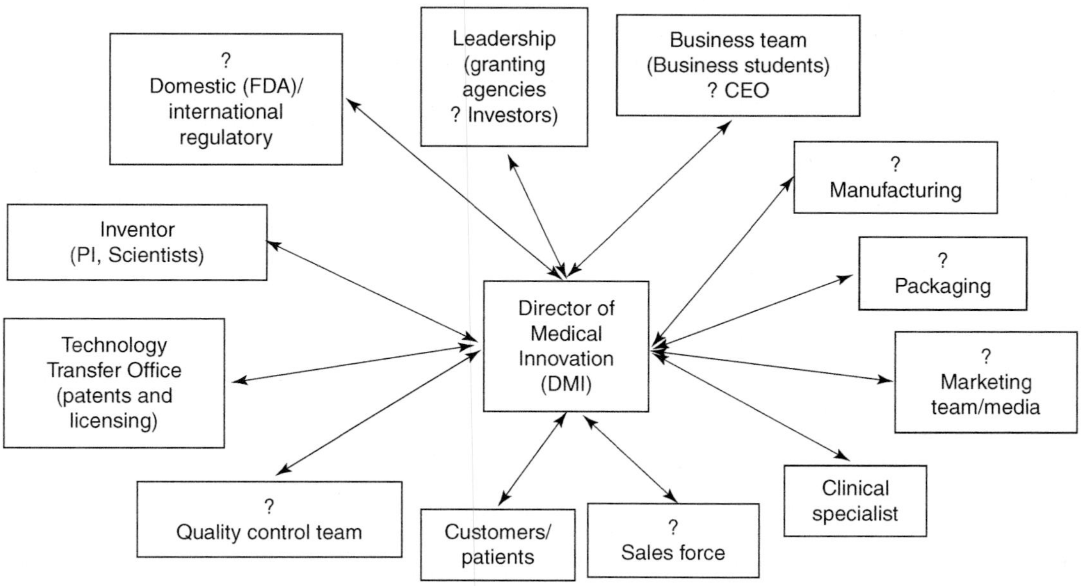

Fig. 17.2 The academic innovation social network (aISN) with a director of medical innovation (DMI). Several early development functions could be covered by academic resources including the product specialist function covered by the DMI, the IP lawyer function covered by the TTO, and the leadership being represented by granting agencies. Yet, many important functions (marked with "?") are still missing from a functional aISN

At present, even in a very small division, there could be a large variation in innovation experience. Some clinicians have a lot of innovation experience with start-up companies and have received funding in the order of tens of millions of dollars, while others are just starting their first spin-off company and struggle to find seed funding. Most clinicians and scientists have never been through the innovation process and do not even know where to start. These discrepancies are more circumstantial than intentional, and, at present, there is no mechanism to share and reproduce a model, because the knowledge is not shared by a common structure. For example, one successful innovator might have contacted an external company who took over the development process, and therefore the clinician might not even be aware of the new product development process that the company is using. The DMI can share the infrastructure within the division, and a lot of the knowledge about the innovation process could be shared, reapplied, and improved with each new project within the IU.

The DMI has many other important roles, depending on their background. With a biomedical engineering and product specialist background, the DMI can help doctors articulate a new clinical need and help generate a patentable solution. For example, one of our innovative products, the portable abdominal insufflator, is designed to address uncontrolled abdominal bleeding. Since abdominal insufflation is performed during laparoscopy procedures, the insufflation function alone is not patentable. Instead the DMI added additional features such as the tissue lifting and needle insertion, which when combined with insufflation, made the new device patentable. Such help is crucial for advancing an idea toward a commercialized product.

The *academic laboratory technicians and students* represent the early development team. The senior clinician or scientist plays many roles: principal investigator for the research project, director of the research laboratory, inventor of the new technology, and manager of the R&D project. In addition, the clinician represents the clinical subject matter expert and the voice of the customer as well. The rest of the laboratory personnel have to play the dual role of scientists and development engineers or even patent lawyers and regulatory experts. This is not always feasible and obviously not based on professional experience in all these areas. Especially for the first-time innovators, the laboratory personnel have no experience with product development, and often this work is confused with the scientific experiments performed during a research project. While a research project is focused on discovery, the development process has to demonstrate technical and commercial feasibility of a solution. Often, a new scientific discovery is not yet commercially viable. Conversely, the commercially viable solutions are not also the most novel, and the scientists lose interest in working on them. For example, the miniaturized insufflator could be a great solution for the market but was abandoned due to not enough novelty.

At the university, the role of the IP lawyers is played by the *technology transfer office* (TTO) for patenting and licensing the new technology. Once a new invention is generated in the laboratory or clinical practice, the inventors file out an invention disclosure form with the TTO for patentability analysis and provisional patent filing. Very often right after filing a provisional patent application, the TTO starts to "shop around" for potential licensees for the technology. Most of the time, the technology is not yet developed enough to be licensed. The patent has not been issued yet, so overall, the industry licensee is presented as a very weak proposal (no patent and no proven technology). Therefore, in the majority of cases, the technology is not licensed under favorable terms. This is perceived as a failure by the inventors who in turn lose interest in innovation, and the patent application is abandoned.

The business team consists of outside business professionals or, as an intermediary step, a group of business students/interns. The senior business students guided by their faculty have the necessary knowledge to study the market opportunity and develop an early business plan. One of the main limitations of these resources is the lack of practical commercialization experience of the students. The academic inventor guiding the students might also not have practical entrepreneurial experience yet. Other limitations are the duration of the academic year and the scope of the course. A better alternative is to involve an experienced business team, although that is usually cost prohibitive for an academic team. A colleague with entrepreneurial experience or an outside friend can act as acting CEOs temporarily to provide early guidance until appropriate funding is raised to hire a professional CEO. A professional CEO with a track record in medical innovation is desired and required by venture capital investors at the later stages of development.

The leadership team are not the inventors but those who bring in the money, i.e., private investors or research-granting agency sources. The most natural funding source for early academic innovation is a granting agency. The capital investment firms finance the more advanced development stages in exchange usually in exchange for a part of the business. The investors do not only bring funds but also process knowledge and business experience.

There is an important distinction between research grant funding and venture capital investing in terms of what is required from the development team. While the granting agencies want to know what the team *can do in the future*, the investors want to know what the team *can do now*. This is a fundamental difference which is sometimes not easily understood by scientists and can result in inappropriate staffing of the project. Most often, the scientists propose to also be the business and engineering experts. They assume that a scientific presentation is the same thing as a business pitch or that the early prototype solution is similar to a solution which is ready for production. Although they could become business and technical experts in the future, for investors, the present credentials are all that matters. Therefore, sometime the investor will hire a professional CEO and engineering team to run the project, which might be hard to accept by the inventor.

An aISN can be built in the academic environment. The available experts need only cover the early innovation until the new products can be licensed to industry which can cover the entire product cycle all the way to commercialization. Still, even during early innovation, some pieces are usually still missing from the aISN but if present could make a big difference in accelerating the translation to market.

The Missing Pieces of the Academic Innovation Puzzle

In addition to the invention and early development resources, there are also several essential functions which are almost always missing in the academic ISN. For example, there rarely is appropriate regulatory support for academic innovation. This is especially important since most of academic innovation is very novel (a critical condition for research grant funding). Therefore, academic innovators aim for the most novel ideas making future translation a particularly long process (an average of 15 years, [7]). An advantage of early regulatory guidance is that it helps identify the regulatory pathway (equivalence with an existing product vs. new clinical trials) and the safety and effectiveness testing that needs to be done before the product can be used clinically. These tests are straightforward and well described in the FDA regulations. They could be run in the academic laboratories (not necessarily the inventor's laboratory) and can turn a research project into an FDA-approved medical product.

The other missing parts are the manufacturing, packaging, quality control, sales, and marketing perspective. Although they seem to be important only in later stages of development, not having early feedback from these additional angles can compromise later success. For example, even if technically feasible, the new product might not be very cost-effective or even possible to manufacture (e.g., if it includes electronic or biological components) or might not sell because it does not fit the customer's need or it will be too expensive for a specific market. Often, the academic development team considers the clinical opinion of the lead clinician as representative for both the sales and the customer perspective. In other words, if the clinician said it is a good idea, it is assumed that there is a market for the new product, and it will be adopted by the customers. Often, without direct market research to back it up, this is the wrong assumption and will result in project failure or require costly design and business strategy adjustments later on.

Knowledge and Information for Innovation

There is a large volume of scientific and clinical knowledge being generated every day in academia. A lot of the knowledge is stored in the form of clinical data, published papers, and presentations. Those can be accessed with the required permissions. The clinical data is a description of the patient care. The information is very detailed and can be accessed via appropriate channels that protect patient privacy. Numerous clinical research studies are based on recorded clinical data, and the majority focus on improving clinical practice rather than the medical device or the medication.

The published basic research data rarely cover all the performed research; rather, it usually just satisfies the requirements for a particular publication. As a matter of fact, the higher the impact factor of the scientific publication, the higher the volume of data that is required but the shorter and more compact the article is, and therefore only a summary of the large amount of data can be included in the text of the paper. The work of a large group of people is sometimes summarized in only 3–4 pages and as many figures. Also, in basic research, the papers reflect the scientific discovery, whereas the innovation/translational potential is rarely addressed in more than one or two sentences in the introduction and/or the conclusion sections.

Besides what gets published (either in a single or a series of papers), there is still a large volume of unpublished data including data from secondary or failed experiments that never gets published or accessed. These additional data are stored on individual computers and other media and may or may not be used for later analysis. Often, the unpublished data are regarded as useless and not monitored. From an innovation perspective, data from failed experiments are as important as data from successful experiments, as can define the narrow specifications of a new product and avoid an expensive optimization study later. In industry, all early experiments and prototype versions are documented in the design history file to be used later to avoid similar mistakes or help narrow the product specifications. A similar solution as an experiment history file should be implemented to keep track and make use of the entire data set.

Clinical data are stored and closely monitored usually in centralized data management system such as the EPIC system, but critical innovation information is absent from such systems. From this database, all the recorded clinical information related to a specific clinical procedure can be accessed and analyzed [8]. Unfortunately, there are no comments about the difficulty of the procedure or shortcomings related to patient recovery or convenience, cost of the procedure, physician ease of use, or physician/facility productivity. This information would be crucial for identifying an unmet clinical need which will be the basis of future innovation. Instead of having this information recorded for every procedure and every clinician, the DMI will have to interview each individual doctor who performs a particular procedure, which is a time-consuming process and rarely happens. Often, a doctor will contact the DMI with a clinical need which is assumed to be encountered by all doctors. This is rarely the case, but currently there is no easy way to extract the same clinical need information from a large number of doctors unless they are interviewed in person by the DMI.

The knowledge and information required for successful academic innovation exist either as clinical patient records or research data but is not easily accessible. A centralized electronic system which keeps track of the shortcomings of each clinical or experimental procedure could be a great resource for future innovation in that field.

The Academic Solution: Trauma and Emergency Medicine Innovation (TEMI) Program

We were aware of the lack of coordination of the academic resources for innovation. In our own division, there were several separate successful innovation projects, but overall everybody felt that there is a need for a more focused approach. In particular we identified problems with both the innovation process and its execution. The first author of this chapter was hired as the director of medical innovation (DMI) and initiated the Trauma and Emergency Medicine Innovation Program (TEMI). TEMI started in May 2015 to accelerate academic innovation by providing specialized faculty-to-faculty intradepartmental support during the innovation process and execution. Overall, we have evaluated 37 new biomedical innovation ideas, filed 5 new patents, wrote over 10 research grant applications, and did over 10 VC funding presentations. We have advanced one project to the start-up phase and obtained seed funding to advance the proof of concept. There are several specific features that set the TEMI program apart from other academic innovation initiatives:

1. *Transparency*. Each step of the innovation process, from defining the clinical need and formulating a solution for prototyping, writing the patent, to pitching for funding, is transparent to the clinician inventor.
2. *Focus on the clinical field*. In our case trauma surgery and emergency medicine. Without focus on a clinical field, the specific innovation needs of the clinical subspecialty could be ignored in favor of other medical specialties with a larger business potential. In our case, the patient population for trauma and emergency medicine (TEM) is much smaller than cancer and cardiovascular disease. A university level approach to innovation will likely place TEM second over other specialties. Also, the investors who are focused on cancer or cardiovascular disease treatment would not see trauma innovation as an opportunity. Instead, we reached out to specialized investors (often the clinicians who work in the same field) and industry departments which are focused on trauma to advance our projects.
3. *Co-PI collaborative work*. It was very important for the DMI to be a faculty member rather than administrative support. In this position, the DMI can collaborate on research grants, co-write publications (such as the present chapter), provide innovation education/training, and be an active part of the entrepreneurship system.
4. *Commercialization focus*. Generally, the goal of academic innovation is to license the technology. Due to the technology transfer office (TTO) culture, this could be perceived as the next step after patent protection. In contrast, we set the goal to commercialize the technology that we develop. In this way we are addressing the entire process of commercialization in our model rather than just patent protection which is rarely enough for licensing.
5. *Process and execution support*. The key to changing the innovation culture is process and execution support. Currently, there is a lot of emphasis on advising and education. Even with a lot of knowledge about the innovation process, in the present academic environment where clinicians and scientists are busy with clinical practice or writing the next research grant, it is practically impossible to execute any of the work without additional resources. That results in less enthusiasm and involvement in innovation despite the knowledge.
6. *Information and knowledge management*. The vast amount of new information and knowledge that is generated during the innovation process (i.e., new ideas, design of prototypes, manufacturing specifications, business plans, vendor contracts, investor pitches, etc.) requires a new management system that can be easily shared among the aISN.

TEMI Innovation Process Support

Our process support is educational and operational. At the education level, we have organized introductory lectures to educate faculty, residents, and fellows on the innovation process. The topics discussed include a description of the innovation resources within the university, the intellectual property protection process, and the regulatory requirements.

Besides six introductory lectures about the innovation process, we have offered a start-up boot camp where residents and clinicians can participate in one of our ongoing innovation projects as clinical experts or another business function that they might want to perform. While we make sure that the activities are coordinated and follow the commercialization goal, the residents help with creating a clinical customer profile, analyzing the potential market, predicting the sales prices, and creating 5-year sales forecasts. We have applied this concept with great success to the portable abdominal insufflator and two other projects with clinicians from the Master of Public Health Program at the Harvard School of Public Health.

At the operational level, we first created a simplified six-step innovation development sorting system to identify the most advanced projects. The six steps focus on:

Step 1. Clinical need ideas. Record all new medical product ideas which are based on a real clinical need and can be described in detail during a 1-hour interview with clinicians. Although one might think that everybody has many ideas, the clinicians and scientists usually only mention the ideas that they have been thinking for a while about. The maximum number of ideas we got from one clinician during a 1-hour session was four, and only one was considered the most promising.

Step 2. Working prototype. Sort out all ideas without an engineering solution or a functional prototype. Although many ideas could result into a prototype, if there are some ideas for which the team has already built a working prototype, those projects are further along the development path.

Step 3. Patentability. Sort out all engineering solutions which are not patentable. Often, the clinicians or scientists focus on improving an existing solution. The "me too" ideas, although useful in clinical practice, will not generate a strong IP, and therefore the licensing potential is reduced.

Step 4. Business case. Sort out patents which are not economically feasible because of lack of freedom to operate or other economic reasons (the market is too small to justify the investment, the distribution channels are unclear, there are no available reimbursement codes).

Step 5. Trauma and emergency medicine (TEM) focus. Pick the projects which have a TEM focus to take advantage of the clinical expertise in our group. Some projects might apply to a larger population of patients than trauma. For example, the portable abdominal insufflator might apply to all laparoscopic surgeries. Although it is tempting to add as many clinical applications as possible, expanding the product use to other a larger application where the main clinical consultant is not a specialist might make the entire project less fit for the initial application (e.g., the portability is not an issue for OR laparoscopic procedures) and less credible.

Step 6. Licensing potential. Evaluate the licensing potential and sort out the projects which are not ready for licensing. There could be many reasons for low licensing potential depending on the requirements for licensing from industry. Currently, the medical device companies require significant de-risking to be performed before they license. This includes the product design to be finished and an FDA application to be filed or even approved.

Although this sorting process is not comprehensive, it is feasible for limited academic resources and aligned with the current practice of the TTO.

Secondly, we put together a professional service support structure which spanned outside the academic environment. In addition to the existing academic structure, we needed to involve IP, FDA, and business consultants. We also needed a network of prototype development companies and venture capital investors specialized in the trauma field. Each project required a different prototype manufacturer (i.e., catheters vs. complex electronic devices) even if they address the trauma market. For funding, it is necessary to involve a large number of investors for every opportunity as their specialty and appetite for investment vary.

Equally important, if not more important than any other resources, we needed to create a funding structure for early development. Generally, the traditional granting agencies do not sponsor early development work. One new program at NIH, the National Center for Accelerated Innovation, offers small grants for feasibility ($50,000) and commercial plan development ($200,000). These funds do not cover the development costs which are in the order of millions of dollars for the simplest medical device.

Even so, research grants are not easily available, and other more creative funding infrastructure had to be developed. One such structure could involve first-time investing clinicians, their family and friends. Most clinicians are legally qualified to be accredited investors (annual individual income over $200,000 over the last 2 years) and should be encouraged to invest as they understand the clinical needs the best. It is also problematic for external investors to contribute when there are a lot of potential accredited investors among the clinicians and their close circle of friends, but they do not invest in their own ideas.

TEMI Execution Support

Besides defining a process and a network of resources, the key component which is missing in academia is execution support. It is not sufficient to have the knowledge and a process in place; the most critical part for getting things done is execution. The physicians and senior scientists do not have the necessary time to execute the many steps of the innovation process on their own. Some of the execution tasks that the DMI performed to support the physicians were:

- *Idea mining*. One-hour one-on-one discussion with 22 doctors. These sessions are the first step in identifying the most significant clinical needs and possible solutions that the clinician thought of. The result was that 37 clinical needs and initial solutions were generated as the basis for future innovation. They included old and new problems that the doctors were facing in their practice and wanted to solve.
- *TTO interaction*. The interaction with the TTO includes filing the innovation disclosure, responding to patentability issues, and assisting with the patent text editing. We have filed 12 new invention disclosures, 6 provisional patents, and 3 patents. After IP filing, the licensing process involves interaction with outside companies (two licensing negotiations are ongoing).
- *Grant writing and management*. Several grants are available for funding early developments. We have filed seven Boston Biomedical Innovation Center/National Institute for Accelerated Innovation grants, six NIH STTRs, and three PHI-IDGs (innovation development grant). The DMI was either a PI or co-PI on all these grant applications.
- *Research and development*. Besides applying for grants, the DMI or members of the innovation team assisted with the development of ten new prototypes, two benchtops, two animals, and one clinical testing project.
- *Consultant management*. A significant amount time is necessary to manage the vendor network. We interacted with over 20 people including interviews, product presentations, site visits, and consultant contract negotiation.
- *Industry licensee interaction*. As mentioned before, the licensing process requires the involvement of the inventor/innovation team to provide technical and marketing assistance to the PHI associates.

TEMI Information and Knowledge Management

Within the TEMI program, in order to manage the vast amount of new information and knowledge created during the innovation process, we have created a standard electronic folder system for each innovation project and for each doctor. Each project folder contains sub-folders for the clinical need, the design inputs (general functional requirements), IP, design output (solution), technical specifications, prototype execution, testing, business plan, and fund raising. The result was over 400 folders to be managed individually by the DMI. In contrast to the traditional way where each inventor is managing their innovation projects in a different way, this new management system is superior since it applies the same process to all projects. Even so, managing so many projects and folders manually turned out to be very time-consuming and not practical. Another limitation was that the results cannot be easily shared to each individual team member or external consultants. A more open-shared electronic resource was needed.

The Academic-Industry Solution: The Academic Innovation Management System (AIMS)

We have developed AIMS as an academic and industry collaboration to organize the science, knowledge, and information generated in the academic innovation environment and connect them with the outside industry [9]. AIMS contains a complex management system of the entire life cycle of innovation with a special emphasis on being academia friendly. AIMS allowed us to complement all the functions which were missing in the aISN with external resources such as investors, regulatory consultants, IP lawyers, and sales and marketing experts (Fig. 17.3).

The first step in introducing a new project in AIMS is a seven-step "Idea" flow sequence from defining the idea, creating a SWOT analysis, inputting the preliminary studies, performing a preliminary patent and FDA analysis, and ending with the idea summary which explains the main benefit of the new solution.

The next sequence of six questions, the "Pitch," contains a preliminary analysis of the market that could easily be performed by a clinician with minimal knowledge of the patient population and incidence of the disease as well as existing competitive product currently used in their field. The Pitch also contains information about the team members and projected expenses for development. This information is similar to

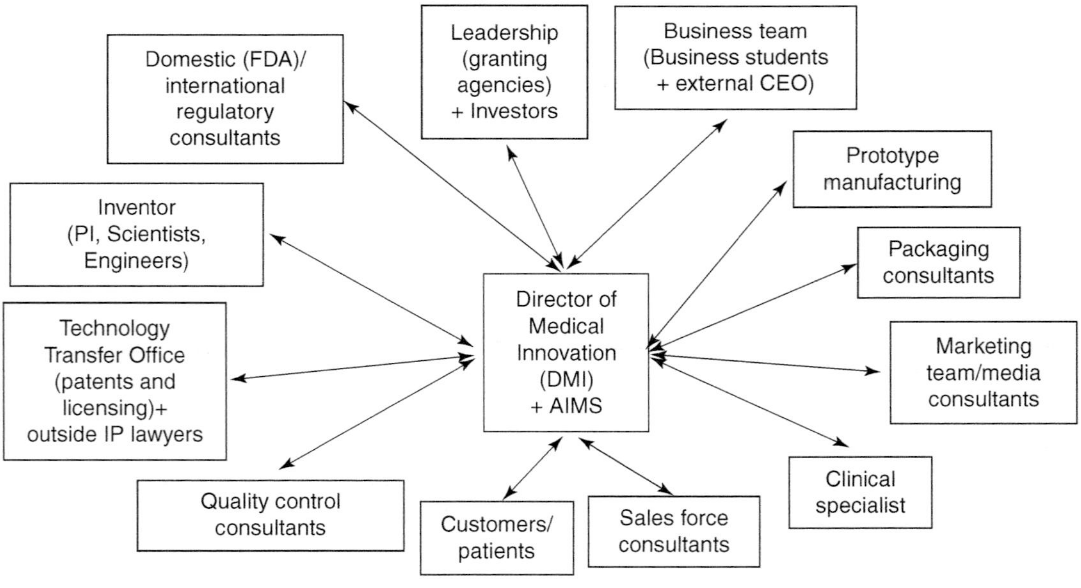

Fig. 17.3 Improved academic innovation social network (aISN) with director of medical innovation (DMI) and the external network, academic innovation management system (AIMS). The missing functions of the aISN are complemented by external resources including investors and expert consultants which have been selected and prescreened by the AIMS network. The collaboration with the industry and investment worlds is greatly accelerated when the aISN is complemented with AIMS

describing the team and projected budget for a scientific grant.

The third component is the "Launch" module, which contains the marketing plan, the budget, and the schedule for launch. This is a later step in the process, but usually the capital investors require early plans to figure out the total cost of the project, the estimated sales and expenses, and a time schedule for launch and commercial sales.

The result of the initial three-phase (Idea, Pitch, and Launch) questionnaire is a PDF document of a business pitch which can be used by clinician inventor to present to investors. Currently most clinician pitches contain a detailed description of the clinical need and little to no information about the business opportunity which is ultimately what investors are interested in.

The other functions of AIMS include idea ranking, idea funnel, project management tools, brainstorming platform, and customer and prospects management. A significant resource is the partner section where the academic partner can find and engage industry partners for rapid feedback or long-term project help. At present the AIMS platform is available free of cost to academic programs who want to start an innovation program and connect to external resources.

Conclusions

Currently, the academic innovation social network (aISN) is segmented and ineffective. On the other hand, the industry R&D network (RDN) is well established and use a time-tested process for turning innovative ideas into products. For each new product, at the center of the RDN, there is a product specialist who makes sure that new product is fit for use from a technical, business, regulatory, and commercialization.

In contrast, the aISN is made primarily of the inventors and their academic laboratory personnel. The technology transfer office (TTO) helps with intellectual property protection and licensing the technology. Some help can be provided by business school on the business development side.

In order to accelerate innovation, there is an urgent need to better organize the entire process. A recent initiative in trauma and emergency medicine innovation (TEMI) illustrates solutions for creating a winning academic innovation infrastructure in a specific clinical field. In addition, an industry-academia partnership developed a complex electronic resource package for academic innovation management system (AIMS) to mine innovative ideas, manage the innovation process, sort promising projects, and connect the academic worlds with capital investors and service providers. Both the academic programs, TEMI and the private e-resource platform AIMS, are adaptable to any academic specialty and industrial environment. Only by applying similar solutions to a large number of innovative ideas at many academic units and universities, we can learn to create a robust system that addresses all challenges and dramatically advances academic innovation.

Acknowledgments The research leading to these results has received funding from UEFISCDI Romania, under the project "Innovative portable insufflation device to stop uncontrolled abdominal bleeding in military and civilian trauma," contract no. 244PED/2017, PN-III-P2-2.1-PED-2016-1587, and the Competitiveness Operational Program 2014–2020 under the project P_37_357 "Improving the research and development capacity for imaging and advanced technology for minimal invasive medical procedures (iMTECH)" grant, Contract No. 65/08.09.2016, SMIS-Code: 103633.

References

1. Massachusetts General Hospital. Home page. Retrieved from: https://www.massgeneral.org/about/overview.aspx. Accessed on 9 June 2018.
2. Gruionu G, Velmahos G. The lean innovation model for academic medical discovery. In: Latifi R, Gruessner RWG, Rhee PM, editors. Advanced technologies in surgery, trauma and critical care. Heidelberg: Springer Science + Business Media; 2015. p. 73–80.
3. Zenios S, Makower J, Yock P, Denend L, Brinton TJ, Kumar UN, editors. Biodesign: the process of innovating medical technologies. Cambridge: Cambridge University Press; 2010.
4. Aulet B. Disciplined entrepreneuship: 24 steps to a successful startup. Hoboken: Wiley; 2013. p. 272, ISBN 978-1-118-69228-8.
5. Miller JC, Serrato R, Represas-Cardenas JM, Kundahl G. The handbook of nanotechnology: business, policy, and intellectual property law. Hoboken: Wiley; 2005. p. 99.

6. Inside a Grassroots Academic Innovation Community. Inside Higher Ed. April, 11th, 2018. Retrieved from: https://www.insidehighered.com/digital-learning/views/2018/04/11/when-there-no-playbook-building-grassroots-academic-innovation. Accessed on 9 June 2018.
7. Ries E. The lean startup: how today's entrepreneurs use continuous innovation to create radically successful businesses. New York: Crown Business; 2011.
8. Steffens TG, Gunser JM, Saviello GM. Perfusion electronic record documentation using epic systems software. J Extra Corpor Technol. 2015;47(4):237–41.
9. AIMS – Academic Innovation Management. Home page. Retrieved from: www.acadinno.com. Accessed on 10 June 2018.

18

Modern Hospital as Training Grounds Dealing with Resident Issues in New Era

Saju Joseph, Amy Joseph, Leslie S. Forrest, Jane S. Wey, and Andrew M. Eisen

New Learners

Education at every level is facing new challenges. The technology and breadth of information available on our phones today are 10X greater than that which was required to send Neil Armstrong to the moon in 1969 [1]. Learners today have access to extraordinary amounts of data in the palms of their hands. Previous generations of learners spent most of their time absorbing facts and assimilating these data into the day-to-day aspects of their career. Mastery of one's career came from practice and the experience of connecting knowledge to a situation, being efficient, and optimizing the outcome.

In medicine, residency is the key to acquiring foundational experience, ideally in an environment that facilitates exponential learning. Residency forces trainees to develop efficiency in their workflow to allow for the time required to process large amounts of data created through patient care. This immersion technique creates active learners who are engaged in both the process and the outcome. Yet, as not all students learn optimally using this technique, tailoring training to the individual learner allows for the highest likelihood of success.

Modern hospitals have been quick to adopt new technologies to improve patient outcomes and experiences. Many hospitals have advanced electronic medical records (EMR), and patients are able to view their results soon after, or even concurrently with, their providers. These systems can seamlessly interface with external systems throughout the world. Providers may have immediate access to the health records of patients even when services had been provided outside of their network.

While these EMR advances have improved the patient experience within the healthcare system, the true breakthrough has been for the providers and administrators. Physicians can access patient records prior to initiating care. Administrators can track costs, lost time, and workflow issues with minimal effort. Residents can complete some of their work from any location and have access to significant repositories of data for research.

In the operating room, new technology continues to advance surgical care. Surgeons who employ these innovations do so with a solid foundation in "conventional" open surgical techniques. This foundation was developed in surgical training with repetition, coaching, mentorship, and time. Advances like laparoscopy, robotic surgery, and catheter-based surgery have expanded the range of proficiencies expected of the modern surgeon. Unfortunately, training time for residents has not increased to allow experiential learning opportunities in these skills. With

S. Joseph (✉) · A. Joseph · L. S. Forrest · A. M. Eisen
Graduate Medical Education, The Valley Health System, Las Vegas, NV, USA
e-mail: saju.joseph@uhsinc.com

J. S. Wey
Department of Surgery, Riverside Health System, Newport News, VA, USA

R. Latifi (ed.), *The Modern Hospital*, https://doi.org/10.1007/978-3-030-01394-3_18

the evolution of these techniques, the foundations of traditional open surgery have weakened within the workforce.

Graduate medical education has lagged behind the modern hospital in the adoption of new technologies and training techniques. Residents today have improved efficiency of time, data acquisition, and analytics to better assess patient conditions. They can also access tremendous amounts of current medical literature with minimal time or effort. Modern residency training isn't about the effort needed to gather and compile data, but rather the integration of massive amounts of available data to improve patient outcomes on the individual, institutional, community-wide, national, and even global scales. That process also requires extensive training in communication and problem-solving. Residents are no longer just finding answers to questions but instead are identifying problems from the existing data and developing solutions.

Educational Moments and Feedback

The most important job training hospitals have is educating residents to be successful physicians. However, these institutions have negligible guidance as to the best way to achieve that goal and even less feedback regarding the success or failure of their graduates.

Feedback for learners during training has been formalized for quite some time. The ACGME includes the core competencies as a foundation by which residents can receive feedback and measure their professional preparedness. Informal feedback and teachable moments are the areas in which most educational leaders focus their energy. Technology has expanded the acuity and enhanced the benefit of these moments for the learner. Faculty can provide formal and informal feedback instantaneously, while also capturing the details and specifics that make this type of feedback valuable. Feedback is more useful for the learner when it is provided as close to the teachable moment as possible. Ultimately, feedback serves to educate the learner and helps to develop the mentor/mentee relationship.

Time has been the greatest challenge in the changing healthcare landscape. Physicians are required to do more in less time to generate sufficient revenue to stay fiscally viable. This "time crunch" has affected academic medicine as well, particularly with respect to teaching. While educational content has evolved alongside advances in technology, clinical decision-making within the hospital remains relatively static. Thus, as faculty have less time to dedicate to education, learners have less time to grasp the nuances of applied medicine.

Fitting education into the framework of today's care necessitates using short intervals of time for condensed instruction, usually relevant to the situation at hand. These "educational moments" are incorporated into the usual flow of the workday. While these moments are often spontaneous and of high impact, they do not necessarily follow a preconceived curriculum and vary greatly by the individuals involved. Modern resident training couples these instrumental on-the-spot moments of learning with a more structured curriculum but still requires residents to be self-directed in the completion of their training. Therefore, graduate medical education programs must ensure resident self-directed learning is effective and the residents are not "losing the forest for the trees." Finally, training programs must prepare faculty to identify these educational moments and modify teaching techniques as needed for a varied group of learners to maximize success.

Identifying Resident Issues

Training residents involves much more than preparing them to provide innovative care to patients. The goal of a successful GME program is to develop students into professionals who are prepared to practice the art and science of medicine for the betterment of their patients. Mastery of the following skills is critical to achieve this end:

1. Medical knowledge and experience
2. Medical decision-making (ability to aptly apply knowledge and experience)

3. Exposure to new technologies and their application
4. Communication
5. Teamwork and the healthcare delivery models
6. Financial training
7. Leadership training
8. Wellness vs stress and burnout

The transition from student to professional is not uniform and requires active learning by the resident to achieve mastery. Currently, training programs may achieve excellence in some aspects of preparation but may fail in others. This incomplete mastery of all aspects of healthcare knowledge leaves gaps in a physician's skill set, leaving them ill prepared to practice on their own (Fig. 18.1). This struggle to practice, especially early in one's career, has been shown to result in high burnout rates, poor patient outcomes, and increased costs [2]. In the following sections, we outline our approach to each component of resident training and highlight areas of innovation that may change the approach in the future.

Medical Knowledge and Experience

The foundation of resident training is teaching medical knowledge and providing opportunities to acquire hands-on experience. While this has not changed over time, the methods used are changing dramatically. In the past, didactic lectures, textbooks, and journals taught medical knowledge. Advances in care were slowly assimilated into hospitals through new providers, sometimes driven by patient demand, after careful consideration by the hospital system and peer review.

Today, medical knowledge circulates in an instant. Conferences and medical associations have active social media campaigns that engage physicians worldwide with scientific developments and innovations faster than ever before.

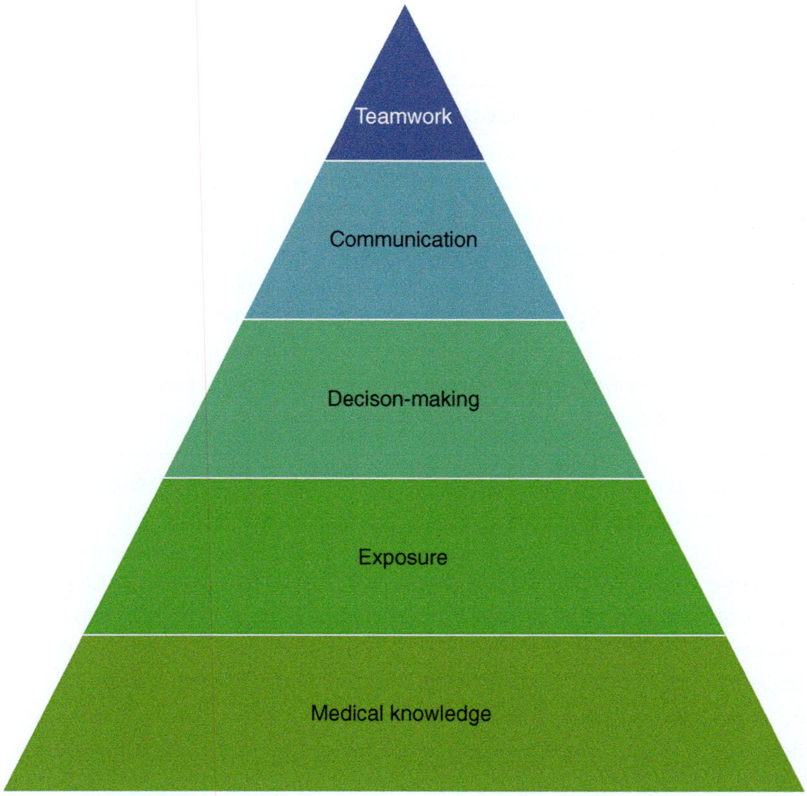

Fig. 18.1 Historical training goals

Simultaneously, advances in medications and procedures are marketed directly to patients, with hospitals and physicians scrambling to keep up. Unfortunately, many of these "advances" do not necessarily produce better outcomes and often significantly increase costs.

The paradigm of young faculty advancing care is becoming obsolete as technology is outpacing training. New techniques and innovations often require faculty to spend more time caring for their patients as they acquire the skill set needed to perform novel procedures. This shift often results in a more limited training experience for the resident as hospitals balance innovation with patient safety.

Simulation is a safe alternative for resident training, especially with respect to innovations. Simulation allows residents to train in a consequence-free environment while still gaining valuable feedback from faculty. While simulation does not replace direct patient care, it does provide a dynamic platform to teach core competencies, as well as pioneering techniques to which residents might otherwise have limited access during their training.

Medical Decision-Making

Resident exposure to clinical care allows for the development of clinical decision-making. There are six basic components to this process [3]:

- Medical knowledge base
- Data gathering
- Correlation to the clinical situation
- Applications and limitations of the medical literature
- Costs and outcomes of different interventions
- Medical decisions

While most medical students are taught elements at the top of this decision tree, residents are required to incorporate all of the components, including considering the socioeconomic impact of medical care. As residents progress, they develop a more multifaceted and nuanced approach to making medical decision while keeping abreast of the ever-growing body of medical literature. Modern training programs must incorporate the added step of factoring in the cost/benefit analysis of a given clinical course or treatment to the resident decision tree.

New Technologies

As discussed above, advances in technology are constantly impacting healthcare delivery, costs, and outcomes. While residents may be exposed to these new technologies in both the hospital and the simulation lab, achieving clinical mastery of new techniques, in addition to basic skills, can be difficult within the residency period. Furthermore, coaches/experts are integral to the development of these new skills. As noted earlier, physicians have minimal time to train residents on new technologies and/or may be just learning themselves. Additionally, incorporating new techniques sporadically may detract from a resident's exposure to a procedure done in the standard fashion.

Robotic surgery is an excellent example of this paradigm. Surgeons began training on the robot with other faculty as assistants. As robotic technology evolves, surgeons continue to be active learners. While in certain situations, this may benefit patients and improve outcomes; the resident training experience has suffered. Currently, a minority of surgical graduates are masters of robotic surgery, while simultaneously hospital systems respond to patient demands by marketing and promoting robotics. This has led to unsafe surgical practices demonstrating the need for further training.

Communication and Teamwork

The process of healthcare delivery has many complex working parts. During the course of patient care, multiple small errors can be made which, in and of themselves, are largely inconsequential. However, the cumulative effect of compounded errors can result in varying degrees of undesirable consequences. This concept, known as the Swiss cheese model, has been well documented in healthcare [4]. In many of these circumstances, the mistakes are related to a failure in communication and are nearly always preventable if team members are effective communicators. Resident training has identified that communication training and multidisciplinary team building are integral to patient outcomes and a positive work culture [5].

Modern hospitals strive for a positive work environment for all employees. This environment translates to a more positive patient experience and may improve patient outcomes. The "culture of safety" concept was borrowed from the airline industry's mandate for flight safety [6, 7]. Training residents in the "culture of safety" philosophy encourages the diffusion of this ethos throughout the hospital setting.

Modern training programs strive to support multidisciplinary teamwork, collegial culture, and open communication. This collaboration must incorporate all healthcare providers, such as nursing, physical therapy, and respiratory therapy. Additionally, as healthcare delivery becomes more complex, a greater number of specialists can become involved in a single patient's care. While this has allowed for greater specificity, it also increases the chance for errors. Thus, communication and teamwork are of paramount importance.

Financial Training

Increasingly, financial concerns play a role in patient care decisions from both the patient's and the provider/hospital's perspective. Patients often struggle with healthcare expenses, forcing them to choose between paying their medical bills and paying for basic needs such as food and shelter. Even when a patient is insured, the cost of the insurance, co-pays, and other out of pocket expenses can become financially overwhelming. Some patients end up considering treatment options based on cost, choosing a generic medication over a brand name, foregoing a costly chemotherapy option, or delaying or avoiding a needed surgery due to projected work time/income loss. Unfortunately, patients and providers must deal with these financial realities. Today's clinicians must incorporate consideration of a patient's finances into their healthcare decision-making.

Globally speaking, the burden of costs associated with health overall affects the economy in a myriad of ways. In the past, hospitals were relatively financially secure because of multiple solid revenue streams such as research grants, private insurance reimbursement, Medicare funding, and state and federal tax revenue. However, more recently, there has been a significant reduction in research funding and both Medicare and private insurance reimbursement. Compounding this loss of revenue is a significant increase in expenditures for operating costs, pharmaceuticals, resident education, and caring for an aging population. Hospitals are forced to make difficult decisions about spending in an effort to balance fiscal viability with appropriate patient care. It is clearly important that residents gain understanding of the financial considerations of treatment decisions while in training, including the importance of counseling patients on the potential financial impact of treatment options, while also being aware of the effect various decisions may have on the hospital costs and operational margins.

Trainees must be taught the economics of their practices and how to survive within the changing financial environment. As healthcare finances change, physician lifestyle and compensation are directly affected. Physicians today are more likely to be employed by a corporation, leading to a loss of autonomy. Non-physicians, with little clinical experience, may oversee physicians in these entities. Even academic faculty face the challenge of balancing revenue generation with research and education in a constantly changing healthcare landscape. With the loss of autonomy, reduced compensation for work product, and bureaucracy of healthcare, many physicians are feeling disenfranchised. In this environment, it is not surprising that millennial learners are less willing to sacrifice their work/life balance for a marginal return.

Financial training in residency is a necessity. It should educate trainees about the costs of running a practice, understanding and maximizing reimbursement, recognizing downstream revenue and external revenue sources, comprehending the financial implications of all healthcare decisions, and achieving fiscal transparency by the GME department within the healthcare system. Understanding the cost and institutional goals of resident training allows residents to be active participants in their learning and the financial decisions that affect their educational environment. A successful program trains residents to understand their value, teaches them the financial implications of their care, appreciates their contributions, prepares them financially, and provides mentorship throughout their careers.

Leadership Opportunities

Changes in healthcare have put a premium on leadership. The traditional hospital management paradigm of expanding growth, increasing volume, and extending service lines does not always lead to success in today's healthcare market. It is important to recognize that not all care is profitable, service lines require a significant up-front investment, and growth outside of the service area has a deleterious effect on both the community and the hospital system. Furthermore, as more quality and patient initiatives are linked to reimbursement, modern hospitals increasingly benefit from clinical leadership to optimize patient outcomes and minimize waste. While physicians are highly trained for clinical work, few have developed the leadership skills necessary to succeed in healthcare/hospital management. As more physicians pursue these roles as a means to continue service, maintain financial solvency, and advocate for their communities, there is an increase in physicians seeking leadership courses or master's degrees in business administration or public health.

As with clinical practice, adequate exposure to leadership skills provides an opportunity for residents to develop these skills themselves. Ultimately, leadership training for residents allows the learner to develop acumen, as well as emotional intelligence, the latter of which is increasingly emphasized in developing physician leaders [8]. Connecting the clinical practice of medicine to the everyday choices that administrators make illuminates the often complex nature of even the simplest decisions in the hospital system. For residents, the recognition that their skill set is applicable to nonclinical situations is enlightening and may provide additional options for professional development and career choice.

Dr. Spence Taylor, in his presidential address to the Southern Surgical Society in 2015, said the most valuable lesson he learned about leadership was "Things are the way they are because someone wants it that way [9]." In order to institute change, it is crucial to identify who that "someone" is and either address their concerns about change or force the change in spite of their objections. Neither technique is right all the time, but knowing when to use one versus the other is the key to good leadership. From a resident perspective, this same skill set is important in many clinical interactions. Whether faced with a patient who is resistant to medical advice or another provider disagreeing with a clinical decision, the approach and leadership style is the same in achieving the desired understanding. Ultimately, these skills enable residents to educate and encourage patients to make healthy decisions personally and globally.

Stress and Wellness

Physicians and residents are similar to highly trained professional athletes. There are only minor differences between success and failure in both healthcare and athletics. Repetition, adaptability, extensive training, and a great deal of physical, mental, and emotional strength are required to succeed in both fields. There may be limited opportunity to analyze outcomes to improve performance as both must move their concentration to the next game/patient.

Unlike an athlete, there is no off-season for physicians. The physical, mental, and emotional strain of providing healthcare is continuous and occurs around the clock. Residents are involved in the most complex life and death decisions while working long hours with minimal pay. Compounding the situation, they often feel isolated from the rest of society and have minimal education on coping with stress. Ultimately, the closest similarity between physicians and athletes is in the resiliency required to continue functioning at the highest level after failing moments earlier. In sports, it is described as having a "short memory."

While stress in resident training is not new, our understanding of how that stress affects performance is [2]. Wellness, work/life balance, and resiliency are becoming integral parts of resident education. By teaching time efficiency along with recognition and management of stress, encouraging participation in inter-professional teams, providing loss counseling, and emphasizing the importance of life outside of the hospital, residents are empowered to reach their potential and develop as physicians and people. Hospitals and patients also benefit from a physician workforce that has lower stress, reduced anxiety, and a better ability to cope with loss and failure [2]. While these wellness programs are still in their infancy, the success of these programs in other settings shows great promise for their application in GME.

Conclusions

Modern hospitals are dynamic in their approach to patients and resident training. The leadership within these institutions must balance patient outcomes and experiences, innovation and technology, and physician work/life balance with resident education and preparation for practice. The new paradigm of educational needs for residents continues to change as healthcare delivery changes (Fig. 18.2). Adding to the complexity of this model are the financial implications that now affect healthcare directly. Training programs focus their training on educational moments, effective communication, multidisciplinary teamwork, and exposure to new technology. They strive to allow the residents to develop independent decision-making skills while minimizing risks to patients.

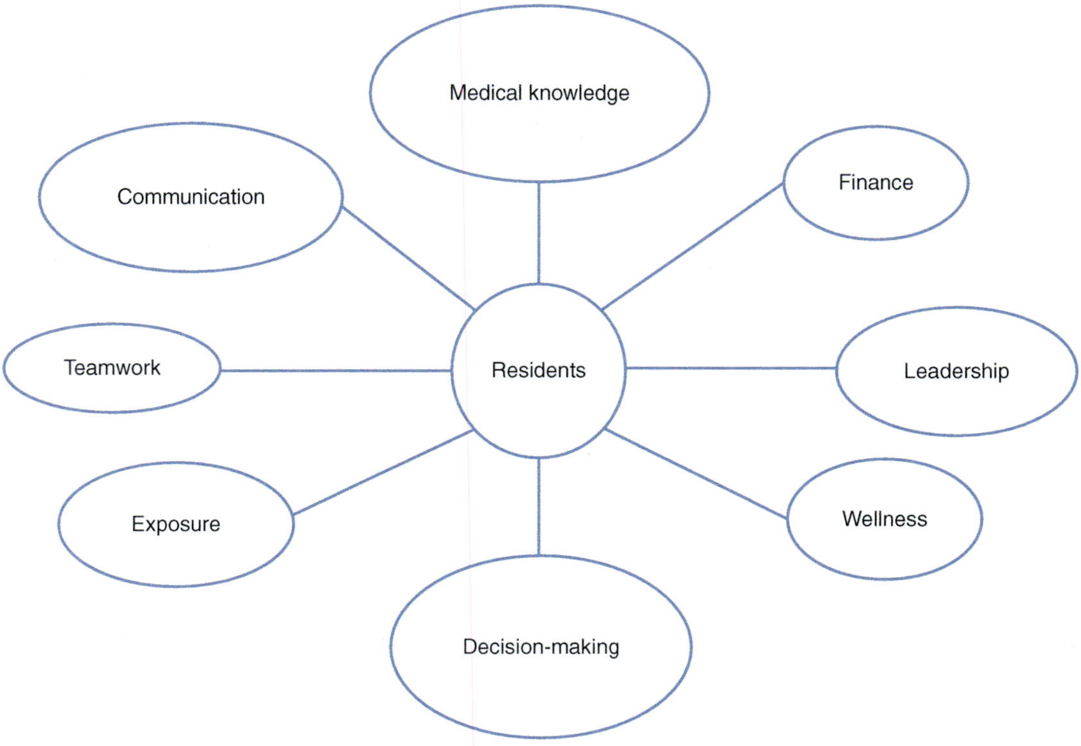

Fig. 18.2 Modern training paradigm

While most modern hospitals succeed in this model, the higher-functioning institutions include wellness in resident training to provide stronger and more resilient future physicians. Furthermore, these programs prepare residents for the financial environment of healthcare that will influence their personal and professional life. Finally, preparing residents for leadership allows trainees the opportunity to develop skills that are applicable to many different careers, while also enhancing their clinical care. Ultimately, the goal of modern training programs is to provide a comprehensive learning environment capable of training students with different learning styles and prepare residents for a successful career.

References

1. Apollo 11: The computers that put man on the moon. ComputerWeekly.com. July 2009. Retrieved from: www.computerweekly.com/feature/Apollo-11-The-computers-that-put-man-on-the-moon
2. Steenhuysen J. Counting the costs: U.S. hospitals feeling the pain of physician burnout. November 21, 2017. Reuters.com. Retrieved from: https://www.reuters.com/article/us-usa-healthcare-burnout/counting-the-costs-u-s-hospitals-feeling-the-pain-of-physician-burnout-idUSKBN1DL0EX
3. Agency for Healthcare Research and Quality (AHRQ). Evidence-based decisionmaking. Retrieved from: http://www.ahrq.gov/professionals/prevention-chronic-care/decision/index.html
4. Reason J. Human error: models and management. BMJ. 2000;320:768.
5. Sirriyeh R, Lawton R, Gardner P, et al. Coping with medical error: a systematic review of papers to assess the effects of involvement in medical errors on healthcare professionals' psychological well-being. Qual Saf Health Care. 2010;19:e43.
6. Brown RL, Holmes H. The use of a factor-analytic procedure for assessing the validity of an employee safety climate model. Accid Anal Prev. 1986;18(6):455–70.
7. Gill G, Shergill G. Perceptions of safety management and safety culture in the aviation industry in New Zealand. J Air Transp Manag. 2004;10:233–9.
8. Mintz LJ, Stoller JK. A systematic review of physician leadership and emotional intelligence. J Grad Med Educ. 2014;6(1):21–31.
9. Taylor S. Presidential address. Southern Surgical Society; 2015.

19 Healthcare Provider-Centered: Ergonomics of Movement and Functionality

Priya Goyal, Elizabeth H. Tilley, and Rifat Latifi

Introduction

The word ergonomics is derived from the Greek *ergon* (work) and *nomos* (laws) to denote the science of work. It is defined as "the scientific discipline concerned with the understanding of interactions of humans and other elements of a system, and the profession that applies theory, principles, data and methods to design in order to optimize human well-being and overall system performance [1]." The term occupational ergonomics is more appropriate, as it intends to promote health, efficiency, and well-being of employees by designing safe, satisfying, and productive work environments and applies to all occupations, including healthcare providers, with healthcare as one of the fastest-growing sectors of the US economy. Jobs in healthcare are growing substantially compared to other sectors. Between 2010 and 2020, jobs in the healthcare sector are projected to grow by 30%, more than twice as fast as the general economy. Registered nurses, home health aides, and personal healthcare aides are among the occupations nationally projected to have the largest job growth between 2010 and 2020, adding more than two million jobs and with another 700,000 job openings due to vacancies from attrition [2].

There is a close and dynamic relationship between working life and health, where health affects work life and work life affects health. Workplace injuries and illnesses harm the worker—not only in terms of physical injury and disability but also mentally and emotionally. Ergonomics focuses on the appropriate design of workplaces, systems, equipment, work processes, and environments to accommodate workers. In the hospital industry, this number consists of millions of employees. Providing an environment with proper ergonomics and functionality and free of work-related injury is of outmost importance. This chapter will highlight the importance of the application of ergonomics in the healthcare sector and emphasize the necessity of how it can improve patient and staff safety.

Magnitude of the Problem

The World Health Organization/International Labour Organization (WHO/ILO) has reported that of all fatalities in industrial countries, 5–7% are attributed to work-related illnesses and occupational injuries [3]. Work-related injuries and illnesses account for an estimated loss of $250 billion annually in medical expenses, and reduced productivity is another big loss. According to an estimate

P. Goyal · E. H. Tilley
Department of Surgery, Westchester Medical Center, Valhalla, NY, USA

R. Latifi (✉)
New York Medical College, School of Medicine, Department of Surgery and Westchester Medical Center, Valhalla, NY, USA
e-mail: rifat_latifi@nymc.edu; rifat.latifi@wmchealth.org

R. Latifi (ed.), *The Modern Hospital*, https://doi.org/10.1007/978-3-030-01394-3_19

by Leigh, these losses are 12% more than the cost of all cancers and 30% more than costs for diabetes [4]. The Association of American Medical Colleges' 2014 Physician Specialty Data Book states that at-risk physicians comprise 20.4% (175,955 of 860,939 physicians) of the active physician workforce. This workforce is expected to face a shortage by 2025, with a loss of 25,200–33,200 surgeons alone, and disability is one contributing factor [5]. The American Nurses Association (ANA) predicts that there will be more registered nurse jobs available through 2022 than any other profession in the United States. The US Bureau of Labor Statistics (2018) projects that 1.1 million additional nurses are needed to avoid a further shortage. Similarly, a crisis looms in the field of laboratory workers. The US Department of Health and Human Services predicted that an additional 138,000 workers will be needed with only 50,000 expected to be trained in areas including phlebotomy and histotechnology [6]. This shortage, along with demanding nature of jobs in hospitals, early retirement, and workplace injuries, has the potential to create a situation of crisis over the span of the next few years. ANA's survey found that patient handling accounted for 25% of all work-related claims incurring financial losses to the hospitals.

Data indicates that the most common causes of workers' compensation claims in hospitals were strains (28%), followed by falls, trips, and slips (17%). More detailed data from the National Council on Compensation Insurance (NCCI) shows that 20% of lost-time injuries were caused by "lifting." This eye-opening data is compelling enough to bring necessary interventions in workplaces. The workers' compensation claims estimate a range from an average of $25,450 to $38,280 per injury [7].

Table 19.1 Ergonomics is multidisciplinary in scope, with three broad domains

Domains	Definition	Components
1. Physical ergonomics	Physical ergonomics relates to physical activity with human anatomical, anthropometric, physiological, and biomechanical characteristics	Working postures Material handling Repetitive movements Work-related musculoskeletal disorders Workplace layout
2. Cognitive ergonomics	Cognitive ergonomics is concerned with interactions among human's mental processes, such as perception, memory, and reasoning with motor response	Mental workload Decision-making Skilled performance Human reliability Work stress quality of training Teamwork, participatory design
3. Organizational ergonomics	Organizational ergonomics is concerned with optimization of sociotechnical systems, including their organizational structures, policies, and processes	Communication and crew resource management Work design and design of working times Cooperative work Virtual organizations, telework, and quality management

Based on data from Ref. [8]

Ergonomics: Physical, Cognitive, and Organizational

Table 19.1 describes the three broad domains of ergonomics: physical, cognitive, and organizational [8]. Physical ergonomics relates to physical activity with human anatomical, anthropometric, physiological, and biomechanical characteristics. Cognitive ergonomics is concerned with interactions among human's mental processes, such as perception, memory, and reasoning with motor response. Organizational ergonomics is concerned with optimization of sociotechnical systems, including their organizational structures, policies, and processes.

Application of Physical Ergonomics

Surgeons, interventional medical specialists, nurses, nursing aides, and radiographers all are at the highest risk of occupation-related injuries. A report published by the Institute of Medicine (IOM) showed that patient safety is directly linked to medication errors, adverse drug events, duty hours, fatigue, and healthcare worker's working conditions [9]. Human factors and ergonomics (HFE) are the key component in these adverse events [10]. Good ergonomics in the workplace can improve productivity and morale of workers and decrease injuries, sick leave, staff turnover, and absenteeism.

Physical ergonomics is concerned with human anatomical, anthropometric, physiological, and biomechanical characteristics as they relate to physical activity [11]. The Centers for Disease Control (CDC) classifies the ergonomic hazards as physical, chemical, biological, ergonomic, and work-related stress. Physical risks are due to heavy lifting of patients or equipment, postural imbalance, vibration, nonionizing (UV) and ionizing (X-rays) radiation, prolonged duration of surgery, and incorrect posture while operating. Work-related musculoskeletal disorders refer to conditions involving nerves, tendons, muscles, and supporting structures of the body that are caused or exacerbated by workplace conditions or exposures that may impair working capacity. In a recent systematic review of physical complications in 5828 physicians, musculoskeletal disorders (MSDs) were the most common complications with degenerative cervical spine disease seen in 17%, rotator cuff pathology seen in 18%, degenerative lumbar spine disease seen in 19%, and carpal tunnel syndrome seen in 9% [12]. The chemical risks are exposure to inorganic agents such as mercury; organic agents such as solvents, resins, and anesthetic gases; caustic agents (formaldehyde and hydrogen peroxide); and allergens (latex) [13]. The biological hazards may be caused by airborne microorganisms as well as via body-fluid transmission; the most common pathogens are bacteria, viruses (HIV, HBV, HCV), and fungi [14]. The main objective of HFE-based system design is to improve the well-being (e.g., clinician and patient satisfaction) and overall system performance which includes patient safety. Table 19.2 details guidelines to avoid various workplace injuries.

Application of Technologies to Improve Ergonomics and Safety

The Occupational Safety Healthcare Act (OSHA's 1970) strives to "assure safe and healthful working conditions for working men and women..." and mandates that "each employer shall furnish to each of his/her employers employment and a place of employment which are free from recognized hazards that are causing or are likely to cause death or serious physical harm to his/her employees." Applying ergonomics to day-to-day activities of healthcare personnel and the healthcare facility will help healthcare providers and administrators to move forward in attaining safer outcomes. The OSHA has issued comprehensive guidelines on how to apply HFEs in hospitals.

It is extremely important that leadership demonstrates the commitment to reduce or eliminate patient handling hazards by establishing the program that addresses continued training of employees in injury prevention. There should be procedures in place for reporting early signs and symptoms of back pain and other musculoskeletal injuries.

Employees should participate in workplace safety programs by being fully cognizant of unsafe working conditions if any are present and should promptly report signs and symptoms of injuries.

Ergonomics in the Operating Room

Factors that cause work-related MSD in surgeons are awkward posture, repetitive movements, and excessive force [15]. The signs of musculoskeletal symptoms are muscle pain,

Table 19.2 Guidelines to avoid injuries

Type of guidelines	Who can apply	What to do
Lifting guidelines	Nurse assistants, licensed practical nurses, registered nurses, and dispatch team	Never transfer patients/residents when off balance Lift loads close to the body Never lift alone, particularly fallen patients/residents; use team lifts or use mechanical assistance Limit the number of allowed lifts per worker per day Avoid heavy lifting especially with spine rotated Training on when and how to use mechanical assistance
Patient handling	Nurse assistants, licensed practical nurses, registered nurses, and dispatch team	Devices such as shower chairs that fit over the toilet, using this device can eliminate multiple transfers performed directly by healthcare workers Toilet seat risers: equalize the height of wheelchair and toilet seat, making it a lateral transfer rather than a lift up and back into wheelchair Mechanical lift equipment to help lift patients/residents who cannot support their own weight Overhead track mounted patient lifters: a tract system built into the ceiling that sling lifts attach to. This system provides patient/residents mobility from room to room without manual lifting Lateral transfer devices: devices used to laterally transfer a patient/resident, for example, from bed to gurney. This type of device helps prevent staff from back injuries Sliding boards: A slick board used under patients/residents to help reduce the need for lifting during transfer of patient/residents
		Slip sheets/roller sheets: help to reduce friction while laterally transferring patients/residents or repositioning patients/residents in bed Height-adjustable electric beds that have height controls to allow for easy transfers from bed height to wheelchair height Walking belts or gait belts (with handles) that provide stabilization for ambulatory patients/residents by allowing workers to hold onto the belt and support patients/residents when walking
Medical management	Program, supervised by a person trained in the prevention of musculoskeletal disorders, should be in place to manage the care of those injured	The program should have: Accurate injury and illness recording Early identification and treatment of injured employees "Light duty" or "no lifting" work restrictions during recovery periods Systematic monitoring of injured employees to identify when they are ready to return to regular duty

discomfort, numbness down, burning, tenderness, swelling, limited range of motion, and loss of power. Open, laparoscopic, or microsurgery has all been equally shown to cause work-related MSD. Teaching correct working methods and using proper seats and ergonomic equipment are the best strategies to reduce musculoskeletal symptoms in the surgical profession. Adjustability of the table height and the optimal placement of the monitor during laparoscopic surgery are other important interventions to be considered [16].

Application of Integrated Cognitive and Organizational Ergonomics

The study of cognitive human factors is concerned with mental processes such as perception, memory, reasoning, and motor response, as they affect interactions among humans and other elements of a system [17]. High cognitive demands have been shown to influence physical capabilities, and physical demands definitely influence cognition. Compared with nonmedical personnel, medical employees are more likely to experience negative emotions from their job due to high workload, high pressure, higher expectations, and patient complaints [18]. There is mounting evidence that occupational psychosocial risk factors, such as high psychosocial demands, low job control, or low social support, have a role in causing MSD in doctors, allied health professionals, nurses, and aides [19, 20].

Effective solutions are multifaceted and include training, engineering changes, application of information, and technologies to create effective human-computer interaction and adjustments to agency policies.

The National Institute for Occupational Health (NIOSH) has published important guidelines which are helpful in tackling workplace stress. Figure 19.1 considers important milestones in applying cognitive ergonomics.

One way in which employers can reduce workplace stress is to clearly assign roles according to capabilities. This involves clearly defining an employee's role and responsibility, allowing them the opportunity to participate in the decision-making process, and reducing uncertainty about career development. Finally, it is

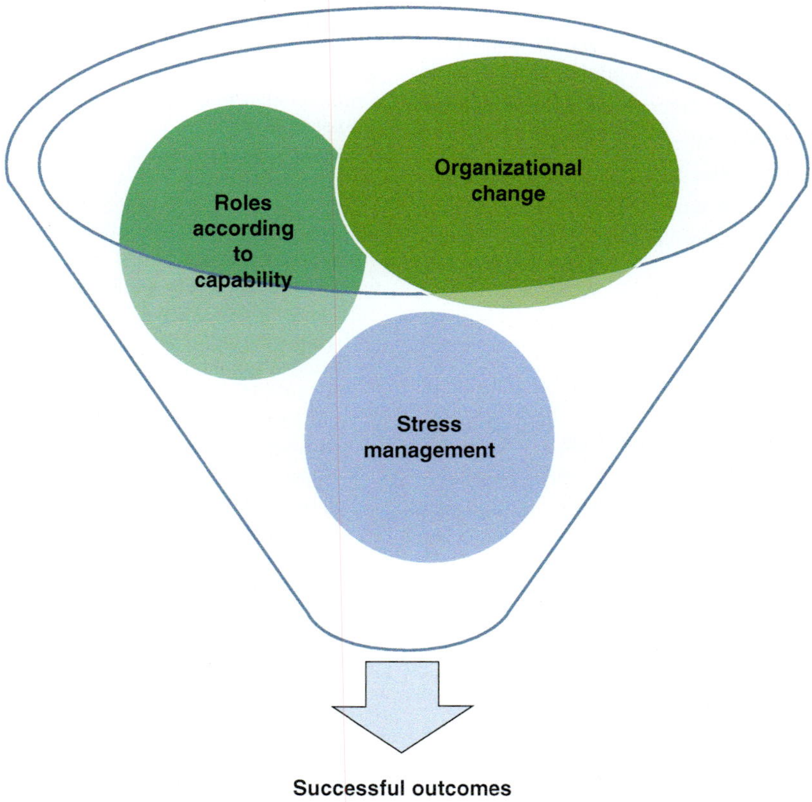

Fig. 19.1 Successful management of employee's health [1]

important to, as best as possible, provide job security by clear expectation.

Some of the elements of organizational ergonomics overlap with cognitive and physical ergonomics. Organizational ergonomics is concerned with optimization of organizational structures, policies, and processes. Various risk factors leading to dissatisfaction in an organization are work stress and training, lack of effective communication, workplace violence, and human conflict.

Organizational Change

Studies have shown that interventions based on team-based approaches (e.g., composed of doctors, nurses, managers, pharmacists, psychologists, etc.) for patient care delivery have been successful in improving job satisfaction and reducing job stress. Team-based care is defined by the National Academy of Medicine as "the provision of health services to individuals, families, and/or their communities by at least two health providers who work collaboratively with patients and their caregivers—to the extent preferred by each patient—to accomplish shared goals within and across settings to achieve coordinated, high-quality care" [21]. This approach allows services to be delivered efficiently, saving time.

Stress Management

Stress management at a workplace goes a long way in improving the healthcare professional's stress level. Stress management techniques include the following:

- Training in coping strategies
- Progressive relaxation
- Biofeedback
- Cognitive-behavioral techniques
- Time management
- Developing interpersonal skill

Conclusion

The application of ergonomics in healthcare has been getting the proper attention in recent decades. With advancing technologies, we are in a much better position to study the subject and intervene to reduce to severe consequence of improper repeated positional standing, lifting, and injuries.

References

1. International Ergonomics Association. The discipline of ergonomics http://iea.cc/browse.php?contID=what is ergonomics. Published August 2000. Accessed 16 Feb 2018. https://www.iea.cc.
2. Bureau of Labor Statistics. Employment projections. Table 2.7: Employment and output by industry. Retrieved from: www.bls.gov/emp/ep_table_207.htm. Updated January 2012. World Health Organization (WHO).
3. World Health Organization. Global strategy on occupational health for all: The way to health at work, WHO. 2014. Available from: http://www.who.int/occupational_health/publications/globstrategy/en/index4.html.
4. Leigh JP. Economic burden of occupational injury and illness in the United States. Milbank Q. 2011;89:728–72. https://doi.org/10.1111/j.1468-0009.2011.00648.x.
5. Center for Workforce Studies, Association of American Medical Colleges. 2014 physician specialty data book. https://members.aamc.org/eweb/upload/Physician%20Specialty%20Databook%202014.pdf. Published November 2014. Accessed 6 May 2018.
6. Haddad LM, Toney-Butler TJ. Nursing, shortage. [Updated 2018 May 13]. In: StatPearls [Internet]. Treasure Island (FL): StatPearls Publishing; 2018.. Available from: https://www.ncbi.nlm.nih.gov/books/NBK493175.
7. Aon Risk Solutions. 2013. Personal communication from the authors of 2012 Health Care Workers Compensation Barometer to ERG, an OSHA contractor.
8. Carayon P, Xie A, Kianfar S. Human factors and ergonomics as a patient safety practice. BMJ Qual Saf. 2014;23(3):196–205.
9. Ulmer C, Wolman DW, Johns ME. Resident duty hours: enhancing sleep, supervision and safety. 1st ed. Washington, DC: The National Academied Press; 2008.
10. Quoted in Institute of Medicine. To error is human: building a safer health system. 1st ed. Washington: National Academy Press; 2000.

11. NRC (National Research Council). Musculoskeletal disorders and the workplace: low back and upper extremities. Washington, DC: National Academy Press; 2001.
12. Epstein S, Sparer EH, Tran BN, et al. Prevalence of work-related musculoskeletal disorders among surgeons and interventionalists. A systematic review and meta-analysis. JAMA Surg. 2018;153(2):e174947.
13. Mehta A, Gupta M, Upadhyaya N. Status of occupational hazards and their prevention among dental professionals in Chandigarh, India: a comprehensive questionnaire survey. Dent Res J. 2013;10(4):446–51.
14. Goniewicz M, Włoszczak-Szubzda A, Niemcewicz M, Witt M, Marciniak-Niemcewicz A, Jarosz MJ. Injuries caused by sharp instruments among healthcare workers—international and Polish perspectives. Ann Agric Environ Med. 2012;19(3):523–7.
15. Aghilinejad M, Ehsani AA, Talebi A, Koohpayehzadeh J, Dehghan N. Ergonomic risk factors and musculoskeletal symptoms in surgeons with three types of surgery: open, laparoscopic, and microsurgery. Med J Islam Repub Iran. 2016;30:467.
16. Janki S, Mulder EEAP, IJzermans JNM, et al. Ergonomics in the operating room. Surg Endosc. 2017;31:2457.
17. Jahncke H, Hygge S, Mathiassen SE, Hallman D, Mixter S, Lyskov E. Variation at work: alternations between physically and mentally demanding tasks in blue-collar occupations. Ergonomics. 2017;60(9):1218–27.
18. Zhou C, Shi L, Gao L, et al. Determinate factors of mental health status in Chinese medical staff: a cross-sectional study. Dang Y, ed. Medicine. 2018;97(10):e0113.
19. Bernal D, Campos-Serna J, Tobias A, et al. Work-related psychosocial risk factors and musculoskeletal disorders in hospital nurses and nursing aides: a systematic review and meta-analysis. Int J Nurs Stud. 2015;52:635–48.
20. Anderson SP, Oakman J. Allied health professionals and work-related musculoskeletal disorders: a systematic review. Saf Health Work. 2016;7:259–67.
21. Mitchell P, Wynia R, Golden B, et al. Core principles and values of effective team-based health care. Discussion Paper. Washington, DC: Institute of Medicine; 2012. https://www.nationalahec.org/pdfs/VSRT-Team-Based-Care-Principles-Values.pdf.

Ergonomics in Minimal Access Surgery

20

Selman Uranues, James Elvis Waha, Abe Fingerhut, and Rifat Latifi

Introduction

In the empirical sense, ergonomics – the study of human efficiency in the workplace – began about the time that the first man attached his handstone to a stout wooden shaft with a thong (Fig. 20.1a). The result was a more efficient tool or weapon that gave him more reach and leverage.

In the following millennia, humans continued to invent and then develop and improve all manners of tools, weapons, instruments, and machines to make them more useful and efficient (Fig. 20.1b), but it was only in 1857 that Wojciech Jastrzebowski coined the term "ergonomics" in his *Outline of Ergonomics* and laid the foundation for a formal science of the human being in the workplace [1]. The field of ergonomics flourished with industrialization during the two World Wars and is with us today in virtually every field of human endeavor, including surgery, in a continuing effort to find the optimal compromise between fitting a human being to a working environment and fitting a working environment to a human being.

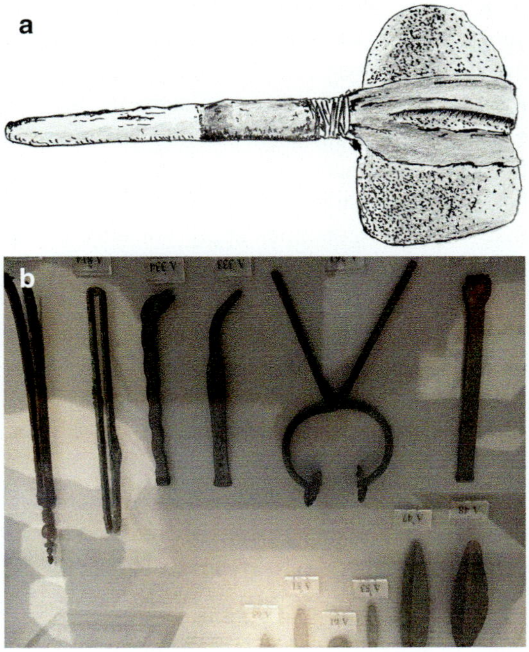

Fig. 20.1 (**a**) Stone Age hammer, a kautaq, an Inuit hammer used to crush the bones which is made of an oblong stone mounted on a short slightly curved handle. (**b**) Historic surgical instruments (Archaeological Museum of Athens, Greece)

S. Uranues (✉)
Department of Surgery, Section for Surgical Research, Medical University of Graz, Graz, Austria
e-mail: selman.uranues@medunigraz.at

J. E. Waha
Department of Surgery, Division of General Surgery, Medical University of Graz, Graz, Austria

A. Fingerhut
Surgical Research, Surgical Department, University of Graz, Graz, Austria

R. Latifi
New York Medical College, School of Medicine, Department of Surgery and Westchester Medical Center, Valhalla, NY, USA

R. Latifi (ed.), *The Modern Hospital*, https://doi.org/10.1007/978-3-030-01394-3_20

No one can say exactly when people began using instruments to peer into the human body, starting with its natural openings, but the earliest descriptions of endoscopy were recorded by Hippocrates (460–375 BCE) as rectal speculum similar to those still in use today [2]. For more than two millennia, scientists and surgeons have developed a great variety of evermore sophisticated equipment, not only to peer into the body but also to treat problems they encountered while they were at it.

Surgeons go into their field to improve patients' health, but probably no individual has ever chosen surgery as a profession for the sake of his or her own health. Surgery subjects the surgeon to stress, often in its most extreme forms, mentally and physically. Accordingly, high priority must be given to providing surgeons with an ergonomically optimized working environment that will allow them to do their job well with the best possible results. It must be noted, however, that surgical ergonomics apply not only to the operating surgeon but also to the entire surgical team and the complete infrastructure. First and foremost, the patient's safety must be assured at all times: *primum non nocere*. In this chapter we will describe ergonomics in minimal access surgery.

From Endoscopy to Laparoscopy and the Emergence of Ergonomics in Minimal Access Surgery (MAS)

Probably nothing besides anesthesia, analgesia, antisepsis, and antibiosis has so revolutionized surgery as did the advent of laparoscopy with Kurt Semm's appendectomy in 1980 and Erich Mühe's cholecystectomy in 1985. Initial skepticism and opposition gave way to acceptance as young surgeons eagerly took to the new and promising technique. The larger 5 mm and 10 mm instruments were replaced by 2 mm and 3 mm instruments as ever smaller instruments were introduced for increasingly complicated surgeries. In the meanwhile, there is no organ in the trunk – thorax, abdomen, and pelvis – that is not accessible to laparoscopic surgery, and as with the classical gallbladder, laparoscopic surgery has come to be the state-of-the-art gold standard for many organs and diseases.

As we now have generations of children and young adults who have never known a world without information technology (IT), there are now generations of surgeons who were introduced to endoscopy/laparoscopy/minimal access surgery (MAS) as early as medical school. Today, no doctor can expect to become board certified in surgery without a degree of mastery of MAS techniques. In the initial phase, however, there were major challenges to be met since the new technique meant that the old rule book for surgery had been thrown away and replaced with an entirely new one. However, before ergonomics could be seriously tackled, surgeons had to adapt to the many novelties of laparoscopic surgery: instruments that lie on a fulcrum point, loss of depth perception, impaired peripheral vision, absence of surgical assistants to manipulate instruments, and the presence in an already crowded operating room (OR) of additional equipment that must be so accommodated as to minimize the risk of accidents and mishaps in an OR that is often only dimly lit. According to Cutner et al., the movement of heavy equipment around a theatre complex together with increased theatre clutter increases the hazards for all staff and adds to inefficiencies [3].

Once laparoscopy had become established, attention could be turned to the ergonomics involved, and numerous good descriptions of the ergonomics of basic laparoscopy are available [4]. After laparoscopic surgery had been standardized, a search began for improved and innovative ways to access the human body, with laparoscopy as the starting point. Related subtechnologies now include NOTES (natural orifice transluminal endoscopic surgery), SILS (single-incision laparoscopic surgery), LESS (laparoendoscopic single-site surgery), and, in a category of its own, robotic and robotic-assisted surgery.

Surgical Ergonomics and the Surgeon's Health

Surgery is painful, not only to the patient but also to the surgeon. Since surgeons have always been susceptible to work-related musculoskeletal disorders (MSD) even with conventional open surgery, it has only been fairly recently that attention has been drawn to the relationship between the ergonomics of open surgery, MAS in all its varieties, robotic surgery, and the surgeon's health.

Historically, surgical strain from MAS was thought to affect only some 15% of surgeons practicing it, but more recent data suggest as much as 88% of traditional MAS surgeons and 45% of robotic surgeons. Franasiak and Gehrig in fact speak of a "strain epidemic" in MAS [5].

Along these same lines, Park et al. described an "impending epidemic" among MAS surgeons [6]. Since there was little evidence to support the widely held belief that laparoscopy puts greater strain on surgeons than open surgery, they surveyed 317 laparoscopic surgeons who completed a comprehensive questionnaire. Almost 90% reported physical symptoms or discomfort. High case volume was the strongest predictor of symptoms, with the exception of eye and back symptoms, which were regularly reported even with low case volumes. A recent systematic review and meta-analysis focused on surgeons and interventionalists as at-risk physicians and also spoke of an "impending epidemic" of MSD, but did not differentiate between surgical specialties and technical approaches [7]. The main findings are nonetheless relevant: a high prevalence of MSDs among at-risk physicians, with no overarching intervention to improve the situation, and less attention to physicians' physical well-being than to psychological factors such as burnout and suicide, important as they are [7].

A systematic review and meta-analysis by Stucky et al. are enlightening [8]. A search of the literature from 1980 to 2014 produced 40 articles evaluating MSD and ergonomic outcomes in 5152 surveyed surgeons. Sixty-eight percent reported generalized pain. Approximately half reported pain in the back, neck, and arm or shoulder, while 71% reported fatigue. Numbness was reported by 37% and stiffness by 45%. When compared with surgeons performing open surgery, MAS surgeons were significantly more likely to have pain in the neck, arm, shoulder, hands, and legs and to be more susceptible to fatigue.

In contrast, a much smaller study by Janki et al. [9] of surgeons affiliated with the Dutch Society for Endoscopic Surgery, Gastrointestinal Surgery, and Surgical Oncology, as well as surgeons, gynecologists, and urologists at a cluster of training hospitals in the Netherlands, covered 127 respondents, almost half of whom suffered from MSD and a quarter of whom had symptoms in the past but no longer did. So a significant proportion of this small population had relevant complaints, but the authors failed to find a significant difference between surgeons who predominately performed laparoscopic or open surgery. Stucky et al. [8] suggest that MAS is in fact more harmful to the surgeon than open surgery.

There is yet another wild card to consider: robotic surgery. In a pig study by Hubert et al., surgeons performed standard and robot-assisted surgeries with recording of electromyography (EMG), heart rate, and physical and mental workloads to evaluate muscular strain and cognitive stress induced by the two techniques [10]. Physical workload and perception of effort invested were statistically significantly greater during standard laparoscopies, though mental stress was identical. Increased heart rate during standard laparoscopy confirmed greater physical expenditure.

Elhage et al. undertook an in vitro study with urological surgeons who performed a simulated vesicourethral anastomosis using robotic, laparoscopic, and open approaches and found that robot-assisted surgery combined the accuracy of open surgery while causing the surgeon less discomfort than laparoscopic surgery and maintaining minimal access conditions [11]. With conventional laparoscopy, however, the surgeons took longer than with the robotic system and made more errors.

Pierhoples et al. [12] noted that in spite of increasing interest in understanding the toll that operating takes on the surgeon's body, the effect of robotic surgery on the surgeon had not been studied. A 26-question online survey was sent to 19,866 surgeons from all specialties trained in the use of robots, and 1407 (7%) responses were received. The data analysis was based on 1215 surgeons who practiced all 3 techniques.

Of those, 871 (71.6%) had complaints attributable to performing surgery, of whom 55.4% attributed their complaints to laparoscopic surgery, 36.3% to open surgery, and 8.3% to robotic surgery. A higher case load predicted increased symptoms for open and laparoscopic surgery, but not for robotic surgery. With robotic surgery, neck, back, hip, knee, ankle, foot, and shoulder pain were less likely to occur than with the other two methods, while elbow and wrist pain were less likely with robotic than with laparoscopic surgery. Eye pain, however, was more likely with robotic surgery than with the two other approaches, and finger pain was more likely with robotic than with open surgery. Nearly a third of respondents noted that they considered their own comfort when choosing a surgical modality, and there appears to be a tendency for surgeons to increasingly take their own health into account.

Besides subjective surveys based on questionnaires, objective performance studies have been made to assess ergonomics of conventional laparoscopic and robotic surgeries. Lee et al. [13] examined the hypothesis that the unique features of robotic surgery would demonstrate skill-related results in both a lower physical and cognitive workload and uncompromised task performance. MAS surgeons grouped by experience with robotic surgery performed training tasks using both techniques: the physical workload was assessed with electromyography from eight muscles and the cognitive workload with the NASA Task Load Index (NASA-TLX). Their results showed that physical and cognitive ergonomics with robotic surgery were statistically significantly less challenging than with tasks performed with conventional laparoscopic equipment. Unsurprisingly, surgeons with the highest level of experience in robotic surgery had the greatest ergonomic benefit from the system, highlighting a need for well-structured training and well-defined ergonomic guidelines for robotic surgery.

In 2017, Francisco and Juan Sanchez-Margallo [14] reviewed the status of ergonomics in laparoscopy, LESS, and robot-assisted surgery, based on the literature and their own experience. They too found that experience was a determinant of ergonomics during laparoscopic surgery and that better ergonomics improved task performance. LESS was found to be more physically demanding than conventional and hybrid approaches, making more demands on the back and arm muscles, but providing a better wrist position than traditional laparoscopy. In accordance with Lee et al., they found that physical and cognitive ergonomics were significantly less challenging with robotic assistance than with conventional laparoscopy. Besides conventional photogrammetry and video recordings, new methods for ergonomic assessment have evolved for application in the OR based on kinematic analysis, muscle activity, and/or mental stress. These include 3D motion tracking, electrogoniometry, data gloves, electromyography, and force platforms. Besides the NASA-TLX, a special Surgery Task Load Index (SURG-TLX) has been available since its validation in 2011. As the equipment for MAS, whether robotic or not, becomes ever more sophisticated, so do the means of assessing its ergonomics.

The demand for MAS, in whatever form, continues to increase: it promises good or better patient outcomes, less pain, quicker recovery, and better cosmetic results. Healthcare providers and hospital administrators welcome this and shorter hospitalizations. Unfortunately, the size of the pool of MAS surgeons is not increasing fast enough to meet the growing demand, meaning that they will have to handle ever larger caseloads, to the detriment of their health, which in some cases may lead to early retirement, contributing to a healthcare supply problem [5].

What About the Operating Room Itself?

In the operating room, the transition from conventional to MAS or robotic surgery is not universal. In some institutions, it is still in progress or has not even begun. Since many hospitals do not have the resources to optimally accommodate new technologies in modern, dedicated ORs, many MASs are still performed in conventional operating rooms, with all the hazards and inconvenience of squeezing even more equipment into a small and crowded OR and loss of time that set up and subsequent dismantling entail. The better solution would seem to be an integrated OR, a state-of-the-art system with boom-mounted laparoscopic equipment and monitors permanently installed for on-demand use. In an integrated OR, all the surgical and room equipment is linked via an interface and can be controlled remotely [3]. The integrated OR in and of itself could make a major contribution to the solution of many of the ergonomic problems confronting the surgical team. There is no, however, universal agreement on the superiority of the integrated OR. Blikkendaal et al. used video recordings to compare laparoscopic hysterectomies performed in a conventional cart-based OR and in a dedicated integrated OR with regard to the incidence and effect of equipment-related surgical flow disturbances (e.g., malfunctioning, intraoperative repositioning, device setup) and found that the integrated OR failed to offer any advantage [15]. Since they underscored that the surgical team should be aware of different potential sources of disruption in the integrated OR, this suggests that when the team is thoroughly familiar with the integrated OR, the problems may decrease and the advantages come to the fore.

Since MAS is no longer restricted to tertiary centers and other major hospitals, an integrated OR can be economically feasible for hospitals that do not have the resources or even the need of other high-end options such as the hybrid or digital OR.

Where Are the Guidelines?

Authors often mention ergonomics guidelines and the need for same. Lee et al. emphasized the need for well-structured training and well-defined ergonomics guidelines to maximize the benefits to be attained from using robotic surgery [13]. Shankar et al. undertook a questionnaire survey of 150 laparoscopic surgeons that covered, in addition to physical distress associated with ergonomic problems in the OR, their awareness of the ergonomic guidelines for laparoscopy, finding a high degree of unawareness of the existence of such guidelines [16]. Most of the respondents had never received any specific training or education related to ergonomics. van Det et al. offered brief guidelines for positioning of the monitor, patient, laparoscopic equipment, and surgical team but these, as in other works [4], did not take the newer varieties of MAS and robotic surgery into account [17].

Much of the training in techniques appears to be informal: when the new "toy" is carted into the OR, the only available information on its use is provided by the company representative. Surgeons line up to try it out and learn mostly by trial and error. If they experience discomfort or pain, they will try to alleviate it themselves as best they can, changing positions of the equipment or their bodies; they generally are not eager to seek treatment for their ailments. Information, recommendations, and suggestions will be passed on by word of mouth. This is, after all, how surgery has always been practiced and, to a large degree, taught. Nonetheless, it would certainly be advantageous to have validated practice guidelines and training programs, even though, with the current speed of technological progress and innovation, they would regularly need to be updated.

Operating Table, Positioning the Patient, and Positions of the Surgical Team

The patient must be so positioned on the operating table so as not to incur temporary or permanent physical harm. Fixation must ensure that the patient will not slip and that there will be no pressure on sensitive areas. Since the table can be tilted in any direction in laparoscopic surgery, secure fixation is an important consideration. The operating surgeon and the members of the surgical team should all be able to view the monitor without constantly turning the head or body or adopting an uncomfortable position to do so. The height of the monitor and its angle are important ergonomic factors: the gaze down position (the height of the monitor is below eye level) is best. Poor adjustment of the monitor can lead to muscle tension in the neck and shoulders, fatigue, tremor, and inaccurate motion sequences. The height of the table should allow the surgeon's elbow to bend between 90° and 120° (Fig. 20.2a). The rest of the team should adjust in favor of the principal surgeon.

Trocar Positioning

The intra-abdominal working area should determine the direction in which the trocars are inserted, and the direction of all trocars should focus on the surgical field. Only those trocars causing the least tissue damage should be preferred. It has not been clearly shown that bladeless trocars are better than cutting trocars. The angle of the trocar axis to the body surface is important; this *elevation angle* should be between 40° and 60°. Freedom of motion is best when the trocar does not penetrate more than 1–3 cm beyond the peritoneum. Trocars that are not optimally directed to the target organ with an out-of-range elevation angle force the surgeon to work against torque, increasing the effort needed for manipulations and leading to early fatigue and tremor.

The positioning of the trocars determines the effectiveness of the camera and the freedom of

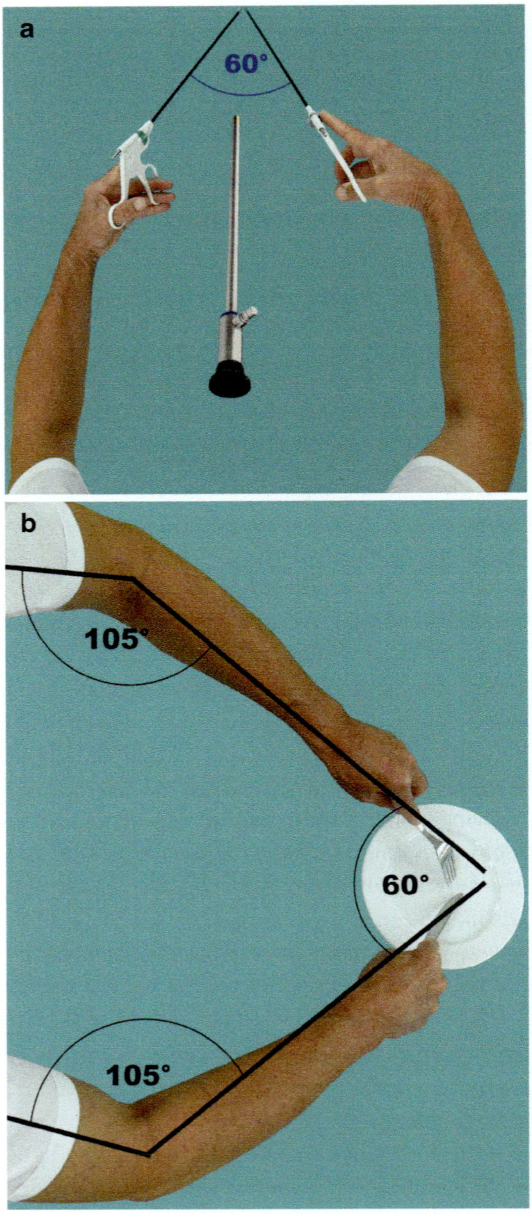

Fig. 20.2 Showing the physiologic triangulation during eating (**a**) which is the most used physiologic brain-eye-hand control axis. The same triangulation setup during laparoscopic surgery (**b**) leading to the best result

instrument mobility. Ideally, the optic should be at the center point of the triangulation (Fig. 20.2a,b). The optimal setup is when the two working trocars are on the left and right at equal distance from the optic; this is called the "in-axis" position (Fig. 20.2a). When both of the

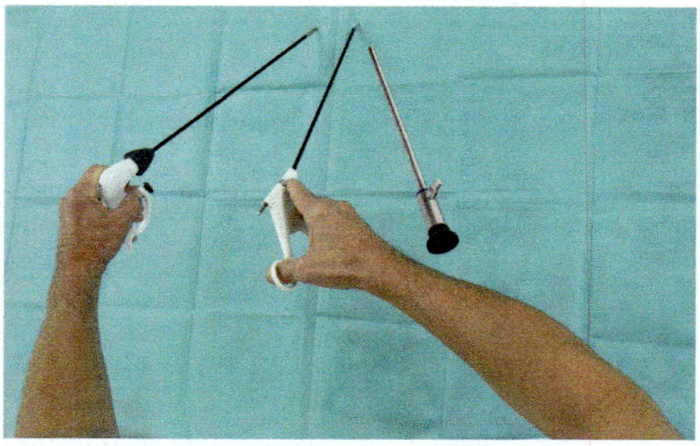

Fig. 20.3 Off-axis working setup with instruments nearly parallel to each other, and the optic is out of the brain-eye-hand axis

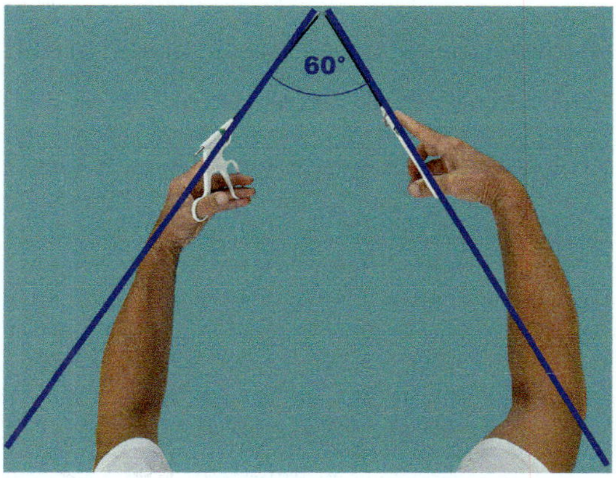

Fig. 20.4 Optimal manipulation angle of 60° ensures best results in suturing and intracorporeal knotting

working trocars are to the left or to the right of the optic, this is called "off axis" (Fig. 20.3), which for longer procedures is tiring and impede smooth manipulation.

With ideal triangulation of the trocars, the angle between the two working instruments (*manipulation angle*) should be 45°–60° (Fig. 20.4). If the angle is smaller, the instruments are nearly parallel, rending suturing and knotting unnecessarily difficult and not infrequently leading to an unsatisfactory result. If the manipulation angle is greater than 75°, manipulation will be increasingly difficult. The diameter and angle of view of the optic should be chosen to suit the planned procedure. Optics with the brightest and best vision are 10/11 mm in diameter. Optics with smaller diameters provide weaker light. View angles of 0°, 30°, and 45° are most commonly chosen. Angular optics provide the best axis-to-target view (OATV). They prevent distortion due to an oblique angle of view and accordingly false distance perception when the target organ is not directly in the optic axis.

Surgeon-Assistant Interactions

Surgery requires teamwork, regardless of the technique involved. The interaction between the principal and assisting surgeons is of utmost importance, demanding optimal harmony. This can only be achieved when at least the most important steps in the operation are discussed in advance and tasks assigned to each and every member of the team, with the assistant having a major role [18]. The more experienced the assistant and the longer the team has worked together, the smoother the workflow and the better the outcome will be.

Ergonomics in MAS: Quo Vadis?

Jacques Marescaux, the innovative French researcher and surgeon, states in his essay, "Looking at the future with an augmented eye [19]," that "The current evolution of MAS, endoluminal and percutaneous surgery, taken individually, seems to reach a natural plateau, with little incremental developments generating only small added value for patients." He then goes on to project something like a quantum leap, a merger of interventional radiology, gastroenterology, and MAS into a hybrid image-guided therapeutic approach. As he sees it, the next steps in surgery will be directed toward a transdisciplinary hybrid use of robotics, advanced imaging systems, and sources of energy. If he were to be asked what he sees as the long-term future of surgery, his answer would be, "Hopefully, the future will lead to the end of surgery…and nobody will miss it."

Until that happens – if it happens – ergonomics in MAS will continue to search for a good comprise between fitting the surgeon to the OR and fitting the OR to the surgeon.

Acknowledgment The authors gratefully acknowledge the assistance of Eugenia Lamont in performing the literature search and drafting the text.

Further, the authors thank Martin Stelzer, medical photographer and illustrator at the Medical University of Graz, for illustrations and for providing Fig. 20.1a for this chapter.

References

1. Jastrzębowski WB. An outline of ergonomics, or the science of work based upon the truths drawn from the Science of Nature: 1857. Central Institute for Labour Protection. Warsaw: Central Institute for Labour Protection; 2000.
2. Shah J. Endoscopy through the ages. BJU Int. 2002;89:645–52.
3. Cutner A, Stavroulis A, Zolfaghari N. Risk assessment of the ergonomic aspects of laparoscopic theatre. Gynecol Surg. 2013;10:99–102.
4. Fingerhut A, Hanna GB. Ergonomics of the minimally invasive operating theatre. In: Bonjer HJ, editor. Surgical principles of minimally invasive procedures: Springer International New York City; 2017. https://doi.org/10.1007/987-3-319-43196-3.
5. Franasiak JM, Gehrig PA. Ergonomic strain in minimally invasive surgery: addressing the strain epidemic. JCOM. 2015;22(6):267–73.
6. Park A, Lee G, Meenaghan N, Dexter D. Patients benefit while surgeons suffer: an impending epidemic. J Am Coll Surg. 2010;210(3):306–13.
7. Epstein S, Sparer EH, Tran BN, Ruan QZ, Dennerlein JT, Singhai D, Lee BT. Prevalence of work-related musculoskeletal disorders among surgeons and interventionalists: a systematic review and meta-analysis. JAMA Surg. 2018;153(2):e174947.
8. Stucky CCH, Cromwell KD, Voss RK Chaing YJ, Woodman K. Surgeon symptoms, strain and selections: systematic review and meta-analysis of surgical ergonomics. Ann Med Surg. 2018;27:1–8.
9. Janki S, Mulder EEAP, IJzermans JNM. Ergonomics in the operating room. Surg Endosc. 2017;31:2457–66.
10. Hubert N, Gilles M, Desbrosses K, Meyer JP, Felbinger J, Hubert J. Ergonomic assessment of the surgeon's physical workload during standard and robotic assisted laparoscopic procedures. Int J Med Robot. 2013;9(2):142–7.
11. Elhage O, Challacombe B, Shortland A, Dasgupta P. An assessment of the physical impact of complex surgical tasks on surgeon errors and discomfort: a comparison between robot-assisted, laparoscopic and open approaches. BJU Int. 2015;115:274–81.
12. Pierhoples TA, Hernandez-Boussard T, Wren SM. The aching surgeon: a survey of physical discomfort and symptoms following open, laparoscopic, and robotic surgery. J Robot Surg. 2012;6(1):65–72.
13. Lee GI, Lee MR, Clanton T, Sutton E, Park AE, Marohn MR. Comparative assessment of physical and cognitive ergonomics associated with robotic and traditional laparoscopic surgeries. Surg Endosc. 2014;28:456–65.
14. https://www.intechopen.com/books/laparoscopic-surgery/ergonomics-in-laparoscopic-surgery. Accessed 26 July 2018.
15. Blikkendaal MD, Driessen SRC, Rodrigues SP, Rhemrev JPT, Smeets MJGH, Dankelman J, van den Dobbelsteen JJ, Jansen FW. Measuring surgical safety during minimally invasive surgical procedures: a validation study. Surg Endosc. 2018;32(7):3087–95.
16. Shankar M, Manjunath K, Krishnappa R. Ergonomics in laparoscopy: a questionnaire survey of physical discomfort and symptoms in surgeons following laparoscopic surgery. Int Surg J. 2017;4:3907–14.
17. van Det MJ, Meijerink WJHJ, Hoff C, Totté ER, Pierie JPEN. Optimal ergonomics for laparoscopic surgery in minimally invasive surgery suites: a review and guidelines. Surg Endosc. 2009;23:1279–85.
18. Chui A, Bowne WB, Sookraj KA, Zenilman ME, Fingerhut A, Ferzli GS. The role of the assistant in laparoscopic surgery: important considerations for the apprentice-in-training. Surg Innov. 2008; 15:229–36.
19. Marescaux J, Diana M. Looking at the future with an augmented eye. Ann Laparosc Endosc Surg. 2016;1:36–42.

Part III

Clinical Aspect of Modern Hospital: The Back Bone of Modern Transformation

Emergency Department of the New Era

21

Alejandro Guerrero, David K. Barnes, and Hunter M. Pattison

Abbreviations

APP	Advanced practice provider
BPA	Best practice alert
CDS	Clinical decision support
CPOE	Computerized physician order entry
ECG	Electrocardiogram
ED	Emergency department
EHR	Electronic health record
EMR	Electronic medical record
EMS	Emergency medical services
FOAM	Free open-access medical education
HIE	Health information exchange
MI	Myocardial infarction
POC	Point of care
QT	Queuing theory
STEMI	ST-segment elevation myocardial infarction
TLP	Triage liaison provider
t-PA	Tissue plasminogen activator
US	Ultrasound
WCD	Wearable computing device

A. Guerrero (✉)
Acute Care Surgery, InterTrauma Medical, New York, NY, USA
e-mail: guerrero@InterTrauma.com

D. K. Barnes
Department of Emergency Medicine, UC Davis Health, UC Davis Medical Center, UC Davis School of Medicine, Sacramento, CA, USA

H. M. Pattison
Department of Emergency Medicine, UC Davis Medical Center, Sacramento, CA, USA

Availability of Patient Data

Until recently, an efficient and practical mechanism for transferring useful patient care information between healthcare providers seemed elusive. Conventional medical records, paper-based amalgamations of clinical and non-clinical information, were often redundant, frequently physically damaged, and missing vital information which were funneled into unwieldy folders stored in filing cabinets remote from the clinical setting. Physical records were cumbersome, took time to retrieve and review, and offered access that was limited to the individual practitioner or medical office in possession of the file. Facsimile machines closed part of the time gap but replaced one problem with another, reams of documentation with varying relevance and legibility.

The need for accurate and timely communication of patient data is particularly obvious in the dynamic environment of the emergency department (ED) where patient arrivals are unscheduled, acuity is stochastic, diagnoses are broad and undifferentiated, and care is decentralized [1]. Patients, representing the full spectrum of age, comorbidity, and chief complaint, expect and demand that their providers will have access to meaningful data upon which to make careful and informed treatment decisions. Archaic storage and transfer of patient information hampered emergency physicians from delivering optimal, individualized treatment, ultimately altering clinical trajectories and jeopardizing patient safety [2].

R. Latifi (ed.), *The Modern Hospital*, https://doi.org/10.1007/978-3-030-01394-3_21

Patient-Centered Shareable Data

The ubiquity of computers and widespread access to the Internet gradually spurred a critical transition to electronic medical records (EMRs). Physician adoption of EMRs spiked accordingly from 18% to 57% from 2001 to 2011 [3]. In their most rudimentary form, EMRs offered the same information as paper records but in an inherently more structured, accessible, and sharable framework. Used in isolation, however, EMRs do not automatically solve information gaps for patients arriving to the ED [4, 5].

Even when institutions are utilizing their own EMR, 32% of referrals to the ED contain at least one information deficit, approximately half of which are considered essential to patient care [6]. One-third of referrals lack information as crucial as an up-to-date medication list or past medical history. Only one in ten referrals includes pertinent contraindications such as a record of life-threatening allergies [7]. Inconvenient or delayed access to information from a transferring institution leads time-constrained ED physicians to favor old discharge summaries from their own EMR as a source of critical information [7]. Information deficits in the emergency setting are a significant contributor to adverse drug events [8].

Networked Health Information Exchange

EMRs have naturally evolved into interconnected electronic health records (EHRs) to address issues with information exchange. EHRs are distinguished by the ability of healthcare providers to share, manage, and consult across multiple healthcare organizations. Single EHRs function as real-time, patient-centered databases that support the ability of the provider to access, review, interpret, and unify an abundance of information from sources such as emergency departments, past and present primary and specialty care physicians, urgent care facilities, pharmacies, laboratories, and imaging facilities [9]. While most systems are currently limited to facilities using the same EHR vendor, the ultimate goal is universal and unrestricted health information exchange (HIE) across all facilities regardless of vendor or geographic location. Table 21.1 lists some of the examples of widely used EHRs (Table 21.1).

Table 21.1 List of ten most widely used EHRs

Most common
Epic
Cerner
Less commonly used
Allscripts
NueMD
NextGen
Centricity
eClinicalWorks
Meditech
Soarian
T-System

HIEs have the potential to dissipate healthcare boundaries and have demonstrated a number of key benefits for EDs when tested on a community-sized scale. Unsurprisingly, emergency medicine providers utilize HIEs more often when presented with complex patients [10]. The most common area for which HIEs provide vital information unavailable from other sources concerns home medications [11]. Additionally, accessing an HIE within 90 days of an imaging study resulted in a significant decrease in the chance imaging was repeated in the ED [12]. Overall, HIEs decreased the odds of patients being admitted to the hospital by 24–30% [13, 14] by reducing the number of avoidable admissions [15]. Patients who are admitted while when an HIE is available have significantly shorter lengths of stay [16] as well as a 57% lower chance of readmission within 30 days of discharge [17]. Through these means, as well as an overall reduction in hospital resource utilization, HIEs have translated into significant cost savings [18]. One study spanning 11 EDs indicated that patients with information available in an HIE experienced a reduction in Medicare-allowable reimbursements by an average of $1,947 (US) [19]. Annual savings associated with HIE usage were estimated to be $357,000 (US) from unnecessary admissions [13] and over $600,000 (US) from avoided readmissions [17].

Technology at the Bedside

As EHRs become increasingly enmeshed into the ED workflow, physicians have been shown to spend as much as 65% of their time on documentation during an ED patient visit [20]. Within the chaotic and hectic emergency environment, even minimal disruptions of physician attention can have important consequences to ED workflow and efficiency. With Internet-capable cell phones and tablets increasingly commonplace, comprehensive integration of EHR functionality and other clinical support services into mobile devices has helped quell this potential pitfall [21].

When used in combination with an EHR, mobile devices have been shown to improve overall productivity [22]. The ability to access medical records at the bedside leads to improved efficiency and more face time with patients [23]. The greatest benefit from handheld devices is demonstrated during time-sensitive situations requiring rapid response and decision-making [24]. Tablets are associated with fewer logins and less time spent on computer workstations which in one study resulted in 38 fewer minutes per ED shift [25]. Despite some apprehension that handheld devices unnecessarily distract providers, the majority of patients whose physicians use handheld devices in the examination room report positive perceptions [26]. Physicians report equally high degrees of satisfaction with tablet use and endorse their use as a means to optimize data gathering, streamline their clinical workflow, and improve communication with both their peers and patients [27]. These uses encompass only the most perfunctory utilizations of mobile devices in the ED, with others actively exploring radiologic study interpretation [28] and complex patient-centered decision support [29].

Portable Health Information

Patients who are actively engaged in managing their health receive better overall medical care [30]. Surveys indicate that over 10% of cell phone users have downloaded an application to help them track or manage their health [31]. With patient-centered care, one of the care domains of the Academy of Medicine, and patient engagement on the rise, several avenues of patient-centered and portable health information have been explored as an interim solution to closing information gaps in the ED. Mobile health information brings with it numerous benefits, particularly while HIE implementation remains in its infancy. Patient data files on a personal smartphone or tablet could theoretically be instantly accessed anywhere in the world. Similar benefits have also been highlighted for those living in predominantly rural or impoverished regions [32]. There are however significant risks and security concerns associated with maintaining private health information on mobile storage media, the most apparent of which is the potential for breach of protected health information [33].

Portability has been explored through both expected and abstract modalities each with advantages and disadvantages. In one example of simple portability, patients were provided with USB memory cards or portable hard drives containing their health information [33]. Another combined compact storage devices with logging of physician encounters into a web-based electronic health portal retrievable through SMS text messaging at the patients' request. While the system proved helpful in facilitating quick retrieval of medication lists in geriatric patients, its success was hampered by the need to consistently update information in the web-based portal [32]. More sophisticated approaches have leveraged cloud-based integration and identity validation for EHR access from any location with an added element of security [34].

Patient Flow

Emergency department overcrowding with its associated protracted wait times is a mounting concern for healthcare organizations globally [35]. The turn of the century saw wait times continue to surge, even for conditions in which clinical outcomes are known to be dependent on prompt detection and treatment [36, 37]. Various studies have validated that crowding in the ED portends lower patient satisfaction, more patients having leaving without treatment, higher complication rates, and increased mortality [38–41]. With such dire consequences for healthcare quality and patient safety, there exists the need to identify operational interventions that can mitigate crowding and promote efficient patient throughput.

ED crowding is the result of numerous factors that conspire to create a supply and demand mismatch [42]. First, ED utilization has been on a continual upward trajectory, reaching a record of 141 million visits in the USA in 2014 in the midst of a tumultuous healthcare landscape [43]. In addition to higher volume, EDs face patients who present with high acuity and increasingly complex comorbidities necessitating complex evaluation and management [44, 45]. Elevated demand unfortunately coincides with reduced supply as the number of EDs, especially in rural areas, has declined over the last two decades [46]. Finally, the allocation of inpatient resources, most often outside the direct control of the ED, contributes substantially to ED boarding as patients wait for inpatient bed assignments held up by prolonged hospital discharged, understaffed units, and backlogged operating rooms [47, 48].

Queuing Theory

Queuing theory (QT) is a branch of operation research methodology that employs mathematical modeling to predict performance metrics as they pertain to waiting in line, particularly the average idle time, queue length, and customer detriment [49]. Implementation of QT has gained prominence throughout service-oriented industries, including healthcare, as a method for quickly analyzing the response of resource-limited systems to varying levels of demand while also facilitating direct comparison of process alternatives to pinpoint areas for improvement [50, 51].

While the ED is similar to other service-oriented organizations (i.e., the goal is to minimize the wait time), it also projects a number of unique characteristics that make it more challenging to implement QT. First, patient influx into the ED varies with time [52], introducing a fluctuating demand typically mitigated in other healthcare settings by wait lists or appointment systems [53]. Patients are also prioritized based on urgency rather than arrival time, an unpredictable characteristic [54]. Next, the extent and variability of services provided by the ED far surpass other business providers [55], with physicians spending longer periods of time providing a service [56]. Even the most routine procedures may incur a high degree of individual variability in performance time and required resources [49, 56]. Numerous externalities, such as intra- and inter-hospital resources, further compound ED wait times because of similar independent variables such as utilization of catheterization labs, availability of radiology services, and even the status of crowding in other EDs [49].

Despite these limitations, application of QT, particularly when used in combination with discrete-event simulation, has shown promising results. In one study, reallocation of providers as predicted by QT translated into 21.7% fewer patients leaving without being evaluated [57]. Similarly, strategic scheduling of senior emergency medicine residents based on QT modeling decreased average length of stay by 15 min. The same study found optimizing laboratory staff could reduce length of stay by 90 min, while addition of another EKG technician during peak hours could reduce the time from order to completion by 8 min [58]. Queue-based simulations further demonstrate the addition of a fast track with an extra nurse can reduce overall median wait times by more than 35 min while reducing overall nursing resource demand [59]. Finally, adding flexibility to allocating beds for low- and high-acuity patients also proved capable of significantly reducing wait times for patients [60].

Lean Methodology

Lean methodology is a quality improvement strategy for operating principles first pioneered by the automobile manufacturing industry in the 1950s and since adapted by the healthcare

Table 21.2 Basic principles of lean methodology in healthcare

The goal of lean methodology
Remove all non-value-added activity from the care of the patient
The principles of lean methodology
Monitor for *defects*, which in healthcare is defined as anything that prevents perfect care
Standardize workflow
Real-time problem-solving
Continuous adjustments in workflow based on detailed monitoring for *defects*
Workflow is adjusted in a standardized manner
In concept, these principles *are* the work, not in addition to the work

industry for use in hospitals [61, 62]. Lean strategy focuses on identifying and eliminating process steps that lack value starting with the determination of the root cause for an issue or process as viewed by individuals entrenched within the system (e.g., frontline assembly people in the car industry) (Table 21.2). Dissection of the inner workings of a complex process then facilitates a detailed understanding of how the process can be amended. Over the last decade, Lean has been used to improve the efficiency of healthcare delivery in hospitals around the world [63–65].

Using lean methodology, inefficient processes have been identified in the ED including time spent waiting to see providers, turnaround time for lab results, and transport time to and from the radiology suite—which contribute to increased length of stay and worsening patient satisfaction scores [66]. A systematic review applying lean methodology to ED patient flow found improvement in eight of the nine cases across a multitude of metrics. EDs were able to increase patient volume and satisfaction while reducing length of stay, patients leaving without being seen, and overall costs. Within these studies, EDs reported success with a human-centered approach that placed a focus on both employees and patients. Changes included increasing support from high-level management, allocating resources based on local community needs, and work standardization to streamline major bottlenecks including initial triage and decisions to admission [67].

Diversion of Low-Acuity Patients

Nonurgent visits to the ED are defined by presentation for a condition for which a delay in management is not likely to increase the risk of an adverse outcome [68]. Some studies report that visits in this category account for up to 30% of all ED visits in the USA [69, 70]. Utilization of the ED for issues that could be managed in a primary care office results in superfluous treatment, poor primary care provider relationships, and inflated healthcare costs [71–73]. Combined with the burden of increasingly high patient volumes, methods for safely diverting lower-acuity patients have become a priority.

There have been several interventional strategies to reduce the number of low-acuity presentations to the ED. One study found prehospital telephone triage appropriately identified patients appropriate for the ED, with phone-triaged patients significantly more likely to require admission. In contrast, only 15% of cases referred to alternative care pathways ultimately presented to the ED, of whom fewer than 10% were determined to be appropriate for the ED [74]. In another approach, bedside patient registration was found to decrease the time from triage to bed for nonurgent patients. However, this effect was most pronounced in the morning, when there were typically more ED beds available [75]. Others have explored the possibility of managing minor injuries in the ED on an appointment basis reporting 79% of patients firmly in favor of this system, especially when able to book from their phone or home computer [76].

Clinical Documentation

High patient volume, limited downtime, and frequent interruptions place ED physicians at high risk for medical errors, inefficient billing, and malpractice claims [77]. Critically ill patients at high risk for poor clinical outcomes elicit a unique degree of scrutiny and require clear and accurate documentation. These challenges have propelled ED physicians to adopt novel charting modalities.

EHRs and computerized physician order entry (CPOE) were both posited as solutions to medical documentation errors caused by poorly legible handwritten records and inconsistent use of medical abbreviations [78–80]. While providing a plethora of benefits, EHR implementation also introduced entirely new challenges for physicians as they learned new billing codes and spent more time charting patient encounters [81, 82]. Early experience suggested EHRs lead to lower productivity, barriers to patient interaction, and lower provider and patient satisfaction [83, 84].

Medical Scribes

The birth of the medical scribe promised to alleviate some of this new charting burden ushered onto ED physicians by EHR implementation. Scribes permit thorough documentation of physicians' evaluation and assessment of patients as they occur, theoretically decreasing the opportunity for lost or forgotten clinical data due to time constraints or information overload. Scribe presence facilitates a more direct and attentive interaction between physicians and patients by eliminating the need to chart and take a patient history simultaneously [85]. A meta-analysis demonstrated scribes can significantly increase the number of patients seen per hour by ED physicians [86]. However, singular hospital ED studies have shown the potential for substantially greater benefits. One community hospital-based study reported a significant improvement in all patient throughput metrics, total work RVUs per hour, patients seen per hour, and patient satisfaction [87]. Others have described notable benefits to physician productivity, patient-clinician interaction, documentation time, and billing parameters [85, 88–90]. One novel variation on the use of scribes involves using a wearable computing device (WCD) to stream the entire physician-patient interaction to scribes located remotely. While this approach has captured the imagination of the public, the effectiveness and practicality of this approach have yet to be determined.

Speech-to-Text Conversion

Speech recognition software translates spoken clinical information into text ideally improving documentation speed by circumventing typing inefficiencies and other difficulties with the EHR interface. Commercially available speech recognition software for medical charting was first introduced over 20 years ago [91]. Early iterations of were plagued by documentation errors including word substitution and outright omissions, inaccuracies that could propagate dramatic clinical consequences [92]. Fortunately, speech recognition software has matured substantially with improvements to translation coding that replaced rigid language and grammar constraints with more inclusive probability-based models [93] that have been further enhanced by sophisticated acoustic modeling sensitive to distinct phonemes and advanced signal processing [94, 95].

When compared to traditional transcription services in the ED, speech recognition software demonstrated slightly worse accuracy (98.5% versus 99.7%) and more error corrections per chart (2.5 versus 1.2) while significantly decreasing the overall turnaround time from 39.6 to 3.65 min [96]. Other studies have shown speech recognition software increased documentation speed by 26% [97] and resulted in fewer workflow interruptions [98].

Accurate and reliable speech recognition certainly has the potential to streamline ED documentation greatly. Despite increasing promise, current language models have not managed to overcome errors completely and have a learning curve [99]. A comprehensive review spanning multiple medical disciplines demonstrated accuracy ranging from 88% to 96%, appearing to improve by 0.03% per year in tandem with technology [100]. One random sample of ED notes using the latest speech recognition for documentation discovered an average of 1.3 errors per record of which 14.8% were considered critical. Enunciation errors were exceedingly the most common, accounting for 53.9% of the total [101].

Visual Documentation

There are some aspects of medical care that are better evaluated through visualization regardless of the detail provided through text documentation. Wounds, rashes, and dyskinesias all exemplify cases in which embedment of photos or video into the EHR could positively influence clinical decision-making. While important, photo or video documentation of patients should not be managed haphazardly due to the inherent risk to patient privacy and confidentiality.

Novel technologies exist to add photo and video technology to the ED record. Secure, EHR-linked mobile applications have been at the forefront of integration. One hospital implemented a camera application that converted an image into a PDF that was then seamlessly integrated into the corresponding patient's EHR documentation. Nine out of ten ED physicians who used the application found it to be useful in their clinical practice and easy to use [102]. Similar concepts have been successfully implemented for consultation with dermatologists and pathologists [103, 104]. Wearable smart technology is also being explored as a potential source for capturing important clinical events. One study found video of simulated cardiopulmonary resuscitation events recorded by a WCD provided slightly better global visualization and audio compared to stationary video cameras. Furthermore, significantly fewer of the WCD videos suffered from limitations in interpretability [105].

Access to Clinical Management Guidance

Traditionally, practitioners delivered medical care in isolation. Individual patient results were highly variable and frequently suboptimal and relied heavily on the treating physicians' personal experience or local expertise [106]. Resident physician education, based on a model of apprenticeship, was derived primarily from bedside teaching parlayed by senior clinicians with the inevitable inheritance of scientifically outdated management paradigms and general acquiescence of knowledge passed down over time. The healthcare system has since eschewed this cottage industry of nonintegrated, wholly autonomous practitioner in favor of evidence-based standardization and defragmentation. This transition has resulted in a gradual shift toward improved access to clinical management guidance, a change crucial to the ED model where quick and decisive management has major implications for critically ill and injured patients.

Embedded Clinical Decision Support

Clinical decision support (CDS) is an indelible result of health information technology, encompassing software that judiciously supplies clinical information pertinent to the patient to streamline and strengthen evidence-driven healthcare delivery [107]. Embedded CDS, typically in the form of electronic reminders (also known as best practice alerts, BPAs), is capable of enhancing patient care through several delivery processes [108, 109]. Marked reductions in medication errors and adverse events associated with theophylline [110] and antibiotics have been reported [111, 112]. Physicians also adhere to guideline-based care more frequently [113] such as in the use of head imaging after mild traumatic brain injury [114] or prophylaxis for sexual assault victims [115].

Despite an array of improvements to clinical performance, the impact of CDS on patient outcomes in the ED has not been extensively cataloged [116]. One prospective trial found an electronic CDS with guideline-recommended decision support for diagnosis, severity, disposition, and antibiotic selection in pneumonia patients significantly reduced mortality for community-acquired, but not healthcare-associated, pneumonia [117]. Meta-analysis has also shown CDS can marginally lower mortality by improving the adequacy of antibiotic coverage, increasing compliance with antibiotic guidelines, and reducing resistance [118]. As CDS becomes more common, questions as to the liability of their use arise. For example, if a CDS made an inappropriate recommendation or failed to make an appropriate recommendation, how would that be judged in the event of a negative outcome? While the final decision and responsibility rest with the provider, in the opinion of this author, great care should be placed on training this next generation of providers so that they will use CDS responsibly and not rely on it too heavily. Ultimately, the ability of CDS tools to translate into better patient outcomes will be dependent on the quality of the guidelines on which the CDS is based, its ability to accurately provide appropriate information, and the provider's judicious use of the technology [119].

Online Supplemental Education

Free open-access medical education (FOAM, or FOAMed) has proliferated within emergency medicine in recent years. Table 21.3 lists some common FOAM resources (Table 21.3). FOAM is a living, evolving collection of medical resources and tools created to engage trainees and to facilitate lifelong learning among a new generation of social media-adept resident physicians. Within the specialty of emergency medicine alone, the FOAM movement has spawned hundreds of blogs, podcasts, and online resources to disseminate information useful to everyday practice in the ED [120]. With the persistent gap between cutting-edge research and clinical practice, FOAM has been posited as a bridge for hastening the transition of knowledge from the lab to the bedside [121]. Studies have already demonstrated that spreading research on social media can both increase the number of future citations [122] and result in the article being downloaded more frequently [123]. Several breakthrough studies in emergency medicine have attributed their rapid spread to the power of social media including the use of tranexamic acid for trauma, delayed sequence intubation, and NODESAT approach to oxygenation [120].

Table 21.3 FOAM resources

Websites/groups
Life in the Fast Lane
www.lifeinthefastlane.com
Emergency Department Critical Care & Resuscitation
www.EMCrit.org
R.E.B.E.L. EM (Rational Evidence-Based Evaluation of Literature in Emergency Medicine)
www.REBELEM.com
Conference
SMACC (Social Media & Critical Care)
www.SMACC.net.au

With the ubiquity of smartphones and computers, FOAM has found a growing role as a portable adjunct to resident education through asynchronous learning [124]. While FOAM continues to develop into a go-to resource for clinicians-in-training, some have cautioned learners regarding its popularity. In 2016, a review of FOAM resources reported that only 71.5% of required core content for emergency medicine could be found in the current material and concluded that FOAM is imbalanced and not comprehensive [125]. Another assessment of the available resources urged learners to engage in the critical appraisal of each piece of content and to evaluate for a credentialed author, reliable references, and overall accuracy [126].

Telemedicine and Consulting in the ED

Telemedicine encompasses the utilization of telecommunication technology for collaborative, real-time patient management. Telecommunication facilitates the provision of medical services to sites corporeally distant from the provider delivering care. While some healthcare systems have built their own telemedicine platforms from scratch, most telemedicine requires either a service to manage the technologic infrastructure or involves entire practices that outsource both the technology and the clinical service. Table 21.4 lists some of the popular vendors that provide this service to in the ED setting (Table 21.4). Telemedicine communication has evolved from basic telephone service

Table 21.4 Telemedicine uses

Radiology
Stroke neurology
Non-stroke neurology
Neurosurgery
Burn surgery
Dermatology
Cardiology with remote interpretation of ECGs

to fiber optic and even satellite transmission of digital signals [127]. Telemedicine is an ideal adjunct for the ED allowing isolated emergency physicians to access management support from specialists otherwise unavailable in their local environment.

One regional assessment demonstrated the use of telemedicine was more common in rural EDs without continuous access to a variety of neurological and surgical specialties. Stroke and other neurological presentations accounted for 68% of total uses of telemedicine resources [128]. The use of telemedicine has been shown to reduce the ED door-to-provider time by an average of 6 min and length of stay by 22.1 min for transferred patients. Furthermore, patients first encountered a provider 14.7 min earlier than they would have without telemedicine [129]. Review of the currently available literature indicates telemedicine can be readily incorporated into existing referral frameworks with the potential to minimize unnecessary patient transfers and optimize the care of patients within their local environments [130]. While telemedicine is a rapidly evolving field, some implementation barriers and unresolved issues have been identified including uncertainties about provider liability, hardware expenses, licensing and credentialing, and the ability to capture charges associated with the service.

Prehospital Information

Prehospital care is comprised of all medical interventions from bystander-initiated interventions (e.g., cardiopulmonary resuscitation) through emergency medical service (EMS) activation and hospital transfer. In high-acuity patients, the management and interventions throughout the prehospital period can dramatically alter patient outcomes [131]. One study in a high-income country found up to one-third of trauma-related deaths were potentially preventable with optimized prehospital management [132]. While the actions taken before and during transportation to the hospital are essential, the transfer of care to the ED team is equally important.

Traditionally, the collaboration between the EMS and the ED was surface level, consisting primarily of the ED being alerted a critically ill or injured patient was inbound by the transporting ambulance crew. Information brevity was the rule, limited to a one-liner or brief summary of the suspected condition, but in the most complex cases could be as esoteric as a single symptom. Inadequate, incomplete, or inaccurate information during EMS to ED transitions jeopardizes time-sensitive conditions. Mobile diagnostic and treatment strategies have continued to evolve allowing for time-sensitive diagnostic tests to be performed during transit rather than waiting for arrival to the ED. These interventions have the potential to dramatically impact triage, patient flow, and ultimately clinical outcomes for many time-sensitive conditions [133].

Prehospital Electrocardiogram

Acute, outpatient cardiovascular events are potentially lethal, inexpensive to screen based on physical exam findings, and frequently amenable to time-sensitive interventions. Patients with ST-segment elevation myocardial infarction (STEMI) experience significantly improved clinical outcomes and reduced mortality when reperfusion is performed within a narrow window [134]. Performance of 12-lead electrocardiogram (ECG) by EMS with pre-arrival transmission to the receiving ED maximizes the time for cardiologist notification and cardiac catheterization lab activation. This process has translated to a reduction in door-to-balloon time by an average of 16.3 min in one national registry [135]. Another study found that the target "door-to-balloon time less than 90 min" increased from 44% in the control group to 76% in the intervention group for which the prehospital ECG was provided to the receiving ED [136].

Prehospital Head Imaging for Stroke

During large-vessel ischemic strokes, neuronal damage is directly proportional to the time left untreated [137]. Despite the well-established practice of tissue plasminogen activator (t-PA) in ischemic stroke [138], fewer than one-third of eligible patients receive it during the acceptable treatment window [139, 140]. While EMS transportation has been associated with reduced door-to-imaging time for ischemic stroke [141], the ability of EMS to accurately diagnose stroke is highly variable [142–144]. To counteract this and provide accurate diagnostic information to the receiving ED provider, mobile stroke units have been developed. Mobile stroke units are ambulances equipped with a CT scanner facilitating timely diagnosis of acute stroke—and importantly radiographic contraindications and alternate diagnoses—to promote rapid delivery of t-PA or thrombectomy after arrival [145]. Studies of the mobile stroke unit concept have demonstrated a reduction in median time from first medical notification to treatment decision by 41 min and time to t-PA infusion by 35 min [146].

Prehospital Ultrasound for Trauma

Ultrasound (US) is a critical diagnostic tool used for evaluation of trauma patients with suspected hemorrhage on arrival to the ED [147]. The use of point-of-care US has resulted in reduced time to surgical intervention [148]. With the miniaturization and increased portability of ultrasound technology, prehospital ultrasound has garnered significant attention for its potential role in identifying injuries frequently missed by physical exam by EMS providers [149]. Studies have shown prehospital ultrasound can be useful in early diagnosis of several difficult-to-evaluate conditions including intraabdominal hemorrhage, pericardial effusion, and pneumothorax. Early diagnosis and communication to the receiving hospital translated into increased preparedness and resource allocation by the ED [150, 151]. Because of the training requirements, and inter-operator variability in the best of circumstances, its utility on a large scale has yet to be determined.

Accurate Triage Systems

Integral to improving patient flow and preventing ED overcrowding is the implementation of accurate and effective triage systems. Triage—the process of sorting and assigning patients to determine priority of care and evaluation—continues to evolve due to increased utilization of ED services by the public despite stagnant improvements to infrastructure and resources [152]. Traditionally performed by an experienced nurse or medical assistant at the point of first contact with patients, implementation of newer triage models and screening processes has led to significant improvements in selected performance metrics [153].

Triage Liaison Providers

Historically, triage focused on getting the right resources to the right patient at the right time. In this older model, nurses served a purpose (triaging patients), while physicians served another (treating patients). More recently, in order to mitigate the effects of overcrowding and increase ED throughput, there has been a significant focus on the involvement of physicians and advanced practice providers (APP) in the triage and screening of ED patients. Despite a persistent increase in ED patient volumes, the incorporation of a senior physician as the triage liaison provider (TLP) has been shown to improve ED performance metrics including wait times, LOS, and overall throughput efficiency [154, 155]. A systematic review examining the impact of using a senior physician as a TLP demonstrated decreased ED length of stay decreased by an average of more than 30 min and also a significant reduction in the percentage of patients who left without being treated [156].

Incorporation of physicians into triage systems, while potentially yielding measurable benefits to triage accuracy, efficiency, and patient satisfaction, must be balanced against the added cost of staffing a physician provider in that role and the loss of that provider in providing direct patient care. Some institutions have examined the use of resident physicians and APPs as triage providers instead of senior physicians. One retrospective study found that both resident and attending physician TLPs improved door-to-provider time and median LOS. Not surprisingly, models using resident physicians were more cost-effective [157]. The use of APPs (e.g., physician assistants) in the role of a TLP was also found to reduce LOS and wait times. Further studies comparing different providers in triage are needed to assess the overall financial implications of this strategy [158].

Risk Stratification

In addition to the utilization of physicians and APPs in directing triage, the use of risk stratification algorithms helps facilitate the triage of emergency department patients. The most commonly utilized system is the Emergency Severity Index (ESI) score, a five-level triage scale developed by ED physicians using the patient's clinical status as a surrogate for their urgency of care and needed resources [159]. Using ESI, lower-acuity patients, who would receive a score of level 4 or 5, may be triaged to lower-acuity areas (e.g., fast track) and be assessed by more cost-effective providers, while higher-acuity level 1 or 2 patients may be taken directly to critical treatment areas and receive higher levels of care. Adoption and standardization of the ESI triage system into hospital workflow strongly correlate with decreased ED LOS and patient mortality [160] and are valid predictor of hospital admissions, resource utilization, and ED LOS in the pediatric emergency population [161].

Table 21.5 List of commonly used POC tests

Pregnancy test
Urine strip testing
Capillary blood glucose
Arterial blood gas
Lactate
Chemistry panel
Hemoglobin
B-type natriuretic peptide
Cardiac enzymes
Fecal occult analysis
Influenza screening
Rapid strep test

Diagnostic Testing and Regionalization of Care

In addition to triage algorithms, EDs have adapted the use of point-of-care (POC) diagnostic tests to rapidly identify patients needing higher levels of care and resources, including specialty care and transfer if those resources are unavailable [162]. Table 21.5 lists some of the most common POC tests used in the ED (Table 21.5). The use of a screening electrocardiogram for patients with a chief complaint of chest pain is associated with increased identification of patients with acute myocardial infarction (MI) and decreased delays in the administration of thrombolytic agents and percutaneous coronary intervention (PCI) [163]. Both POC D-dimer and troponin assays have also been used to screen patients for whom pulmonary embolism and myocardial infarction, respectively, are possible diagnoses. However, only POC D-dimer was found to significantly decrease average ED LOS and hospital admission [164, 165]. While the sensitivity in identifying patients with pneumonia was poor, the use of a chest radiograph triage protocol decreased time to antibiotic administration for patients admitted to the hospital with community-acquired pneumonia [166].

References

1. Rothenhaus T, et al. Information systems for emergency care: American College of Emergency Physicians; 2009.
2. Kerr K, Norris T. Improving health care data quality: a practitioner's perspective. Int J Inf Qual. 2008;2(1):39–59.
3. Hsiao C, et al. Electronic medical record/electronic health record systems of office-based physicians: 2009 and preliminary 2010 state estimates. National Center for Health Statistics, November 2011.
4. Ben-Assuli O. Electronic health records, adoption, quality of care, legal and privacy issues and their implementation in emergency departments. Health Policy. 2015;119(3):287–97.
5. Miranda ML, Ferranti J, Strauss B. Geographic health information systems: a platform to support the 'triple aim'. Health Aff. 2013;32(9):1608–15.
6. Stiell A, et al. Prevalence of information gaps in the Emergency Department and the effect on patient outcomes. CMAJ. 2003;169(10):1023–8.
7. Remen VM, Grimsmo A. Closing information gaps with shared electronic patient summaries: how much will it matter? Int J Med Inform. 2011;80(11):775–81.
8. Jensen SA, et al. Erroneous drug charts: a health hazard? Tidsskr Nor Laegeforen. 2003;123:3598–9.
9. Evans RS. Electronic health records: then, now, and in the future. Yearb Med Inform. 2016;Suppl 1:S48–61.
10. Vest JR, et al. Factors motivating and affecting health information exchange usage. J Am Med Inform Assoc. 2011;18(2):143–9.
11. Bahous MC, Shadmi E. Health information exchange and information gaps in referrals to a pediatric emergency department. Int J Med Inform. 2016;87:68–74.
12. Vest JR, Kaushal R, Silver MD. Health information exchange and the frequency of repeat medical imaging. Am J Manag Care. 2014;20(11):eSP16–24.
13. Vest JR, et al. Association between use of a health information exchange system and hospital admissions. Appl Clin Inform. 2014;5(1):219–31.
14. Wilcox AB, Shen S, Dorr DA. Improving access to longitudinal patient health information within an emergency department. Appl Clin Inform. 2012;3(3):290–300.
15. Ben-Assuli O, Shabtai I, Leshno M. Using electronic health record systems to optimize admission decisions: the Creatinine case study. Health Informatics J. 2015;21(1):73–88.
16. Flaks-Manov N, et al. Health information exchange systems and length of stay in readmissions to a different hospital. J Hosp Med. 2016;11(6):401–6.
17. Vest JR, Kern LM, Silver MD. The potential for community-based health information exchange systems to reduce hospital readmissions. J Am Med Inform Assoc. 2015;22(2):435–42.
18. Carr CM, et al. Observational study and estimate of cost savings from use of a health information exchange in an academic emergency department. J Emerg Med. 2014;46(2):250–6.
19. Saef SH, Melvin CL, Carr CM. Impact of a health information exchange on resource use and Medicare-allowable reimbursements at 11 emergency departments in a midsized city. West J Emerg Med. 2014;15(7):777–85.
20. Neri PM, Redden L, Poole S. Emergency medicine resident physicians' perceptions of electronic documentation and workflow: a mixed methods study. Appl Clin Inform. 2015;6(1):27–41.
21. Dexheimer JW, Borycki EM. Use of mobile devices in the emergency department: a scoping review. Health Informatics J. 2015;21(4):306–15.
22. Schooley B, et al. Impacts of mobile tablet computing on provider productivity, communications, and the process of care. Int J Med Inform. 2016;88:62–70.
23. Fleischmann R, Duhm J, Hupperts H, Brandt SA. Tablet computers with mobile electronic medical records enhance clinical routine and promote bedside time: a controlled prospective crossover study. J Neurol. 2015;262(3):532–40.
24. Prgomet M, Georgiou A, Westbrook JI. The impact of mobile handheld technology on hospital physicians' work practices and patient care: a systematic review. J Am Med Inform Assoc. 2009;16(6):792–801.
25. Horng S, et al. Prospective pilot study of a tablet computer in an Emergency Department. Int J Med Inform. 2012;81(5):314–9.
26. Strayer SM, et al. Patient attitudes toward physician use of tablet computers in the exam room. Fam Med. 2010;42(9):643–7.
27. Duhm J, Fleischmann R, Schmidt S, et al. Mobile electronic medical records promote workflow: physicians' perspective from a survey. JMIR Mhealth Uhealth. 2016;4(2):e70.
28. O'Connell TW, Patlas MN. Mobile devices and their prospective future role in emergency radiology. Br J Radiol. 2016;89(1061):20150820.
29. Singh N, et al. Tablet-based patient-centered decision support for minor head injury in the emergency department: pilot study. JMIR Mhealth Uhealth. 2017;5(9):e144.
30. Finn NB. Collaboration, communication and connection: fostering patient engagement in health care. J Participat Med. 2012;4:e20.
31. Purcell K. Half of adult cell phone owners have apps on their phones. [Online] Pew Internet Research, 2011. http://pewinternet.org/Reports/2011/Apps-update.aspx.
32. Radhakrishna K, et al. Electronic health records and information portability: a pilot study in a rural primary healthcare center in India. Perspect Health Inf Manag. 2014;11:1b.
33. Huang LC, Chu HC, Lien CY, et al. Privacy preservation and information security protection for patients' portable electronic health records. Comput Biol Med. 2009;39(9):743–50.
34. Coats B, Acharya S. Leveraging the cloud for electronic health record access. Perspect Health Inf Manag. 2014;11:1g.

35. Institute of Medicine. Hospital-based emergency care: at the breaking point. Washington DC: National Academies Press; 2006.
36. Wilper AP, Woolhandler S, Lasser KE. Waits to see an emergency department physician: U.S. trends and predictors, 1997-2004. Health Aff. 2008;27:w 84–95.
37. Horwitz LI, Bradley EH. Percentage of US emergency department patients seen within the recommended triage time: 1997 to 2006. Arch Intern Med. 2009;169:1857–65.
38. McCarthy ML, Zeger SL, Ding R. Crowding delays treatment and lengthens emergency department length of stay, even among high acuity patients. Ann Emerg Med. 2009;54:492–503.
39. Pines JM, Iyer S, Disbot M, Hollander JE, Shofer FS, Datner EM. The effect of emergency department crowding on patient satisfaction for admitted patients. Acad Emerg Med. 2008;15:825–31.
40. Pines JM, Pollack CV Jr, Diercks DB, et al. The association between emergency department crowding and adverse cardiovascular outcomes in patients with chest pain. Acad Emerg Med. 2009;16:617–25.
41. Chalfin DB, Trzeciak S, Likourezos A, et al. Impact of delayed transfer of critically ill patients from the emergency department to the intensive care unit. Crit Care Med. 2007;35:1477–83.
42. Hoot NR, Aronsky D. Systematic review of emergency department crowding: causes, effects, and solutions. Ann Emerg Med. 2008;52:126–36.
43. Rui P, Kang K. National Hospital Ambulatory Medical Care Survey: 2014 Emergency Department Summary Tables. Center for Disease Control. [Online] [Cited: February 19, 2018.] https://www.cdc.gov/nchs/data/nhamcs/web_tables/2014_ed_web_tables.pdf.
44. Peters ML. The older adult in the emergency department: aging and atypical illness presentation. J Emerg Nurs. 2010;36:29–34.
45. Pines JM. Trends in the rates of radiography use and important diagnoses in emergency department patients with abdominal pain. Med Care. 2009;47:782–6.
46. Hsia RY, Kellermann AL, Shen YC. Factors associated with closures of emergency departments in the United States. JAMA. 2011;305:1978–85.
47. Bullard MJ, Villa-Roel C, Bond K. Tracking emergency department overcrowding in a tertiary care academic institution. Healthc Q. 2009;12:99–106.
48. Pines JM, Batt RJ, Hilton JA, Terwiesch C. The financial consequences of lost demand and reducing boarding in hospital emergency departments. Ann Emerg Med. 2011;58:331–40.
49. Gupta, D. Queueing models for healthcare operations. [book auth.] BT Denton. Handbook of healthcare operations management: methods and applications. New York : Springer, 2013.
50. Cochran JK, Roche KT. A multi-class queueing network analysis methodology for improving hospital emergency department performance. Comput Oper Res. 2009;36:1497–512.
51. Lakshmi C, Sivakumar AI. Application of queueing theory in health care: a literature review. Operations Research for Health Care. 2013;2:25–39.
52. McCarthy ML, et al. The challenge of predicting demand for emergency department services. Acad Emerg Med. 2008;15:337–46.
53. Gupta D, Denton BT. Appointment scheduling in health care: challenges and opportunities. IIE Trans. 2008;40(9):800–19.
54. Moll HA. Challenges in the validation of triage systems at emergency departments. J Clin Epidemiol. 2010;63:384–8.
55. Konrad R, et al. Modeling the impact of changing patient flow processes in an emergency department: insights from a computer simulation study. Operations Research for Health Care. 2013;2:66–74.
56. Green LV, Kolesar PJ, Whitt W. Coping with time-varying demand when setting staffing requirements for a service system. Prod Oper Manag. 2007;16:13–39.
57. Green LV, et al. Using queueing theory to increase the effectiveness of emergency department provider staffing. Acad Emerg Med. 2006;13(1):61–8.
58. Alavi-Moghaddam M, Forouzanfar R, Alamdari S, et al. Application of queuing analytic theory to decrease waiting times in emergency department: does it make sense? Arch Trauma Res. 2012;1(3):101–7.
59. Fitzgerald K, Pelletier L, Reznek MA. A queue-based Monte Carlo analysis to support decision making for implementation of an emergency department fast track. J Health Eng. 2017;4:1–8.
60. Laker LF, et al. The flex track: flexible partitioning between low- and high-acuity areas of an emergency department. Ann Emerg Med. 2014;64(6): 591–603.
61. Fujimoto T. The evolution of a manufacturing system at Toyota. New York: Oxford University Press; 1999.
62. Andersen H, Rovik KA, Ingbrigsten T. Lean thinking in hospitals: is there a cure for the absence of evidence? A systematic review of reviews. BMJ Open. 2014;4:e003873.
63. De Koning H, et al. Lean six sigma in healthcare. J Healthc Qual. 2006;28:4–11.
64. Brandao De Souza L. Trends and approaches in lean healthcare. Leadersh Health Serv. 2009;22:121–39.
65. Villeneuve C. Fujitsu's Lean Solutions Group - Lean Healthcare in Canada. Fujitsu Sci Tech J. 2011;47:41–8.
66. Migita R, et al. Emergency department overcrowding: developing emergency department capacity through process improvement. Clin Pediatr Emerg Med. 2011;12:141–50.
67. Bucci S, de Belvis AG, Marventano S. Emergency Department crowding and hospital bed shortage: is Lean a smart answer? A systematic review. Eur Rev Med Pharmacol Sci. 2016;20:4209–19.
68. Young G, Wagner M, Kellermann A, Bouley E. Ambulatory visits to hospital emergency departments. Patterns and reasons for use. 24 Hours in the ED Study Group. JAMA. 1996;276(6):460–5.

69. Durand A, Gentile S, Devictor B, et al. ED patients: how nonurgent are they? Systematic review of the emergency medicine literature. Am J Emerg Med. 2010;29(3):333–45.
70. Northington W, Brice J, Zou B. Use of an emergency department by nonurgent patients. Am J Emerg Med. 2005;23:131–7.
71. Carret M, Fassa A, Kawachi I. Demand for emergency health service: factors associated with inappropriate use. BMC Health Serv Res. 2007;7:131.
72. Phelps K, Taylor C, Kimmel S, Nagel R, Klein W, Puczynski S. Factors associated with emergency department utilization for nonurgent pediatric problems. Arch Fam Med. 2000;9:1086–92.
73. Redstone P, Vancura J, Barry D, Kutner J. Nonurgent use of the emergency department. J Ambulatory Care Manage. 2008;31(4):370–6.
74. Eastwood K, Morgans A, Smith K, et al. Appropriateness of cases presenting in the emergency department following ambulance service secondary telephone triage: a retrospective cohort study. BMJ Open. 2017;7(10):e016845.
75. Takakuwa KM, Shofer FS, Abbuhl SB. Strategies for dealing with emergency department overcrowding: a one-year study on how bedside registration affects patient throughput times. J Emerg Med. 2007;32(4):337–42.
76. Roberts L, Dykes L. Emergencies by appointment: would patients with minor injuries prefer a booked appointment at their local emergency department to the current walk-in service provision. Emerg Med J. 2014;31(9):786.
77. Yu KT, Green RA. Critical aspects of emergency department documentation and communication. Emerg Med Clin North Am. 2009;27(4):641–54.
78. Velo GP, Minuz P. Medication errors: prescribing faults and prescription errors. Br J Clin Pharmacol. 2009;67(6):624–8.
79. Awan S, Abid S, Tariq M. Use of medical abbreviations and acronyms: knowledge among medical students and postgraduates. Postgrad Med J. 2016;92:721–5.
80. Yu FB, Menachemi N, Berner ES. Full implementation of computerized physician order entry and medication-related quality outcomes: a study of 3364 hospitals. Am J Med Qual. 2009;24(4):278–86.
81. Howard J, Clark EC, Friedman A. Electronic health record impact on work burden in small, unaffiliated, community-based primary care practices. J Gen Intern Med. 2013;28(1):107–13.
82. Payne TH, Corley S, Cullen TA. Report of the AMIA EHR-2020 Task Force on the status and future direction of EHRs. J Am Med Inform Assoc. 2015;22(5):1102–10.
83. Basanti A, Walch R, Todd B. Computerized prescriber order entry decreases patient satisfaction and emergency center physician productivity. Ann Emerg Med. 2010;56(3):s83–4.
84. Farber NJ, Liu L, Chen Y. EHR use and patient satisfaction: what we learned. J Fam Pract. 2015;64(11):687–96.
85. Shultz CG, Holmstrom HL. The use of medical scribes in health care settings: a systematic review and future directions. J Am Board Fam Med. 2015;28(3):371–81.
86. Heaton HA, Nestler DM, Lohse CM. Impact of scribes on emergency department patient throughput one year after implementation. Am J Emerg Med. 2017;34(10).
87. Shuaib W, Hilmi J, Caballero J, Rashid I, Stanazai H, Tawfeek K, Amari A, Ajanovic A, Moshtaghi A, Khurana A, Hasabo H, Baqais A, Szczerba AJ, Gaeta TJ. Impact of a scribe program on patient throughput, physician productivity, and patient satisfaction in a community-based emergency department. Health Informatics J. 2017;35(2):311–4.
88. Bastani A, Shagiri B, Palomba K, Bananno D, Anderson W. An ED scribe program is able to improve throughput time and patient satisfaction. Am J Emerg Med. 2014;32(5):399–402.
89. Hess JJ, Wallenstein J, Ackerman JD, Akhter M, Ander D, Keadey MT, Capes JP. Scribe impacts on provider experience, operations, and teaching in an academic emergency medicine practice. West J Emerg Med. 2015;16(5):602–10.
90. Heaton HA, Nestler DM, Jones DD, Varghese RS, Lohse CM, Williamson ES, Sadosty AT. Impact of scribes on billed relative value units in an academic emergency department. J Emerg Med. 2017;52(3):370–6.
91. Johnson M, Lapkin S, Long V, et al. A systematic review of speech recognition technology in health care. BMC Med Inform Decis Mak. 2014;14(1):94.
92. Bliss MF. Speech recognition for the health professions: (using Dragon naturally speaking). Upper Saddler River, NJ: Prentice Hall; 2005.
93. Paulett JM, Langlotz CP. Improving language models for radiology speech recognition. J Biomed Inform. 2009;42(1):53–8.
94. Gales M, Young S. The application of hidden Markov models in speech recognition. Found Trends Signal Process. 2008;1(3):197–203.
95. Eddy SR. What is a hidden Markov model? Nat Biotechnol. 2004;22(10):1315–6.
96. Zick RG, Olsen J. Voice recognition software versus a traditional transcription service for physician charting in the ED. Am J Emerg Med. 2001;19(4):295–8.
97. Vogel M, Kaisers W, Wassmuth R, Mayatepek E. Analysis of documentation speed using web-based medical speech recognition technology: randomized controlled trial. J Med Internet Res. 2015;17(11):e247.
98. Dela, JE, Shabosky, JC, Albrecht, M, Clark, M, Milbrandt, JC, Kegg, JA. Typed Versus Voice Recognition for Data Entry in Electronic Health Records: Emergency Physician Time Use and Interruptions. West J Emerg Med. 2014;15(4):541–74.
99. Hodgson T, Magrabi F, Coiera E. Efficiency and safety of speech recognition for documentation in the electronic health record. J Am Med Inform Assoc. 2017;24(6):1127–33.

100. Hodgson T, Coiera E. Risks and benefits of speech recognition for clinical documentation: a systematic review. J Am Med Inform Assoc. 2016;23(e1):e169–79.
101. Goss FR, Zhou L, Weiner SG. Incidence of speech recognition errors in the emergency department. Int J Med Inform. 2016;93:70–3.
102. Landman A, et al. A mobile app for securely capturing and transferring clinical images to the electronic health record: description and preliminary usability study. JMIR Mhealth Uhealth. 2015;3(1):e1.
103. Pecina JL, Wyatt KD, Comfere NI, Bernard ME, North F. Uses of mobile device digital photography of dermatologic conditions in primary care. JMIR Mhealth Uhealth. 2017;5(11):e165.
104. Hartman DJ, Parwani AV, Cable B, Cucoranu IC, McHugh JS, Kolowitz BJ, Yousem SA, Palat V, Reden AV, Sloka S, Lauro GR, Ahmed I, Pantanowitz L. Pocket pathologist: a mobile application for rapid diagnostic surgical pathology consultation. J Pathol Inform. 2014;5(1):10.
105. Kassutto SM, Kayser JB, Kerlin MP, Upton M, Lipschik G, Epstein AJ, Dine CJ, Schweickert W. Google glass video capture of cardiopulmonary resuscitation events: a pilot simulation study. J Grad Med Educ. 2017;9(6):748–54.
106. Swensen SJ, et al. Cottage industry to postindustrial care — the revolution in health care delivery. N Engl J Med. 2010;362:e12.
107. Osheroff J, Teich J, Levick D, et al. Improving outcomes with clinical decision support: an implementer's guide. 2nd ed. Chicago: HIMSS; 2012.
108. Damiani G, Pinnarelli L, Colosimo SC, et al. The effectiveness of computerized clinical guidelines in the process of care: a systematic review. BMC Health Serv Res. 2010;10:2.
109. Bright TJ, Wong A, Dhurjati R, et al. Effect of clinical decision-support systems: a systematic review. Ann Intern Med. 2012;157(1):29–43.
110. Hurley SF, Dziukas LJ, McNeil JJ. A randomized controlled clinical trial of pharmacokinetic theophylline dosing. AJRCCM. 1986;134(6):1219–24.
111. Evans RS, Pestotnik SL, Classen DC, et al. A computer-assisted management program for antibiotics and other antiinfective agents. N Engl J Med. 1998;338:232–8.
112. Burton ME, Ash CL, Hill DP. A controlled trial of the cost benefit of computerized bayesian aminoglycoside administration. Clin Pharmacol Ther. 1991;49:685–94.
113. Chaudhry B, Wang J, Wu S, et al. Systematic review: impact of health information technology on quality, efficiency, and costs of medical care. Ann Intern Med. 2006;144:742–52.
114. Gupta A, Ip IK, Raja AS, et al. Effect of clinical decision support on documented guideline adherence for head CT in emergency department patients with mild traumatic brain injury. J Am Med Inform Assoc. 2014;21:e347–51.
115. Britton DJ, et al. Impact of a computerized order set on adherence to Centers for Disease Control guidelines for the treatment of victims of sexual assault. J Emerg Med. 2013;44:528–35.
116. Garg AX, et al. Effects of computerized clinical decision support systems on practitioner performance and patient outcomes. JAMA. 2005;293(10): 1223–38.
117. Dean NC, et al. Impact of an electronic clinical decision support tool for emergency department patients with pneumonia. Ann Emerg Med. 2015;66(5):511–20.
118. Curtis CE, Bahar FA, Marriot JF. The effectiveness of computerised decision support on antibiotic use in hospitals: a systematic review. PLoS One. 2017;12(8):e0183062.
119. Landman AB. The potential for clinical decision support to improve emergency care. Ann Emerg Med. 2015;66(5):521–2.
120. Nickson CP, Cadogan MD. Free Open Access Medical education (FOAM) for the emergency physician. Emerg Med Aust. 2014;26(1):76–83.
121. Young PJ, Nickson CP, Gantner DC. Can social media bridge the gap between research and practice? Crit Care Resp. 2013;15:257–9.
122. Eysenbach G. Can tweets predict citations? Metrics of social impact based on Twitter and correlation with traditional metrics of scientific impact. J Med Internet Res. 2011;13:e123.
123. Allen HG, et al. Social media release increases dissemination of original articles in the clinical pain sciences. PLoS One. 2013;8:e68914.
124. Reiter DA, Lakoff DJ, Trueger NS, et al. Individual interactive instruction: an innovative enhancement to resident education. Ann Emerg Med. 2013;61: 110–3.
125. Stuntz R, Clontz R. An evaluation of emergency medicine core content covered by Free Open Access Medical Education resources. Ann Emerg Med. 2016;67(5):649–653.e2.
126. Grock A, Paolo W. Free open access medical education: a critical appraisal of techniques for quality assessment and content discovery. Clin Exp Emerg Med. 2016;3(3):183–5.
127. Physicians, American College of Emergency. Emergency medicine telemedicine. Ann Emerg Med. 2016;67(5):687–9
128. Zachrison KS, Hayden EM, Schwamm LH. Characterizing New England emergency departments by telemedicine use. West J Emerg Med. 2017;18(6):1055–60.
129. Mohr NM, Young T, Harland KK. Emergency department telemedicine shortens rural time-to-provider and emergency department transfer times. Telemed J E Health. 2018;24(8):582–93.
130. du Toit, M, Malau-Aduli, B and Vangaveti, V. Use of telehealth in the management of non-critical emergencies in rural or remote emergency departments: a systematic review. J Telemed Telecare. 2017.

131. Wilson MH, et al. Pre-hospital emergency medicine. Lancet. 2016;387(10020):2526–34.
132. Chiara O, Scott JD, Cimbanassi S. Trauma deaths in an Italian urban area: an audit of pre-hospital and in-hospital trauma care. Injury. 2002;33:553–62.
133. Kyriacou E, et al. Emergency health care information systems. Conf Proc IEEE Eng Med Biol Soc. 2011;2011:2501–4.
134. Antman EM, Anbe DT, Armstrong PW, et al. CC/AHA guidelines for the management of patients with ST-elevation myocardial infarction: a report of the American College of Cardiology/American Heart Association Task Force on Practice Guidelines. Circulation. 2007;115(15):296–329.
135. Curtis JP, et al. The pre-hospital electrocardiogram and time to reperfusion in patients with acute myocardial infarction, 2000–2002: findings from the national registry of myocardial infarction-4. JACC. 2006;47(8):1544–52.
136. Chen KC, et al. Effect of emergency department in-hospital tele-electrocardiographic triage and interventional cardiologist activation of the infarct team on door-to-balloon times in ST-segment-elevation acute myocardial infarction. Am J Cardiol. 2011;107(10):1430–5.
137. Saver JL. Time is brain—quantified. Stroke. 2006;37(1):263–6.
138. Group, The National Institute of Neurological Disorders and Stroke rt-PA Stroke Study. Tissue plasminogen activator for acute ischemic stroke. N Engl J Med. 1995;333(24):1581–7.
139. Fonarow GC, Smith EE, Saver JL, et al. Timeliness of tissue-type plasminogen activator therapy in acute ischemic stroke: patient characteristics, hospital factors, and outcomes associated with door-to-needle times within 60 minutes. Circulation. 2011;123(7):750–8.
140. Fassbender K, Balucani C, Walter S. Streamlining of prehospital stroke management: the golden hour. Lancet Neurol. 2013, 12(6):585–96.
141. Minnerup J, et al. Effects of emergency medical service transport on acute stroke care. Eur J Neurol. 2014;21(10):1344–7.
142. Buck BH, et al. Dispatcher recognition of stroke using the National Academy Medical Priority Dispatch System. Stroke. 2009;40(6):2027–30.
143. Jones SP, et al. The identification of acute stroke: an analysis of emergency calls. Int J Stroke. 2013;8(6):408–12.
144. Ramanujam P, Guluma KZ, Castillo EM. Accuracy of stroke recognition by emergency medical dispatchers and paramedics--San Diego experience. Prehosp Emerg Care. 2008;12(3):307–13.
145. Mason J. Mobile stroke units for prehospital care of ischemic stroke. CADTH Issues in Emerging Health Technologies. 2017.
146. John S, et al. Brain imaging using mobile CT: current status and future prospects. J Neuro Img. 2015;26(1):5–15.
147. Spahn DR, Bouillon B, Cerny V, et al. Management of bleeding and coagulopathy following major trauma: an updated European guideline. Crit Care. 2013;17(2):R76.
148. Melniker LA, et al. Randomized controlled clinical trial of point-of-care, limited ultrasonography for trauma in the emergency department: the first sonography outcomes assessment program trial. Ann Emerg Med. 2006;48(3):227–35.
149. Hasler RM, et al. Accuracy of prehospital diagnosis and triage of a Swiss helicopter emergency medical service. J Trauma Acute Care Surg. 2012;73(3):709–15.
150. Walcher F, et al. Prehospital ultrasound imaging improves management of abdominal trauma. Br J Surg. 2006;93(2):238–42.
151. Mazur SM, et al. Use of point-of-care ultrasound by a critical care retrieval team. Emerg Med Australas. 2007;19(6):547–52.
152. Fernandes CM, Tanabe P, Gilboy N, et al. Five-level triage: a report from the ACEP/ENA Five-level Triage Task Force. J Emerg Nurs. 2005;31:39–50.
153. Oredsson S, Jonsson H, Rognes J, et al. A systematic review of triage-related interventions to improve patient flow in emergency departments. Scand J Trauma Resusc Emerg Med. 2011;19:43.
154. Holroyd BR, et al. Impact of a triage liaison physician on emergency department overcrowding and throughput: a randomized controlled trial. Acad Emerg Med. 2007;14:702.
155. Rogg JG, et al. A long-term analysis of physician triage screening in the emergency department. Acad Emerg Med. 2013;20(4):374–80.
156. Abdulwahid MA, et al. The impact of senior doctor assessment at triage on emergency department performance measures: systematic review and meta-analysis of comparative studies. Emerg Med J. 2016;33(7):504–13.
157. Weston V, Jain S, Gottlieb M, et al. Effectiveness of resident physicians as triage liaison providers in an academic emergency department. West J Emerg Med. 2017;18(4):577–84.
158. Nestler DM, Fratzke AR, Church CJ, et al. Effect of a physician assistant as triage liaison provider on patient throughput in an academic emergency department. Acad Emerg Med. 2012;19(11):1235–41.
159. Wuerz R, Milne LW, Eitel DR, Travers D, Gilboy N. Reliability and validity of a new five-level triage instrument. Acad Emerg Med. 2000;7(3):236–42.
160. Wuerz R. Emergency Severity Index triage category is associated with six-month survival. ESI triage study group. Acad Emerg Med. 2001;8(1):61–4.
161. Green NA, Durani Y, Brecher D, DePiero A, Loiselle J, Attia M. Emergency Severity Index version 4: a valid and reliable tool in pediatric emergency department triage. Pediatr Emerg Care. 2012;28(8):753–7.
162. Rooney KD, Schilling UM. Point-of-care testing in the overcrowded emergency department: can it make a difference? Crit Care. 2014;18:692.

163. Graff L, Palmer AC, Lamonica P, et al. Triage of patients for a rapid (5-minute) electrocardiogram: a rule based on presenting chief complaints. Ann Emerg Med. 2000;36(6):554–60.
164. Lee-Lewandrowski E, Nichols J, Van Cott E, et al. Implementation of a rapid whole blood D-dimer test in the emergency department of an urban academic medical center: impact on ED length of stay and ancillary test utilization. Am J Clin Pathol. 2009;132(3):326–31.
165. Koehler J, Flarity K, Hertner G, et al. Effect of troponin I Point-of-Care testing on emergency department throughput measures and staff satisfaction. Adv Emerg Nurs J. 2013;35(3):270–7.
166. Cooper JJ, Datner EM, Pines JM. Effect of an automated chest radiograph at triage protocol on time to antibiotics in patients admitted with pneumonia. Am J Emerg Med. 2008;26(3):264–9.

Trauma Room: "A Minute Man" Operating Room – Managing the Chaos Using Technologies

22

Muhammad Zeeshan and Bellal Joseph

Introduction

Trauma is a major public health problem worldwide. It accounts for one out of every ten mortalities, leading to an annual death toll of almost 6 million[1], a number that is predicted to rise to 10 million by 2030 [2]. Despite the advent of novel resuscitation strategies and improved surgical and critical care, trauma remains one of the leading causes of morbidity and mortality in the United States [1]. Annually 26.9 million people with trauma are managed in emergency room; 2.5 million are admitted to hospital. Additionally, these people often have life-long physical, psychological, and occupational disabilities resulting in total medical and work loss cost of $671 billion [3].

Evolution of Technology and Integration in Healthcare Sector

Over the recent years, there have been tremendous innovations in information technology (IT) which resulted in successful integration of technology in healthcare sector. From the electronic medical records to online prescriptions, computed tomographic (CT) scans to magnetic resonance imaging (MRI), a trauma room to the state-of-art hybrid operating rooms, and minimally invasive endoscopic procedures to robotic surgeries, technological advancements have revolutionized the healthcare sector. It has improved the organizational efficiency of hospitals resulting in improved patient safety and patient satisfaction [4, 5]. The advanced diagnostic and therapeutic modalities have particularly increased the standard of care for time-sensitive ailments especially trauma. A trauma surgeon should have the latest armament to manage patients presenting in the trauma bay.

Managing Chaos Using Technology in Trauma Room

Trauma victims present with multiple undiagnosed injuries, emergent evaluation and definitive management of these traumatic injuries can improve the survival. Every 3 min delay in the management of these patients can increase mortality by 1% [6]. The advent of latest technology and tremendous research has resulted in the development of best practice guidelines that can be adopted today to prevent the delays in definitive management of trauma patients and improve the outcomes. After initial primary and secondary survey, each patient undergoes a plain X-ray of the chest and pelvis and focused on assessment with sonography for trauma (FAST) of the

M. Zeeshan · B. Joseph (✉)
Division of Trauma, Critical Care, Emergency Surgery, and Burns, Department of Surgery, University of Arizona, Tucson, AZ, USA
e-mail: bjoseph@surgery.arizona.edu

R. Latifi (ed.), *The Modern Hospital*, https://doi.org/10.1007/978-3-030-01394-3_22

abdomen followed by a CT scan. Below we will discuss the management of major injuries in detail.

Trauma Resuscitation

In the United States, trauma is the main cause of mortality and years of life lost, and over the last decade, deaths from trauma have increased significantly. Over 20–40% of trauma, deaths after hospital admission are attributable to massive hemorrhage [7]. These trauma deaths can be prevented with rapid resuscitation and improved hemorrhage control strategies. During the initial management, patients should be assessed for any external wounds, and bleeding should be controlled with direct pressure. In trauma bay, every patient with hemorrhage should get two large IV cannulas according to ATLS guidelines [8]. The mechanism of injury, initial vitals, and FAST examination can guide the need for resuscitation. Over the last decade, innovative diagnostic modalities and research have resulted in evidence-based and patient-centered resuscitation strategies. Previously, crystalloids were used as a primary therapy for initial resuscitation, but they can lead to dilutional coagulopathy, hypothermia, and volume overload [9]. The emerging literature is supporting initial resuscitation with blood products, i.e., packed red blood cells (PRBCs), fresh frozen plasma (FFP), and platelets. The famous Pragmatic, Randomized Optimal Platelets and Plasma Ratios (PROPPR) trial has concluded that trauma patients should receive initial resuscitation in 1:1:1 ratio to improve outcomes [10].

Massive Transfusion Protocols

For the management of severe hemorrhage, the hospitals should have a massive transfusion protocol (MTP) which should be initiated in anticipation of the need for large-scale transfusion. Determining when to initiate MTP has been a topic of great debate. There are multiple scores that can predict the need for massive transfusion. Currently, the assessment of blood consumption (ABC) score is used at various institutes. It relies on four parameters (penetrating mechanism of injury, positive FAST, systolic blood pressure [SBP] ≤90 mmHg, heart rate [HR] ≥120 bpm); each positive parameter has a score of 1, and a total score of ≥2 predicts the need for massive transfusion [11]. In an analysis of patients with high-level trauma activations, we modified the ABC score and concluded that replacement of hypotension and tachycardia with shock index and addition of pelvic fracture resulted in enhanced discriminatory power of ABC score. We proposed the Revised Assessment of Bleeding and Transfusion (RABT) score which has four parameters as shown below:

- Penetrating mechanism of injury
- Shock index (HR/SBP) >1.0
- Positive FAST
- Pelvic fracture of X-ray

Each positive parameter has a score of 1, and a total score of ≥2 predicts massive transfusion with better accuracy, sensitivity, and specificity compared to ABC score [12].

Factor Replacement and Tranexamic Acid

Hemorrhage is the most common preventable cause of death in patients with trauma and every one out of four hemorrhagic patients develop coagulopathy, which exponentially increases the mortality [13]. With an increased understanding of the pathophysiology of coagulopathy, there is a paradigm shift toward more goal-directed resuscitation strategies with early antifibrinolytic therapy and factor replacement that are tailored toward the individual needs of each patient. Hyper-fibrinolysis is an important component of coagulopathy and directly correlates with mortality in trauma patients. An earlier intervention with antifibrinolytic agent such as tranexamic acid (TXA) can improve survival as shown in the famous CRASH-2 trial which was a randomized clinical trial (TXA vs placebo) and included over 20,000 trauma patients in 274 hospitals across 40 countries. CRASH-2 trial concluded that TXA administration within 3 h of injury was associated with lower mortality (14.5% vs 16%, RR: 0.91[0.85–0.97]) [14].

The utility of factor replacement with coagulation factors VIIa, factor IX, and prothrombin complex concentrate (PCC) for reversal of trauma-induced coagulopathy (TIC) is well established in the military. However, over the recent years, factor replacement has emerged as an important adjunct therapy in resuscitating hemorrhagic patients in civilian settings [15]. Multiple studies have shown the efficacy and safety of factor replacement. In a recent study, Jehan et al. concluded that the use of four-factor PCC as an adjunct for trauma resuscitation not only improved the survival but also decreased the blood products required for optimal resuscitation of injured trauma patients with evidence of TIC [16]. The goal of trauma resuscitation should be minimum crystalloid transfusion with earlier blood product resuscitation in 1:1:1 ratio and factor replacement. All patients should receive TXA within 3 h of injury to decrease the rate of TIC and improve survival.

Viscoelastic Testing Modalities

Over the recent years, viscoelastic testing such as thromboelastography (TEG) and rotational thromboelastography (ROTEM) has revolutionized resuscitation in trauma. TEG was introduced in 1948 by Hertert, while ROTEM is a modified version of TEG technology. Both of them are the point of care tests to analyze hemostasis in trauma patients. They provide a real-time visual assessment of clot initiation, strength, and clot lysis [17]. The primary clinical use of TEG/ROTEM lies in the rapid turnover of the results. The traditional laboratory measurements (prothrombin time, activated partial thromboplastin time, international normalized ratio) usually take longer compared to TEG/ROTEM that generally provide the results in 15–20 min. Additionally, multiple studies have shown the superiority of TEG/ROTEM over the conventional parameters to predict the hemostatic status of patients. Tapia et al. in their analysis of trauma patients have concluded that TEG-based resuscitation is superior to massive transfusion in penetrating trauma, while it is equivalent in blunt trauma [18]. The viscoelastic testing in trauma consensus panel has issued its recommendations for TEG-ROTEM-based resuscitation [19]. The American College of Surgeons has clear guidelines for TEG/ROTEM-based transfusion protocol, and they have provided clear-cut points to initiate transfusion of specific blood components as shown in Table 22.1. TEG/ROTEM should be readily available in trauma bay where they can guide the need for resuscitation. They not only identify patients who require massive transfusion but also minimize the unnecessary transfusion of blood products and save hospital resources.

Table 22.1 Transfusion triggers based on TEG/ROTEM

TEG cut point	ROTEM cut point	Transfuse
r-value >9 min	CT exTEM >100 s CT inTEM >230 s	Plasma
k-time >4 min	–	Plasma and/or cryoprecipitate
α-Angle <60°	MCF fibTEM <8 mm	Cryoprecipitate and/or plasma
mA <55 mm	MCF exTEM <45 mm MCF fibTEM >10 mm	Platelets
LY 30 >7.5%	ML exTEM >15%	TXA

Abbreviations: TEG thromboelastography, *ROTEM* rotational thromboelastography, *TXA* tranexamic acid

Noninvasive Blood Flow Monitoring

Post-traumatic hemorrhage is usually manifested as a shock, which is defined as a state of inadequate perfusion and delivery of oxygen to tissues. The inadequate perfusion causes secondary inflammatory- and immune-related events which subsequently contribute to multi-organ failure and death. Recognizing shock at the earliest possible stage and preventing its progression are the two important strategies to prevent this horrific sequela. However, unfortunately, the traditional vital signs (i.e., capillary refill, heart rate, systolic blood pressure, and pulse pressure) are not a sensitive indicator of tissue perfusion. Therefore, the traditional vital signs may not be used as a clear endpoint for trauma resuscitation. Over the last decade, an intense research and evolution of technology have resulted in the development of more sensitive and noninvasive methods to serve as resuscitation endpoint.

Near-Infrared Spectroscopy (NIRS)

Near-infrared spectroscopy (NIRS) was first pioneered by Jobsis and Millikan. Since its development, it has been an exciting prospect for the noninvasive monitoring of blood flow and tissue oxygenation in trauma patients. It not only provides information about intravascular oxygenation status of hemoglobin (Hb) but also the oxygen utilization in the cell. This technology uses light with wavelengths ranging from 600 to 1000 nm. The dispersion pattern of light waves in blood and biological tissue provides information about the oxygen concentration. NIRS can be used in devastating trauma-related pathologies including hemorrhagic shock, compartment syndrome, sepsis, and multi-organ failure to monitor oxygen delivery and consumption at the cellular level [20]. Additionally, NIRS is being investigated as a potential tool for noninvasive monitoring of brain tissue oxygenation, intracranial pressure, and cerebral perfusion pressure in patients with traumatic brain injury [21].

Pulse CO-Oximeter (Masimo)

Hemoglobin level is one of the most important laboratory test ordered in patients with trauma and shock. It helps guide the therapeutic plan of managing these patients. However, the traditional method of measuring Hb involves invasive blood sampling which is time-consuming and has a potential risk of biohazards. Noninvasive methods of continuous Hb monitoring have been proposed as an alternative to the traditional Hb measurement. The Pulse CO-Oximeter (Masimo Rainbow SET, Masimo, Irvine, CA) is an FDA-approved device which is capable of measuring Hb continuously using a spectrophotometric sensor. Multiple studies have analyzed the accuracy and predictive ability of this device. Macknet et al. in their case series of patients undergoing surgery have shown a good correlation of Masimo measured Hb to the traditional invasive Hb measurements [22]. In another study, we evaluated the accuracy of the Masimo device in severely injured trauma patients and concluded that in patients with Hb < 8 mg/dL, Masimo has an accuracy of 88% to predict Hb level. Additionally, it continuously monitors Hb level that can provide real-time data about the response of trauma patients to blood transfusion and help us tailor the resuscitation strategies according to the needs of patients [23].

Traumatic Brain Injuries

Traumatic brain injury (TBI) is one of the leading causes of death and disability. According to the Centers for Disease Control and Prevention (CDC), 2.8 million people sustain a TBI annually. About 2.5 million of these injured individuals are treated in an emergency department, with approximately 282,000 hospitalizations and 56,000 deaths resulting in an estimated financial burden of $76.5 billion [24]. Patients presenting with a traumatic brain injury (TBI) are initially treated and assessed according to the Advanced Trauma Life Support (ATLS) protocol. Patients are intubated and resuscitated according to their hemodynamic status. The initial management focuses on keeping an adequate oxygenation and blood pressure.

Role of CT Scan

CT scan is currently the preferred imaging procedures for initial evaluation and detection of skull fractures, head bleeds, and edema. All the patients presented with moderate or severe TBI that is defined as GCS < 14 undergo a non-contrast CT scan. However, the patients who have mild TBI, i.e., GCS 14–15, may not need a CT imaging. There are two major tools that can guide the use of CT scan for initial evaluation of patients presenting with a mild TBI. Canadian CT head rule and New Orleans's criteria (Table 22.2) can be used to identify patients who require a CT scan of the head [25–27]. Both of these tools have a sensitivity of almost 100% to identify clinically significant injuries. In pediatric population, the concern of radiation exposure limits the use of CT scans as children are more sensitive to radiation as compared to adults, and it increases the lifetime risk of cancer significantly. Pediatric Emergency Care Applied Research Network

(PECARN) head rule can be used to identify patients who require a CT scan of the head in pediatric trauma patients [28].

Initial physical examination, CT scan findings, and previous medical history dictate the hospital course and need for a repeat head CT scan in these patients. At our institution, we have developed brain injury guidelines (BIG) that can guide the further management of patients with TBI (Table 22.3). The patients are divided into three categories: BIG-1, BIG-2, and BIG-3. Patients in BIG-1 and BIG-2 are managed by acute care surgeons without a neurosurgical consultation and repeat CT scan of the head [29]. Clinical deterioration of neurological status prompts a neurosurgical consultation and repeat CT scan of the head in these patients. Patients in BIG-3 category undergo repeat head CT scan, neurosurgical consultation and neurosurgical intervention at the discretion of neurosurgeon. This practice has resulted in a significant decrease in the rate of neurosurgical consultation, repeat head CT scans, hospital costs, and hospital length of stay without any change in mortality [30]. The safety and efficacy of BIG have been validated in the pediatric population as well as institutions with limited resources [31, 32].

Table 22.2 Criteria to predict the need for head CT scan in TBI

New Orleans's criteria	Canadian CT head rule
Age >60 Vomiting Headache Drug or alcohol intoxication Persistent anterograde amnesia Visible trauma above clavicle Seizures	*High risk for neurosurgical intervention:* Age >65 Two or more episodes of vomiting GCS < 15 at 2 h after injury Suspected open or depressed skull fracture Any sign of basal skull fracture *Medium risk of brain injury detection on CT scan:* Retrograde amnesia >30 min Dangerous mechanism (pedestrian struck, ejection from vehicle during crash, fall from height >5 ft or >5 stairs)

Evaluation of Cervical Spine Injuries

In North America, annually 13 million trauma patients with a suspicion of cervical spine injury are presented to the ED [33]. Every patient with TBI should be suspected to have a cervical spine injury, and a cervical collar should be placed in the ED. A detailed physical examination can further guide the requirement of radiographic imaging of the cervical spine. Currently, two specific criteria have been developed which can help

Table 22.3 Brain injury guidelines

Variables	BIG-1	BIG-2	BIG-3
LOC	Yes/no	Yes/no	Yes/no
Neurologic examination	Normal	Normal	Abnormal
Intoxication	No	No/yes	No/yes
CAMP	No	No	Yes
Skull fracture	No	Non-displaced	Displaced
SDH	≤4 mm	5–7 mm	≥8 mm
EDH	≤4 mm	5–7 mm	≥8 mm
IPH	≤4 mm, 1 location	5–7 mm, 2 locations	≥8 mm, multiple locations
SAH	Trace	Localized	Scattered
IVH	No	No	Yes
Therapeutic plan			
Hospitalization	Observation (6 h)	Yes	Yes
RHCT	No	No	Yes
NSC	No	No	Yes

Abbreviations: *BIG* brain injury guidelines, *CAMP* Coumadin, aspirin, Plavix, *EDH* epidural hemorrhage, *IVH* intraventricular hemorrhage, *IPH* intra-parenchymal hemorrhage, *LOC* loss of consciousness, *NSC* neurosurgical consultation, *RHCT* repeat head computed tomography, *SAH* subarachnoid hemorrhage, *SDH* subdural hemorrhage decide the need for CT imaging in suspected cervical spine trauma. According to the National Emergency X-Radiography Utilization Study (NEXUS) Low-Risk Criteria (NLC), CT scan of the cervical spine is indicated in trauma patients unless they meet all of the following criteria [34]:

- No posterior midline tenderness
- No evidence of intoxication
- A normal level of alertness
- No focal neurological deficit
- No painful distracting injuries

The Canadian C-Spine Rule (CCR) can also be used to evaluate the need for CT imaging in suspected cervical spine injury. It is based upon multiple high-risk and low-risk factors and the ability of the patients to rotate the neck [35]. Stiell et al. performed a prospective observational study to compare the NEXUS and CCR and concluded that CCR has better sensitivity and specificity to identify C-spine injuries, and its use would have decreased unnecessary radiographic imaging [36].

Evaluation of Cerebrovascular Injuries

Carotid and vertebral artery injuries are collectively called as cerebrovascular injuries. Trauma to the neck can cause an intimal tear that can result in dissection, intraluminal hematoma, occlusion, or complete transection of the vessel. The incidence of cerebrovascular injuries is as low as 1% in blunt trauma. However, these injuries are associated with high rates of morbidity and mortality [37]. Due to the improvement of CT technology and advent of 64, 128 and 256-slices CT scan, CT angiography (CTA) is the screening test of choice for emergent evaluation of patients with suspected cerebrovascular injuries. The Eastern Association for the Surgery of Trauma and Western Trauma Association have provided specific guidelines for the indication of CTA in these patients. According to these guidelines, all patients with symptoms of arterial hemorrhage from the head to neck, cervical hematoma, cervical bruit in <50y, neurological deficit, the severe facial trauma of midface, basilar skull fracture, and fracture of C1–C3 vertebrae should undergo a CTA for the screening of cerebrovascular injuries. An earlier diagnosis and timely intervention can prevent the mortality and severe neurological deterioration associated with cerebrovascular injuries [38, 39].

Penetrating Head Injuries

Penetrating injuries to the head are less prevalent than blunt injuries; however, they carry a worse prognosis. The American Association of Neurological Surgeons and the Brain Trauma Foundation have created evidence-based best practice guidelines for the management of penetrating TBI [40]. The initial management should follow the standardized ATLS protocol, and the patients should undergo aggressive resuscitation. After initial evaluation and stabilization of patients' hemodynamic status, the site of injury should be inspected meticulously for CSF leaks, bleeding, and oozing of brain parenchyma [41]. Currently, the CT scan is the primary modality of evaluation, and all patients with a penetrating TBI (pTBI) should undergo a CT scan as a part of initial evaluation protocol. Previous literature supported an expectant management of patients with pTBI especially those who present with low GCS and bilateral hemispheric injuries [42]. However, the emerging evidence advocates for an "aggressive" approach to manage all patients with pTBI. At our institution, we adopted a policy of aggressive resuscitation with blood products and hyperosmolar therapy even in patients with low GCS and bi-hemispheric injuries, and it led to an improved survival from 10% in 2008 to 46% in 2011 [43]. Additionally, an aggressive management not only improves survival but also increases the rate of organ donation in lethal brain injuries [44]. If surgery is deemed necessary, it should be performed within 1 h after the hemodynamic stability of patients. Patients with pTBI are particularly prone to infectious complications, and the rate varies from 5 to 23% [45]. There is no consensus regarding the use of prophylactic antibiotics. Lin et al. in their study of pTBI recommend the use of prophylactic antibiotics for 2–3 days [46]. The recent US military guidelines recommend prophylaxis with cefazolin for 5–7 days [47]. However, other studies

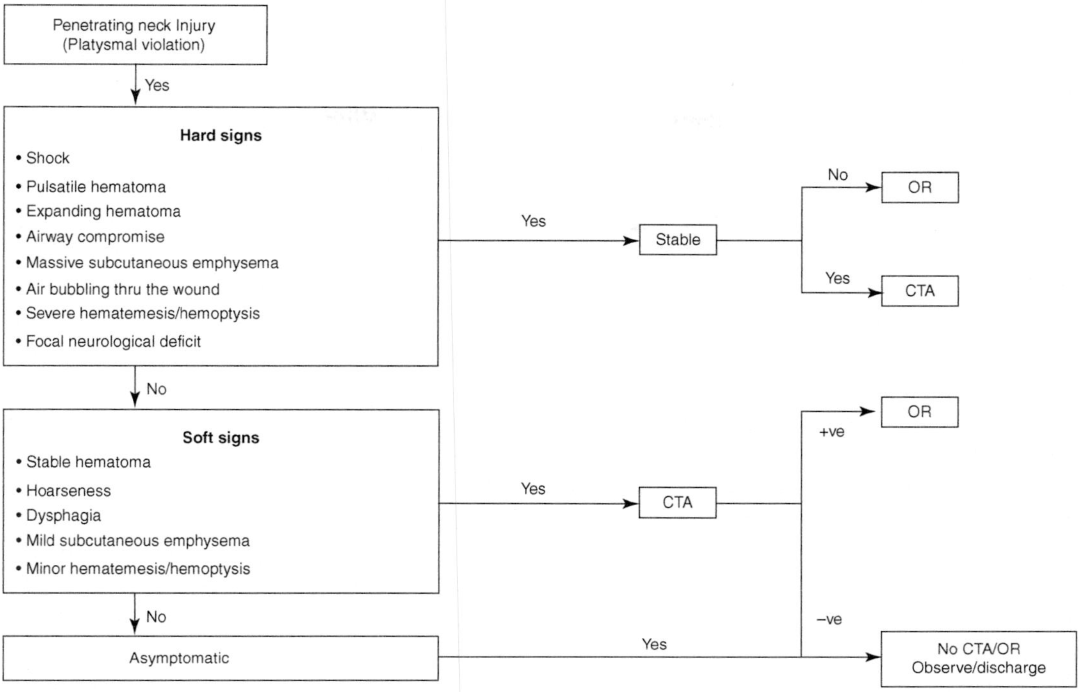

Fig. 22.1 No zone approach for evaluating penetrating neck injuries

report that there is inadequate evidence to support the use of prophylactic antibiotics [48]. The need for starting prophylaxis antibiotics should be determined on an individual basis, and if deemed necessary the antibiotics should be started as soon as possible in these patients [41].

Penetrating Neck Injuries

Penetrating neck injuries (PNI) account for 5–10% of trauma-related admissions in adults. Carotid artery is the most common structure injured, and exsanguination is the main cause of death in patients with PNI [49]. All the patients with PNI should undergo timely hemodynamic evaluation and management of injuries as they can decompensate rapidly. The hard and soft signs of injuries should be identified. Previously, the need for CTA and surgical exploration was determined by the zone of injury. However, the emerging literature is supporting a no-zone approach for the evaluation of PNI. Prichayudh et al. and Ibraheem et al. analyzed the sensitivity of physical examination to identify patients requiring CTA for evaluation of PNI and concluded that physical examination alone can guide the requirement of CTA and following a no-zone approach would lead to lower rates of unnecessary CTA and negative explorations [50, 51]. PNI can be evaluated with a no-zone approach as shown in Fig. 22.1.

Traumatic Thoracic Injuries

The chest is the 3rd most commonly injured region of the body, 1 out of every 3rd trauma patient is admitted secondary to chest trauma, and thoracic injuries account for 25% of trauma deaths. Blunt mechanism accounts for 60–75% of thoracic injuries, while penetrating mechanism of injury causes 24–40% of thoracic injuries [52]. The most common mechanism of thoracic trauma is motor vehicle collision followed by falls [53]. The chest wall constitutes the rib cage, intercostal muscles, and costal cartilage. The thoracic cavity houses vital organs of the body including the aorta, heart, lungs, and esophagus. Injuries to these organs can lead to devastating outcomes. These injuries should be identified and treated immediately in the trauma room. The aortic injuries alone have a high mortality of 95%; earlier detection and treatment can save 70% of these patients [54].

Role of Ultrasonography Modalities

Ultrasonography (USG) was first introduced in trauma in 1990s as the focused assessment with sonography for trauma (FAST). Since its inception, FAST has been incorporated as an integral component for the evaluation of trauma patients. Over the last decade, its utility has been extended to evaluate the pneumothorax and hemothorax in patients who present with chest trauma. Addition of USG imaging of the chest has resulted in extended FAST (eFAST) [55]. eFAST has been shown to have a higher sensitivity for diagnosing pneumothorax and hemothorax compared to CXR. To diagnose hemothorax on chest X-ray, 50–100 mL fluid is required, while eFAST can detect as little as 20 mL of fluid in pleural space. Currently, eFAST is performed to rule out cardiac tamponade, hemothorax, and pneumothorax. The sliding lung and "comet tail" artifact signs can reliably rule out pneumothorax. Additionally, USG view of the inferior vena cava can help define the type and a tailored management of shock in trauma patients [56].

Role of X-Ray

Poster-anterior chest X-ray (CXR) is one of the most valuable diagnostic tests for the evaluation of chest trauma. It can easily diagnose rib fractures, hemo-/pneumothorax, and lung contusions. Specific signs, e.g., mediastinal widening, pneumomediastinum, and emphysema, can further guide the diagnostic and treatment strategies in these patients [57]. It is cheap, easily available, and can be performed rapidly, making it the tool of choice for the initial evaluation of in chest trauma.

Role in CT Scan

The diagnostic accuracy of CT scan is much better than CXR, and it allows for detailed evaluation of intrathoracic structures. Currently CT scans is an integral part of the diagnostic protocols for evaluation of injuries to the area of the chest, and patients admitted secondary to high-energy trauma rapidly undergo CT scan of the chest [58]. With latest MDCT and three-dimensional (3D) reconstruction, we can examine the vital structures in the chest including major vessels with a sensitivity and specificity approaching 100% [59]. The history and physical examination at presentation guides the requirement for CT scan in patients with chest trauma. The NEXUS group has created criteria to identify patients that require a CT for evaluation of chest trauma. They identified following signs which can be related to intrathoracic injuries:

- Chest wall tenderness
- Distracting painful injury
- Rapid deceleration injury (fall >20 feet; MVC > 40mph)
- Abnormal chest radiograph
- Sternal tenderness
- Thoracic spine tenderness
- Scapular tenderness

The absence of all of the abovementioned signs indicates a very low risk for intrathoracic injuries, and a CT scan is not warranted [60].

Managing Blunt Thoracic Injuries

The patients presented with blunt chest trauma should be resuscitated initially according to the ATLS guidelines. The further management is guided by the hemodynamic status of the patients as shown in Fig. 22.2. Hemodynamically stable patients are usually evaluated with eFAST, CXR, and ECG. In case of high mechanism injury, they usually require chest CT or angiography to rule out aortic injuries. The utility of cardiac enzymes remains controversial for the diagnosis of blunt cardiac injury [61]. Patients with unstable hemodynamic status should undergo rapid assessment with eFAST, CXR, and ECG to identify any life-threatening conditions including pneumothorax, hemothorax, and cardiac tamponade. Patients with a pneumothorax and hemothorax should undergo a rapid decompression with a tube thoracostomy. A chest tube or a pigtail catheter can be used for this purpose. The safety and effectiveness

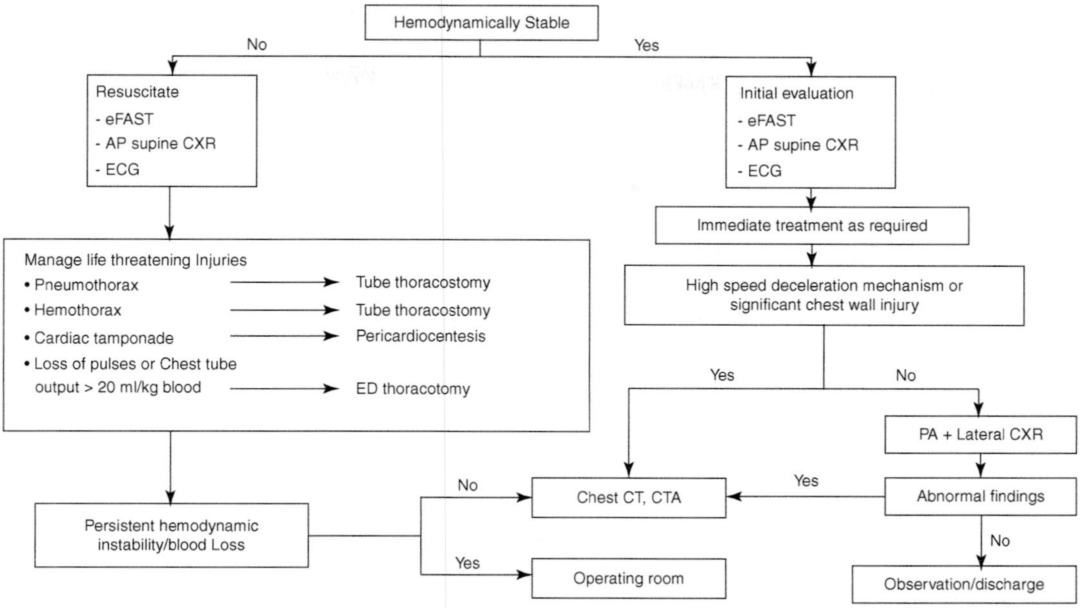

Fig. 22.2 Management of blunt thoracic trauma

of small-caliber pigtail catheter for traumatic hemo- and pneumothorax are well established [62, 63]. Bauman et al. in their 7-year prospective analysis concluded that 14-French pigtail catheter had similar failure rate, tube insertion-related complications, and drainage output compared to large 32–40 French chest tube [64]. Pigtail catheters are small caliber and can be placed percutaneously with less tissue trauma and pain at the site of insertion. Patients with cardiac tamponade should undergo rapid pericardiocentesis, and an ED thoracotomy can be performed for further resuscitation in these patients. After stabilization of hemodynamic status, all patients should undergo chest CT scan.

Managing Penetrating Thoracic Injuries

Penetrating thoracic injuries are rare but have worse outcomes compared to blunt thoracic trauma. Three percent of all trauma-related deaths can be attributed to penetrating chest trauma. Most of these injuries are managed non-operatively with serial examination and tube thoracostomy; however, 15–30% of penetrating thoracic injuries will eventually need a surgical management [65]. The hemodynamically stable patients should undergo a rapid evaluation with eFAST and CXR. A large pneumothorax and hemothorax should be managed by a tube thoracostomy [66]. CT scan should be performed in high-risk patients. The indications for CT scan are

- Trajectory crossing the mediastinum
- Signs and symptoms of major thoracic injury (vascular, tracheobronchial, esophageal)
- Persistent symptoms that are not explained with a CXR

The initial evaluation and resuscitation strategy in hemodynamically unstable patients is similar to hemodynamically stable patients. However, patients with cardiac tamponade undergo a rapid pericardial drainage or sternotomy to decompress the heart [67]. If there are signs of posterior/lateral hemothorax, an anterolateral thoracotomy should be performed to identify the underlying thoracic injury, and damage control closure should be done [68].

ED Thoracotomy

ED thoracotomy is performed in trauma room to resuscitate patients who are on the verge of cardiac arrest. It is a very high-risk procedure.

Hospitals should have clear policies to determine the need for this high-risk procedure. The Eastern Association for the Surgery of Trauma (EAST), Western Trauma Association (WTA), and American College of Surgeons Committee on Trauma (ACS-COT) have evidence-based guidelines and indications of ED thoracotomy as summarized below [69–71].

- Patients with blunt chest trauma who lost vital signs in transit or in the ED or patients with cardiac tamponade diagnosed with eFAST and do not have any severe lethal injuries (e.g., massive traumatic brain injuries, severe polytrauma). ED thoracotomy is contraindicated in patients who have no signs of life at the scene, who have massive lethal injuries, and those who require >10 min prehospital CPR.
- Patients with penetrating chest trauma who lost vital signs in transit or in the ED and are hemodynamically unstable despite initial resuscitation or pulseless for <15 min.
- Patients with penetrating injuries to the neck or extremity and having CPR for <5 min.

Abdominal Trauma

Abdominal is the 2nd most common region injured in trauma patients, and it accounts for 7–10% of trauma deaths. Every one out of four patients with abdominal trauma needs surgical exploration for the injuries [72]. Blunt mechanism accounts for 80% of abdominal trauma seen in the trauma bay, and the most mechanism of injury is motor vehicle crash followed by pedestrian struck. Almost 13% of these patients have intra-abdominal organ injuries [73]. The most common organ injured is the spleen followed by the liver and hollow viscus. On the other hand, 20% of all abdominal injuries are attributable to penetrating mechanism, with stab wounds and gunshot wounds as the most common causes of injury. The most common organs injured in penetrating abdominal trauma are the small bowel followed by the colon and liver [73].

Role of Ultrasonography

Previously, diagnostic peritoneal lavage was used as a decision-making tool to evaluate the requirement for laparotomy in trauma patients. However, FAST has replaced this invasive test. The traditional FAST includes a simple sonographic imaging with a low-frequency ultrasound probe to assess fluid in pericardial, peri-hepatic, peri-splenic, and pelvic areas. It is portable, readily available, easy to learn, and can be performed in <1 min in the trauma bay. FAST is primarily used to detect hemoperitoneum in patients with abdominal trauma. Currently, it is the point of care test which is usually performed alongside the secondary survey of trauma patients.

Role of X-Ray

Plain radiographs of the abdomen are not very helpful in the evaluation of blunt abdominal trauma (BAT). In GSW and stab wounds, plain radiographs are usually performed to evaluate the trajectory of wound. Presence of lower rib fractures, free air under diaphragm, violation of diaphragm, and pelvic fractures on X-ray are important findings that indicate presence of intra-abdominal injuries and indicate further evaluation.

Role of CT Scan

Since its inception in clinical medicine by Dr. Hounsfield and Dr. Ambrose in 1972, computed tomographic technology has underwent significant evolution resulting in remarkable innovations. These advances have substantially improved the diagnostic ability of CT scans, and it is currently the modality of choice for evaluating intra-abdominal injuries in trauma patients. After an initial physical examination and USG evaluation, patients with suspected injuries are taken to a CT scan which can identify intra-abdominal injuries with a high sensitivity and specificity of 97–98% and 97–99%, respectively [74, 75]. In trauma patients, time is of great essence, and delay of even a single minute increases the risk of adverse outcomes. With the advent of latest CT scans, the imaging time has been reduced to a mere few seconds. With CT imaging, we can define and grade the specific

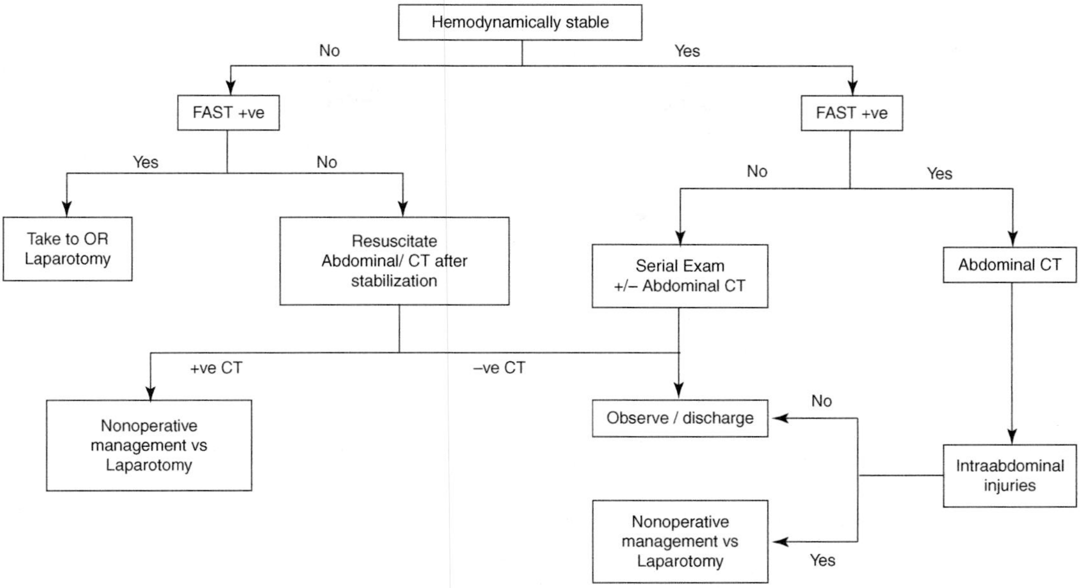

Fig. 22.3 Management of blunt abdominal trauma

injuries to the solid and hollow viscus organs; detect the site of active bleeding; assess the retroperitoneal space and vertebral column for traumatic injuries; and evaluate the integrity of the pelvis. However, CT scans have a very low sensitivity to detect mesenteric and pancreatic duct injuries. Additionally, CT scans require IV contrast, which can cause contrast nephropathy in already deteriorating hemorrhaging patients, and there is a potential risk for radiation exposure.

Managing Blunt Abdominal Injuries

Initial management of injuries is focused on rapid stabilization and identification of life-threatening injuries according to ATLS protocols. A physical examination is of immense importance to rule out any major illness. Nishijima et al. reviewed 10,757 patients with BAT and concluded that seat belt sign, hypotension, femur fracture, abdominal distension, guarding, and rebound tenderness on physical examination are most strongly associated with intra-abdominal injuries [76]. The further management of BAT depends upon the hemodynamic status of the patient. Hemodynamically stable patients with a positive FAST should undergo an abdominal CT scan for evaluation of their injuries. Patients with a negative FAST can be managed with serial examination. In hemodynamically unstable patients, a positive FAST indicates an intra-abdominal injury, and they should be taken to the operative room for laparotomy for definitive care. While the patients with negative FAST should undergo resuscitation and taken to CT scan after initial stabilization (Fig. 22.3).

Managing Penetrating Abdominal Injuries

Patients with PAT are at high risk for intra-abdominal injuries especially small bowel injuries. The healthcare providers should have higher suspicion of injuries in these patients. They can go in shock and deteriorate rapidly due to intra-abdominal injuries. Patients with any of the following signs of physical examination should undergo emergent laparotomy [77, 78].

- Hemodynamic instability
- The evisceration of intra-abdominal contents
- Peritonitis
- Impalement
- Signs of gastrointestinal bleeding (frank blood on nasogastric aspiration or rectal exam)

All the patients without an indication of laparotomy should be managed by local wound exploration, X-ray, CT scan, and serial physical examination.

Managing Pelvic Fractures

Pelvic fractures constitute 3% of all skeleton injuries. High-energy impacts, e.g., motor vehicle crash and pedestrian struck, are the major causes of pelvic fractures. Pelvic fractures are associated with higher mortality ranging from 5 to 16% because they cause disruption of the presacral and lumbar venous plexus resulting in life-threatening retroperitoneal hemorrhage [79]. Early detection and control of bleeding can lead to improved survival in these patients. In the trauma room, any patient with a suspicion of pelvic fracture should undergo a pelvic X-ray, and patients should be assessed for the stability of the pelvis; if unstable he/she should receive a pelvic binder. All the hemodynamically stable patients should undergo a rapid CT scan and managed accordingly. Hemodynamically unstable patients should undergo an aggressive resuscitation, and FAST can guide the further treatment strategy in these patients. Patients with FAST positive should be taken to the operative room for laparotomy, pelvic packing, and stabilization. Patients with negative FAST can undergo diagnostic peritoneal aspiration, and they can be managed with angioembolization or peritoneal packing.

Role of Resuscitative Endovascular Balloon Occlusion of the Aorta (REBOA)

REBOA is a resuscitative technique in which a balloon is advanced and inflated in the aorta that obstructs the distal blood flow and increases proximal aortic pressure leading to an increased cerebral and myocardial perfusion. It was first described by Hughes in 1954 [80]. Over the recent years, development of novel endovascular approaches and state-of-the-art technological modifications led to an increased use of REBOA in the resuscitation of trauma patients [81]. REBOA provides a temporary occlusion of distal blood flow and has been advocated as a "physiological bridge" to more definitive care in hemodynamically unstable patients with torso trauma and lower body injuries [82]. REBOA is indicated for hemorrhagic shock in patients with SBP <90 mmHg and transient or no response to initial ATLS resuscitation. The Joint Trauma System Clinical Practice Guideline (JTS CPG) have specific algorithm for REBOA placement in trauma patients [83].

Telemedicine, Telepresence, and Tele-trauma

Over the last three decades, there have been rapid advances in the technology including endoscopic, laparoscopic, and robotic surgeries. The development of state-of-the-art communication technology and virtual and augmented reality has led to the emergence of telemedicine which is defined as the use of medical information shared through technology to improve outcomes. The concept of telepresence and telemedicine is still evolving in trauma. The trauma systems were developed to bring the right patient to the right place at the right time to provide right care. Because of the shortage of trauma centers, tele-trauma has the ability to bring the right specialist using technology to the patients right away. It has transformed the concept of "golden hour" into "now care" [84]. Tele-trauma can help us save healthcare resources by reducing unnecessary transfers and hospital cost. Additionally, through tele-trauma, earlier identification and management of trauma patients in low-income and peripheral areas with limited accessibility to level I trauma centers can improve survival and patients' satisfaction [85, 86]. Currently, multiple programs are underway to streamline the use of virtual reality, augmented reality, and remote robotic surgeries in acute care service.

Conclusion

Despite the advent of latest technology and improved treatment strategies, trauma is still the leading cause of death and disability. Healthcare providers should have a diverse state-of-the-art armament in the trauma room, and they should follow a patient-centered, disease-based, research-oriented, and technology-driven approach to manage these patients.

References

1. World Health Organization. Injuries and violence: the facts. Accessed on 12 July 2018; Available from: http://www.who.int/violence_injury_prevention/key_facts/en/.
2. Mathers CD, Loncar D. Projections of global mortality and burden of disease from 2002 to 2030. PLoS Med. 2006;3(11):e442.
3. Cost of injuries and violence in the United States. Accessed on 12 July 2018; Available from: https://www.cdc.gov/injury/wisqars/overview/cost_of_injury.html.
4. Chasm Q. A new health system for the 21st century. Washington, DC: National; 2001.
5. Gawande A, Bates DW. The use of information technology in improving medical performance. Part II. Physician-support tools. Med Gen Med. 2000;2(1):E13.
6. Clarke JR, et al. Time to laparotomy for intra-abdominal bleeding from trauma does affect survival for delays up to 90 minutes. J Trauma Acute Care Surg. 2002;52(3):420–5.
7. US Centers for Disease Control and Prevention. Injury prevention and control: data and statistics. Accessed on 20 April 2018; Available from: https://www.cdc.gov/injury/wisqars/fatal.html.
8. Subcommittee A, Tchorz KM, I.A.w. group. Advanced trauma life support (ATLS®): the ninth edition. J Trauma Acute Care Surg. 2013;74(5):1363.
9. Spinella PC, Holcomb JB. Resuscitation and transfusion principles for traumatic hemorrhagic shock. Blood Rev. 2009;23(6):231–40.
10. Holcomb JB, et al. Transfusion of plasma, platelets, and red blood cells in a 1: 1: 1 vs a 1: 1: 2 ratio and mortality in patients with severe trauma: the PROPPR randomized clinical trial. JAMA. 2015;313(5):471–82.
11. Nunez TC, et al. Early prediction of massive transfusion in trauma: simple as ABC (assessment of blood consumption)? J Trauma Acute Care Surg. 2009;66(2):346–52.
12. Joseph B, et al. Massive transfusion: the revised assessment of bleeding and transfusion (RABT) score. World J Surg. 2018;42(11):3560–7.
13. Brohi K, et al. Acute traumatic coagulopathy. J Trauma Acute Care Surg. 2003;54(6):1127–30.
14. Collaborators C. The importance of early treatment with tranexamic acid in bleeding trauma patients: an exploratory analysis of the CRASH-2 randomised controlled trial. The Lancet. 2011;377(9771):1096–1101. e2.
15. Kushimoto S, et al. Efficacy and safety of a 4-factor prothrombin complex concentrate for rapid vitamin K antagonist reversal in Japanese patients presenting with major bleeding or requiring urgent surgical or invasive procedures: a prospective, open-label, single-arm phase 3b study. Int J Hematol. 2017;106(6):777–86.
16. Jehan F, et al. The role of four-factor prothrombin complex concentrate in coagulopathy of trauma: a propensity matched analysis. J Trauma Acute Care Surg. 2018;85(1):18–24.
17. Whiting D, DiNardo JA. TEG and ROTEM: technology and clinical applications. Am J Hematol. 2014;89(2):228–32.
18. Tapia NM, et al. TEG-guided resuscitation is superior to standardized MTP resuscitation in massively transfused penetrating trauma patients. J Trauma Acute Care Surg. 2013;74(2):378–86.
19. Inaba K, et al. 2014 consensus conference on viscoelastic test–based transfusion guidelines for early trauma resuscitation: report of the panel. J Trauma Acute Care Surg. 2015;78(6):1220–9.
20. Ward KR, et al. Near infrared spectroscopy for evaluation of the trauma patient: a technology review. Resuscitation. 2006;68(1):27–44.
21. Davies DJ, et al. Near-infrared spectroscopy in the monitoring of adult traumatic brain injury: a review. J Neurotrauma. 2015;32(13):933–41.
22. Macknet MR, et al. The accuracy of noninvasive and continuous total hemoglobin measurement by pulse CO-oximetry in human subjects undergoing hemodilution. Anesth Analg. 2010;111(6):1424–6.
23. Joseph B, et al. Continuous noninvasive hemoglobin monitor from pulse ox: ready for prime time? World J Surg. 2013;37(3):525–9.
24. Traumatic Brain Injury–Related Emergency Department Visits, Hospitalizations, and Deaths — United States, 2007 and 2013. Accessed on 18 July, 2018; Available at https://www.cdc.gov/mmwr/volumes/66/ss/ss6609a1.htm.
25. Haydel MJ, et al. Indications for computed tomography in patients with minor head injury. N Engl J Med. 2000;343(2):100–5.
26. Goldstein J, Loyd L. Abington suspends trauma center. In: Philadelphia inquirer. Philadelphia. Accessed on 12 July 2018; Available from http://articles.mcall.com/2002-12-19/news/3427446_1_trauma-center-trauma-patients-emergency-room.
27. Stiell IG, et al. The Canadian CT head rule for patients with minor head injury. Lancet. 2001;357(9266):1391–6.
28. Nakhjavan-Shahraki B, et al. Pediatric emergency care applied research network (PECARN) prediction rules in identifying high risk children with mild traumatic brain injury. Eur J Trauma Emerg Surg. 2017;43(6):755–62.
29. Joseph B, et al. The BIG (brain injury guidelines) project: defining the management of traumatic brain injury by acute care surgeons. J Trauma Acute Care Surg. 2014;76(4):965–9.
30. Joseph B, et al. Changing paradigms in the management of 2184 patients with traumatic brain injury. Ann Surg. 2015;262(3):440–8.

31. Azim A, et al. Big for small: validating brain injury guidelines in pediatric traumatic brain injury. J Trauma Acute Care Surg. 2017;83(6):1200–4.
32. Martin GE, et al. Safety and efficacy of brain injury guidelines at a level III trauma center. J Trauma Acute Care Surg. 2018;84(3):483–9.
33. Pitts SR, et al. National hospital ambulatory medical care survey: 2006 emergency department summary. Natl Health Stat Rep. 2008;7(7):1–38.
34. Hoffman JR, et al. Validity of a set of clinical criteria to rule out injury to the cervical spine in patients with blunt trauma. N Engl J Med. 2000;343(2):94–9.
35. Stiell IG, et al. The Canadian C-spine rule for radiography in alert and stable trauma patients. JAMA. 2001;286(15):1841–8.
36. Stiell IG, et al. The Canadian C-spine rule versus the NEXUS low-risk criteria in patients with trauma. N Engl J Med. 2003;349(26):2510–8.
37. Biffl WL, et al. The unrecognized epidemic of blunt carotid arterial injuries: early diagnosis improves neurologic outcome. Ann Surg. 1998;228(4):462.
38. Bromberg WJ, et al. Blunt cerebrovascular injury practice management guidelines: the Eastern Association for the Surgery of Trauma. J Trauma Acute Care Surg. 2010;68(2):471–7.
39. Biffl WL, et al. Western Trauma Association critical decisions in trauma: screening for and treatment of blunt cerebrovascular injuries. J Trauma Acute Care Surg. 2009;67(6):1150–3.
40. Carney N, et al. Guidelines for the management of severe traumatic brain injury. Neurosurgery. 2017;80(1):6–15.
41. Kazim SF, et al. Management of penetrating brain injury. J Emerg Trauma Shock. 2011;4(3):395.
42. Kaufman H, et al. Patients with Glasgow Coma Scale scores 3, 4, 5 after gunshot wounds to the brain. Neurosurg Clin Nş Am. 1995;6(4):701–14.
43. Joseph B, et al. Improving survival rates after civilian gunshot wounds to the brain. J Am Coll Surg. 2014;218(1):58–65.
44. Joseph B, et al. Prothrombin complex concentrate use in coagulopathy of lethal brain injuries increases organ donation. Am Surg. 2014;80(4):335–8.
45. Aarabi B, Mossop C, Aarabi JA. Surgical management of civilian gunshot wounds to the head. In: Handbook of clinical neurology. New York: Elsevier; 2015. p. 181–93.
46. Lin DJ, et al. "Time is brain" the Gifford factor-or: why do some civilian gunshot wounds to the head do unexpectedly well? A case series with outcomes analysis and a management guide. Surg Neurol Int. 2012;3:98.
47. United States Army (2012) Institute of Surgical Research. Joint theater trauma system clinical practice guidelines-management of patients with severe head trauma. Accessed on 12 July 2018; Available from http://jts.amedd.army.mil/index.cfm/PI_CPGs/cpgs.
48. Bayston R, et al. Use of antibiotics in penetrating craniocerebral injuries. Lancet. 2000;355(9217):1813–7.
49. Mittal V, et al. Carotid artery injuries and their management. J Cardiovasc Surg. 2000;41(3):423.
50. Prichayudh S, et al. Selective management of penetrating neck injuries using "no zone" approach. Injury. 2015;46(9):1720–5.
51. Ibraheem K, et al. "No zone" approach in penetrating neck trauma reduces unnecessary computed tomography angiography and negative explorations. J Surg Res. 2018;221:113–20.
52. Graber G. Blunt and penetrating injuries of the chest wall, pleura, and lungs. Gen Thorac Surg. 2005;2:951–71.
53. Dongel I, et al. Management of thoracic trauma in emergency service: analysis of 1139 cases. Pak J Med Sci. 2013;29(1):58.
54. Demetriades D, et al. Diagnosis and treatment of blunt thoracic aortic injuries: changing perspectives. J Trauma Acute Care Surg. 2008;64(6):1415–9.
55. Gracias VH, et al. Defining the learning curve for the focused abdominal sonogram for trauma (FAST) examination: implications for credentialing. Am Surg. 2001;67(4):364.
56. Montoya J, et al. From FAST to E-FAST: an overview of the evolution of ultrasound-based traumatic injury assessment. Eur J Trauma Emerg Surg. 2016;42(2):119–26.
57. Ho M-L, Gutierrez FR. Chest radiography in thoracic polytrauma. Am J Roentgenol. 2009;192(3):599–612.
58. Omert L, Yeaney WW, Protetch J. Efficacy of thoracic computerized tomography in blunt chest trauma. Am Surg. 2001;67(7):660.
59. Kea B, et al. What is the clinical significance of chest CT when the chest x-ray result is normal in patients with blunt trauma? Am J Emerg Med. 2013;31(8):1268–73.
60. Rodriguez RM, et al. Derivation and validation of two decision instruments for selective chest CT in blunt trauma: a multicenter prospective observational study (NEXUS Chest CT). PLoS Med. 2015;12(10):e1001883.
61. Joseph B, et al. Identifying the broken heart: predictors of mortality and morbidity in suspected blunt cardiac injury. Am J Surg. 2016;211(6):982–8.
62. Kulvatunyou N, et al. 14 French pigtail catheters placed by surgeons to drain blood on trauma patients: is 14-Fr too small? J Trauma Acute Care Surg. 2012;73(6):1423–7.
63. Kulvatunyou N, et al. Two-year experience of using pigtail catheters to treat traumatic pneumothorax: a changing trend. J Trauma Acute Care Surg. 2011;71(5):1104–7.
64. Bauman ZM, et al. A prospective study of 7-year experience using percutaneous 14-French pigtail catheters for traumatic hemothorax/hemopneumothorax at a level-1 trauma center: size still does not matter. World J Surg. 2018;42(1):107–13.
65. Miniño AM, et al. Deaths: injuries, 2002. Accessed on 12 July 2018; Available from https://stacks.cdc.gov/view/cdc/43296.
66. Meyer DM. Hemothorax related to trauma. Thorac Surg Clin. 2007;17(1):47–55.

67. Nicol AJ, et al. Sternotomy or drainage for a hemopericardium after penetrating trauma: a randomized controlled trial. Ann Surg. 2014;259(3):438–42.
68. Beall AC, et al. Surgical management of penetrating thoracic trauma. Chest. 1966;49(6):568–77.
69. Working G, A. Ad Hoc Subcommittee on Outcomes. Practice management guidelines for emergency department thoracotomy. Working Group, Ad Hoc Subcommittee on Outcomes, American College of Surgeons-Committee on Trauma. J Am Coll Surg. 2001;193(3):303.
70. Burlew CC, et al. Western Trauma Association critical decisions in trauma: resuscitative thoracotomy. J Trauma Acute Care Surg. 2012;73(6):1359–63.
71. Seamon MJ, et al. An evidence-based approach to patient selection for emergency department thoracotomy: a practice management guideline from the Eastern Association for the Surgery of Trauma. J Trauma Acute Care Surg. 2015;79(1):159–73.
72. Fabian TC, et al. Current issues in trauma. Curr Probl Surg. 2002;39(12):1160–244.
73. Isenhour JL, Marx J. Advances in abdominal trauma. Emerg Med Clin. 2007;25(3):713–33.
74. Peitzman AB, et al. Prospective study of computed tomography in initial management of blunt abdominal trauma. J Trauma. 1986;26(7):585–92.
75. Holmes JF, McGahan JP, Wisner DH. Rate of intraabdominal injury after a normal abdominal computed tomographic scan in adults with blunt trauma. Am J Emerg Med. 2012;30(4):574–9.
76. Nishijima DK, et al. Does this adult patient have a blunt intra-abdominal injury? JAMA. 2012;307(14):1517–27.
77. Jansen JO, et al. Selective non-operative management of abdominal gunshot wounds: survey of practise. Injury. 2013;44(5):639–44.
78. Inaba K, et al. Prospective evaluation of the role of computed tomography in the assessment of abdominal stab wounds. JAMA Surg. 2013;148(9):810–6.
79. Vaidya R, et al. Patients with pelvic fractures from blunt trauma. What is the cause of mortality and when? Am J Surg. 2016;211(3):495–500.
80. Hughes CW. Use of an intra-aortic balloon catheter tamponade for controlling intra-abdominal hemorrhage in man. Surgery. 1954;36(1):65–8.
81. Biffl WL, Fox CJ, Moore EE. The role of REBOA in the control of exsanguinating torso hemorrhage. J Trauma Acute Care Surg. 2015;78(5):1054–8.
82. Martinelli T, et al. Intra-aortic balloon occlusion to salvage patients with life-threatening hemorrhagic shocks from pelvic fractures. J Trauma Acute Care Surg. 2010;68(4):942–8.
83. Joint Trauma System Clinical Practice Guideline (JTS CPG) for resuscitative endovascular balloon occlusion of the aorta (REBOA) for hemorrhagic shock. Accessed on 2 April 2018; Available from: http://prytimemedical.com/wp-content/uploads/2017/07/REBOA_-CPG_FINAL.pdf.
84. Latifi R, Rhee P, Gruessner R, editors. Technological advances in surgery, trauma and critical care. New York: Springer Science + Business Media; 2015.
85. Latifi R, et al. Initial experiences and outcomes of telepresence in the management of trauma and emergency surgical patients. Am J Surg. 2009;198(6):905–10.
86. Latifi R, et al. Telemedicine and telepresence for trauma and emergency care management. Scand J Surg. 2007;96(4):281–9.

23 Acute Care Surgical Services: Return to Traditional Surgery as Backbone of the Modern Hospital

James M. Feeney and Rifat Latifi

Introduction

The medical climate around the world and in the USA in the twenty-first century has become very complex. Like no other time in history, financial pressures, medicolegal pressures, educational pressures, academic and research benchmarking pressures, and a more informed populace demand more bedside presence, improved diagnostic accuracy, perfect financial and billing acumen, higher patient satisfaction, exquisitely detailed documentation, efficient and effective continuing education, and mountains of logistical support. These pressures have never been stronger. All these demands must be met, and met on a trajectory of continuous improvement, and all while under continual pressure to reduce the price tag for the services rendered. Additionally, to compound the complexities of running the modern hospital, just as medical professionals look to provide improved access to better, faster, and more precise service, physicians and staff also look to limit work hours, reclaim lifestyle, and decrease workplace burdens in an effort to prevent physician and staff burnout.

J. M. Feeney (✉)
Department of Surgery, Westchester Medical Center, Valhalla, NY, USA
e-mail: james.feeney@wmchealth.org

R. Latifi
New York Medical College, School of Medicine, Department of Surgery and Westchester Medical Center, Valhalla, NY, USA

Redistributing these tensions appropriately and effectively, and thereby meeting the demands listed above, involves reengineering models for the different service provisions. Finding the best model of providing care for trauma, critical care, and emergency surgeries has become an important goal of many hospitals worldwide, but particularly so in the USA. As the model of specialist-based and multispecialty-driven care recedes into a historical footnote, the hospital-based specialist caring for patients based on data-driven best practices emerges as a streamlined and effective care model. Different care models have arisen in the past several years to address these and other forces within modern hospitals, but perhaps none has been as successful as the acute care surgery (ACS) model, a distinctly different model of care for the provision of acutely injured or ill patients with surgical diseases. This model arose initially from dissatisfaction within the trauma and surgical critical care community. Trauma and critical care surgery, as a discipline, was facing somewhat of an identity crisis. Surgeons in the field were dissatisfied with increasingly non-operative scope of practice, and the relegation of operative care to other "consultant" specialties. The culmination, or rather exposure, of the actual depths of this dissatisfaction was laid bare when The Institute of Medicine (IOM) released a report in 2007, which cited a shortage in physicians caring for emergent patients [1], This report noted that trauma surgery and emergency general surgery were unpalatable

R. Latifi (ed.), *The Modern Hospital*, https://doi.org/10.1007/978-3-030-01394-3_23

to residents and medical students, among other reasons, because of long work hours and frequent call requirements. Residents and medical students came to view trauma surgeons as "resuscitation doctors," who abdicated the operative management to other "operating surgeons" [2]. Remuneration for these efforts was significantly lower than other "operating surgeon" efforts. Interdisciplinary coordination, communication, and discharge planning seemed to be the main roles of the trauma surgeon, and this was a stark contrast to the "golden age of trauma surgery," when trauma surgeons were considered master surgeons who operated on the neck, chest, abdomen, and any injured blood vessel; an era when nonoperative management was distinctly unusual [3, 4]. Given all these changes, the search for a new identity began for those once known as 'a trauma surgeon'. In fact, what was apparently happening was a return to the "good old days", when a surgeon could do just about every procedure, could manage any critical care problem, and was immediately available to intervene in all kinds of emergencies.

In 2003, at a joint meeting of the American Association for the Surgery of Trauma (AAST), American College of Surgeons, Western Trauma Association, and Eastern Association for the Surgery of Trauma formed an ad hoc committee to study the situation and make recommendations, under the auspices of the AAST. The efforts of the AAST were finally manifested by the report of the Committee to Develop the Reorganized Specialty of Trauma, Surgical Critical Care, and Emergency Surgery of the American Association for the Surgery of Trauma. The AAST committee sought to clearly identify root causes of the problems facing the specialties of trauma surgery and critical care surgery, and more importanty, to describe and develop the potential training paradigm for a reorganized specialty. In essence, the committee looked to define a career practice model that would be technically and intellectually challenging, lifestyle friendly, and economically sustainable [2]. The committee delivered its recommendation for the formation of a new discipline in March 2005. The call for the reorganization of trauma, critical care, and emergency general surgery was quickly followed by robust discussions of curricula [2, 3], and fellowship requirements [3] for training in the newly organized specialty, to be called Acute Care Surgery (ACS).

How would this new "specialty" be defined? What would be the scope of practice? Could these new surgeons really address the pressing and immediate workforce issues? What would be the financial impacts to hospitals? Would they be positive or negative? Would the new specialty hurt established surgeons' books of business substantially? How, where, and by whom would these new "specialists" be trained? These were just a few of the serious questions that were raised at the very outset of the new undertaking. These questions, debated in meeting rooms and conferences for years before ACS was officially sanctioned and trainees seated, represented the nagging doubts of traditionally trained surgeons, tasked with addressing gaps in patient care, difficulties meeting critically ill or injured surgical patient's needs, and the chronic inability to hire new surgeons into trauma and critical care jobs. These questions, and the thoughtful, deliberate approach taken to answer them, represent a shining example of leadership by many of our master surgeons of this era. Answering these questions would reveal whether ACS had a role in twenty-first-century medicine, or perhaps more precisely, what that role would look like. Answering these questions would determine the feasibility of deliberately and thoughtfully establishing a new nationwide specialty, one that sought to address so many shortfalls in, what was at the time, modern medicine.

Definition and Identity of Acute Care Surgery (ACS)

Defining the new discipline of ACS involved, initially and most pressingly, determining which procedures and patient populations would fall under this new rubric of "acute care surgery." Was this merely to be appendectomies and cholecystectomies, with occasional breast and perirectal abscess drainage? Was this to include orthopedic, neurosurgical, or cardiothoracic procedures such as external fixation of fractures, rib plating, external ventricular drainage, intracranial pressure monitoring, or video-assisted thoracoscopic surgery (VATS)?

Most agreed that trauma surgery, the care of the injured patient, and critical care surgery were the cornerstones of the new discipline [5]. But what would be the differences hospitals and fellow physicians would use to distinguish ACS from other surgical specialties? What would distinguish ACS from general surgery patients? Certainly, general surgery encompasses appendectomies and cholecystectomies, but what about necrotizing fasciitis and dead gut? What about ruptured aortic aneurysms or non-traumatic pericardial tamponade? Who would decide the scope of care, and how could that be codified across the country, in order to establish training benchmarks? Where would the new training occur, and what would be the requirements to teach ACS? Which, if any, neurosurgical or orthopedic procedures would be included in the purview of the ACS surgeon, and who would teach them?

The AAST and the American College of Surgeons, along with other associations including the EAST and Western Trauma Association, each formed committees to study these and other important questions, and to make recommendations. Many of the leaders in surgery served on committees with more than one organization, and the thought leaders quickly came to organize their approach to the de novo creation of a new specialty. Finally, through the efforts of these women and men, a rough shape to the definition of what would constitute ACS came to emerge, and long before the first trainees matriculated, the overarching goals became apparent [2–6]. Momentum toward a new structure for training surgeons was gathering.

In 2008, the first ACS program matriculated students at the University of Nevada School of Medicine hospital. The curriculum established by the AAST, finalized in 2007, mandated 12 months of surgical critical care training and a further 12 months of extensive operative experience in thoracic, vascular, and complex hepatobiliary and pancreatic procedures. Additionally, experience in the diagnosis, management, and operative treatment of neurosurgical injuries was included in the final curriculum, including intracranial pressure monitor placement, and emergency burr hole placement. Experience with the use of interventional radiology techniques was also included in the curriculum, including required prowess in on-table arteriography and IVC filter placement. Finally, competency with diagnostic upper and lower GI endoscopy and bronchoscopy also came to be required.

With the discipline newly defined, and the new fellows lining up to be admitted, the only thing left to do was actually teach the first class of fellows. After the proverbial gates were opened, and the training well begun, a career of measuring results and assessing the various impacts of the newly created fellowship would certainly ensue. Would this new training profile suit the changing needs of hospitals? Would the new career pathway assuage fears of a diminishing workforce? More importantly, would the new model improve patient care, access, satisfaction, and outcomes? The decade that followed would have some answers to these pressing questions, but most importantly, over that decade, acute care surgeons and acute care surgery services became the recognized backbone of the modern hospital. Even the most well-recognized hospitals and hospital systems, where there were no major trauma sections or divisions, created their acute care surgery services to streamline resources, improve lifestyles, and most importantly, improve patient care.

Impacts to Patient Care

Perhaps the most important factor in assessing the success or failure of a reorganized medical delivery system is the impact to patients. For ACS to become an accepted part of any hospital structure, there had to be improved service and immediate access to top level care for surgical emergencies, preferably at a lower cost and preferably with streamlined efficiency.

As lofty as the sentiment of "improved care" is, there are several components to the overarching concept. Improved could mean better outcomes, it could mean more efficiency, or it could simply mean that the patients were more satisfied, despite costs, complication rates, or resource utilization. The initial data from early adopters of acute care surgery have been quite positive.

The easiest and most plentiful among these are the data for improved outcomes. ACS services in many data appear to improve outcomes in such basic surgical emergencies as appendicitis and cholecystitis [7–17] in terms of reduced complications. However, the data support much more than a simple decrease in complication rates, which may in truth be statistically demonstrable due to any number of confounders. The data also suggest that the benefits extend to several other facets of care.

Data also suggest that implementing formal ACS services improves timeliness of operative intervention, meaning that patients experience improved ED to OR times, which in turn leads to decreased perforation rates in appendicitis (with unchanged negative appendectomy rates), decreased operative times (in both appendicitis and cholecystitis), and decreased conversion-to-open rates [10–13]. All of these improvements lend to the durable and sustainable decrease in complication rates but also serve to ease emergency department overcrowding [15], improve operating room utilization (including reductions in nighttime operating room usage) [16, 17], and improve resource allocation, including critical care bed access. Finally, ACS services also decrease overall lengths of stay [7–17]. This wealth of benefits to patient outcomes, access to care, and resource utilization, which appears to be reproducible and durable across different medical systems and types of hospitals, probably, therefore, exposes a very real (i. e. not statistical noise) and distinctly positive benefit to reorganizing the care of the acute surgical patient to a service model such as this [9, 14].

Many of these data were collected in very busy, urban hospital centers. There was a preconceived notion, at the outset of the adoption of the ACS model, that at those hospitals, the trauma surgeon would be unable to break away from the care of the injured patient to care for the emergently ill surgical patient. This also appears not to be the case. Although the trauma surgeons are busy in both emergency general surgery and trauma surgery, there does not appear to be a delay in the care of one or the other type of patient by virtue of the combination of these services. On the contrary, the times from consultation to operative intervention were consistently reduced in both patient presentations [12, 13].

Additionally, the operative resources also appear to be streamlined, especially in cases where ACS surgeons are given block time in the operating rooms. This leads to a reduction in the use of "add-on lists" and improvement in overtime costs [17]. ED overcrowding is also reduced by the institution of an ACS service [15], and the numbers of cases completed during non-peak hours (night) also appear to be reduced, possibly reducing overtime and costs [17].

Still, as good as this care delivery model seems, at the outset, questions immediately arose as to where to find surgeons both capable and interested in performing this myriad of different services. Addressing these issues would require structural changes to surgical training and education, as well as changes to hospitals' credentialling and medical staff bylaws.

Educational Impacts

In the early days of ACS, before the AAST and American College of Surgeons defined (redefined) the concept of acute care surgeons, the erstwhile predominant disciplines of trauma and critical care surgery, as career choices, were distinctly unpopular [5]. In 1992, the resident workforce survey conducted by the American College of Surgeons registered trauma and critical care as having very low desirability for residents, due largely to nonoperative workload and long hours of in-house call [5]. However, there were other reasons. One large dissatisfier in the survey was the consideration that trauma surgeons were "surgical babysitters" for consultant specialty services. Residents also felt that the remuneration for amount of work was, comparitively, very low. Expanding a skill set that had relinquished such procedures as interventional radiology and endoscopy would not be easy, and training surgeons to take business away from other specialists would have to be accomplished, initially at least, by those other specialists. This educational environment would have to arise in a setting of waning interest in caring for surgical emergencies, and resistance from other effected specialties.

These declines in the availability of general surgeons willing or able to care for the acutely ill and injured were first noted in the 1991 Scudder Oration, by Dr. George Sheldon, wherein he prophesied a shortage of surgeons interested in trauma alone [3]. He also suggested that the key to alleviating the workforce problem, and the consequent quality problems that stemmed from the lack of access to trauma care, was a new specialty that incorporated trauma, elective and emergency surgery, and critical care. He also commented that this workforce shortage was at a critical state. It was manifested by critical shortages of surgeons in as many as 1450 counties across the USA [5] and expected to worsen, especially in rural and underserved urban areas.

The unseen question, still understudied and underappreciated, is whether ACS service models impact resident training. No data exist to directly support improvements in general surgery resident training as a result of ACS care model implementation, but there are some indirect data. While several have advocated that "…advances in medicine are often a function of advances in trauma" or that quality advances in medicine in general have stemmed directly from advances in trauma [18], data to directly assess what benefit ACS care models have in the completion of ACGME requirements is still lacking. Prior to the inception of ACS as a service line, critical care cases and trauma cases were increasingly difficult to document for general surgical trainees [19]. Although the effects on resident training are unknown, ACS fellows, in the first year of case logs from accredited ACS fellowships, demonstrated an average of nearly 200 cases per year [19]. This represents a substantial increase in supervised cases over the general surgery residency.

Still, because about 50% of those cases fell outside the list of desirable cases for the fellows, the curriculum was revised in 2014, end of training assessments added, and revised expectations (based on location of intervention and incision type), opting for a less granular and more anatomic approach to difficult cases [20]. This readjustment, based on outcomes and data, is an essential part of programmatic education. This is representative of sustained and formulaic effort toward continuous quality improvement. These data, if trended, followed, and utilized to make substantive and positive changes over the course of years, have the ability to lead to training and education that match the needs of the patient population, hospital, educational discipline, and communities.

This kind of approach to programmatic improvements is certainly scalable to other services. Dr. Mattox also suggested, in his 2000 Scudder Oration, that improvements in trauma care often lead to improvements in medicine in general [19]. Furthermore, he suggested that other service lines can use the technology of continuous improvements in their educational systems to ensure that those educational processes meet the needs of the trainees, change them when they do not, and build on the positive outcomes; other training paradigms can utilize the system of assessment, improvement, and reassessment being directed at ACS to endure that the needs of the hospital and community are met by the established training programs. In this way, the act of establishing, assessing, and adjusting the training modules in an ACS program can serve as a model for other service lines in the hospital. In this way, potentially, the educational impact of an ACS program might ripple throughout an entire hospital system.

Finally, even though the nascent ACS curriculum has yet to yield long-term data, a very high fraction of graduated fellows demonstrate ongoing use of their ACS-acquired skills; a majority continue to practice ACS. Practice elements that were satisfiers included (1) scope of practice, (2) case mix, (3) percentage emergency general surgery, (4) lifestyle, and (5) case complexity (with 3 and 4 tied) [21]. This is in contradistinction to earlier data (1990s) on trauma as a career and on surgical critical care as a career. Graduates agreed that the ACS fellowship prepared them well for practice and was worth the time invested (82%), increased their marketability and self-confidence (80%), and prepared them well for academics (71%) and administration (63%). Of those surveyed, 93%would encourage others to do an ACS fellowship [21–26]. This ringing endorsement of ACS training, even though the specialty is new, is a good indicator that the ACS specialty is an educational success that is both functional and satisfying.

Of course, despite the impacts on education, the structure and improvements in education, and the potential benefits of teaching these skills at all levels of trainees, considerations must be given to the financial risks (and possible benefits) to establishing and maintaining an ACS service line. The cost-benefit ratio exposed by this model of providing emergency surgical care is important in describing the sustainability of ACS service lines insomuch as hospital finances are involved.

Financial Impacts

Certainly, no discussion of modern healthcare should be complete without discussion of the financial impacts of any model of care, whether those impacts be positive or negative. There are several aspects to any care model that will impact the financial sustainability of that given model, but a complete discussion of the intricacies of all of those facets is well beyond the scope of this discussion. Broadly, however, we can consider two general categories: costs or savings from improvements to the efficiency of patient care and downstream costs or revenues (e.g., revenues to other nonacute services).

The data for improvements in streamlining of care are abundant [8–10, 15–17, 19–22]. These data also substantiate improvements in departmental productivity [19], contribution margin [20], and resource utilization [17] while still realizing improvements in patient outcomes, access to care, timeliness of care, ED overcrowding, and lengths of stay. Essentially, these streamlined processes include several specific, well-documented examples. One example is reduced ED overcrowding, improved ED throughput, and improved ED to OR times for acute surgical problems. These improvements could be expected to have wide-ranging effects, including improved patient satisfaction, improved staff utilization, and improved Left-Without-Being-Seen (LWOBS) rates, although these possible effects have not been well studied [15]. In the studies of improved OR utilization, fewer cases are completed at night or on off shifts, which would be expected to reduce call schedule utilization, overtime pay, and improve job satisfaction for all staff involved.

However, again, questions remain. Are these data suggesting that as ACS surgeons take care of more emergent and urgent cases, we are simply shifting the workload from elective general surgeons to the ACS surgeons? Might it not be true that the total numbers of cases does not change but simply frame-shifts to ACS surgeons, to the detriment of elective general surgeons? This question raises an important question about how modern hospitals might distribute workload and whether the ACS care model might favor some surgeons over others. In several studies on productivity, this does not appear to be the case. ACS surgeons' productivity appears to increase, while elective general surgeons' cases do not appear to realize any statistically significant decline [20, 21]. This might be expected to lend to higher job satisfaction for all surgeons and less disruptions to planned surgical schedules because of the events over a 'call period'. Additionally, hospitals appear, at least in this early data, to enjoy a higher contribution margin from ACS cases than from elective cases, and ACS surgeons appear to have a higher job satisfaction, statistically, to go with their higher productivity.

The realignment of surgical resources to include an ACS model, therefore, tends to benefit most, if not all aspects of patient care, resource utilization, financial remuneration, and job satisfaction. Clearly, from a financial standpoint, the reorganization of service lines to an ACS service model represents a financial benefit to hospitals, a sustained improvement in satisfaction for surgeons [23, 24], improvements in resource utilization from emergency departments to operating rooms, improved efficiency for managers [15, 17], and a boon to patient outcomes [7–17]. Even in hospitals that do not offer the full complement of ACS services (e.g., community hospitals or non-trauma centers), this realignment appears to offer sustainable improvements to the patients' outcomes, as well as hospitals' resources, and finances [9, 14]. In this sense, there is little doubt as to the substantial improvements that ACS service lines represent.

Perhaps, more subtly, ACS services also contribute substantially to downstream revenue. Patients who need emergent surgery often need further procedures, close follow-up care, and more intense medical monitoring in the period of time after emergent surgery. Additionally, medical comorbidities are often discovered or exacerbated by emergent surgical care. Specialist care post-hospitalization is often required as a consequence of emergent surgical care. Finally, many people come to the attention of the medical community for the first time in their lives as a consequence of a surgical emergency. Often, patients do not have primary care providers (PCPs), and the follow-up period of care represents an opportunity to enroll patients with PCPs within the same system as the ACS services. All of these care opportunities represent a need for increased access and a potential for increased revenue capture that is a direct result of the presence of ACS services. In one study on the topic, downstream inpatient activity generated from an initial ACS service resulted in another 27% increase in downstream revenue from the revenue generated during the initial acute surgical events [27]. These data, coupled with the improved contribution margins, tend to suggest that ACS services are financially sound and contribute to the overall growth of the hospital and system.

As service lines go, therefore, it seems that there is little financial downside to ACS as a separate service line. Improvements come in many ways besides just the direct revenues from the patients that are receiving the immediate services. Many different service lines, including primary care and consultant specialist services, benefit substantially from the mere existence of an ACS service. Challenges, however, remain.

Challenges to ACS Model

Although the benefits, as described above, clearly exist, as with any new technology or organizational effort, there are still some challenges and pitfalls. Many of these challenges stem from a national shortage of surgeons willing or interested in performing ACS roles. Partially, this is a financial challenge. Reimbursement for ACS surgeons is still, in some places, lower than elective general surgeons who perform similar volumes of work [28]. This is an operational issue that could be solved at the administrative level; however, currently, there is no impetus to do so. Antiquated relative value reimbursement incentives, originally constructed with the elective general surgeon in mind, fail to accurately capture the differences between payor mixes, work flow, nonclinical duties, and nonoperative foci of mature ACS programs as compared with other hospital-based services [28, 29], and therefore, the lack of incentive and reimbursement tailoring to the ACS population and work flow yields inefficient remuneration, billing, and incentivization. This leads, in some quarters, to continued workforce shortages, as surgeons gravitate toward the centers that have successfully married incentivization schemes to the redirected workflows, and not kept to old standards more aligned with private practice or elective surgeons.

Perhaps more importantly, quality of care is still not codified, measured, tracked, and benchmarked as for other specialties. Variations in care both within hospitals and between different centers are not yet studied to a point where data-driven quality metrics are in widespread use to address untoward events [29]. These benchmarking data will be essential to the continued improvements in ACS programs, along the same course as the continuous quality improvement that is the bedrock for the trauma services. As ACS services mature, certification programs and quality databases can be expected to emerge and fill the, as of yet, vacant role of quality assurance and risk-stratified benchmarking.

Finally, the implementation of a de novo ACS service line requires leadership, training, and both organizational structure and infrastructure necessary to the success of the programs [30]. During the implementation phases, there are still relatively few graduates from ACS-accredited programs and fewer still with extensive leadership experience in change management. New leaders in ACS will have to grow, embrace the breadth of their specialty, and model this specialty as hospital, academic, and professional leaders. When that is apparent, ACS will have the tools necessary to mentor the second generation of ACS surgeons and guide them in their professional growth. These pitfalls, however, are essentially simple "growing pains." They should not deter institutions from establishing and maintaining ACS programs and reaping the myriad benefits of this reorganized care model.

Conclusions

The creation of ACS service lines was seen as a possible solution to a confluence of problems including quality, resource utilization, financial declines, workforce atrophy, educational ennui, and job dissatisfaction within the discipline of trauma and critical care. Given that the creation of ACS as a specialty has improved surgeons' perceptions of lifestyle, addressed overhanging educational concerns about decreasing critical care and trauma cases, streamlined resource utilization, improved quality of care for surgical emergencies, and, so far, trended toward improved workforce shortages, the creation has been a success. Early adopters noted some pitfalls, all of which have been addressed on ongoing bases to ensure that the training paradigm and structural issues reflect the needs of the hospitals and patient populations.

In that sense, this thoughtfully engineered specialty has been a success. However, in another, very important way, the success has been even more magnified. The confluence of all of these benefits, taken together, lends a strength and reliability to a hospital's ability to deal with critically injured or ill surgical patients. This new strength in ability leads to substantial downstream improvements on many fronts. This cultural shift, the paradigm that results from this convergence, is what gives the ACS specialty enough strength, enough staying power, to be considered the backbone of the modern hospital.

References

1. Institute of Medicine (of the National Academies). The future of emergency care. Fact Sheet June 2006. Acute Care Surgery: Trauma, Critical Care, and Emergency Surgery.
2. Acute Care Surgery: Trauma, Critical Care, and Emergency Surgery. The committee to develop the reorganized specialty of trauma, surgical critical care, and emergency surgery. J Trauma Acute Care Surg. 2005;58(3):614–6. https://doi.org/10.1097/01.TA.0000159347.03278.E1.
3. Spain DA, Miller FB. Education and training of the future trauma surgeon in acute care surgery: trauma, critical care, and emergency surgery. https://doi.org/10.1016/j.amjsurg.2005.05.014.
4. Moore EE. Trauma surgery: is it time for a facelift? Ann Surg. 2004;240:563–4.
5. Britt LD. Trauma: still the cornerstone of acute care surgery specialty. J Am Coll Surg. 2017;226:211–22.
6. Green SM. Trauma surgery: discipline in crisis. Ann Emerg Med. 2009;53:198–207.
7. Cubas RF, Gómez NR, Rodriguez S, Wanis M, Sivanandam A, Garberoglio CA. Outcomes in the management of appendicitis and cholecystitis in the setting of a new acute care surgery service model: impact on timing and cost. https://doi.org/10.1016/j.jamcollsurg.2012.06.415. Get rights and content.
8. Lau B, DiFronzo LA. An acute care surgery model improves timeliness of care and reduces hospital stay for patients with acute cholecystitis. Am Surg. 2011;77(10):1318–1321(4).
9. O'Mara MS, Scherer L, Wisner D, Owens LJ. Sustainability and success of the acute care surgery model in the nontrauma setting. J Am Coll Surg. 2014;219(1):98–100. https://doi.org/10.1016/j.jamcollsurg.2014.02.022. Get rights and content.
10. Ekeh AP, Monson B, Wozniak CJ, Armstrong M, McCarthy MC. Management of acute appendicitis by an acute care surgery service: is operative intervention timely? https://doi.org/10.1016/j.jamcollsurg.2008.01.016.
11. Earley AS, Pryor JP, Kim PK, Hedrick JH, Kurichi JE, Minogue AC, Sonnad SS, Reilly PM, Schwab CW. An acute care surgery model improves outcomes in patients with appendicitis. Ann Surg. 2006;244:498.
12. Murphy PB, DeGirolamo K, Van Zyl TJ, Allen L, Haut E, Leeper WR, Leslie K, Parry N, Hameed M, Vogt KN. Impact of the acute care surgery model on disease- and patient-specific outcomes in appendicitis and biliary disease: a meta-analysis. https://doi.org/10.1016/j.jamcollsurg.2017.08.026.
13. Khalil M, Pandit V, Rhee P, Kulvatunyou N, Orouji T, Tang A, O'Keeffe T, Gries L, Vercruysse G, Friese RS, Joseph B. Certified acute care surgery programs improve outcomes in patients undergoing emergency surgery: a nationwide analysis. J Trauma Acute Care Surg. 2015;79:60–4.

14. Hameed SM, Brenneman FD, Ball CG, Pagliarello J, Razek T, Parry N, Widder S, Minor S, Buczkowski A, MacPherson C, Johner A, Jenkin D, Wood L, McLoughlin K, Anderson I, Davey D, Zabolotny B, Saadia R, Bracken J, Nathens A, Ahmed N, Panton O, Warnock GL. General surgery 2.0: the emergence of acute care surgery in Canada. Can J Surg. 2010;53:79.
15. Qureshi A, Smith A, Wright F, Brenneman F, Rizoli S, Hsieh T, Tien HC. The impact of an acute care emergency surgical service on timely surgical decision-making and emergency department overcrowding. https://doi.org/10.1016/j.jamcollsurg.2011.04.020.
16. Privette AR, Evans AE, Moyer JC, Nelson MF, Knudson M, Mackersie RC, Callcut RA, Cohen MJ. Beyond emergency surgery: redefining acute care surgery. https://doi.org/10.1016/j.jss.2014.11.012.
17. Britt RC, Weireter LJ, Britt LD. Initial implementation of an acute care surgery model: implications for timeliness of care. J Am Coll Surg. 2009;209:421–4.
18. Sheldon GF. Trauma manpower in the decade of aftershock. Bull Am Coll Surg. 1992;77:6e12.
19. Mattox KL. TraumaLine 2000: a history of change and a vision for the future. Bull Am Coll Surg. 2000;85:24e34.
20. Dente CJ, Duane TM, Jurkovich GJ, Britt LD, Meredith JW, Fildes JJ. How much and what type: analysis of the first year of the acute care surgery operative case log. J Trauma Acute Care Surg. 2014;76(2):329–39. https://doi.org/10.1097/TA.0000000000000114. David A. Spain.
21. Davis KA, Dente CJ, Burlew CC, Jurkovich GJ, Reilly PM, Toschlog EA, Cioffi WG. Refining the operative curriculum of the acute care surgery fellowship. J Trauma Acute Care Surg. 2015;78(1):192–6. https://doi.org/10.1097/TA.0000000000000477.
22. Burlew CC, Davis KA, Fildes JJ, Esposito TJ, Dente CJ, Jurkovich GJ. Acute care surgery fellowship graduates' practice patterns: the additional training is an asset. J Trauma Acute Care Surg. 2017;82(1):208–10. https://doi.org/10.1097/TA.0000000000001309.
23. Barnes SL, Cooper CJ, Coughenour JP, MacIntyre AD, Kessel JW. Impact of acute care surgery to departmental productivity. J Trauma Acute Care Surg. 2011;71(4):1027–34. https://doi.org/10.1097/TA.0b013e3182307146.
24. Procter L, Bernard AC, Korosec RL, Chipko PL, Kearney PA Jr, Zwischenberger JB. An acute care surgery service generates a positive contribution margin in an appropriately staffed hospital. https://doi.org/10.1016/j.jamcollsurg.2012.09.020.
25. Miller PR, Wildman EA, Chang MC, Meredith JW. Acute care surgery: impact on practice and economics of elective surgeons. J Am Coll Surg. 2012;214(4):536–8. https://doi.org/10.1016/j.jamcollsurg.2011.12.045.
26. Lissauer ME, Schulze R, May A, Esposito T, Duane TM. Update on the status and future of acute care surgery: 10 years later. J Trauma Acute Care Surg. 2014;76(6):1462–6. https://doi.org/10.1097/TA.0000000000000226.
27. Taheri PA, Maggio PM, Dougherty J, Neil C, Fetyko S, Harkins DR, Butz DA. Trauma center downstream revenue: the impact of incremental patients within a health system. J Trauma Acute Care Surg. 2007;62(3):615–21. https://doi.org/10.1097/TA.0b013e31802ee532.
28. Sweeting RS, Carter JE, Meyer AA, Rich PB. The price of acute care surgery. J Trauma Acute Care Surg. 2013;74(5):1239–45.
29. Santry HP, Madore JC, Collins CE, Ayturk MD, Velmahos GC, Britt LD, Kiefe CI. Variations in the implementation of acute care surgery: results from a national survey of university-affiliated hospitals. J Trauma Acute Care Surg. 2015;78:60–8. https://doi.org/10.1097/TA.0000000000000492.
30. Kaplan LJ, Frankel H, Davis KA, Barie PS. Pitfalls of implementing acute care surgery. J Trauma Acute Care Surg. 2007;62(5):1264–71. https://doi.org/10.1097/TA.0b013e318053dfd8.

Ambulatory Surgery Services: Changing the Paradigm of Surgical Practice

24

Shekhar Gogna and Rifat Latifi

Introduction

Ambulatory surgery services have become increasingly popular worldwide [1] and are a result of advances in surgical technology and rising financial pressures. There are now nearly 35 million outpatient procedure visits in the USA each year [2].

Ambulatory surgery is also known as outpatient surgery, same-day surgery, day surgery, or day case. Ambulatory surgeries do not require an overnight hospital stay. Essentially, the patient is required to stay in the hospital for less than 23 h [2].

These surgeries are considered "outpatient" because the patients do not need an overnight hospital bed. The purpose of outpatient surgery is to keep hospital costs down and save the patient time. The concept of outpatient surgery was introduced by Dr. James Nicoll who performed pediatric surgeries in a free-standing Day Surgery Unit (DSU); the concept took several years to be accepted [3]. And since then, the range of surgeries as outpatient procedures continues to expand.

S. Gogna
Department of Surgery, Westchester Medical Center, Valhalla, NY, USA

R. Latifi (✉)
New York Medical College, School of Medicine, Department of Surgery and Westchester Medical Center, Valhalla, NY, USA
e-mail: rifat_latifi@nymc.edu; rifat.latifi@wmchealth.org

The main advantages of outpatient surgery are cost containment, early mobilization of the patient, less pain because of minimally invasive surgical techniques, early return to home, reduced risk of hospital-acquired infection, and less loss of pay due to early return to work [4]. The disadvantages of outpatient surgery are that it is not feasible for all patients and procedures. Patients have to have a surgical fitness in order to be eligible for outpatient procedures. There may be unanticipated readmissions which may lead to increase in treatment cost and emotional trauma. There is an increasing need for more operating rooms and increased skill among health staff as well as better communication skills [5]. Table 24.1 depicts common ambulatory surgeries.

Worldwide Practice of Ambulatory Surgery

Surgery is a foundational component of all healthcare systems. Surgical needs vary through regions of the world depending on disease prevalence, economic growth, population, healthcare structure, and perception of policy makers. Increasing access to ambulatory surgery is critical for meeting rising demand. In developed countries, increasing the rate of ambulatory surgery is an important objective in order to maximize the utilization of limited economic resources while still providing high-quality care for patients [6]. In undeveloped countries, ambulatory surgery may

R. Latifi (ed.), *The Modern Hospital*, https://doi.org/10.1007/978-3-030-01394-3_24

Table 24.1 Common ambulatory surgeries

Plastic surgery Dupuytren's contracture or carpal tunnel syndrome surgery Arthroscopy Arthrodesis of the finger joints, Ganglion removal Operations for carpometacarpal joint arthrosis Blepharoplasty	**Breast surgery** *Benign breast surgery* Cyst/fibroadenoma excision Biopsies of palpable/non-palpable lesions, duct excision Correction of gynecomastia *Malignant breast surgery* Sentinel lymph node biopsy Lumpectomy Partial/simple mastectomy
Gynecology Diagnostic hysteroscopy Operative hysteroscopy for lesions protruding into the uterine cavity (fibroids) endometrial ablation by hysteroscopy and resectoscope Uterine fibroid embolization using angiography, diagnostic laparoscopy Hydrolaparoscopy Operative laparoscopy	**Ophthalmic surgery** Cataract surgery Oculoplastic surgery Squint surgery Glaucoma
Oral and maxillofacial surgery Cyst enucleation dentigerous cysts, follicular cysts, or keratocysts Marsupialization of mucous retention cysts in the floor of mouth Excision of salivary gland Hemithyroidectomy	**Pediatric surgery** Inguinal hernia Hydrocoele Umbilical hernia Orchidopexy Circumcision
Urology Vasectomy, hydrocelectomy, varicocelectomy, vasectomy reversal, circumcision Minimally invasive procedures Transurethral resection of bladder tumors, ureteroscopic interventions for ureteric stones ESWL for stone treatment	**Vascular surgery** Vasectomy, hydrocelectomy, varicocelectomy, vasectomy reversal, circumcision Minimally invasive procedures Transurethral resection of bladder tumors, ureteroscopic interventions for ureteric stones ESWL for stone treatment
Orthopedic surgery *Shoulder* Arthroscopi rotator cuff surgery Stabilization of acromioclavicular dislocation Open anterior shoulder stabilizations (e.g., Bankart repair, Bristow-Latarjet) *Elbow* Extensor tendon release for treatment of the tennis elbow Ulnar nerve transposition Removal of screws and plates and/or cerclages *Spine* Percutaneous stabilization of a limited number of motion segments Percutaneous balloon vertebroplasty Implantation of devices *Hip* Hip replacement (THA) *Knee* Knee replacement (TKA) Arthroscopic anterior cruciate ligament Removal of osteosynthesis material *Ankle* Arthroscopy-assisted arthrodesis Ankle joint replacement Ligament reconstruction	**Robotics in ambulatory surgery** Total hysterectomy and sacrocolpopexy Cholecystectomy Inguinal, umbilical, and ventral hernia repair Adrenalectomy Antireflux procedures such as fundoplication, achalasia

be the only feasible treatment for a large number of surgical patients [7]. The International Association of Ambulatory Surgery (IAAS) surveyed the trend of growth of ambulatory surgery in participating countries. The results of the report were encouraging – in nearly all of the countries studied, the percentage of outpatient surgery has grown significantly over the time [8].

The variation in activity between countries is vast, with the USA and Canada performing the highest percentage of outpatient surgeries and Scandinavian countries performing the highest percent in Europe. Outpatient surgery is a success in the USA because of two important reasons. One is a focus on efficiency, quality, and cost of care. The second is a focus on the patient and the role of humanism in medicine [6].

Advantage of Ambulatory Surgery

The health system is continuously evolving to meet new health challenges. Escalating healthcare costs and increase in demand for health services are some of the issues which are posing serious stress to healthcare providers and policy makers alike. Ambulatory surgery is an innovative approach to surgical care which discharges patients within hours of surgical procedures.

Ambulatory surgery can be an advantage to the patient. It ensures shorter hospital stays and early mobilization. Ambulatory surgery reduces rates of hospital-acquired infection and venous thromboembolism. There are shorter wait times and a lower risk of cancelation [9]. Cohort studies and clinical experiences indicate that the practice is safe. Major morbidity is rare, discharge is successful on the day of the operation, readmission to the hospital is seldom required, and overall patient satisfaction is high [10].

Hospitals also reap advantages from ambulatory surgery. It costs less than inpatient surgery due to shorter hospital stays and staff reduction. Overnight staffing is unnecessary for ambulatory surgical patients, which decreases the financial burden on the hospital.

From a managerial perspective, ambulatory surgery allows modes of employment preferred by nurses like part-time positions or jobs not requiring night shifts. Such arrangements facilitate retention of nurses, a key resource currently in short supply [11].

Patient and Procedure Selection

Ambulatory surgery is now considered the standard of elective operative care. When a patient needs surgery, ambulatory surgery is the default option, unless major surgery is planned.

The selection criteria differ from country to country; however IAAS has formulated the following guidelines [9]. Some of the salient features of selection criteria are as follows.

1. Type of surgical intervention required: Abdominal and thoracic cavities should only be opened with minimally invasive techniques. Procedure itself should not have significant postoperative risk of hemorrhage and cardiovascular instability. Patient's pain should be able to control with oral analgesia.
2. Medical factors: Patients with stable chronic medical conditions are better managed with day surgery. Patients with unstable medical conditions such as unstable angina or diabetes are unlikely to be appropriate for day surgery. There is no upper age limit for day-case surgery. Full-term infants over 1 month are generally appropriate for day surgery procedures.
3. Social conditions: Patients should have a responsible adult to accompany them home and remain with them for 24 h after surgery. Patient should be able to understand risks, benefits, and alternatives of ambulatory surgery. A well-informed patient is essential for achieving good day surgery outcomes.

Setting Up an Ambulatory Surgery Center

Efficient planning and design of an ambulatory surgery center is essential for successful outcomes. The proximity of an ambulatory surgery center to the hospital is of the upmost importance as the patient should be able to be rapidly transported in case of a medical emergency. There is no ideal design for ambulatory surgery center. However, there are two basic models for the design of a day unit, namely, "racetrack" and "non-racetrack" [8]. "Racetrack" design, is also known as unidirectional model. The advantages of this model are that pre- and postoperative patients are not mixed and there is no potential congestion. However, this design needs larger space, hence extra cost to set up.

On the other hand, in the "non-racetrack" model, the flow of patients is mixed. This model requires less area and less staff. However, there is potential mix up and nurses have to take care of more patients at a given time.

Operational systems such as billing, materials management, and marketing should all be established early in the process. This way, front office employees, opening surgeons, and management will experience ease in scheduling surgeries, billing, and performing case costing which will ensure a stress-free environment for patients [12]. ASCs should be accredited by the Joint Commission, the Accreditation Association for Ambulatory Healthcare (AAAHC), or Accreditation of Ambulatory Surgery Facilities (AAAASF) [13]. Accreditation ensures that ASCs are Medicare-certified, and performance is measured against national standards, thus improving the quality of their care.

Table 24.2 Outcome indicators for ambulatory surgery

Cancelation rates and reasons
Central or peripheral nervous system new deficit
Need for reversal agents: narcotic, benzodiazepine
Reintubation
Unplanned transfusion
Aspiration pneumonitis
Pulmonary embolus
Local anesthetic toxicity Anaphylaxis Possible malignant hyperthermia
Infection
Return to operating room
Unplanned post-procedural treatment in physician's office or emergency department
Unplanned admission to hospital or acute care facility
Cardiopulmonary arrest or death
Nausea and pain not controlled within 2 h in recovery advice (PONV)
Postoperative vomiting rate Prolonged PACU stay (>2 h)
Medication error
Injuries, e.g., eye, teeth
Time to return to light activities of daily living
Common postoperative sequelae, e.g., sore throat, muscle pain, headache
Postdural puncture headache or transient radicular irritation
Discharge without escort or against medical
Patient satisfaction

Outcome Indicators

Recently there has been an increase in the number and complexity of procedures performed at ambulatory surgery centers. There is greater onus on the ASCs to ensure the safety of patients. The Centers for Medicare & Medicaid Service (CMS) require ambulatory surgery centers (ASCs) to carry out a quality assessment and performance improvement (QAPI) program [13]. Morbidity, mortality, unplanned hospital admission/prolonged hospital stay, and readmission rate are traditional measures of outcome related to ambulatory anesthesia/surgery. Table 24.2 summarizes the important outcome indicators for office-based and ambulatory surgery formulated by American Society of Anesthesia task force. There are follow-ups both 1 day and 14 days post-op. Day 30 is meant to document and manage possible complications.

Minor adverse events, such as pain and postoperative nausea and vomiting (PONV), are common. The management of these minor adverse events is the major area of quality assessment and improvement can be easily attained.

Ambulatory Surgery: Changing the Paradigm of Surgery

Over the last three decades, there has been a substantial increase in ambulatory surgery practice. The volume of ambulatory surgery has more than tripled to nearly 54 million procedures annually [14]. There are over 5000 Medicare-certified

ASCs in the USA. The advent of modern surgical equipment, developments in anesthesia in the form of short acting anesthetic, improvements in regional anesthesia, and use of supra-laryngeal airways have led to the rise of ambulatory surgery. New approaches in perioperative pain management (multimodal analgesia and preemptive analgesia) have ensured better patient comfort which later translates into better outcomes. There are a vast number of types of surgeries which are done in ambulatory setting. Table 24.1 depicts most but not all cases done in ambulatory setting.

Managing the Postoperative Pain

The advent of multimodal analgesic techniques for the prevention of pain in the ambulatory setting is one of the great keys to success of ambulatory surgery. The multimodal analgesia approach involves a combination of opioid and non-opioid analgesics that act at different sites within the central and peripheral nervous systems [15]. Figure 24.1 depicts the universal multimodal analgesia scheme and shows the escalation of drugs required.

Pain and nausea are the two most common reasons for delayed discharge and unexpected admissions to the hospitals after ambulatory surgery. Pain control after surgery is vital since ineffective pain control can lead to increased morbidity and mortality. Management of perioperative pain in ambulatory settings starts with anticipation and knowledge of the factors that are more likely to increase or cause the pain. Studies have shown that orthopedic patients had the highest incidence of severe pain, at 16.1%, followed by urologic, general, and plastic surgery at 13.4%, 11.5%, and 10%, respectively [16].

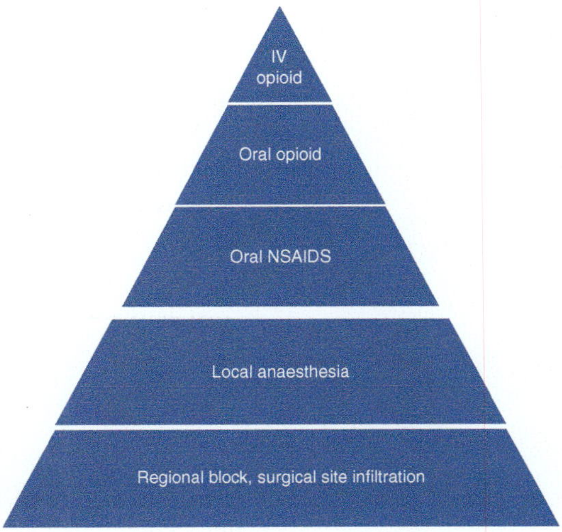

Fig. 24.1 Multimodal analgesia; the basic and escalation of drug

Preoperative planning of risk stratification plays an important role as younger male patients, patients with a high body mass index, and patients with a longer duration of anesthesia have a higher incidence of severe pain. These patients are premedicated with opioid-sparing analgesia. The American Society of Anesthesiologists recommends acetaminophen, gabapentin, or diclofenac with a sip of water before surgery to decrease the need for intravenous medications. Regional anesthesia provides excellent analgesia without the side effects of opioids. Upper and lower extremity blocks like femoral or sciatic blocks all help to provide long-lasting analgesia that can last up to 24 h [17]. Because pain has a subjective component, breaking the vicious cycle of preoperative anxiety leading to increased postoperative pain helps in better pain management after surgery. Controlling severe anxiety with medications such as gabapentin preoperatively and benzodiazepines perioperatively helps with postoperative pain management [18]. Multimodal analgesia is a safe and effective way for the management of pain following major surgery.

Summary

Ambulatory surgery improves quality of care and life with low morbidity. The number and type of surgeries performed at ambulatory centers are increasing. Surgeons and anesthetics alike are acquiring more skills which allowed an impressive worldwide growth in ambulatory surgery over the last few years. Patients prefer ambulatory surgery because they want to be back to normal sooner rather than later. Improved regional anesthesia techniques and multimodal analgesia are promising methods to ensure adequate pain management after surgery. Ambulatory surgery is becoming the standard of care.

References

1. Healthcare Cost and Utilization Project (HCUP). Statistical Brief #188. 2016. Agency for Healthcare Research and Quality, Rockville. Retrieved from: https://www.hcup-us.ahrq.gov/reports/statbriefs/sb188-Surgeries-Hospital-Outpatient-Facilities-2012.jsp.
2. Suskind AM, Zhang Y, Dunn RL, Hollingsworth JM, Strope SA, Hollenbeck BK. Understanding the diffusion of ambulatory surgery centers. Surg Innov. 2015;22(3):257–65.
3. Odhiambo MA, Njuguna S, Waireri-Onyango R, Mulimba J, Ngugi PM. Utilization of day surgery services at Upper hill Medical Centre and the Karen hospital in Nairobi: the influence of medical providers, cost and patient awareness. Pan Afr Med J. 2015;22:28.
4. Gangadhar S, Gopal T, Sathyabhama PK. Rapid emergence of day-care anaesthesia: a review. Ind J Anaesth. 2012;56(4):336–41.
5. Dodaro CA, Grifasi C, Lo Conte D, Romagnuolo R. Advantages and disadvantages of day surgery in a department of general surgery. Ann Ital Chir. 2013;84(4):441–4.
6. Philip BK. Day care surgery: the United States model of health care. Ambul Surg. 2012;17:81–2.
7. Vijayakumar C, Elamurugan T, Sudharsanan S, Jagdish S. Factors hindering practice of day care surgery in a tertiary care centre in southern India: a patient's perspective. J Clin Diagn Res JCDR. 2017;11(6):05–7.
8. Lemos P. Day surgery. Development and practice. London: International Association for Ambulatory Surgery; 2006.
9. Quemby D, Stocker M. Day surgery development and practice: key factors for a successful pathway. Contin Educ Anaesth Crit Care Pain. 2014;14:256–61.
10. Mattila K, Lahtela M, Hynynen M. Health-related quality of life following ambulatory surgery procedures: assessment by RAND-36. BMC Anesthesiol. 2012;12:30.
11. Castoro C, Bertinato L, Baccaglini U, Drace CA, McKee M, with the collaboration of IAAS Executive Committee Members: Policy brief. Day surgery: making it happen. Brussels: WHO European Centre for Health Policy; 2007.
12. Cascardo D. Guidelines for setting up an ambulatory surgery center. Podiatry Manage. 2014;33(8): 127–32.
13. State operations manual appendix Ldguidance for surveyors: ambulatory surgical centers. Centers for Medicare & Medicaid Services https://www.cms.gov/Regulations-and-Guidance/Guidance/Manuals/downloads/som107ap_l_ambulatory.pdf. Updated April 1, 2015. Accessed 12 May 2018.
14. American Society of Anesthesiologists website. Outcome indicators for office-based and ambulatory surgery. October 16, 2013. Retrieved from: http://www.asahq.org/quality-and-practice-management/standards-guidelines-and-related-resources/outcome-indicators-for-office-based-and-ambulatory-surgery.
15. Schug S, Chong C. Pain management after ambulatory surgery. Curr Opin Anaesthesiol. 2009;22:738–43.
16. Vadivelu N, Kai AM, Kodumudi V, Berger JM. Challenges of pain control and the role of the ambulatory pain specialist in the outpatient surgery setting. J Pain Res. 2016;9:425–35.
17. Elvir-Lazo OL, White PF. Postoperative pain management after ambulatory surgery: role of multimodal analgesia. Anesthesiol Clin. 2010;28:217–24.
18. Griffith JP, Whiteley S, Gough MJ. Prospective randomized study of a new method of providing postoperative pain relief following femoropopliteal bypass. Br J Surg. 1996;83(12):1735–8.

Cardiac Surgery in the Modern Hospital

25

Steven L. Lansman, Joshua B. Goldberg, Masashi Kai, Ramin Malekan, and David Spielvogel

Abbreviations

ECMO Extracorporeal membrane oxygenation
VAD Ventricular assist device

Introduction

There are three things that characterize the modern hospital when it comes to cardiac services, and these include the incorporation of enabling technologies, the adoption of databases, and the coalescence of institutions into networks. Each of these has impacted substantially current cardiac surgical programs, as they matured from coronary bypass franchises to "full service stations." Technological advances have given rise to entirely new treatment modalities, such as mechanical assist devices for heart failure, minimally invasive cardiac surgery, and endovascular approaches to structural heart disease. Internal and national cardiac surgical databases have been adopted that monitor, analyze, and disperse outcome data, to provide transparency and improve results. The coalescence of institutions into networks has given rise to efficiencies, allowing more support for primary care physicians in the community and the centralization of high-risk, resource-intense services, such as cardiac surgery. This chapter will discuss the impact of each of these developments to cardiac surgery programs.

Technology

Cardiac surgery programs in the current era span a broad scope of practice, as compared with two decades ago when coronary bypass surgery comprised over 90% of cases. With the advent of preventative measures, such as antihypertensives and statins, and invasive catheter procedures, the volume of coronary bypass surgery has dropped precipitously, approaching one third of its heyday volume. In New York State, for example, the volume of isolated coronary bypass procedures decreased from a peak of 20,220 cases in 1997 to 8356 in 2015, the first uptick in almost 20 years (Fig. 25.1). Successful, modern cardiothoracic programs have grown other aspects of the specialty, including surgical approaches to heart failure, minimally invasive approaches to standard procedures, and endovascular approaches that avoid open surgical approaches altogether. New, enabling technologies have played a critical role in each of these areas.

S. L. Lansman (✉) · J. B. Goldberg · M. Kai
R. Malekan
Department of Surgery, Westchester Medical Center, Valhalla, NY, USA
e-mail: Steven.Lansman@WMCHealth.org

D. Spielvogel
Department of Radiology, Westchester Medical Center, Valhalla, NY, USA

R. Latifi (ed.), *The Modern Hospital*, https://doi.org/10.1007/978-3-030-01394-3_25

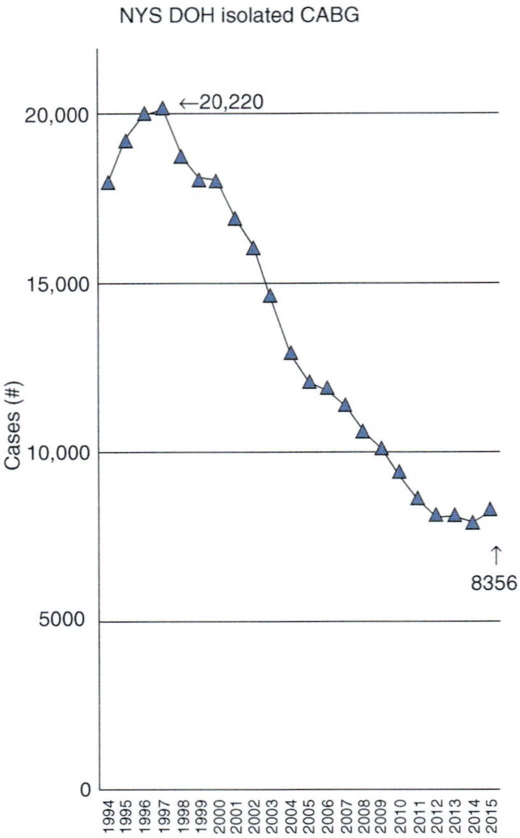

Fig. 25.1 Case volume of isolated coronary bypass surgeries in New York State from 1994 to 2015. (Reprinted from Health NYSDo [12])

Heart Failure

Over the past decade, key advances in heart failure – apart from preventative strategies, a better understanding of pathophysiology, novel drug therapies, and gene-based therapies – include the expanded use of mechanical circulatory support devices. In the short term, these devices have been used as a "bridge to recovery," providing temporary support during transient cardiac failure, and as a "bridge to decision," providing support while observing whether recovery is possible or whether more advanced heart failure therapy will be required. In the long term, these devices have been used as a "bridge to transplant," supporting the failing heart while the patient waits on a transplant list, or not as a "bridge" but as permanent or "destination" therapy.

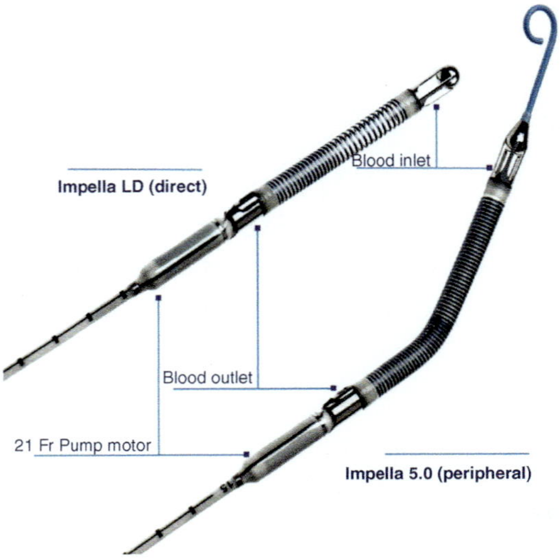

Fig. 25.2 The Impella axial-flow rotary assist device. (Reprinted from Griffith et al. [13]. With permission from Elsevier)

Percutaneous Axial Flow

The Impella CP (Fig. 25.2) is a percutaneous, trans-arterial, continuous axial flow, rotary device, capable of flowing up to 4.3 liters/minute, that is useful as a first-line treatment for the immediate, rapid support of patients in cardiogenic shock [1]. The device comprises the distal part of a catheter that is placed across the aortic valve, and like many rotary devices, it has a rapidly spinning rotor that impels blood through the device, taking blood from the left ventricle and ejecting it into the aorta. The Impella CP is approved for 6-day support, so plans should be in place for weaning the device or progressing to a more advanced level of support.

ECMO

If longer support is required, ECMO (extracorporeal membrane oxygenation) has become an important intervention (Fig. 25.3). A decade ago this option was most often fatal for adults. But with the development of small, efficient oxygenators and compact, extracorporeal rotary pumps, such as the CentriMag device, ECMO has emerged as a "game-changing," lifesaving therapy for patients with

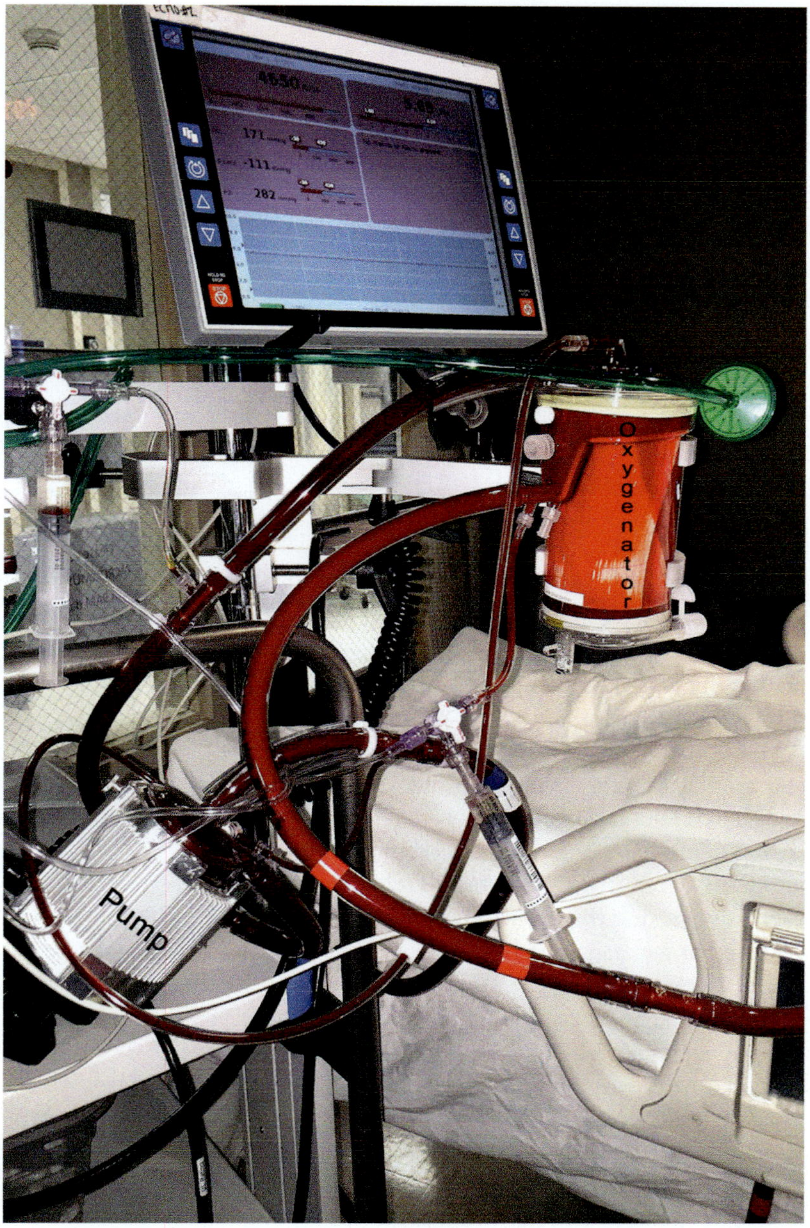

Fig. 25.3 ECMO at bedside. A centrifugal pump receives a patient's venous blood and propels it back to the patient's arterial system. En route, unoxygenated, dark blood from the patient passes through an oxygenator, becoming bright red

cardiogenic shock [2]. The CentriMag is a continuous flow, centrifugal pump that features a bearingless motor, capable of flowing up to 9.9 liters/min, although that level is rarely reached clinically.

For respiratory failure, ECMO can be established in a veno-venous configuration, drawing from the venous circulation and returning oxygenated blood to the venous circulation. For cardiogenic shock, however, an arteriovenous configuration is required to support blood pressure and supplement cardiac output. ECMO can be established via peripheral cannulation, generally with inflow to the device from the right atrium, by cannulating the femoral or jugular vein, and outflow into the femoral or axillary artery. If the femoral artery is used, it is important to ensure that distal flow to the lower extremity is not compromised, and often an additional cannula is required to provide antegrade flow to the leg.

The Impella and ECMO devices constitute a paradigm shift in the treatment of cardiogenic shock.

These devices can be implanted relatively rapidly, reestablishing systemic pressure and perfusion, and thereby can reverse metabolic derangements and avoid end-organ damage. As compared to the Impella, ECMO may take somewhat longer to implant but provides more flow and may be more appropriate for severe shock. Although ECMO support can be maintained longer than the Impella, it is still a temporary solution, and if sufficient myocardial recovery does not occur to permit weaning support, one must consider progressing to an implantable ventricular assist device or cardiac transplantation.

Ventricular Assist Device (VAD)

Implantable ventricular assist devices have undergone incremental changes and improvements since the 1960s. A major change in design has been the shift from pulsatile devices, which were necessarily large because of the need for volume displacement, to continuous, non-pulsatile, rotary devices. Rotary VADs, which include axial-flow and centrifugal-flow devices, have fewer moving parts and do not need valves to prevent backflow during pump diastole, which has permitted progressive size reduction yet increased reliability in successive models (Fig. 25.4).

A recent generation, implantable, rotary VAD is the HeartMate III (Fig. 25.5), a continuous flow, centrifugal pump, capable of flowing up to 10 liters/minute that was designed for circulatory support for 10 years or longer. This device features a bearingless, magnetically levitated impeller, which may improve device durability and reduce blood trauma, promoting lower levels of hemolysis and thrombogenicity. Early results showed better outcomes than an axial-flow pump, primarily due to fewer reoperations for pump failure [3].

Minimally Invasive

Another area in cardiothoracic surgery that technology has revolutionized is minimally access surgery. Enabling technology has included devices

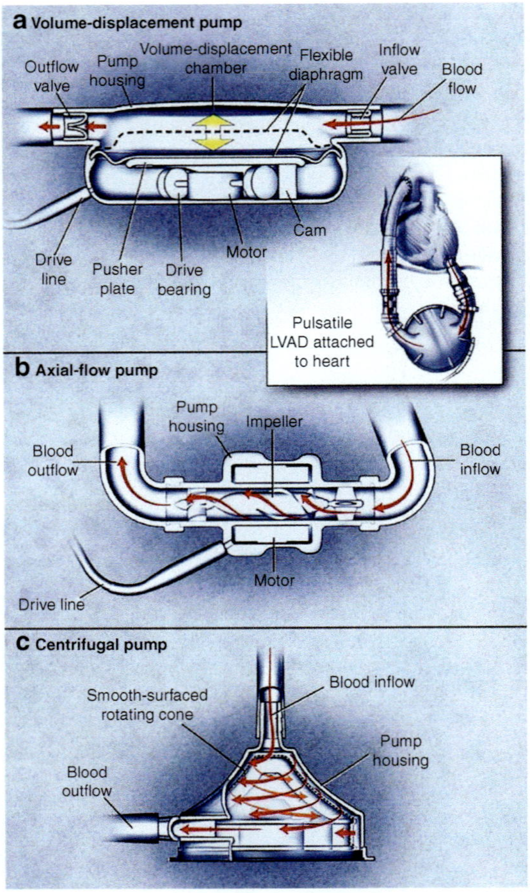

Fig. 25.4 Mechanisms of action of various types of cardiac support devices. (Reprinted from Baughman and Jarcho [14]. With permission from Massachusetts Medical Society)

designed to be used via minimal access incisions, such as tissue retractors, videoscopic imaging, and port access robotic surgery, all of which have application in many branches of surgery.

Sutureless Aortic Valves

More specific to cardiac surgery is the recent FDA approval of "sutureless" aortic valves, designed for more rapid implantation via minimal access approaches, such as the Perceval and the Intuity valves. The Intuity valve is a bovine pericardial, bioprosthetic aortic valve that was

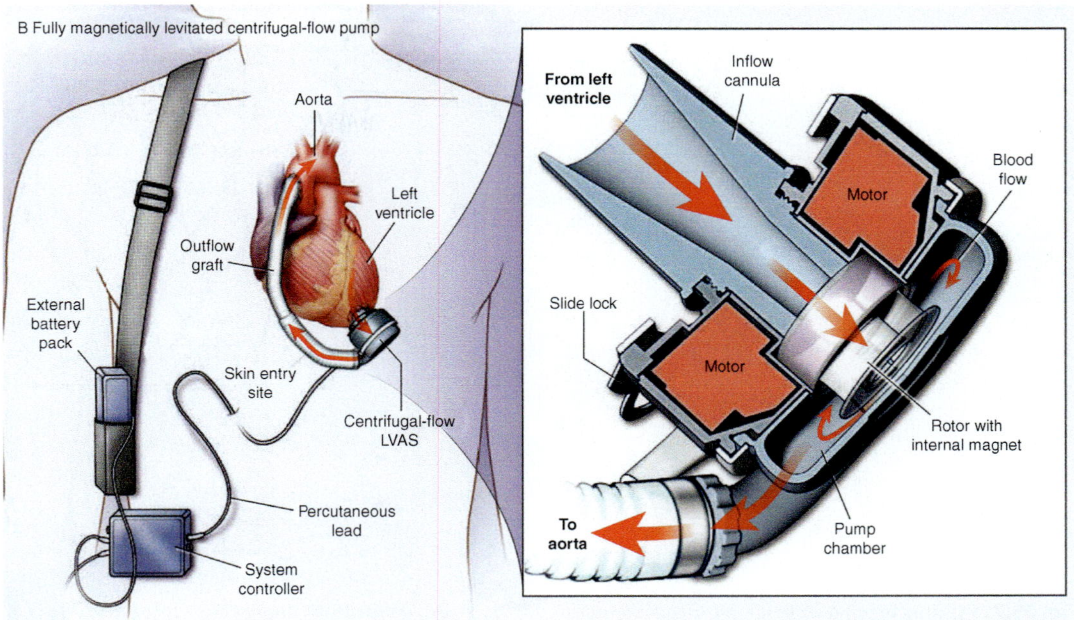

Fig. 25.5 Centrifugal-flow ventricular assist device. (Reprinted from Mehra et al. [15]. With permission from Massachusetts Medical Society)

designed to be rapidly implantable via a small incision (Fig. 25.6). The prosthesis is mounted on a balloon applicator and is guided into position at the level of the aortic annulus, where it is deployed by expanding the balloon. Early [4] and midterm [5] results confirm the performance and safety of these devices.

Endovascular Approach to Cardiac Surgery

Perhaps the minimally invasive approach to the heart, the endovascular approach, avoids a chest incision altogether. Via percutaneously introduced transvenous and transarterial catheters, devices have been developed to address coronary ischemic disease and structural cardiac pathology, such as atrial septal defects, aortic stenosis, and mitral insufficiency.

Transcatheter aortic valve replacement has been shown to be safe and effective in large, well-conducted, prospective, randomized trials for patients at high and intermediate risk for open

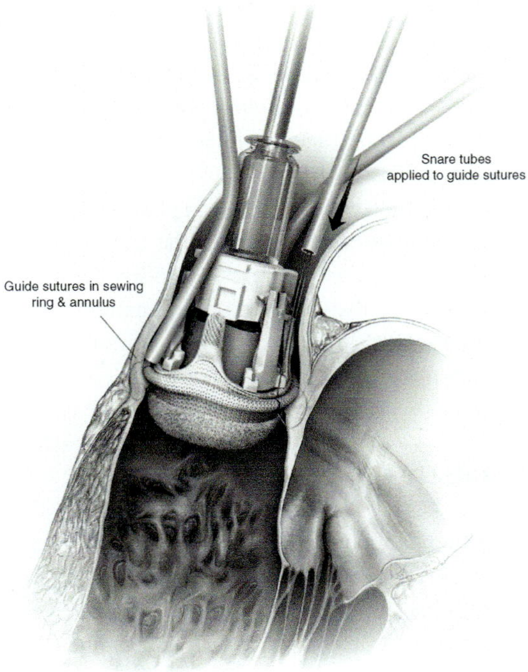

Fig. 25.6 Sutureless aortic valve implantation. (Reprinted from Eudailey and Borger [16]. With permission from Elsevier)

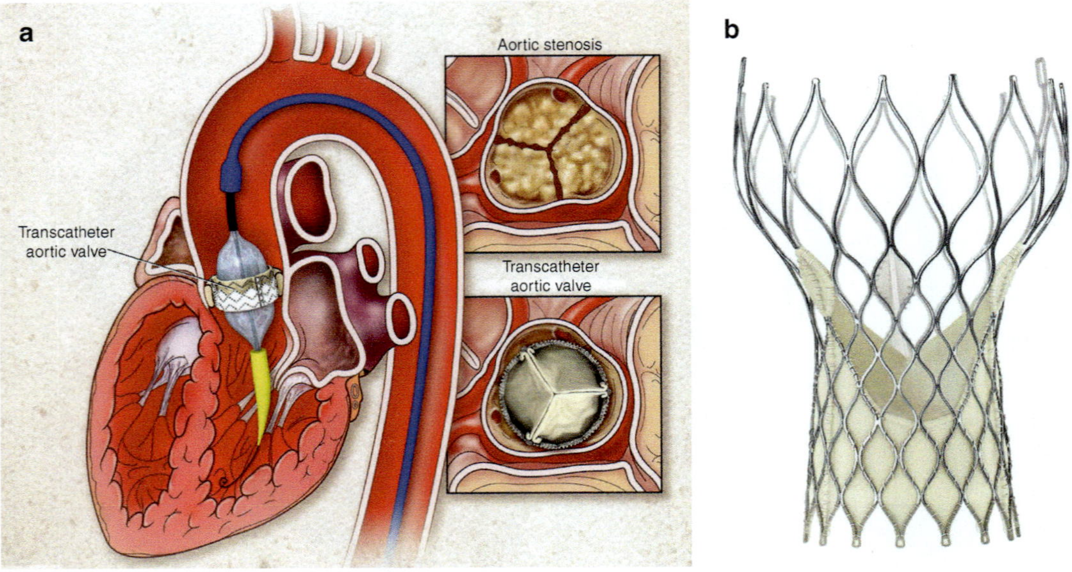

Fig. 25.7 (**a**) Implantation of balloon-expandable transcatheter aortic valve. (**b**) Transcatheter valve with self-expanding Nitinol frame. (**a**: Reprinted from Smith et al. [6]. With permission from Massachusetts Medical Society.) (**b**: Reprinted from Popma et al. [17]. With permission from Elsevier.)

surgery [6, 7]. Presently, the two most commonly used transcatheter aortic valves include a balloon-expandable bovine pericardial valve (Fig. 25.7a) and a Nitinol, self-expanding porcine pericardial valve (Fig. 25.7b) incorporated onto the tip of a catheter delivery system.

Transcatheter aortic valve replacement technology dramatically decreases the trauma of an open procedure, expanding the ability to safely treat aortic stenosis in elderly, frail patients, who are not surgical candidates and for whom therapy was not previously possible.

Databases

A second hallmark of modern cardiothoracic programs is the adoption of internal and multi-institutional registries that monitor, analyze, and disperse data, to improve outcomes and help inform patients.

Departmental Database

Maintaining internal databases is becoming a widespread practice among cardiac surgical programs. A "dashboard," presenting weekly or monthly volume and mortality data, is a good method of tracking "real-time" trends, enabling surgeons to notice and take early action for any disturbing trends. However, by their nature, internal databases are not large enough to risk-adjust and establish benchmarks.

Public Databases

State Level: New York State Department of Health

New York State was one of the first to establish a statewide adult cardiac surgery registry, allowing risk stratification of preoperative comorbidities and leading to release of hospital-specific and, eventually, surgeon-specific outcomes. Long-term monitoring and publication of this data led to decreases in risk-adjusted mortality, in part by identifying low-volume, high mortality participants [8].

National/International: Society of Thoracic Surgeons Database

The Society of Thoracic Surgeons established a voluntary national database for cardiac surgical procedures in 1989 [9]. Currently, there are over 1000 participating sites, and the registry has accumulated approximately 3 million cases, with over 500 fields each, permitting reliable risk-adjusted outcomes. Apart from quality monitoring, the wealth of data made possible a risk model, permitting prospective patient-specific operative risk estimation, based on demographic and clinical data [10]. Other side benefits of such a rich database have been its use as a research tool and, related, the establishment and widespread acceptance of standard definitions for the many variables that comprise the database.

Networks

This is the era of healthcare consolidation, with the merging of institutions into networks, often centered on a large academic institution. A number of financial and quality efficiencies and benefits are obtained from this type of organization, including economies of scale, the centralization of purchasing policies and leverage, the promulgation and oversight of quality protocols throughout the network, and the centralization of resource-intensive services, such as cardiac surgery. For low-volume, expensive, highly specialized services, such as cardiac mechanical assist device and transplantation programs, this arrangement allows one central group to build a team, develop and manage quality protocols, and gain the experience necessary to have good outcomes.

A technological advance that greatly improved efficiency is the advent of telemedicine [11]. For cardiac surgical services, in the context of networks, "tele-morbidity-and-mortality" conferences and "tele-cath" conferences have made it possible to expedite patient care delivery to the network communities while being able to frequently review quality issues throughout the network.

References

1. Vetrovec GW, Anderson M, Schreiber T, et al. The cVAD registry for percutaneous temporary hemodynamic support: a prospective registry of Impella mechanical circulatory support use in high-risk PCI, cardiogenic shock, and decompensated heart failure. Am Heart J. 2018;199:115–21. https://doi.org/10.1016/j.ahj.2017.09.007.
2. Tang GHL, Malekan R, Kai M, et al. Peripheral venoarterial extracorporeal membrane oxygenation improves survival in myocardial infarction with cardiogenic shock. J Thorac Cardiovasc Surg. 2013;145:e32–3. https://doi.org/10.1016/j.jtcvs.2012.12.038.
3. Mehra MR, Goldstein DJ, Uriel N, et al. Two-year outcomes with a magnetically levitated cardiac pump in heart failure. N Engl J Med. 2018;378:1386. https://doi.org/10.1056/NEJMoa1800866.
4. Wahlers TCW, Haverich A, Borger MA, et al. Early outcomes after isolated aortic valve replacement with rapid deployment aortic valve. J Thorac Cardiovasc Surg. 2016;151:1639–47. https://doi.org/10.1016/j.jtcvs.2015.12.058.
5. Meuris B, Flameng WJ, Laborde F, et al. Five-year results of the pilot trial of a sutureless valve. J Thorac Cardiovasc Surg. 2015;150:84–8. https://doi.org/10.1016/j.jtcvs.2015.03.040.
6. Smith CR, Leon MB, Mack MJ, et al. Transcatheter versus surgical aortic-valve replacement in high-risk patients. N Engl J Med. 2011;364:2187–98. https://doi.org/10.1056/NEJMoa1103510.
7. Leon MB, Smith CR, Mack MJ, et al. Transcatheter or surgical aortic-valve replacement in intermediate-risk patients. N Engl J Med. 2016;374:1609–20. https://doi.org/10.1056/NEJMoa1514616.
8. Hannan EL, Cozzens K, King SB 3rd, et al. The New York State cardiac registries: history, contributions, limitations, and lessons for future efforts to assess and publicly report healthcare outcomes. J Am Coll Cardiol. 2012;59:2309–16. 2012/06/16. https://doi.org/10.1016/j.jacc.2011.12.051.
9. Ferguson TB Jr, Dziuban SW Jr, Edwards FH, et al. The STS National Database: current changes and challenges for the new millennium. Ann Thorac Surg. 2000;69:680–91. https://doi.org/10.1016/S0003-4975(99)01538-6.
10. Vassileva CM, Aranki S, Brennan JM, et al. Evaluation of the Society of Thoracic Surgeons online risk calculator for assessment of risk in patients presenting for aortic valve replacement after prior coronary artery bypass graft: an analysis using the STS adult cardiac surgery database. Ann Thorac Surg. 2015;100:2109–16. https://doi.org/10.1016/j.athoracsur.2015.04.149.
11. Latifi R, Olldashi F, Dogjani A, et al. Telemedicine for Neurotrauma in Albania: initial results from case series of 146 patients. World Neurosurg. 2018;112:e747–53.
12. Health NYSDo. Adult Cardiac Surgery in New York State Reports. Source: New York State Department of Health Website
13. Griffith BP, Anderson MB, Samuels LE, et al. The RECOVER I: a multicenter prospective study of Impella 5.0/LD for postcardiotomy circulatory support. J Thorac Cardiovasc Surg. 2013;145:548–54.
14. Baughman KL, Jarcho JA. Bridge to life — cardiac mechanical support. N Engl J Med. 2007;357:846–9.
15. Mehra MR, Naka Y, Uriel N, et al. A fully magnetically levitated circulatory pump for advanced heart failure. N Eng J Med. 2017;376:440–50.

16. Eudailey KW, Borger MA. Intuity Elite Valve Implantation Technique. Oper Tech Thorac Cardiovasc Surg. 2016;21:306–21.
17. Popma JJ, Adams DH, Reardon MJ, et al. Transcatheter aortic valve replacement using a self-expanding bioprosthesis in patients with severe aortic stenosis at extreme risk for surgery. J Am Coll Cardiol. 2014;63:1972–81.

Transplant Services: The Surgery Is the Least of It

26

Thomas Diflo, Gregory Veillette, and Vaughn Whittaker

History

Reports of transplantation of organs and tissues reach back into antiquity. One of the miracles that the twin brother physicians Cosmas and Damian were credited with on their road to sainthood involved transplanting the lower leg of a recently deceased Moor onto the gangrenous stump of a Roman church officer, with apparent good graft function (Fig. 26.1).

In the 1930s, YY Voronoy, a Soviet surgeon, used a temporary kidney transplant in a patient who had gone into renal failure from mercury poisoning, in order to reverse the patient's anuria [1]. The modern era of transplantation began on December 23, 1953, when Dr. Joseph Murray and his team at the Peter Bent Brigham Hospital performed the first successful living donor kidney transplant between two identical twins, the Herrick brothers.

It was for this that Dr. Murray received the Nobel Prize in Medicine and Physiology in 1990. Given the small number of identical twin pairs, one of whom required transplantation, there were not many transplants performed during this era. Once the intricacies of the immune response were better understood, and appropriate medications to blunt or eliminate that response were discovered or developed, transplantation became more widely successful.

The first successful human liver transplant was performed by Dr. Thomas Starzl and his team at the University of Colorado in 1963. Their first patient, a 3-year-old with biliary atresia, died during the transplant operation [1]. Four more patients transplanted in 1963 survived the surgery but subsequently died from infectious complications [ibid]. The Colorado team subsequently placed a moratorium on liver transplantation for 3 years, until better surgical and immunosuppressive techniques could be developed.

Throughout the 1960s and 1970s, immunosuppression consisted of steroids and 6-mercaptopurine or, its synthetic analog, azathioprine. In 1977, Jean Borel presented his studies of cyclosporine A (CyA) at the British Society of Immunology [2], and Sir Roy Calne began his experimental work with CyA at the University of Cambridge [3]. The introduction of CyA for transplantation was nothing short of revolutionary, and 1-year patient and graft survival after kidney transplantation virtually doubled overnight. In addition, long-term survival in liver transplantation and that of other organs was seen for the first time.

T. Diflo (✉)
Department of Surgery, Section of Intra-abdominal Organ Transplantation, Westchester Medical Center, New York Medical College, Valhalla, NY, USA
e-mail: Thomas.Diflo@WMCHealth.org

G. Veillette
New York Medical College, Westchester Medical Center, Valhalla, NY, USA

V. Whittaker
Department of Surgery, Westchester Medical Center and New York Medical College, School of Medicine, Valhalla, NY, USA

R. Latifi (ed.), *The Modern Hospital*, https://doi.org/10.1007/978-3-030-01394-3_26

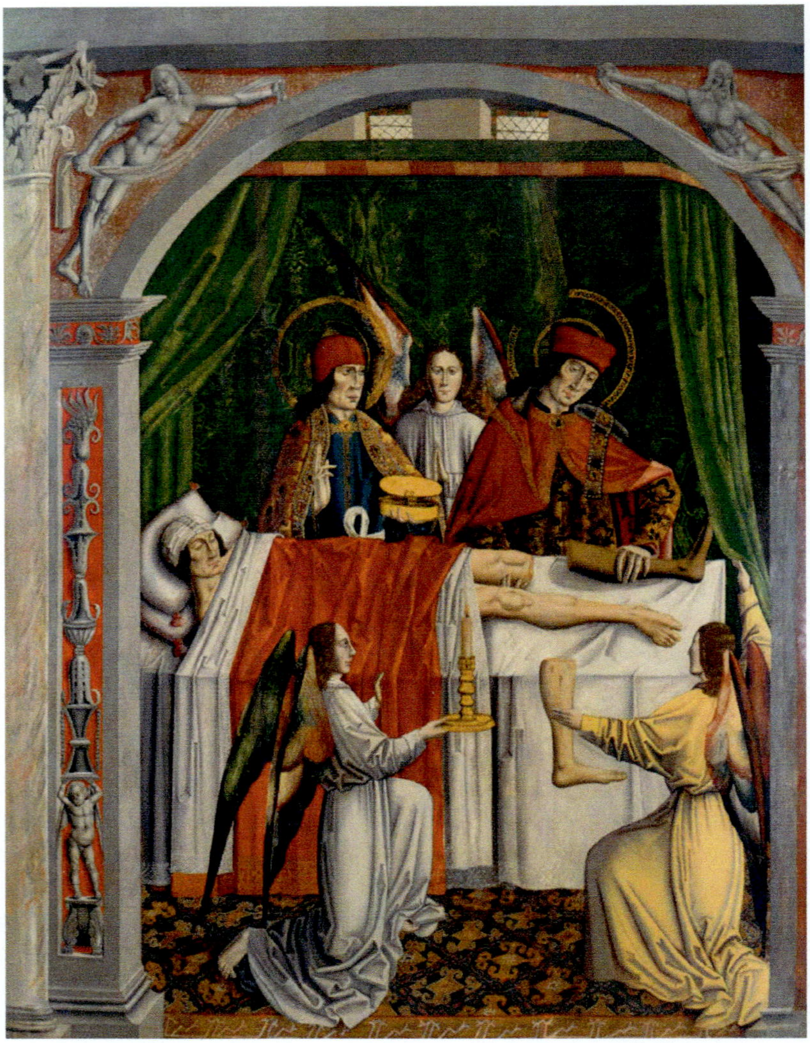

Fig. 26.1 Saints Cosmas and Damian. (Reprinted from "A verger's dream: Saints Cosmas and Damian performing a miraculous cure by transplantation of a leg. Oil painting attributed to the Master of Los Balbases." By Master of Los Balbases. Credit: Wellcome Collection: https://wellcomecollection.org/works/ttutmamh. With permission from Creative Commons License 4.0: https://creativecommons.org/licenses/by/4.0/)

Since then, there have been numerous other medications introduced into the posttransplant armamentarium, including tacrolimus, mycophenolic acid, sirolimus, and several monoclonal antibodies that work against specific portions of the immune response. Each of these introductions has allowed incremental improvements in patient and graft survival, but none have been as earthshaking as the introduction of cyclosporine.

Regulatory Matters

In the 1960s and 1970s, transplantation was essentially unregulated. The 1968 Uniform Anatomical Gift Act (UAGA) allowed the donation of organs or tissues for transplantation as a gift [4]. That same year, a group was convened at Harvard University to define brain death [5]. The 1980 Uniform Determination of Death Act defined death: "…an individual who has sustained either (1) irreversible cessation of circulatory or respiratory functions, or (2) irreversible cessation of all functions of the brain, including the brain stem, is dead" [4]. This allowed the procurement of viable organs from heart-beating cadavers.

In 1984, Public Law 98-507, the National Organ Transplant Act (NOTA), was passed (its original sponsor was Al Gore, then senator from Tennessee). Among other things, this Act established the Organ Procurement and Transplantation Network (OPTN), which is run by the Secretary of Health and Human Services, and the Scientific Registry of Transplant Recipients (SRTR), the main data clearinghouse for all transplant programs in the country. In addition, the law prohibited "the exchange of organs for transplantation for valuable consideration" [4], which is generally interpreted to mean money or property. The OPTN conducts the day-to-day management of transplantation, and, since its inception, the only OPTN has been the United Network for Organ Sharing (UNOS).

Since then, there have been numerous additional laws, amendments, and changes to the rules that govern transplantation. From a practical point of view, all current regulatory policies are maintained by UNOS. The Unites States has been split up into 11 regions for the purpose of organ allocation and sharing.

This regional arrangement has become a contentious issue in the transplant community, as the artificial boundaries have led to significant disparities in organ availability in different parts of the country. This issue has been extremely difficult to remedy, for complex reasons. Suffice it to say that this is an active topic of debate.

The federal government, particularly its insurance endeavors, is represented by the oversight of the Centers for Medicare and Medicaid Services (CMS). CMS's interest in transplantation intensified after Public Law 92-603 amended the Social Security Act to provide Medicare coverage for most end-stage renal disease patients [ibid]. Once the Medicare program became responsible for dialysis and renal transplantation services, CMS took a keen interest in the finances of transplantation and the oversight of transplant centers.

Many of the personnel and other requirements for transplant programs which we will discuss in this chapter are defined and required by UNOS and CMS.

Starting a Transplant Program

Not surprisingly, starting a transplant program requires more than hanging up a sign and seeing patients. Crucial in this endeavor is the strong support of a medical center's administration. Transplant programs represent a huge and expensive undertaking in personnel, materials, organization, and software, so a medical center needs to fully commit to such an undertaking.

The application form from UNOS for establishing a new transplant program is some 288 pages long, so a comprehensive checklist of all that is required is beyond the scope of this chapter. Rather, we will summarize the broad requirements. Historically, transplant programs have been run by surgeons. Obviously, having capable transplant surgeons is a necessary but by no means a sufficient requirement. Years ago, many transplant surgeons felt that they were the best at managing all aspects of transplantation, including pre-, peri-, and postoperative care, as well as immunosuppression and short- and long-term complications. Many still think so. Medicine and transplantation have evolved, however, and there are many talented transplant nephrologists, hepatologists, pulmonologists, and cardiologists working now. UNOS has recognized the importance of these specialists, and these organ-specific personnel are required for any transplant program. Any new transplant surgeon is required to have additional transplant-specific training after completion of residency, usually through one of the numerous American Society of Transplant Surgeons (ASTS)-approved fellowships in the United States or Canada or equivalent international training programs. Similarly, nephrologists, hepatologists, pulmonologists, and cardiologists are required to complete additional transplant fellowships after their internal medicine and fellowship training. Interestingly, the only specialty that has additional examination requirements for certification through the American Board of Internal Medicine is Transplant Hepatology, with no similar requisites for surgeons or other medical personnel.

In many states, there is a requirement to apply for a certificate of need (CON) to justify opening a transplant program. Originally, the CON regulations were directed at limiting the number of new hospital or nursing home beds in the state by requiring the applying institutions to justify such additions. Currently, 34 states, Puerto Rico, the US Virgin Islands, and the District of Columbia have CON requirements [6]. These requirements vary from state to state. As time has gone on, the CON process has been expanded to include the opening of transplant and other high-cost specialty centers.

In addition to transplant centers' hospital, state, and UNOS locations, all transplant centers must be affiliated with an organ procurement organization (OPO). These organizations coordinate all of the deceased donor activity in their respective areas, known as donor service areas (DSAs). There are 58 OPOs in the United States, some of which serve a single transplant institution and some of which serve dozens. Each OPO undergoes oversight by UNOS and CMS, similar to transplant centers.

The sticky topic of finances complicates the requirements for new transplant programs. As mentioned before, the vast majority of transplant patients (essentially all renal failure/kidney transplant patients and many of the other organs' patients) are insured by Medicare. CMS will not approve a new program for Medicare participation until ten patients are transplanted in a 12-month period with each organ for which approval is sought. This leads to the possibility that the medical center will not be paid for any transplant activity until after ten patients are transplanted, which means that the institution must be willing to potentially absorb millions of dollars of loss in the short term. Private insurers frequently follow Medicare's lead, and many private insurers have more stringent participation requirements (e.g., the need to perform 50 annual transplants with acceptable patient and graft survival in order to qualify for a "Center of Excellence" designation).

Personnel and Institutional Requirements

At the bare minimum, UNOS requires the following personnel in order to open a transplant program:

- Transplant surgeon
- Transplant physician
- Physician extenders (nurse practitioners and/or physician assistants)
- Transplant pathologist
- Transplant coordinator
- Nutritionist/dietitian
- Financial counselor
- Social worker
- Administrator
- Data coordinator
- Transplant pharmacist
- Transplant psychiatrist or psychologist

For the physicians and surgeons, UNOS has volume requirements in order to be the surgical or medical directors – the number of transplants performed, the number of transplant patients managed, and the like. There are also time constraints as well. Twenty pancreas transplants performed 15 years ago will not fulfill UNOS regulations to qualify as a pancreas transplant surgical director.

The transplant operations have been refined and improved over the decades. The perioperative mortality rates for kidney and liver transplants are difficult to find, but they should be around 1% for kidneys and less than 5% for livers. While special surgical teams and anesthesiologists are not required for kidney transplantation (although desirable), liver transplant surgery benefits from dedicated liver anesthesiologists (required by UNOS) and committed OR teams. The introduction of new surgical technology, especially intraoperative blood salvage, and availability of veno-venous bypass and hemostatic tools like the argon coagulator and Aquamantys® (Medtronic) bipolar sealer have made transplant surgery easier and safer.

Organ Allocation

The national clearinghouse for organ offers is the computerized UNET system (https://portal.unos.org/) run by UNOS. Kidneys are generally allocated in the local DSA, based on a combination of factors, such as blood type, human leukocyte antigen (HLA) matching between donors and recipients, degree of sensitization (percent of anti-HLA antibodies), and waiting time. There are also mechanisms for broader geographical allocation, based on HLA "zero mismatched" donors and recipients, very high sensitization

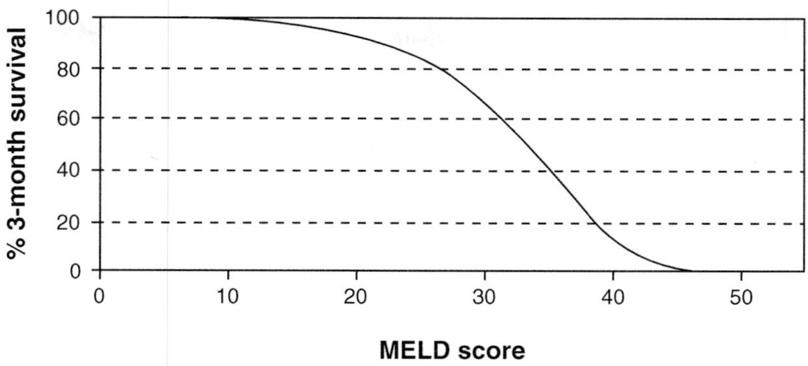

Fig. 26.2 Three-month survival by MELD score. (Reprinted from Wiesner et al. [17]. With permission from Elsevier)

(>98%), and lack of interest in the local DSA for a particular kidney.

Livers are allocated within the DSA based on the Model for End-Stage Liver Disease (MELD) score, which is calculated using the patient's total bilirubin, INR, and serum creatinine (MELD = 3.8*$\log_e$(serum bilirubin [mg/dL]) + 11.2*$\log_e$(INR) + 9.6*$\log_e$(serum creatinine [mg/dL]) + 6.4). More recently, MELD-Na is calculated to include serum sodium as one of the variables. The MELD score runs from 6 to 40, with calculated values above 40 capped at that score. MELD was originally developed as a prognostic score to predict 3-month mortality without transplantation (Fig. 26.2).

Potential recipients under the age of 11 use a different scoring system – PELD – which uses the same criteria as MELD (with the exception of serum creatinine), with the addition of age, weight, height, and serum albumin and the presence or absence of growth failure.

Livers are allocated to the local DSA first, then to the UNOS region, and then nationally if there is no local or regional interest (although there are variances that allow automatic regional allocation in certain areas, such as Region 9). Allocation is to the patients in the DSA with the highest MELD/PELD scores, with some exceptions. An adult or pediatric patient can be declared a "Status 1A" if he or she fulfills certain criteria, such as acute fulminant liver failure without prior liver disease, primary nonfunction of a transplanted liver, hepatic artery thrombosis of a transplanted liver, or acute decompensated Wilson's disease. A child can be declared a "Status 1B" if he or she has nonmetastatic hepatoblastoma, has certain inborn errors of metabolism, or fulfills other clinical requirements (https://optn.transplant.hrsa.gov/governance/policies/). Status 1A and Status 1B patients are allocated organs before those stratified by MELD/PELD. Additionally, UNOS instituted a "Share 35" system a while ago, which allocates livers *regionally* (as opposed to the local DSA) when a patient is listed with a MELD score ≥ 35.

Deceased Donation

The majority of organs for transplantation in the United States come from deceased donors. A single deceased donor can potentially save up to nine lives (two lungs, heart, two kidneys, pancreas, intestine, and liver split into two pieces). If someone is formally registered as an organ donor, that serves as first person consent for donation. If someone is not formally registered, then the OPO will discuss the option of donation with the potential donor's family or healthcare proxy to try and make a decision about his or her wishes to donate.

Once someone is deemed an organ donor, the OPO continues to maintain the viability of the body through mechanical and artificial means. This allows time for allocation of the organs that will be procured from each donor. After a battery of tests to evaluate the quality of the various organs, the OPO performs a match-run to see which recipient will receive that organ (UNET, *v.s.*). The OPO then contacts the respective transplant centers to notify them of the posting of the match runs. This then sets into motion the arduous task of setting up the transplant procedure. The intended recipient is brought into the hospital, and a surgical team is sent to procure the organs. This frequently requires long-distance travel and many hours of work to get the organ from the donor to the intended recipient. The cost of this process is substantial and includes all of the medical and surgical costs of maintaining donors from the time of brain death declaration through the time of procurement, as well as all of the transportation and delivery costs. The sum of costs for obtaining an organ for transplantation is termed the organ acquisition fee, which is then covered by the recipient's insurance as part of the transplant procedure package.

Living Donation

Because of the vast imbalance between the availability of deceased donor organs and the number of patients in need of transplantation, living donation is a reasonable and necessary option. In the United States, a plurality of kidney transplants (and at some centers a majority) are done using living donors. Because of the similarly dire situation in liver transplantation, living donation is a (less common) technique in that arena.

The field of living donation complicates the ethical and technical aspects of transplantation by orders of magnitude. First is the apparent violation of the Hippocratic dictum of primum non nocere. Living donors are healthy people who are undergoing a major surgical procedure that they don't need. Obviously, there are benefits to both the donor and recipient – psychological value to the donor in saving or improving a life and improved health in a recipient. Kidney recipients in particular derive great advantages from living donation, in that living donor kidneys work better, function almost twice as long as deceased donor kidneys, and may allow the recipient to avoid dialysis altogether.

The NOTA prohibitions against trading organs for "valuable consideration" must be an absolute. This requires careful psychological evaluation of the donor to probe for motivations and even the faintest hint of fraud. An Independent Donor Advocate Team (IDAT) is required for the multidisciplinary evaluation of potential donors and to protect their lives and well-being.

The surgical care of the donor must be impeccable: some have observed that living donation is one procedure where there is a possibility of 200% mortality. As with transplantation in general, the evolution and advancement of surgical techniques, especially the introduction of laparoscopic organ recovery, have made the procedures safer and better tolerated by the patients.

Building an Innovative Transplant Program

High-functioning transplant centers are aided in managing the regulatory framework that is imposed on them by hiring full-time, well-trained quality officers whose sole function is to monitor the regulatory environment and ensure that the center is reaching all the desired outcomes. In addition, these officers are key in proactively monitoring outcomes in continuous updatable risk-adjusted techniques [7]. These analyses can anticipate opportunities for improvement and avoid expensive and painful regulatory reprimands in the future. In addition, this will inspire confidence from institutional leadership that the programs are being good stewards of the resources that are being allocated to them.

One of the features of a high-functioning transplant center is to recognize the long-standing donor shortage that is an endemic problem in transplantation. Transplant centers recognize the problem that is created by the exponential growth in the national waiting list but also see an opportunity to grow their programs and serve the wider community in an effort to be responsive to the needs of the patient population. Modern transplant centers take a leadership role in establishing and promoting programs and activities at the local, regional, state, and national levels concerned with increasing donor awareness. These programs are primarily working to increase donor participation by engaging and participating in lobbying efforts with the legislatures and through working with organizations such as New York State Liver and Kidney Consortia and local OPOs. These centers can have outreach clinics and programs which enhance and promote live donation. The investiture of manpower and financial and human resources must be as efficient and comprehensive as possible in identifying and addressing factors that reduce the barriers to successful organ donation. The programs also identify disincentives and remove these barriers to donation and patient access to transplantation. In so doing, these programs convert a challenge into an opportunity for growth and innovation.

In addition, centers that promote and invest resources in living donation are able to build programs [8] which have quality outcomes and volumes that are sustainable. They are involved in programs that increase organ sharing, such as paired donor exchanges at the national level: through the UNOS national paired donation program and some of the various commercial programs, such as the Alliance for Paired Kidney Donation. In addition, they innovate in removing barriers from using some living donors by performing desensitization protocols, ABO-incompatible transplants, and other methods of overcoming immunologic barriers. These must be done, however, while keeping in mind that the regulatory framework may create barriers to innovation by punishing centers for inferior outcomes [9].

A modern transplant center is characterized by effectively providing access to the patient population that it serves. Most transplant centers are midsized, while a significant number are low volume. There are always concerns whether low-volume centers can have the same quality outcome as high-volume centers [10–15].

In order to overcome this barrier, centers are encouraged to have robust quality improvement programs [7].

Preoperative Management

While most kidney transplant patients are admitted electively or semi-electively from home for their transplant operations, a significant number of liver patients are hospitalized or ICU-bound before their transplants. There is little argument that patients in liver failure can be some of the sickest and most difficult patients to manage, with fluid overload, variceal bleeding, hepatic encephalopathy or coma, renal dysfunction, and coagulopathy being common in many of these patients. The care of these patients requires close coordination between hepatologists, surgeons, and intensivists. Patients will frequently require mechanical ventilation, endoscopy, renal replacement therapy, and even intracranial pressure monitoring.

Surgical Procedures

Kidney Transplantation

The kidney transplant operation is done under general anesthesia, usually with a central venous line for fluid and medication administration and venous pressure monitoring. It is our practice to place a three-way Foley catheter with bacitracin-containing solution attached to the irrigation port to aid in bladder dissection. The kidney can be placed extraperitoneally on either the right or left side, although the right external iliac vein is more superficial than that on the left and so is a little easier to dissect and use for anastomosis. The only time when it is strongly recommended to place the kidney on the left is in type 1 diabetic patient who is also getting a pancreas transplant at the same time or is planned for one in the future. There is a higher incidence of thrombosis of the pancreas graft when it is placed on the left side.

The retroperitoneum is entered through a Gibson incision at the junction of the rectus and oblique muscles. The peritoneal sac is reflected cephalad by dividing the filmy attachments from the peritoneum to the psoas muscle and external iliac vessels. A self-retaining retractor such as the Bookwalter® is then used to provide exposure. The external iliac vessels are surrounded with lymphatics, which must be ligated and divided to expose the vessels and to prevent the formation of postoperative lymphoceles. After the vessels are fully dissected, they are controlled with vascular clamps, and the kidney is brought onto the field. The venous and arterial anastomoses are then carried out end to side to the iliac vessels with 5-0 and 6-0 Prolene, respectively. Prior to releasing the clamps, the patient is given 500 mg of methylprednisolone and whatever induction agent (usually thymoglobulin or basiliximab) the center prefers. In addition, mannitol and Lasix are given to stimulate rapid diuresis. After the clamps are removed and hemostasis attained, the Foley tubing is clamped and the bladder inflated with the bacitracin solution. The bladder is identified and the musculature at the appropriate area divided, exposing the mucosa. A small hole is made in the mucosa and the Foley clamp removed. After the ureter is trimmed to the appropriate length, a Lich-Grégoire extravesical ureteroneocystostomy is created with running stitches of 5-0 or 6-0 PDS, with or without the use of a ureteral stent. A short anti-reflux tunnel is created by approximating the bladder musculature around the anastomosis. The kidney is placed in the retroperitoneal pocket and the incision closed in two layers, with or without the use of a closed-suction drain.

Liver Transplantation

After induction of anesthesia, a Swan-Ganz catheter is placed, as well as a second large-bore internal jugular catheter for the rapid infusion of fluids and blood products or for venous return if venovenous bypass is used. The abdomen is entered through a bilateral subcostal incision with a midline xiphoid extension. There are basically three phases of this operation: the hepatectomy phase, the implantation phase, and the mopping-up phase. The hepatectomy is generally the most difficult part of the operation. The left lateral segment is taken down and the gastrohepatic omentum divided. The hilum is then dissected, ligating and dividing the branches of the hepatic artery and common bile duct. The portal vein is left intact until the liver is ready for removal.

The right triangular ligament is taken down and the lateral border of the retrohepatic inferior vena cava identified. All of the short hepatic veins are ligated and divided or just divided with the LigaSure® device. The right hepatic vein is encircled with a vessel loop. At this point, the only remaining attachments of the liver are the portal and hepatic veins. If the choice is to do the transplant with the piggyback technique, the right hepatic vein is divided with a vascular stapler. The portal vein is doubly clamped and divided. The middle and left hepatic veins are clamped with a large Satinsky or German clamp. Because this technique leaves the IVC intact and allows venous return from the lower part of the body, the patients tend to be more hemodynamically stable than with full caval clamping. After the hepatic veins are clamped, the liver is dissected off of them and removed from the field. The middle and left hepatic veins are opened together, and the suprahepatic caval anastomosis is fashioned with running 3-0 Prolene. The preservative solution is flushed out of the liver with a liter or two of lactated Ringers into the portal vein, which is vented from the infrahepatic IVC, which is then ligated. An end-to-end portal vein anastomosis is then performed with running stitches of 5-0 or 6-0 Prolene. The liver is then reperfused by removing the hepatic venous and portal venous clamps.

After hemostasis is attained, the native hepatic artery is dissected back to the origin of the gastroduodenal artery, clamped proximal to this, and divided. An end-to-end hepatic artery anastomosis is done with 6-0 Prolene. When the clamps are removed, the liver is fully reperfused. It is not unusual at this point for the patient to have some "medical" bleeding, and correction of the specific factor or platelet deficiencies is facilitated through the use of thromboelastography (TEG®) or rotational thromboelastometry (ROTEM®). Once the bleeding is controlled, biliary continuity is reestablished with either an end-to-end choledochocholedochostomy or a Roux-en-Y hepaticojejunostomy. The patient's abdomen is closed in two layers after the placement of closed-suction drains.

Immediate Postoperative Care

Managing these patients in the perioperative period can be extremely challenging: what Dr. Bud Shaw has referred to as "The Specter of Postoperative Care" [16]. Because this care is so complex, it is necessary to have protocols and order sets to assure that everything gets done properly. While it is generally unnecessary that kidney recipients go to the intensive care unit after surgery, they generally require a higher level of care than a floor bed – perhaps a "post-op" or "step-down" unit. Liver recipients require ICU care. An otherwise healthy liver recipient who has a well-functioning allograft and uncomplicated surgery is no more difficult to care for than any other patient who has had a major abdominal operation. Such patients are unfortunately rare. More common are patients who are quite debilitated going into surgery, with underlying cardiac, renal, and endocrine dysfunction, and who frequently have had massive transfusions and hemodynamic instability during their surgery.

Careful and effective communication between the transplant team and the intensivists and other ICU personnel is crucial. To that end, we have found it useful to summarize our protocols for postoperative management, including the peculiarities inherent in liver and kidney transplantation, for inclusion in our ICU's treatment guideline manuals. It is important that the surgical team not "cut and run," dumping the patient in the ICU and abandoning the care of the patient exclusively to the ICU team.

The surgical ICU at our institution is a "closed" unit, under the direction of our surgical intensivist team. It is crucial that there be a good relationship between the transplant team and the ICU team to facilitate communication and optimize postoperative care. Mutual respect and appreciation of each group's particular strengths greatly benefit the patients.

We have a comprehensive set of postoperative guidelines which cover all aspects of the care of our transplant patients, including but not limited to care plans for each day postoperatively, immunosuppressive management, prophylactic antimicrobial medications, and management principles for rejection or other complications. There is too much for anyone to remember, so as the Old Testament prophet Habakkuk (2:2) says, "Write the vision, and make it plain upon tablets, that he may run that readeth it." Or, in other words, "The shortest pencil beats the longest memory."

Conclusion

Organ transplantation in the twenty-first century is an immensely complex and expensive undertaking. The regulatory requirements are onerous. Nevertheless, it is also an overwhelmingly rewarding field. The economic and quality of life advantages of transplantation are unequivocal. The surgical and medical advances in the past 60 years have converted transplantation from a Nobel-winning oddity to a routine method of managing end-stage organ failure to the great benefit of tens of thousands of patients.

References

1. Starzl TE. My thirty-five year view of organ transplantation. History of transplantation: thirty-five recollections. UCLA Tissue Typing Laboratory. 1991;145–79.
2. Borel JF, Feurer C, Magnee C, et al. Effects of the new antilymphocyte peptide Cyclosporin A in animals. Immunology. 1977;32:1017.
3. Calne R. Recollections from the laboratory to the clinic. History of transplantation: thirty-five recollections. UCLA Tissue Typing Laboratory. 1991;227–41.
4. US Department of Health & Human Services. Organdonor.gov. Retrieved from: https://organdonor.gov/about-dot/laws/history.html
5. A definition of irreversible coma. Report of the Ad Hoc Committee of the Harvard Medical School to examine the definition of brain death. JAMA. 1968;205(6):337–40.
6. National Conference of State Legislatures (NCSL). Con-Certificate of Need State Laws. August 25, 2016. Retrieved from: http://www.ncsl.org/research/health/con-certificate-of-need-state-laws.aspx.
7. Axelrod D, Guidinger M, Metzger R, et al. Transplant center quality assessment using a continuously updatable, risk-adjusted technique (CUSUM). Am J Transplant. 2006;6(2):313–23.
8. Habbous S, Arnold J, Begen MA, et al. Duration of living kidney transplant donor evaluations: findings from 2 multicenter cohort studies. Am J Kidney Dis. 2018; in print. Habbous S, Garg AX, Lam NN. Optimizing efficiency in the evaluation of living donor candidates: Best Practices and Implications. Current Transplant Rep. 2018;5(1):55–63.
9. Abecassis M, Burke R, Klintmalm G, et al. American society of transplant surgeons transplant center outcomes requirements—A threat to innovation. Am J Transplant. 2009;9(6):1279–86.
10. Edwards EB, Roberts JP, McBride MA, et al. The effect of the volume of procedures at transplantation centers on mortality after liver transplantation. N Engl J Med. 1999;341(27):2049–53.

11. Finks JF, Osborne NH, Birkmeyer JD. Trends in hospital volume and operative mortality for high-risk surgery. N Engl J Med. 2011;364(22):2128–37.
12. Hosenpud JD, Breen TJ, Edwards EB, et al. The effect of transplant center volume on cardiac transplant outcome: a report of the United Network for Organ Sharing Scientific Registry. JAMA. 1994;271(23):1844–9.
13. Rana A, Pallister Z, Halazun K, et al. Pediatric liver transplant center volume and the likelihood of transplantation. Pediatrics. 2015;136(1):e99–e107.
14. Reese PP, Yeh H, Thomasson AM, et al. Transplant center volume and outcomes after liver retransplantation. Am J Transplant. 2009;9(2):309–17.
15. Tracy ET, Bennett KM, Danko ME, et al. Low volume is associated with worse patient outcomes for pediatric liver transplant centers. J Pediatr Surg. 2010;45(1):108–13.
16. Shaw BW. Starting a liver transplant program. Semin Liver Dis. 1989;9(3):159–67.
17. Wiesner R, Edwards E, Freeman R, et al. Model for end-stage liver disease (MELD) and allocation of donor livers. Gastroenterology. 2003;124:91–6.

The Imaging Department of the Modern Hospital

27

Zvi Lefkovitz, Michael J. Seiler, and Angelo Ortiz

Introduction

Numerous breathtaking technological innovations have occurred in the past two decades in every facet of imaging technology that have transformed the field of diagnostic imaging. Today, in the modern hospital, imaging plays a seminal role in the diagnosis and treatment of a vast number of diseases. The imaging department in the modern hospital therefore functions as a key diagnostic hub that must provide safe, reliable, highly efficient, advanced imaging services to patients and referring physicians [1]. In fact numerous referring services have come to rely on the radiologist as an invaluable member of the diagnostic and therapeutic team caring for the patient. Radiologists must provide high-quality subspecialty consultation services to referring physicians, 24/7/365, and many of the department's services must be available 24 h a day. In order for this ideal to be reached, the imaging department must be effectively designed, structured, and managed; must feature advanced, reliable, imaging equipment and information technology infrastructure; and must have a highly trained and dedicated technical, nursing, and physician staff to provide imaging services.

Z. Lefkovitz (✉) · M. J. Seiler · A. Ortiz
Department of Radiology, Westchester Medical Center, Valhalla, NY, USA
e-mail: zvi.lefkovitz@wmchealth.org

Departmental Hierarchy, Organization, Management, and Training

Departmental Hierarchy and Organization

Given the enormous demands placed on the modern imaging department, it must be directed, managed, and organized effectively [2–4]. Accordingly, the department must be managed by a horizontally integrated leadership team designed to foster teamwork. In fact teamwork, not only among the management team but also among all staff members, is the most critical element in assuring the effectiveness of the entire imaging enterprise [5–7]. The members of the management team of the imaging department of the modern hospital are ideally as follows:

1. Medical Director/Chairman: Ideally a radiologist who serves as the senior medical officer of the department, is responsible for all of the imaging services provided by the department, develops and implements the department's strategic plan, assures the department maintains state-of-the-art technology, and assures the department meets or exceeds national quality, efficiency, and productivity standards. The medical director/chairman also serves as the "liaison in chief" for the imaging department.

R. Latifi (ed.), *The Modern Hospital*, https://doi.org/10.1007/978-3-030-01394-3_27

2. Administrative Director: Assists the medical director/chairman in implementing the strategic plan of the department; is responsible for developing and executing the departmental budget and business plans; oversees all equipment purchases, installation, and equipment service; and oversees all radiology clerical and technical staff.
3. IT Director: Is responsible for assuring optimal organization and implementation of the Imaging IT enterprise and day- to-day IT operations; develops and implements comprehensive, ongoing IT training program for all radiology staff, particularly radiologists and technologists; and serves as radiology's "IT liaison" to the hospital IT department.
4. Quality Assurance/Performance Improvement Director: Is responsible for compliance with all regulatory requirements, equipment, and program accreditation, assures comprehensive departmental preparation for all regulatory body surveys, assures all departmental policies are up to date, and serves as radiology's liaison with the institutional quality and safety department.
5. Nursing Director: Manages all day-to-day nursing operations of the department, assures ongoing nursing training for all nursing personnel in radiology, and serves as radiology's liaison with the Department of Nursing.
6. Medical Physicist: Assures the department and institution meet all radiation safety and MRI safety requirements, is responsible for technical analysis and evaluation of all proposed new equipment, and provides acceptance testing of all newly installed imaging equipment.
7. Operational Manager: Oversees and manages the day-to-day technologist operations for all imaging modalities.

With these members of the management team, working jointly toward a unified vision with clear goals and in a fully integrated fashion, the department can function in a highly efficient and productive manner. The members of the management team must be held fully accountable for all activities within their domain. The goal of such a hierarchy is to foster all-important teamwork and to optimize every facet of the department, resulting in a team that functions as a whole that is much greater than the sum of its parts (Fig. 27.1).

Department Committee Structure

Another important organizational component of the modern imaging department is the departmental committee structure. The purpose of these imaging committees is to oversee, foster, and maintain highly innovative and advanced imaging

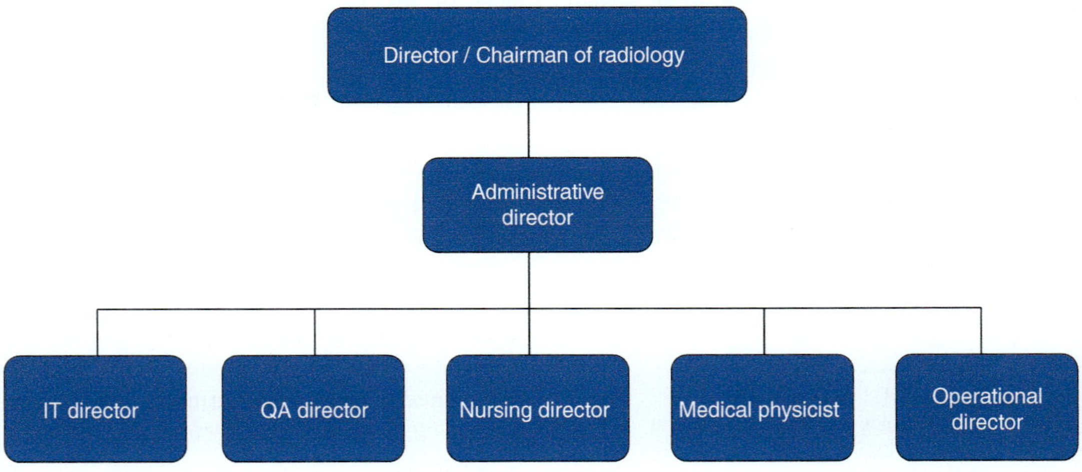

Fig. 27.1 Imaging department hierarchy in the modern hospital

technologies in a safe environment. Key multidisciplinary committees that are necessary for the maintenance of the highest-quality care, operational standards, imaging equipment, and IT standards are as follows:

1. Quality assurance/performance improvement committee: reviews adherence to the key departmental indicators; addresses the full gamut of occurrences and complaints and reviews all procedural complications; and oversees adherence to all imaging equipment accreditation requirements [8, 9]
2. Radiation safety committee: assures adherence to all required radiation safety standards and reviews all radiation safety events and maintains oversight over all radiation safety initiatives and training [10]
3. MRI safety committee: develops and maintains MRI safety standards and policies in conjunction with national standards [11], assures strict hospital-wide adherence to MRI safety standards, and oversees MRI safety training programs
4. Radiology information technology and management committee: oversees the entire Imaging IT enterprise operation and assures IT innovations and upgrades are developed and implemented [12]
5. Imaging equipment and service committee: oversees the planning and implementation of all equipment purchases and projects and assures optimal equipment maintenance and servicing [13]

Training and Education

The advanced imaging technologies of the modern hospital must be operated by a highly trained and skilled workforce to assure optimal operational efficiency and patient care [1]. As technology continues to advance at a rapid pace, it is important that all members of the imaging team maintain cutting-edge skills especially for the operation of advanced CT, ultrasound, MRI, SPECT, and interventional radiology (IR) equipment. Therefore the development and implementation of a comprehensive applications training program for all imaging staff are a critical component of the modern imaging department. Intensive, continual on- and off-site staff training for technologists, Imaging IT personnel, and radiologists, especially for those utilizing advanced applications in Imaging IT, ultrasound, CT, MRI, SPECT scanning, and IR, is critical for assuring optimal utilization of these advanced technologies. Accordingly, in addition to the preliminary training routinely provided by equipment vendors, continual, specialized in-service applications training should be planned for at the time of every equipment purchase or lease.

Imaging Information Technology (IT)

The Imaging IT department plays a seminal role in supporting and maintaining the essential infrastructure of the modern imaging department. The Imaging IT enterprise system in the modern hospital fundamentally allows for maximal flexibility in the storage, transmission, retrieval, and interpretation of imaging studies. The system also allows for the images and interpretations to be rapidly available to referring physicians anytime and anyplace. The Imaging IT system must be closely integrated to the hospital EMR (electronic medical record). Single log-on for all EMR and radiology IT users is a necessary component for the efficiency of the Imaging IT system.

For Imaging IT to provide this critical support for the imaging department, it is vital, from the organizational and operational standpoint, that the Imaging IT team be embedded within the imaging department. Accordingly, the Imaging IT director must report directly to the medical director of radiology with a "dotted line" reporting structure to the director of hospital IT. In this manner, IT priorities for the imaging department can be kept in focus, Imaging IT can be maintained at the cutting edge of technology, and IT issues in the imaging department can be addressed rapidly with the guidance and support of the director of hospital IT [13].

An important function of the Imaging IT team is to develop and enhance efficient workflows while maintaining high quality. This requires a thorough understanding of the imaging department processes, equipment, staff roles, imaging data, and images. Accordingly the Imaging IT team should consist largely of IT specialists with previous experience as radiologic technologists.

The IT department must also be able to provide extensive real-time managing metrics [14–16]. These metrics provide the department's management team with an accurate, up-to-date view of departmental operations and allow for timely well-informed operational and equipment decisions.

The following are the key IT components of the modern imaging department:

1. *Radiology Information System (RIS)*: The RIS is the software that is the electronic management infrastructure of the modern imaging department. The RIS is responsible for the core workflow within the department. The picture archiving and communication system (PACS), voice recognition (VR), and EMR (electronic medical record) systems are closely integrated with the RIS so that all data passes seamlessly through each system providing consistent records. The RIS provides numerous critical electronic operational functions including patient scheduling and billing, examination tracking, study interpretation and distribution, and electronic forms. The RIS serves as the gateway for referring physicians to order and view imaging studies and reports and provides appropriateness criteria to the ordering provider. In addition the RIS provides mission-critical metrics regarding departmental productivity and efficiency that form the basis for the departmental dashboards.
2. *Picture Archiving and Communication System (PACS)*: PACS is critically tied to the RIS (radiology information system) and hospital EMR (electronic medical record).

   PACS is the system with which images are obtained, transmitted, interpreted, and stored electronically. Images from all imaging modalities are interpreted by the radiologists using high-resolution monitors with advanced workstations. This system obviates the need for the processing, retrieval, delivery, and storage of film and allows imaging studies to be interpreted almost immediately after they are obtained. Moreover, prior archived studies can be automatically retrieved for comparison with current studies, thereby significantly enhancing the accuracy of the radiologist's diagnosis [17, 18].

   PACS technology dramatically increases the radiologist's efficiency and diagnostic accuracy [19] and allows access to images electronically without any geographic barriers.

   In addition the introduction of cloud technology allows rapid image sharing from diverse external sources ensuring the continuity of care and enhancing communication among providers. PACS allows for the easy importing of outside images for comparison purposes as well as the exporting of images to patients and referring physicians. Image sharing also reduces redundant or duplicative imaging which in the modern hospital must be kept to a minimum. This not only significantly reduces the unnecessary cost of duplicative imaging but, in the case of X-ray or CT studies, also reduces radiation dose.
3. *VR (Voice Recognition)*: Radiologists in the modern imaging department interpret studies using voice recognition dictation software [20–22] that is fully integrated and intimately tied into the RIS and PACS systems. The VR system must be augmented by artificial intelligence software to assure a very high level of reporting accuracy and reliability. Like the RIS, VR can be mined for mission-critical metrics.
4. *3D Software*: 3D post-processing software is utilized for advanced CT and MRI applications. This system, embedded in PACS and available on the enterprise system, allows radiologists to perform mission-critical 3D analytics on any workstation without any geographic constraints. The use of advanced 3D software includes neurology applications such as perfusion imaging for stroke and quantitative analysis of anatomic changes in the brain, cardiovascular applications such as TAVI analysis and advanced vessel analysis, as well as oncology applications such as lung nodule assessment and tumor tracking.

5. *CAD (Computer-Aided Detection)*: This software identifies and highlights specific abnormalities such as calcifications in mammography [23], detection of lung nodules on CT examinations [24], and polyp detection in the colon on CT colonography (virtual colonoscopy) examinations [25].
6. *AI (Artificial Intelligence)*: AI, currently in its infancy, will undoubtedly, in the short term, play a major role in streamlining the radiologist's workflow and ultimately will play a vital role in assisting the radiologist in identifying abnormalities and in the interpretation of studies [26] (Fig. 27.2).

Imaging Technologies

Imaging technologies that must be available in the modern hospital include both fixed and portable DR radiography, digital fluoroscopy, ultrasound, computed tomography (CT), magnetic resonance imaging (MRI), single-plane and biplane interventional radiology (IR), C-arms for the operating room, and nuclear medicine SPECT imaging. In the modern hospital, imaging technology must be placed in three key locations: the main radiology suite, the emergency department, and the operating room. Portable DR X-ray unit and ultrasound units must be available for bedside imaging for the critically ill patient who cannot be safely transported.

Imaging in the Main Department

The main imaging department must be located in a central hub of the modern hospital, easily accessible from anywhere in the hospital. The modalities that must be available include direct X-ray radiography, both fixed and portable, DR fluoroscopy, CT, MRI, ultrasound, SPECT scanning, and IR.

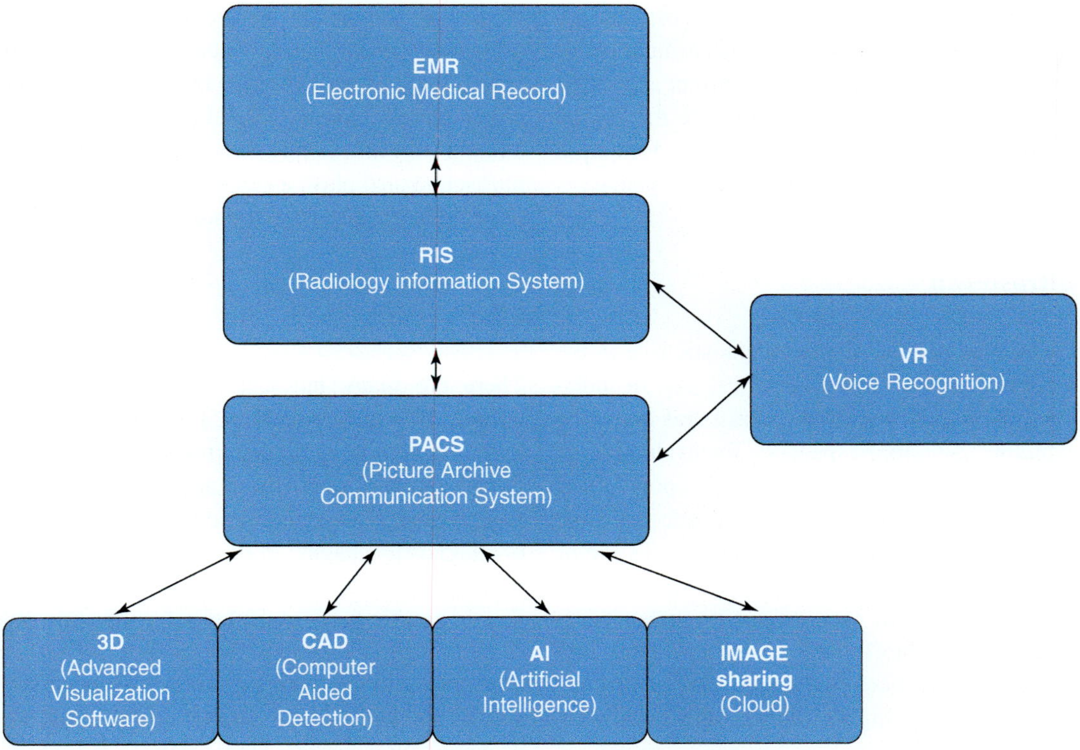

Fig. 27.2 Imaging IT infrastructure in the modern hospital

DR Radiography and Fluoroscopy

Direct X-ray radiography (DR) units, both fixed and portable, are an essential component of the modern imaging department. DR radiography must be immediately available 24/7/365. DR portable units should be deployed in or adjacent to the hospital's intensive care units (ICUs) especially the neonatal ICU and in the operating room. DR radiography is an advanced low-dose X-ray technology that exposes patients to one half of the radiation dose of older analogue computerized radiography [27]. Fixed radiography units must be designed with an upright chest wall stand to assure upright chest and abdominal imaging can be obtained. Fixed DR imaging provides higher-quality diagnostic imaging than portable DR and is primarily utilized for the evaluation of the chest, abdomen, and axial and appendicular skeleton. DR fluoroscopy is utilized primarily for the detection of gastrointestinal leaks or fistulas, particularly postoperatively, and is utilized to evaluate the pharynx and esophagus for leaks following esophageal surgery, trauma, or endoscopy. Fluoroscopy of the oropharynx and esophagus is critical for the evaluation of swallowing impairments and recurrent aspiration [28]. Software is now available for the digital conversion of fluoroscopic images for rapid review via PACS by the speech pathologist.

Ultrasound

Ultrasound plays a pivotal diagnostic role in the modern imaging department [29]. As an indispensable diagnostic tool, ultrasound must be available 24/7/365, especially for evaluation of the pediatric and obstetrical population. Ultrasound provides superb diagnostic real-time imaging without the ionizing radiation of CT or radiography and without the safety hazards associated with MRI. Accordingly, ultrasound is uniquely valuable for the obstetrical, fetal, and pediatric evaluation. Advanced ultrasound units are lightweight, highly mobile, and maneuverable and ideally suited for bedside examinations in the critically ill patient. Diagnostic ultrasound studies are performed by ultrasound technologists utilizing advanced ultrasound technology in the imaging suite. The images are then evaluated and interpreted by radiologists. Since ultrasound, unlike CT or MRI, is far more operator dependent, the ongoing training and supervision of the ultrasound technologists to assure adherence to high imaging standards are paramount [30, 31].

Real-time ultrasound is highly valuable for the evaluation of the abdominal organs [32] including the hepatobiliary system, pancreas, spleen, genitourinary system, and bowel and for the evaluation of abdominal or pelvic masses or collections. Ultrasound is frequently utilized for the evaluation of neck masses and thoracic collections in children and adults. Ultrasound is extremely useful for the evaluation of the brain, spinal cord, hips, and bowel in neonates. Ultrasound is routinely utilized for image guidance for a host of procedures, especially for vascular access.

Advanced ultrasound Doppler technology provides highly accurate evaluation of blood flow and blood vessels, allowing for the diagnosis of blood clots, especially deep vein thrombosis, vessel stenosis, aneurysm, and increased or decreased blood flow in various organs or masses. Doppler ultrasound is extremely useful for vascular evaluation in liver and kidney transplantation. Doppler ultrasound also plays a key role in the evaluation of testicular and ovarian torsion [33].

CT

There are many inherent advantages that are unique to CT and that make CT an invaluable tool in the modern imaging department. CT scanning is painless and noninvasive and requires only a few seconds of scanning time for the acquisition of diagnostic images. Portable CT scanners are now available that can be deployed for bedside imaging particularly of the brain for the critically ill neurosurgical patient that cannot be safely transported to the imaging suite. Advanced CT scanners deliver highly detailed images that are exceptionally accurate. Unlike ultrasound which is limited by air in the lung, by intestinal gas, as well by bone, CT provides precise cross-sectional and three-dimensional images of the brain, spine, musculoskeletal system, neck, chest, abdomen, pelvis, and extremities and is the critical noninvasive and preferred modality for the evaluation of a host of acute and chronic symptoms and diseases, especially abdominal and pelvic pain. These include evaluation of the brain, lungs, heart, vascular tree, abdominal organs, gastrointestinal system, genitourinary system, and musculoskeletal system [34]. CT imaging is a superb, widely utilized tool for the guidance of minimally invasive percutaneous diagnostic procedures including needle biopsies of the lungs, mediastinum [35], and abdominal organs and for therapeutic aspirations and drainages of abdominal and pelvic collections. It is also utilized to provide highly accurate guidance for therapeutic procedures such as microwave and radiofrequency ablations of tumors [36]. Modern CT scanners are designed to significantly reduce radiation dose and, with the introduction of spectral scanning, can also significantly reduce the dose of intravenous contrast [37, 38].

MRI

MRI is a unique modality in the modern imaging department that has revolutionized imaging and is utilized for numerous neurological, musculoskeletal, cardiac, vascular, visceral, and soft tissue applications. MRI is a noninvasive imaging modality that does not use ionizing radiation to obtain diagnostic images. Images can be directly acquired in the coronal, axial, sagittal, or oblique planes without the need to reposition the patient. MRI demonstrates superior soft tissue contrast as compared to other modalities and is an essential tool for the evaluation of the brain, spine, joints, heart, and abdominal pelvic organs [34]. Advanced MRI applications such as diffusion and [39] perfusion imaging also can add functional information in addition to the anatomical information obtained on conventional MRI sequences. In this manner extremely accurate soft tissue characterization can be obtained. This is best demonstrated by MRI's unique ability to identify acute ischemic injury of the brain [40]. Functional MRI provides visualization of the brain during certain activities and can be extremely useful in presurgical planning [41]. Because MRI is radiation-free, it is an ideal modality for the evaluation of pediatric and pregnant patients [42, 43]. Another advantage of MRI is its ability to obtain vascular images without the use of intravenous contrast.

The major disadvantages of MRI as compared to CT are as follows:

1. Relatively slower scanning that is susceptible to motion artifacts. Accordingly, children frequently require general anesthesia for MRI scanning. This requires additional coordination that inevitably results in scheduling delays that are rarely encountered with CT.
2. Safety concerns related to metal implants, foreign bodies, tattoos containing metal, and the potential for ferromagnetic objects to become missiles in the MRI room. The MRI suite therefore must be designed to maximize MRI safety. A comprehensive MRI safety program must be in place to assure all patients are properly screened before entering the MRI suite and that all MRI staff and outside staff such as anesthesiologists are properly trained in MRI safety [44].

Nuclear Medicine SPECT Imaging

Nuclear medicine (NM) is a physiological rather than anatomical imaging modality. In nuclear medicine, radiopharmaceuticals also known as radiotracers or radionuclides are administered intravenously, orally, or by inhalation. The mode of radiotracer administration depends on the disease process that is being studied. In the modern hospital, NM studies are performed by single-photon emission computed tomography (SPECT) cameras. SPECT cameras detect the gamma-ray emissions in three dimensions from the radiotracers that have been administered to the patient. The introduction of advanced CT, MRI, and ultrasound imaging technology has largely supplanted nuclear medicine as a diagnostic modality for many clinical indications. However, NM remains an important modality for a number of important applications [45]: assessment of myocardial perfusion, detection of bone metastases, thyroid and parathyroid imaging, detection of infection, renal function study, detection of gastrointestinal bleeding, evaluation of gastric emptying, neuroectodermal studies, somatostatin receptor studies, and cerebral radionuclide angiography for the confirmation of brain death, which is particularly important for a transplant donor program. Therapeutic radiopharmaceuticals are also utilized including the use of I-131 for the treatment for thyroid cancer and hyperthyroidism, yttrium Y-90 Zevalin treatment for non-Hodgkin's lymphoma, and yttrium Y-90 for treatment of liver cancer [46, 47].

PET-CT technology is an advanced molecular imaging modality utilized most frequently for the diagnosis, staging, and restaging of certain cancers and utilized almost exclusively for outpatients and therefore is generally not deployed in the modern hospital.

Interventional Radiology

Interventional radiology (IR) has become the critical modality for the minimally invasive treatment of numerous disorders. Interventional radiologists perform a myriad of minimally invasive procedures utilizing imaging guidance including fluoroscopic, ultrasound, and CT guidance for targeted treatments. Advanced 3D software is utilized for accurate and rapid catheter vessel navigation. Fusion imaging [48] that utilizes previous imaging that is referenced to the procedural imaging modality can provide highly accurate diagnostic information to assure optimal device localization for numerous applications including biopsies and tumor ablations. In the modern imaging department, the IR suite is ideally designed to treat the most critically ill patients in the hospital in the most efficient manner [49]. The suite should be equipped with an advanced single plane angio-room, biplane angio-room for neurological applications, and ultrasound units utilized for image guidance in vascular access procedures and nephrostomies and fusion ultrasound. Electronic inventory of all supplies with adequate maintenance of par levels particularly for catheters, guidewires, and stents in the IR suite is mandatory.

Interventional radiologists perform a host of procedures [50] including biopsies; drainages of collections; gastrointestinal, hepatobiliary, genitourinary, and vascular interventions; pelvic and splenic embolization; chemoembolization; central venous access; dialysis interventions; thrombolysis; IVC filter placement; kyphoplasty; and vertebroplasty. In many hospitals, the IR suite is also utilized by vascular surgeons for a host of minimally invasive vascular procedures and endovascular neurosurgeons who perform stroke interventions, cerebral aneurysm treatment, and treatment of AVMs. Anesthesiologists performing minimally invasive pain management procedures also routinely utilize the IR suite.

Imaging in the Modern Emergency Department

Imaging support for the emergency department (ED) is critical for the rapid diagnosis and treatment of the emergency patient. To assure rapid decision-making regarding patient admission to the hospital, observation, or treatment and release, imaging must be available either directly in the ED or in an adjacent imaging suite and must be manned by technologists 24/7. The key imaging modalities that must be placed either in the ED or immediately adjacent to the ED are as follows:

1. DR radiography (fixed and portable)
2. Ultrasound
3. CT

DR Radiography

Direct X-ray radiography (DR) is the most frequently utilized modality in the ED. DR radiography provides low-radiation dose imaging that is available almost instantaneously for interpretation by the ED physicians and radiologists. DR radiography is available on portable bedside DR units utilized for chest radiography of critically ill, unstable patients who cannot be transported to the imaging suite, for intubated patients, and for patients after undergoing lifesaving thoracic procedures and after central line insertions. Fixed DR imaging provides higher-quality diagnostic imaging than portable DR and is most frequently utilized for the evaluation of the axial and appendicular skeleton following trauma and for the evaluation of the chest and abdomen.

Ultrasound

Ultrasound performed at the bedside by ED physicians, also known as point-of-care ultrasound (POCUS), is considered an important adjunct to the physical examination [51]. POCUS is routinely performed in the emergency department utilizing inexpensive lightweight and mobile ultrasound technology for the evaluation of patients with cardiac, thoracic, and vascular symptoms and as a screening tool for evaluating the abdomen. POCUS is also routinely utilized for procedural guidance in the ED. For trauma patients focused assessment with sonography for trauma (FAST scanning) is routinely performed [52]. When POCUS identifies an abnormality that requires further clarification, a diagnostic ultrasound examination is frequently required. The advanced diagnostic ultrasound units located in the ED imaging suite are more expensive and technologically advanced than POCUS units, provide a markedly enhanced diagnostic capability, are lightweight, and, when necessary, can be used as portable equipment at the bedside.

CT

CT in the ED is critical for the evaluation of acute trauma, severe headache, chest pain, shortness of breath, and abdominal pain [53]. CT in the ED must be immediately available 24/7 with technologists on-site around the clock [54]. Advanced CT scanners offer very low radiation dose and high speed imaging that reduces motion artifact. This is especially valuable for cardiac and thoracic imaging, trauma patients [55–57], and the pediatric population. This technology also provides extended patient coverage for perfusion imaging, especially in the brain, critical for the evaluation of acute stroke as well as submillimeter imaging that provides exceptional diagnostic accuracy. Recently with the advent of highly advanced spectral scanning [58, 59], available in only a few centers, even greater diagnostic accuracy can be achieved especially for the diagnosis of vascular disease, pulmonary embolus (PE), mesenteric ischemia, and even myocardial infarction. With spectral imaging intravenous iodinated contrast dose can be reduced by 50% without reducing image quality.

Because MRI is a far slower modality than CT (three CT studies can be completed in the time it takes to perform one MRI study) and MRI also has considerable safety constraints, it is not used as the primary modality in the ED except for the following indications:

1. Spinal cord compression
2. Evaluation of appendicitis in the pregnant or pediatric patient
3. Hip fracture not detected by radiography or CT
4. Detection of acute stroke

Accordingly MRI must be available to the ED patient 24/7 but does not necessarily need to be located in or adjacent to the ED suite. Furthermore on-site technologists are not absolutely necessary as long as technologists are available on-call within a 45-min time frame.

Imaging in the Modern Operating Room

Imaging in the operating room typically consists of portable C-arm units that provide intraoperative real-time and static fluoroscopic imaging. C-arms are typically operated by X-ray technologists and are primarily used for surgical navigation and localization by orthopedic surgeons, vascular surgeons, urologists, general surgeons, and anesthesiologists for pain management applications. Intraoperative ultrasound is also frequently performed to assist the surgeon in localization and for intraoperative biopsy guidance. Operating rooms utilized for complex cardiovascular surgery now frequently feature advanced hybrid imaging rooms that combine an angiographic room with an operating room. Operating rooms also utilize portable CT scanners utilized for highly accurate 3D image guidance for hardware placement and localization by orthopedic surgeons and neurosurgeons [60]. In select centers intraoperative MRI (iMRI) units are utilized to enhance the safety and accuracy of neurosurgical procedures of the brain [61].

Conclusion

The modern imaging department is truly a technologic marvel that has revolutionized the practice of medicine. Exceptionally accurate three-dimensional submillimeter imaging with advanced tissue characterization, obtained in a matter of seconds by spectral CT scanners, is now a reality. Highly accurate diagnosis and minimally invasive treatment of complex diseases are now possible utilizing a vast array of imaging technologies. Advances in ultrasound, CT, and low-radiation dose X-ray technologies allow for highly accurate imaging that can be deployed at the bedside for the most critically ill patients. Recent advances in information technology allow unlimited image accessibility to radiologists, referring physicians, and patients, anytime, anyplace. As advances in diagnostic imaging technologies such as spectral CT, advanced MRI, and ultrasound as well as information technologies such as artificial intelligence and computer-aided detection continue to develop and mature, they will, no doubt, have a profoundly positive effect on patient care and outcomes. Furthermore, advances in catheter and guidewire design and angiographic imaging and navigation technologies will further enhance the scope, utilization, and value of the minimally invasive interventions provided in the IR suite.

References

1. European Society of Radiology 2009. The future role of radiology in healthcare. Insights Imaging. 2010;1(1):2–11.
2. Sharpe RE, Mehta TS, Eisenberg RL, Kruskal JB. Strategic planning and radiology practice management in the new health care environment. Radiographics. 2015;35(1):239–54.
3. Muroff LR. Implementing an effective organization and governance structure for a radiology practice. J Am Coll Radiol. 2004;1(1):26–32.
4. Krestin GP. Maintaining identity in a changing environment: the professional and organizational future of radiology. Radiology. 2009;250:612–7.
5. Coburn AF, Croll ZT. Improving hospital patient safety through teamwork: the use of teamstepps in critical access hospitals. Portland: Flex Monitoring Team; 2011. (Policy Brief #21).
6. Baker DP, Day R, Salas E. Teamwork as an essential component of high-Reliability organizations. Health Serv Res. 2006;41:1576–98.
7. The Royal College of Radiologists and the Society and College of Radiographers. Team Working in Clinical Imaging. London: The Royal College of Radiologists and the Society and College of Radiographers, 2012.
8. Kruskal JB, Eisenberg R, Sosna J, Yam CS, Kruskal JD, Boiselle PM. Quality improvement in radiology: basic principles and tools required to achieve success. Radiographics. 2011;31(6):1499–509.
9. Johnson CD, Krecke KN, Miranda R, Roberts CC, Denham C. Developing a radiology quality and safety program: a primer. Radiographics. 2009;29(4):951–9.
10. Ploussi A, Efstathopoulos EP. Importance of establishing radiation protection culture in radiology department. World J Radiol. 2016;8(2):142–7.
11. Crisp S, Dawdy K. Building a magnetic resonance imaging safety culture from the ground Up. J Med Imaging Radiat Sci. 2018;49:18–22.
12. Walz-Flannigan A, Kotsenas AL, Hein S, et al. Implementing a radiology-information technology project: mobile imaging viewing use case and a general guideline for radiologist-information technology team collaboration. AJR. 2015;204:721–6.
13. Youssem DM, Beauchamp NJ. Radiology business practice: how to Succeed: Philadelphia, Elsevier; 2008.
14. Kaplan RS, Norton DP. The balanced scorecard: measures that drive performance. Harv Bus Rev. 1992;70(1):71–9.
15. Kaplan RS, Norton DP. Putting the balanced scorecard to work. Harv Bus Rev. 1993;71(5):134–47.
16. Donnelly LF, Gessner KE, Dickerson JM, et al. Department scorecard: a tool to help drive imaging care delivery performance. Radiographics. 2010;30(7):2029–38.
17. Branstetter IV. BF: basics of imaging informatics. part 1. Radiology. 2007;243(3):656–67.

18. Branstetter BF IV. Basics of imaging informatics: part 2. Radiology. 2007;244(1):78–84.
19. Joshi V, Narra VR, Joshi K, et al. PACS administrators' and radiologists' perspective on the importance of features for PACS selection. J Digit Imaging. 2014;27:486–95.
20. Mehta A, Dreyer KJ, Schweitzer A, Couris J, Rosenthal D. Voice recognition—an emerging necessity within radiology: experiences of the massachusetts general hospital. J Digit Imaging. 1998;11(4 Suppl 2):20–3.
21. Boland GWL. Voice recognition technology for radiology reporting: transforming the radiologist's value proposition. JACR. 2007;4(12):865–7.
22. Krishnaraj A, Lee JKT, Laws SA, et al. Voice recognition software: effect of radiology report turnaround time at an academic medical center. AJR. 2010;195:194–7.
23. Benedikt RA, Boatsman JE, Swann CA, et al. Concurrent computer-aided detection improves reading time of digital breast tomosynthesis and maintains interpretation performance in a multireader multicase study. AJR. 2018;210(3):685–94.
24. Choi W, Choi T. Automated pulmonary nodule detection based on three-dimensional shape-based feature descriptor. Comput Meth Prog Bio. 2014;133(1):37–54.
25. Robinson C, Halligan S, IInuma G, et al. CT colonography: computer assisted detection of colorectal cancer. Br J Radiol. 2011;84:435–40.
26. Thrall JH, Li X, Li Q, et al. Artificial intelligence and machine learning in radiology: opportunities, challenges, pitfalls, and criteria for success. JACR. 2018;15)3:504–8.
27. Boo D, Wber M, Deurloo EE, et al. Computed radiography versus mobile direct radiography for bedside chest radiographs: impact of dose on image quality and reader agreement. Clin Radiol. 2011;66(9):826–32.
28. Palmer JB, Drennan JC. Evaluation and treatment of swallowing impairments. Am Fam Physician. 2000;61(8):2453–62.
29. Loria K. Imaging adaptability: a look at the latest advancements in ultrasound. Radiology Today. 2017;18(3):12.
30. Pinto A, Pinto F, Faggian A, et al. Sources of error in emergency ultrasonography. Crit Ultrasound J. 2013;5(Suppl 1):S1.
31. Patil P, Dasgupta B. Role of Diagnostic ultrasound in the assessment of musculoskeletal diseases. Ther Adv Musculoskelet Dis. 2012;4(5):341–55.
32. American Institute of Ultrasound in Medicine. Practice Parameters. 2017.
33. Kitami M. Ultrasonography of pediatric urogenital emergencies: review of classic and new techniques. Ultrasonography. 2017;36(3):222–38.
34. American College of Radiology. ACR Appropriateness Criteria.
35. Lal H, Neyaz Z, Nath A, Borah S. CT-Guided Percutaneous Biopsy of Intrathoracic Lesions. Korean J Radiol. 2012;13(2):210–26.
36. Smith SL, Jennings PE. Lung radiofrequency and microwave ablation: a review of indications, techniques and post-procedural imaging appearances. Br J Radiol. 2015;88(1046):article 20140598.
37. Danad I, Fayad ZA, Willemink MJ, Min JK. Recent advances in cardiac computed tomography: dual energy, spectral and molecular CT imaging. JACC Cardiovasc Imaging. 2015;8(6):710–23.
38. Tsang DS, Merchant TE, Merchant SE, et al. Quantifying potential reduction in contrast dose with monoenergetic images synthesized from dual layer detector spectral CT. Br J Radiol. 2017;90:1078.
39. Baliyan V, Das CJ, Sharma R, Gupta AK. Diffusion weighted imaging: technique and applications. World J Radiol. 2016;8(9):785–98.
40. Chalela JA, Kidwell CS, Nentwich LM, Luby M, Butman JA, Demchuk AM, Hill MD, Patronas N, Latour L, Warach S. Magnetic resonance imaging and computed tomography in emergency assessment of patients with suspected acute stroke: a prospective comparison. Lancet. 2007;369:293–8.
41. Glover GH. Overview of functional magnetic resonance imaging. Neurosurg Clin N Am. 2011;22(2):133–9.
42. Kinner S, Pickhardt PJ, Riedesel EL, et al. Diagnostic accuracy of MRI versus CT for the evaluation of acute appendicitis in children and young adults. AJR Am J Roentgenol. 2017;209(4):911–9.
43. Bekiesińska-Figatowska M, Romaniuk-Doroszewska A, Szkudlińska-Pawlak S, et al. Diagnostic imaging of pregnant women – the role of magnetic resonance imaging. Pol J Radiol. 2017;82:220–6.
44. Sammet S. Magnetic resonance safety. Abdom Radiol (New York). 2016;41(3):444–51.
45. Bybel B, Brunken RC, DiFillipo FP, et al. SPECT/CT imaging: clinical utility of an emerging technology. Radiographics. 2008;28:1097–113.
46. Jacobs SA. 90Yttrium ibritumomab tiuxetan in the treatment of non-hodgkin's lymphoma: current status and future prospects. Biologics Targets Ther. 2007;1(3):215–27.
47. Kallini JR, Gabr A, Salem R, Lewandowski RJ. Transarterial Radioembolization with Yttrium-90 for the Treatment of Hepatocellular Carcinoma. Adv Ther. 2016;33:699–714.
48. Abi-Jaoudeh N, Kobeiter H, Xu S, Wood BJ. Image Fusion During Vascular and Nonvascular Image-Guided Procedures. Tech Vasc Interv Radiol. 2013;16(3):168.
49. Baerlocher MO, Kennedy SA, Ward TJ, et al. Society of interventional radiology: resource and environment recommended standards for IR. JVIR. 2017;28(4):513–6.
50. Kandarpa K, Machan L. Handbook of interventional radiologic procedures. 4th ed. Philadelphia: Wolters Kluwer Lippincott Williams & Wilkins. p. 2011.
51. Whitson MR, Mayo PH. Ultrasonography in the emergency department. Crit Care. 2016;20:227.
52. Cohen HL, Langer J, McGahan JP, et al. American institute of ultrasound in medicine. AIUM practice guideline for the performance of the focused

assessment with sonography for trauma (FAST) examination. J Ultrasound Med. 2014;33(11):2047.
53. Pandharipande PV, Reisner AT, Biner WD, et al. CT in the emergency department: a real-time study of changes in physician decision making. Radiology. 2016;278(3):812–21.
54. Raja AS, Ip IK, Sodickson AD, et al. Radiology utilization in the emergency department: trends of the last two decades. AJR Am J Roentgenol. 2014;203(2):355–60.
55. Soto JS, Anderson SW. Multidetector CT of blunt abdominal trauma. Radiology. 2012;265(3):678–93.
56. Hinzpeter R, Boehm T, Boll D, et al. Imaging algorithms and CT protocols in trauma patients: survey of swiss emergency centers. Eur Radiol. 2017;27(5):1922–8.
57. Davies RM, Scrimshire AB, Sweetman L. A decision tool for whole body CT in major trauma that safely reduces unnecessary scanning and associated radiation risks: an initial exploratory analysis. Injury. 2016;47(1):43–9.
58. Silva AC, Morse BG, Hara AK, et al. Dual-energy (Spectral) CT: applications in abdominal imaging. Radiographics. 2011;31:1031–46.
59. Rajiah P, Abbara S, Halliburton SS. Spectral detector CT for cardiovascular applications. Diagn Interv Radiol. 2017;23(3):187–93.
60. Conley DB, Tan B, Bendok BR, et al. Comparison of intraoperative portable CT scanners in skull base and endoscopic sinus surgery: single center case series. Skull Base. 2011;21(4):261–70.
61. Mislow JMK, Golby AJ, Black PM. Origins of intraoperative MRI. Neurosurg Clin N Am. 2009;20(2):137–46.

28 Intensive Care Unit Model of Modern Hospital: Genomically Oriented and Biology-Based

Kartik Prabhakaran and Rifat Latifi

Introduction

"Realization of surgical and medical goals in critically ill patients often requires envisioning the goal in advance. Let us consider a 60-year-old male patient with a history of atrial fibrillation who is involved in a motor vehicle collision sustaining multiple injuries including bilateral rib fractures and pulmonary contusions, and requiring laparotomy with splenectomy, followed by intramedullary nail fixation of bilateral femur fractures. The patient remains mechanically ventilated and is being managed in an intensive care unit within the Critical Care Institute of an academic teaching hospital where, on hospital day # 2, he develops severe sepsis with hypotension secondary to a urinary tract infection as well as signs of progressively worsening ARDS. Genomic analysis of the patient at the time of admission predicts that this patient would benefit from early initiation of high-frequency oscillatory ventilation and also falls into the very small subset of patients that would respond well to corticosteroids as adjunctive therapy for his sepsis. This information is obtained using blood and saliva samples obtained in the trauma bay at the time of presentation, analyzed in a laboratory on a separate floor within the same critical institute, and subsequently shared 4 hours later on the day of admission during multidisciplinary critical care rounds by a geneticist and a bionformatic specialist, both of whom are embedded in the rounding critical care team. Genomic analysis also reveals that his risk of cerebrovascular events is much lower than the general population of patients with atrial fibrillation and therefore therapeutic anticoagulation is deferred until further stabilization. Six hours, after initiation of both of the aforementioned treatment strategies, blood and saliva samples are re-drawn from the patient and analyzed by the critical care team using point-of-care testing devices which identify gene transcription profiles congruent with adequate treatment response to both management strategies. The patient is able to make a full recovery and returns to full activities of daily living, and his genomic profile and treatment responses are stored in a worldwide repository of individual and aggregate patient data that interfaces with a universal electronic health record system."

K. Prabhakaran (✉)
Department of Surgery, Westchester Medical Center, Valhalla, NY, USA
e-mail: Kartik.prabhakaran@wmchealth.org

R. Latifi
New York Medical College, School of Medicine, Department of Surgery and Westchester Medical Center, Valhalla, NY, USA

The increasing complexity of disease and critical illness creates an environment where standardized approaches to therapy are conceptually less attractive when compared to individualized, patient-centered treatment plans. Genomic heterogeneity naturally translates into diverse manifestations of disease processes. Consequently, the heterogeneity of physiologic manifestations of disease processes is a natural limitation to practice management guidelines which favor a "one-size-fits-all" approach. Despite modern advances in technology and our understanding of biology, current critical care can therefore be characterized as imprecise. Although evidence-based clinical outcomes research can serve as a "guide" to best practices in critical care, emerging technology in bioinformatics and the genetic basis of disease must service as a platform upon

R. Latifi (ed.), *The Modern Hospital*, https://doi.org/10.1007/978-3-030-01394-3_28

which critical care treatment plans can be tailored to the individual patient. Enthusiasm and progress in genomically oriented medicine should be modeled after early success observed in other areas of medicine such as oncology, psychiatry, pulmonology, and cardiology where the genetic basis of disease has led to precise algorithms for treatment based upon individualized patient biology as opposed to disease pathophysiology. Developing such an individualized approach to critical care will necessitate a broader interdisciplinary approach to the care of patients in intensive care units with collaboration from those that have expertise in genetics, biology, epidemiology, and bioinformatics. In this chapter, we discuss the evolution of precision medicine, the multidisciplinary nature of the field, and its applications to critical care.

Precision Medicine

Although the practice of medicine has always aimed to be "precise," recent advances in our understanding of the complex interplay between the human genome and disease processes have spurred a movement (termed "precision medicine") that aims to exploit our growing knowledge of individual data in creating personalized treatment plans for a variety of disease processes [1]. The completion of the Human Genome Project was accompanied by worldwide hope for a future of linking disease to gene and therapy to individual patient [2]. Historically, the terminology of this approach began with a movement toward "personalized" or "individualized" medicine. However, when balancing the data gathered from the human genome as well as specific biologic pathways, the goal has shifted from creating unique treatment plans for individual persons to rather treatment plans for groups with tightly associated genomic and biologic features [3]. For example, patients who are diagnosed with a specific type of malignancy can be stratified into subgroups with specific genetic variations in tumor biology that can respond to biology-tailored, as opposed to disease-tailored, therapy. Examples of translational research yielding active examples of precision medicine are abundant in the fields of oncology, psychiatry, and infectious diseases. The linkage between specific genetic mutations and disease processes spans the gamut of care from screening (e.g., newborn screening for alpha-fetoprotein for risk of neural tube defects) to diagnosis (e.g., creatine kinase level testing for Duchenne muscular dystrophy) and further to treatment response (e.g., genetic testing for response to immunosuppressive therapy) and long-term monitoring for disease recurrence (e.g., carcinoembryonic antigen for colon cancer). The molecular targeting of specific gene mutations such as HER2 in breast cancer and EGFR in lung cancer has led to significant advances in clinical oncology [4, 5]. These examples have parallel successes in other fields of medicine as well such as psychiatry and pulmonology [6, 7].

Similarly, the understanding of common disease processes treated in the intensive care unit setting such as sepsis, acute respiratory distress syndrome (ARDS), renal failure, and congestive heart failure has been the subject of significant basic science research that has revealed heterogeneity in the phenotype of these diseases. The concept of using biomarkers to aid in the diagnosis of specific disease states has progressed to studying the genetic variability in disease manifestations and treatment response [8]. Gene expression analysis has been used to define subtypes of sepsis and septic shock as well as variability in the response to therapy [9]. Moreover, genomic studies of sepsis have been used to identify genetic polymorphisms that predict outcomes in sepsis [10]. Similarly, the use of biomarkers and genomics has allowed for differentiation of subtypes of ARDS and favorability in ventilator strategies for management [11].

The concept of precision medicine requires not only precision in diagnosis and prediction of disease processes but also a harmonious integration of this information into tailoring individualized treatment plans. Such a path to integration and implementation is contingent upon much more than increasing our knowledge base on the cellular level. The foundations of critical care (i.e., an evidence-based, interdisciplinary, data-driven, efficient plan of management) must be preserved in order to provide cost-effective, timely care to critically ill patients. Moreover, the complexity of critically ill patients mandates a "bird's eye view" of health and illness whereby providers preserve the ability to understand that most patients have a complex interplay between a wide range of coexisting comorbid conditions that often create a synergistic effect upon the patient's outcome.

Critical Care at Present: A Protocol-Centered Paradigm

The care of critically ill patients with high acuity of index illness compounded by coexisting comorbidities and organ failure requires supplementing sound clinical judgment with evidence-based therapies. In turn, evidence-based medicine has given rise to terminology such as "best practices," "goal-directed therapy," "practice management guidelines," and "protocols." The reliance on such terms has been driven by comparisons to yet other terms such as "usual care" [12]. The pertinent questions are: (1) What is usual care?, (2) Do protocols make a difference?, and (3) Are there any disadvantages to using protocol-based therapy?

Although the concept of "usual care" is a shifting paradigm based on graduated implementation of emerging evidence and technology, studies of common intensive care unit pathologies suggest that many patients do not receive desired care [13]. This concept is highlighted by studies of patients with commonly treated intensive care unit diagnoses such as sepsis and acute respiratory distress syndrome (ARDS). The seminal study by Rivers et al. demonstrated a significant survival benefit when sepsis was treated with early goal-directed therapy [14]. In that study, and several others that followed, the early goal-directed therapy or "protocol" was compared to a non-protocolized treatment regimen termed "standard therapy," akin to "usual care." Similarly, the standardization of optimal ventilator management strategies for the treatment of ARDS was shown to confer a significant benefit for mortality and morbidity among intensive care unit patients [15]. Subsequent studies have not only reinforced the protective effects of such strategies but have also led to the development of specific lung-protective ventilator management protocols employed widely across intensive care units internationally. Another frequently seen example of protocol-driven care exists in the form of sedation management and weaning from mechanical ventilation. The desire to use evidence-based techniques to optimize and standardize the approach to reduce ventilator days and both hospital and intensive care unit length of stays has led to the establishment of protocols to wean sedation and extubate patients in a safe and timely manner [16, 17].

The vast majority of studies that have either developed or evaluated patient care "protocols" in the intensive care unit setting utilize the concept of "standard therapy" or "usual care" as the control group for comparison. Although "standard therapy" or "usual care" can be specified in individual studies as a basis for comparison, the terms are of little value when discussing current practices at large. Due to differences in hospital settings (i.e., teaching versus nonteaching, urban versus rural, community versus academic hospitals, etc.), the wide variation of "standard therapy" and "usual care" across healthcare settings mitigates the meaning of the concept of standard of care. Moreover, the adoption and incorporation of the very same protocols advocated in such studies create for an ever-changing definition of standard therapy. In fact, recent large studies on the management of sepsis such as ProCESS (protocolized care for early septic shock) and ARISE (Australasian resuscitation in sepsis evaluation) failed to demonstrate a benefit to early goal-directed therapy "protocols" [18, 19]. The interpretation of such results does not necessarily negate the benefit of protocolized care itself but raises significant questions as to whether the baseline for comparison (i.e., usual care) has itself now evolved to the point of incorporating the goal-directed and protocolized approach espoused by the original study by Rivers and colleagues [14].

As more and more intensive care units have established a reliance on protocols and guidelines espoused by evidence-based medicine in the form of large clinical trials or alternatively by specialty society consensus statements, questions continue to abound regarding the value of such protocols in improving outcomes. A recent multi-institutional observational study sought to examine exactly such a question and found that while clinical protocols are highly prevalent across intensive care units in the United States, the number of existing protocols was not associated with either protocol compliance or patient mortality [20].

Based on the results of such studies, it is important to distinguish between the utility and limitations of protocols as it relates to intensive care. Standardization of approach and incorporation of evidence are not fatal flaws in intensive care; rather they must be balanced with the understanding that the complexity of critical illness and phenotypic variation in disease presentation leave much to be desired when attempting to create or utilize a "one size fits all" recipe to patient care. By and large, protocols fail to account for individual differences not only in the pathophysiology of disease but also to treatment response. A genomically based, personalized medicine approach to critical care is essential in accounting for these differences. The challenge lies in reconciling the importance and relative contributions of personalized medicine and evidence-based protocols and guidelines.

Critical Care: Prospects for the Future

The creation of a personalized, genomically oriented and biology-based approach to the practice of critical care must rely on accurate prediction of disease onset and severity, early individualized intervention, real-time multidisciplinary data acquisition and analysis, monitoring of treatment response, and constant reassessment of disease progression. Using modern advances in bioinformatics, numerous studies have demonstrated the utility of biomarkers and genetic analysis to predict outcomes in the setting of sepsis [21, 22]. Furthermore, biomarkers and genomic variants have been studied extensively as diagnostic tools and predictors of outcomes in ARDS [23, 24]. Early diagnosis and prediction of clinical outcomes confers an enormous benefit in being able to effectively utilize resources to triage patients to appropriate clinical settings and to communicate effectively with families of critically ill patients regarding expectations and goals of care. The key step in translating these advances into personalized diagnostics and prediction lies in utilizing the information gathered from prediction tools to alter and individualize treatment, at the risk of deviating from established protocols and practice management guidelines. Moreover, it is important to understand that treatments that are effective at one stage of critical illness may not be appropriate for application at later stages [25].

As such, real-time bioinformatics obtained during the course of a critically ill patient's disease course can be used to abandon, modify, or augment the treatment approach based upon the individual's treatment response judged not only by clinical response but rather by genomic prediction and evidence of success or failure. The variation in response to the same pathogen or insult is highlighted by a study of trauma patients which retrospectively identified genes whose expression not only varied over the course of hospitalization but also was significantly different between those with complicated versus uncomplicated recovery. Moreover, the investigators found that a newly developed commercial system to rapidly quantify RNA was a more accurate predictor of outcome when compared to traditional prognostic models such as Acute Physiology, Age, and Chronic Health Evaluation (APACHE) and Injury Severity Score (ISS) [26]. One could naturally extend this application to advocate for genomic analysis not only at the time of insult (i.e., trauma) or diagnosis but also at different points along the course of patient management in order to study treatment effectiveness and to re-stratify patients for expected outcomes. Such stratification of patients by genetic profile, and re-stratification after admission, would allow for prediction of outcomes, appropriate triage of patients to optimize intensive care unit bed utilization, appropriate modification of existing treatment protocols, and assessment of responsiveness to specific treatment strategies.

One does not need to look much further than ARDS to identify a specific area of critical illness that has been the subject of so much investigational effort, yet little in the way of consensus in identifying effective treatment strategies. Aside from the widely accepted value of lung-protective strategies for mechanical ventilation, interventions such as prone positioning, high-frequency oscillatory ventilation, high positive end-expiratory pressure, lung recruitment maneuvers, and extracorporeal membrane oxygenation have all been the subject of studies both heralding and refuting relative merits [27]. The question for future providers is not necessarily to reengage in debate regarding relative merits of the aforementioned strategies but rather to question whether any or all of these strategies have benefits and/or harm for individual patients based on a patient's individual biologic profile. Similar to modern oncologic care where, for example, the presence of the HER2 mutation in certain phenotypes of breast cancer would call for targeted therapy in the form of trastuzumab, it is conceivable to aim toward a model where the identification of specific biomarkers and genetic profiles would call for similarly targeted therapy for certain individuals with ARDS.

A Multidisciplinary and Technology-Driven Approach

Critical care, by definition, is a field that is multidisciplinary in nature to an extent that supersedes most other fields in medicine. The requirements for specific skills sets, the breadth of required knowledge, and the increasing reliance on technology mandate that almost all intensive care unit teams are comprised of a team with varied expertise. A team comprised of, but not limited to, intensivists, consultants, nurses, mid-level providers, nutritionists, pharmacists, respiratory therapists, physical and occupational therapists, and social workers is commonplace in the modern intensive care unit with the interplay between them essential in delivering effective care to the critically ill patient. The cross-fertilization of knowledge between the aforementioned parties creates not only for a rich academic and educational environment for staff but also for a data-driven, comprehensive, and efficient means to provide state-of-the-art care to the patient.

The development of a genomically oriented and biology-based approach to the practice of critical care begins far beyond the bedside in the form of preclinical basic science. The identification and development of biomarkers, novel therapeutics, genetic associations, and mathematical modeling often begins with nonhuman models of disease and is subsequently translated to the bedside after scores of preclinical and clinical testing. The translation of these advances from the bench to the bedside requires a strong connection between preclinical and clinical science; it is this gap that must be bridged on a practical level in order to translate knowledge into practice. In addition to the various disciplines previously described as comprising critical care teams, the creation of a genomic medicine team consisting of individuals with expertise in genetics, bioinformatics, and statistical analysis is crucial in applying advances in genomics to the practice of critical care.

This concept of translational medicine requires commitment on the part of individuals, institutions, and healthcare systems at large. On an individual level, encouraging the career development of physician-scientists to serve at the interface between bench research and clinical delivery of care is essential. The incorporation of genomic medicine into medical training, the expansion of training grants, and the effective recruitment and retention of physician scientists are important in creating a model of biology-based medicine. Additionally, clinical integration of basic science, bioinformatics, and clinical medicine is important on institutional levels, whereby Departments of Critical Care are formed, housing multidisciplinary specialists as previously described.

Commitment to creating a personalized approach to the intensive care unit, and medicine at large, also requires changes in the healthcare system. Implementation of an effective and comprehensive electronic health record which includes the genetic fingerprint of the entire population is integral to creating a user-friendly and cost-effective model of personalized medicine where genomics are no more than a fingertip away from clinicians. A readily accessible and easy-to-use bank of genotypic and phenotypic data would allow providers to access family history data, provide accurate screening, and evaluate treatment responsiveness. Of note, several healthcare systems in the United States have successfully integrated family history and genomic medicine to electronic health records [28]. Of equal importance is the rapidity with which new technology and therapeutics are evaluated in clinical trials and brought to the forefront of clinical medicine. As basic science and genomic research often outpace clinical trials, the lag time between product development and implementation often creates an environment where newly approved diagnostics and therapeutics are rendered ineffective or at best controversial by clinical trials and investigations.

Perhaps most importantly, the dynamic nature of patient care in intensive care units creates a need for rapid data analysis and strategy implementation. Particularly in the intensive care unit, patients are admitted under conditions of acute distress, and clinical status can change rapidly. As a result, optimizing patient outcomes relies heavily on rapid data gathering and assimilation, followed by constant reassessment of patients' clinical status and treatment strategies. To this end, the practice of critical care has been aided substantially by the concept of point-of-care testing. Albeit in limited use in modern intensive care unit medicine, pulmonary artery catheters have evolved to continuous cardiac output monitoring allowing for clinicians to not only obtain real-time data for monitoring but also to guide therapy in the form of intravenous volume and vasoactive medication administration [29]. Similarly, point-of-care testing of arterial blood gas samples has significantly impacted the practice of critical care by allowing clinicians the ability to make decisions in real time with respect to prompt changes in ventilator management, timely extubation, and correction of critical electrolyte disturbances [30]. Yet another important example of point-of-care testing lies in viscoelastic testing as a predictor of hemostasis and a guide for hemostatic resuscitation [31]. Following these examples, genomic analysis of disease severity and prognosis, response to therapeutics, and reassessment of clinical status is best translated into clinical practice with the development of a user-friendly interface that allows for (1) rapid data acquisition, (2) high accuracy, and (3) cost-effectiveness.

Challenges and Barriers to Implementation of Genomics-Based Patient Care

The enthusiasm among the medical community about the implications of genomics for patient care is tempered by the knowledge that significant gaps in knowledge, structure, and function create challenges that must be overcome in order to reap the benefits and realize the promise of genomics and precision medicine. Barriers to implementation of genomics common to most fields of medicine are related to physician and patient perception, ethical considerations, cost-effectiveness, technologic infrastructure and large volume data management, and the need to work within the confines of regulatory requirements.

The complexity and acuity of patients and disease processes in critical care create specific challenges that must be considered when planning for a future of critical care that is driven by genomics and precision medicine. First, although diagnoses within intensive care unit settings are associated with a high degree of morbidity and mortality, their prevalence across populations at large is relatively small. Unlike the unfortunately ubiquitous nature of sepsis, consider the difference in sample size between ARDS and breast cancer across the world's population. Naturally, the number of patients in a given year diagnosed with ARDS is much smaller. A smaller sample size leads to a small "cohort" of patients to study variations in genomic variations. Distilling this approach even further to the individual patient and his/her genomic fingerprint creates for difficulty in adequate sample size for eligibility in study treatment enrollment and to study treatment effects and safety in clinical trials [32]. This specific challenge requires effort on several levels – large-scale data management and sharing among institutions and governments to increase sample size, creation of new regulatory pathways to evaluate treatment safety and efficacy, and modification of clinical trial design adapted to a need for greater specificity and less generalization.

One of the most significant challenges in precision medicine applied to critical care (precision critical care) lies in the very same characteristic that separates critical care from many other fields of medicine – management of "multi-morbidity" [33]. While most adult disease states exist superimposed upon a framework of comorbid chronic medical illness, patients in critical care settings often not only have similar chronic comorbidities such as heart failure and diabetes but also have multiple organ system dysfunction acutely. The constellation of prehospital comorbid conditions compounded with acute multisystem organ dysfunction creates for a population of patients that is more prone to adverse events which may confound the study of treatment effects. Moreover, when the genomic fingerprint of a patient with a specific critical care diagnosis is used to predict outcomes or alter treatment choices, the complex interplay between pre-existing chronic illnesses and multisystem acute organ dysfunction must be accounted for on a biologic level and in real time. For example, if the genomic profile of a specific patient with ARDS indicates that the patient would benefit from a specific ventilator management strategy, how would that conclusion be altered or modified based on the coexistence of acute sepsis and renal failure superimposed on pre-existing immune compromise secondary to solid organ transplantation? This complex interaction between disease states also creates challenges in study design for evaluating treatment efficacy and safety as patients with poor prognoses and "multi-morbidity" are often excluded from study designs for fear of confounding. While lessons learned from the application of genomics to other fields such as oncology hold promise for enhanced diagnostics and targeted therapies, the complexity of critical care will require a higher order of bioinformatics and data analysis to provide accurate, effective, personalized care.

The complexity of both genomics and critical illness when interfaced creates a volume of data that must be acquired, stored, managed, and accessed. Although intensive care units themselves generate large volumes of data in real time, much of this data cannot be adequately stored and managed as it stands today. Bedside vital signs, information from noninvasive cardiac monitoring, and data from mechanical ventilators are acquired at the level of milliseconds in real time, yet the majority of this data is purged on a daily basis as the sheer volume creates difficulties for platforms to store and categorize such data [34]. The data acquired from genomic analysis of critically ill patients not only require storage but also active interface with the real-time intensive care unit data, as previously described, in order to determine treatment efficacy and guide management. This interface highlights another challenge with respect to data management. While the development of biomarkers to aid diagnosis and prognosis of critical care disease states is in some ways genomically targeted cancer therapy with respect to having the luxury of time, the application of genomics to active management and treatment of critically ill patients must take into account the rapidity with which decisions must be made. Patients in acute respiratory failure, sepsis, and other shock states require prompt assessment and implementation of treatment. The timeliness of critical care requires that genomic analysis evolve to real-time data capture and analysis, with point-of-care testing and user-friendly data dissemination. Furthermore, statistical modeling and actuarial science can enhance the power of genomics by predicting algorithms for treatment options and decision trees far in advance, thereby mitigating the urgency for real-time analysis in critical situations.

Conclusions

We clinicians know that not two patients with same disease respond the same to same surgical or medical treatment. Thus, in today's and future intensive care unit of model modern hospital, no longer can one size fit all, but care must be genomically oriented, biology-based, and entirely personalized. The challenges of multi-morbidity, data storage and accessibility, and regulatory barriers will require efforts that begin with an interdisciplinary approach that bridges the gap between preclinical science and the practice of critical care.

References

1. Mirnezami R, Nicholson J, Darzi A. Preparing for precision medicine. N Engl J Med. 2012;366(6):489–91.
2. Lander ES, Linton LM, Birren B, Nusbaum C, Zody MC, Baldwin J, Devon K, Dewar K, Doyle M, FitzHugh W, et al. Initial sequencing and analysis of the human genome. Nature. 2001;409(6822):860–921.
3. Seymour CW, Gomez H, Chang CCH, Clermont G, Kellum JA, Kennedy J, Yende S, Angus DC. Precision medicine for all? Challenges and opportunities for a precision medicine approach to critical illness. Crit Care. 2017;21:257.
4. Piccart-Gebhart MJ, Procter M, Leyland-Jones B, Goldhirsch A, Untch M, Smith I, Gianni L, Baselga J, Bell R, Jackisch C, et al. Trastuzumab after adjuvant chemotherapy in HER2-positive breast cancer. N Engl J Med. 2005;353(16):1659–72.
5. Maemondo M, Inoue A, Kobayashi K, Sugawara S, Oizumi S, Isobe H, et al. Gefitinib or chemotherapy for non-small-cell lung cancer with mutated EGFR. N Engl J Med. 2010;362:2380–8.
6. Nassan M, Nicholson WT, Elliott MA, Rohrer Vitek CR, Black JL, Frye MA. Pharmacokinetic pharmacogenetic prescribing guidelines for antidepressants: a template for psychiatric precision medicine. Mayo Clin Proc. 2016;91:897–907.
7. Rogers GB, Wesselingh S. Precision respiratory medicine and the microbiome. Lancet Respir Med. 2016;4:73–82.
8. Ware LB, Koyama T, Zhao Z, Janz DR, Wickersham N, Bernard GR, et al. Biomarkers of lung epithelial injury and inflammation distinguish severe sepsis patients with acute respiratory distress syndrome. Crit Care. 2013;17:R253.
9. Maslove DM, Tang BM, McLean AS. Identification of sepsis subtypes in critically ill adults using gene expression profiling. Crit Care. 2012;16:R183.
10. Christaki E, Giamarellos-Bourboulis EJ. The beginning of personalized medicine in sepsis: small steps to a bright future. Clin Genet. 2014;86:56–61.
11. Calfee CS, Janz DR, Bernard GR, May AK, Kangelaris KN, Matthay MA, et al. Distinct molecular phenotypes of direct vs indirect ARDS in single-center and multicenter studies. Chest. 2015;147:1539–10.
12. Levy MM. Early goal-directed therapy: what do we do now? Crit Care. 2014;18(6):705.
13. Prasad M, Christie JD, Bellamy SL, Rubenfeld GD, Kahn JM. The availability of clinical protocols in US teaching intensive care units. J Crit Care. 2010;25(4):610–9.
14. Rivers E, Nguyen B, Havstad S, Ressler J, Mussin A, Knoblich B, Peterson E, Tomlanovich M, for the Early Goal-Directed Therapy Collaborative Group. Early goal-directed therapy in the treatment of severe sepsis and septic shock. N Engl J Med. 2001;345:1368–77.
15. Needham DM, Colantuoni E, Mendez-Tellez PA, et al. Lung protective mechanical ventilation and two year survival in patients with acute lung injury: prospective cohort study. BMJ. 2012;344:e2124.
16. Ely EW, Baker AM, Dunagan DP, et al. Effect on the duration of mechanical ventilation of identifying patients capable of breathing spontaneously. N Engl J Med. 1996;335(25):1864–9.
17. Girard TD, Kress JP, Fuchs BD, et al. Efficacy and safety of a paired sedation and ventilator weaning protocol for mechanically ventilated patients in intensive care (Awakening and Breathing Controlled trial): a randomised controlled trial. Lancet. 2008;371(9607):126–34.
18. Investigators PCESS, Yealy DM, Kellum JA, Huang DT, Barnato AE, Weissfeld LA, Pike F, Terndrup T, Wang HE, Hou PC, LoVecchio F, Filbin MR, Shapiro NI, Angus DC. A randomized trial of protocol-based care for early septic shock. N Engl J Med. 2014;370:1683–93.
19. ARISE Investigators; ANZICS Clinical Trials Group, Peake SL, Delaney A, Bailey M, Bellomo R, Cameron PA, Cooper DJ, Higgins AM, Holdgate A, Howe BD, Webb SA, Williams P. Goal-directed resuscitation for patients with early septic shock. N Engl J Med. 2014;371:1496–506. https://doi.org/10.1056/NEJMoa1404380.
20. Sevransky JE, Checkley W, Herrera P, et al. Protocols and hospital mortality in critically ill patients: the United States critical illness and injury trials group critical illness outcomes study. Crit Care Med. 2015;43(10):2076–84.
21. Shi D, Song Z, Yin J, et al. Genetic variation in the tissue factor gene is associated with clinical outcome in severe sepsis patients. Crit Care. 2014;18(6):631.
22. Scherag A, Schoneweck F, Kesselmeier M, et al. Genetic factors of the disease course after sepsis: a genome-wide study for 28 day mortality. EBioMedicine. 2016;12:239–46.
23. Garcia-Laorden MI, Lorente JA, Flores C, et al. Biomarkers for the acute respiratory distress syndrome: how to make the diagnosis more precise. Ann Transl Med. 2017;5(14):283.
24. Meyer NJ, Feng R, Li M, et al. IL1RN coding variant is associated with lower risk of acute respiratory distress syndrome and increased plasma IL-1 receptor antagonist. Am J Respir Crit Care Med. 2013;187(9):950–9.

25. Marini JJ, De Backer D, Ince C, et al. Seven unconfirmed ideas to improve future ICU practice. Crit Care. 2017;21(Suppl 3):315.
26. Cuenca AG, Gentile LF, Lopez MC, et al. Development of a genomic metric that can be rapidly used to predict clinical outcome in severely injured trauma patients. Crit Care Med. 2013;41(5):1175–85.
27. Fan E, Brodie D, Slutsky AS. Acute respiratory distress syndrome: advances in diagnosis and treatment. JAMA. 2018;319(7):698–710.
28. David SP, Johnson SG, Berger AC, et al. Making personalized health care even more personalized: insights from activities of the IOM genomics roundtable. Ann Fam Med. 2015;13(4):373–80.
29. Wiesenack C, Fiegl C, Keyser A, et al. Continuously assessed right ventricular end-diastolic volume as a marker of cardiac preload and fluid responsiveness in mechanically ventilated cardiac surgical patients. Crit Care. 2005;9(3):R226–33.
30. Allardet-Servent J, Lebsir M, Dubroca C, et al. Point-of-care versus central laboratory measurements of hemoglobin, hematocrit, glucose, bicarbonate and electrolytes: a prospective observational study in critically ill patients. PLoS One. 2017;12(1):e0169593.
31. Da Luz LT, Nascimento B, Shankarakutty AK, et al. Effect of thromboelastography (TEG®) and rotational thromboelastometry (ROTEM®) on diagnosis of coagulopathy, transfusion guidance and mortality in trauma: descriptive systematic review. Crit Care. 2014;18(5):518.
32. Chambers DA, Feero WG, Khoury MJ. Convergence of implementation science, precision medicine, and the learning health care system: a new model for biomedical research. JAMA. 2016;315(18):1941–2.
33. Bierman AS, Tinetti ME. Precision medicine to precision care: managing multimorbidity. Lancet. 2016;388(10061):2721–3.
34. Celi LA, Mark RG, Stone DJ, Montgomery RA. "Big data" in the intensive care unit. Closing the data loop. Am J Respir Crit Care Med. 2013;187:1157–60.

Surgeon of the Modern Hospital

29

Allison G. McNickle and John J. Fildes

Introduction

As a part of the modern hospital, the surgeon of the future will face a new set of technologic advances, human dynamics, and challenges compared to a decade ago. Innovation and technologic advancement is ever present making the operating room landscape of even 10 years ago seems obsolete. The field is dynamic with the constant challenge for the surgeon to be cutting edge, engaged with all medical stakeholders, and a leader of a multidimensional team. Rarely is the modern surgeon only a competent clinician but must extend themselves to have skills as a leader, clinical investigator, or educator. This chapter explores areas in which the modern surgeon will be challenged (Table 29.1).

Table 29.1 Challenges for the modern surgeon

1. Leading a high-performance team
2. Bringing leadership to bedside
3. Contributing new knowledge
4. Incorporating new technologies
5. Ensuring high-quality care
6. Overcoming multigenerational and diversity challenges
7. Optimizing the delivery of multidisciplinary care

Demographics

The modern surgeon will find their skills in demand as workforce growth is underpaced for the projected population expansion. Much is made of the overall physician shortage as well as regional limitations, which is also especially true of surgical specialists. The American College of Surgeon (ACS) supports the Ensuring Access to General Surgery Act of 2017 stating "research is necessary to determine exactly what constitutes a surgical shortage area, and subsequently where these areas exist" to ensure access to high-quality healthcare across the United States [1]. The current shortage is forecasted to worsen over the next decade, with shortfall estimates of 20,000–30,000 surgical specialists [2]. Population growth and aging coupled with the associated cancer incidence are similarly projected to increase the demand for oncologic surgeons and outpace the general surgery workforce [3].

The simple answer to this issue would be to produce more physicians and surgeons. In the 1970s there was the belief that a surplus of physicians and surgeons existed resulting in a lack of growth and expansion of training programs through the year 2000 [4]. The Accreditation Council for Graduate Medical Education (ACGME) and the Association of American Medical Colleges (AAMC) have recognized this deficiency and are on pace to increase medical

A. G. McNickle (✉)
UNLV School of Medicine, Las Vegas, NV, USA
e-mail: allison.mcnickle@unlv.edu

J. J. Fildes
Department of Surgery, UNLV School of Medicine, Las Vegas, NV, USA

R. Latifi (ed.), *The Modern Hospital*, https://doi.org/10.1007/978-3-030-01394-3_29

school enrollment by 30% by 2019 [5]. An increase in medical students is the first step toward addressing the physician shortage, and then we must increase the pipeline into surgical fields. Several programs have put forth initiatives, namely, medical student interest groups to enhance early (MS1 and 2) attention toward surgical specialties [6]. Similarly, other strategic pipeline programs have demonstrated early success in recruiting underrepresented groups into procedural specialties [7]. This early exposure may assist in overcoming the stigma of lifestyle, personality, and length of training that are often cited as reasons not to pursue surgical fields.

As of yet, residency positions have not experienced a similar growth. AAMC data as of 2015 reported 8158 residents and fellows in general surgery. First year residency positions in general surgery have grown 5.1% between 2010 and 2015 [8]. Surgical training "deserts" exist especially in the intermountain and rural regions, which represent a potentially untapped resource for graduate medical education (GME) expansion [9]. With increasing numbers of residents pursuing fellowships, the exact impact on the general surgery workforce is unknown. Targeting resident attrition is a second front to address surgical workforce shortages. Pooled estimates of residents leaving surgery are approximately 18% with significant interstudy variation. Attrition occurs more frequently in females and after intern year with residents most frequently switching programs (20%) or to anesthesia (13%) [10]. Not surprisingly, residents with realistic expectations about surgical residency were less likely to quit [11].

The practicing general surgery workforce has declined approximately 25% in the last 25 years, mostly seen in urban areas (8.0–5.9 per 100,000) [12]. The 2015 workforce comprised 25,254 active physicians with 81% male and 46% over the age of 55 years. Across surgical specialties, recent workforce change has been variable from losses in thoracic (−4.2%) and orthopedics (−3.4%) to growth in plastic/reconstructive (+2.9%), neurologic (+5.9%), and vascular surgery (+17.7%) [8]. Beyond quantitative change in surgeon number is the heterogeneous distribution. Large gaps exist in access to even basic emergency general surgery care across rural and underserved communities [13]. Modern medicine will have an ongoing challenge of addressing physician shortages and uneven practitioner distribution to ensure access to care across the nation.

The Surgeon as a Leader of a High-Performance Team

The modern surgeon is not isolated at the top of the chain of command. They must effectively engage and lead all stakeholders to create a high performance team.

The surgeon is the undeniable leader of the team throughout all phases of surgical care; however, the moody domineering style is no longer appropriate or accepted. A great surgeon of the past was often defined by technical acumen or experience – personality be damned – whereas greatness today extends to leadership, educational, and humanistic qualities [14]. The modern surgeon is tasked with creating a high-performance team to optimize patient safety and outcomes. The American College of Surgeons 2010 Statement on High-Performance Teams affirms the "commitment by all team members to teamwork…respectful behaviors, where contributions of all disciplines and providers are valued, recognition and constructive resolution of conflict" [15].

Surgical leadership may vary from transactional (task-focused) to transformational (team-focused). How often have you instructed a more junior staff member in suturing, performing a central line, or draining an abscess? Surgical residency provides an excellent foundation in transactional leadership. Stepping forward, the surgeon in practice must now lead teams across domains (pre-op, operating room, and post-procedural). They must seek to engage a wide variety of staff – nurses, social workers, patient advocates, and therapists as well as all manner of trainees. Effective leadership must adapt to patient factors and team composition. A severely injured patient with an inexperienced or unfamiliar team may benefit from directive leadership; while an experienced team with a less injured patient may benefit from an empowering (or overseeing) leader [16]. Fluidity in leadership style and recognizing the valence (positive or negative balance) of specific behaviors will facilitate team success [17].

Unfortunately, medical education is less effective in instilling the intangibles of surgical leadership than the technical skills of a given procedure. A study of faculty at the University of Michigan identified knowledge gaps, an appetite for self-improvement, and career advancement as major motivations to seek formal leadership training. Specific objectives for these individuals included improved communication skills, team building, and understanding the healthcare context [18]. There are innumerable printed resources that examine leadership styles and techniques for effective team management. More specific manuals such as the ACS book *Optimal Resources for Surgical Quality and Safety* devote whole chapters to surgical leadership [19]. Beyond written information, specialized courses such as the ACS *Surgeons as Leaders: From Operating Room to Boardroom* focus on leadership issues such as navigating operational and human aspects of change, commitment to a shared vision, and leading in difficult environments. Beyond the skill set this training imparts, it connects the surgeon leader with like-minded colleagues. Goals for the modern surgeon should be to understand our own management style, seek opportunities to enhance our skill set, and optimize our leadership of the surgical team.

The Surgeon's Role in Patient-Centered Care and Bringing Leadership to Bedside

The modern surgeon is a champion of patient autonomy and encourages shared decision-making. They engage patients throughout the course of care.

Historically, physicians and surgeons were tasked with "taking care of patients" – identifying and treating their illness in the way the practitioner deemed most appropriate. The relationship was asymmetric, deferential to the surgeon's opinion, with a less attention to the patient's voice. Modern attitudes place more emphasis on patient autonomy. The patient-physician relationship exists along a spectrum from the "paternalistic doctor" to the "informed patient" with the goal to have a middle-of-the-road "shared decision-making" interaction [20].

Take, for example, the common general surgery consult for symptomatic cholelithiasis or recurrent mild diverticulitis. The surgeon's gestalt for operative intervention may be at odds with the patient's perception of the disease or its impact on their lives. The surgeon should facilitate a treatment discussion and elicit the patient's preference without coercion, especially in cases of treatment equipoise, thus taking a patient-centered rather than disease-centered approach. Patient-centeredness is, in essence, a caregiver's recognition of the individual experience of illness and shared decision-making to create a therapeutic alliance. Patient empowerment, which is slightly different, strives to put the individual in control of their health and treatment [21]. It is summed up succinctly by Kravitz and Melnikow: "Most patients want to see the road map, including alternative routes, even if they don't want to take over the wheel" [22]. While working to achieve a patient-centered approach, there will be patients that have no desire to take an active or empowered role in their own care. In these cases, the surgeon, having offered a shared decision-making approach, may reasonably default to a more paternalistic approach.

Decision-making aids such as the ACS NSQIP calculator may foster a dialogue about a plan of care. Based upon patient and procedural characteristics, the calculator estimates the 30-day risk of death, serious complications, and any complication. A recent study comparing medical and surgical residents' estimations of postoperative complications found both groups overestimated morbidity and mortality compared with the NSQIP calculator [23]. Use of such a tool can allow the treatment team to frame a recommendation within realistic expectations. By ensuring patient involvement in their medical care, the modern surgeon becomes a champion of patient autonomy.

The Surgeon's Role in Research and New Knowledge

The modern surgeon should step beyond being a clinician/technician and seek to contribute to current medical knowledge.

Historically, "the surgeon scientist represents the ideal translational scientist who can address important and oftentimes difficult clinical questions at the bench and take these discoveries back to the bedside" [24]. This was epitomized by exceptional role models in surgical history: Dr. Alfred Blalock's work on cyanotic heart disease, Dr. Joseph Murray with the first successful renal allograft transplantation, and Dr. Basil Pruitt's understanding of the care of burn patients to name a few. The current status of the surgeon-scientist is an endangered species, with less than 3% of medical school graduates being MD-PhDs. Surgeons face an uphill battle, more so than even other medical specialties to secure grant funding – with only 13% of grant requests from surgery departments being funded in 2013. Similarly the workforce of surgeon-scientists is aging with over 50% being over the age of 51 years [24]. It has been observed that the quantity of clinical trained (MD or MD-PhD) applicants for National Institute of Health (NIH) grants has not increased with time as compared to the ever-increasing numbers of PhDs [25].

Over half of general surgery residencies offer research time (range, 1–4 years) with approximately 10% requiring a dedicated research block [26]. It is estimated that one-third of US surgical residents pursue formal research training. Participation in a mandatory research curriculum is demonstrated to increase resident academic productivity during training [27] as well as after entering the surgical workforce [28]. The volume and impact factor of publications was highest among those obtaining a PhD degree [25]. Despite the academic impact of research training, lab time is often viewed as "time off" from clinical duties, occasionally as a time for moonlighting or hopefully rarely, servitude to the institution. Not surprisingly, residents undertaking dedicated research time perceive a decline in their clinical aptitude and surgical skill, especially if conducting "basic science" research or spending 2 or more years in the lab [29]. On the other hand, the most beneficial aspects of research for residents was to learn to formulate a research question, critically review the literature, as well as write abstracts and manuscripts [30]. While interested residents should continue to be involved in dedicated research time, all trainees would benefit from a dedicated curriculum focused on teaching investigative skills.

Those individuals that have the aptitude and interest to pursue a career as a surgeon-scientist should be encouraged to join scientifically focused professional groups such as the Society of University Surgeons (SUS) or the Association of Academic Surgery (AAS). Academic productivity and NIH funding for practicing surgeons are significantly higher for members of the SUS and AAS [31, 32]. While not all surgeons will engage in high-volume research, the modern surgeon should be able to critically evaluate their techniques and outcomes as well as be able to engage with colleagues in a scientific forum. "By re-establishing the 'identity' of the modern surgeon to include a scientific background, skills as an educator, and a practice of surgical innovation and advancement, trainees can once again aspire to lead careers similar to the heroes of surgery" [33].

Technology for the Modern Surgeon

The modern surgeon nurtures technological development, seeking safe, cost-effective and efficient improvements for the delivery of care.

At a basic level, "most surgeons innovate on a daily basis, tailoring therapies and operations to the intrinsic uniqueness of every patient and their disease" [34]. Beyond that the modern surgeon faces the challenge of rapid technological growth and change. Previously, a surgeon could practice for 20 plus years with a relatively static skill set;

however, the pace of modern surgical evolution may require a revised skill set less than 10 years out of residency [35]. Residency programs are challenged with training new surgeons on an evolving set of "modern" procedures. Think about the basic technique of hemostasis – from an era of monopolar cautery and clamp-and-tie to having bipolar cautery, ultrasonic, and other advanced energy sources, not to mention the array of topical hemostatics. As an example, most general surgery trainees will learn laparoscopic common bile duct exploration or possibly a combined laparoscopic/endoscopic approach to choledocholithiasis. How many of those trainees will have done open common bile duct explorations as a bailout for the minimally invasive approach? Some would question whether residents in current training are getting enough repetitions to be proficient at both the primary and bailout techniques to be a safe surgeon in practice. On the positive side, the incorporation of training curriculum such as Fundamental Use of Surgical Energy (FUSE), Laparoscopic Surgery (FLS), and Endoscopic Surgery (FES) ensures that junior residents gain a basic skill set. The modern surgical residency, in partnership with the ACGME, will need ongoing evaluation of procedural volumes to ensure success in practice.

The practicing surgeon faces a potentially greater set of challenges in adapting technology, including the lack of access to procedural mentors/preceptors and the time commitment needed to overcome the learning curve. An important question is who is responsible for ensuring adequate training and proficiency. In February 2017, the Washington State Supreme Court ruled on the case of *Taylor v Intuitive* that the device manufacturer is liable for ensuring that its technology (in this case, the da Vinci robot) is safely adopted. While it is clear that approval should rely on proficiency and peer review/proctoring, it is unclear how to best accomplish this [36]. Surgical leaders are tasked with the challenge of privileging new technologies without a clear, established path. Though the Taylor case placed responsibility on the device manufacturer, the inherent conflict of interest creates issues with certifying proficiency. The Society of American Gastrointestinal and Endoscopic Surgeons (SAGES) has provided guidelines for the introduction of new technologies and techniques. These guidelines suggest that specialty societies have a critical role in the assessment of new technologies and techniques as well as training in these methods. The scope of training/retraining is dependent upon the degree of novelty – a more substantial change or modification should undergo stepwise education from cognitive training to models to preceptorship to use with monitoring of outcomes. Most importantly, the surgeon should be ethical in regard to the potential conflict of interest and profile of the device [37].

For a small number of surgeons, the challenge of designing of innovative techniques and technologies will occupy part of their career. The life cycle of creating a device is long – from concept to prototype to preclinical studies to clinical trial to marketing and clinical use. Innovators face many hurdles including time and capital investment, compliance with regulatory guidelines, and management of patents/intellectual property/production. More often the surgeon is engaged as a technique or device is being targeted for commercial use [38]. Above all, the modern surgeon must balance the desire for innovation and new methodologies against the safety of their patients.

Quality and Performance Improvement for the Modern Surgeon

The modern surgeon strives to be better through lifelong learning, assessment and performance review.

The modern surgeon faces improvement challenges on multiple levels – targeting improvement for both themselves and their institution. The American Board of Surgery (ABS) qualifying and certifying exams remain a right of passage after completion of residency training. With approximately 1400 exams given yearly, the passing rate on these exams is 80% each with an additional 1400 or more recertifying at greater than 94% passing rate per year [39]. In recent years, the challenge of ensuring up-to-date knowledge has been a hot topic. Surgeons are tasked with obtaining continuing medical education (CME) credit, including a fraction with self-assessment activities. The ABS is seeking to move beyond the once-a-decade high-stakes exam covering the breadth of general surgery – much of which is beyond the scope of a given surgeon's practice to a more pertinent and clinically applicable method. The move to a more frequent and focused exam mirrors the wishes of the diplomates and the rapidly evolving world of surgery. These requirements allow the modern surgeon to be more flexible with their personal improvement and hone in on learning that is germane to their everyday practice.

As noted previously, residents and fellows receive supervised training allowing them to perform at a high level. Once in practice, surgeons generally lack a structure for feedback and may experience a performance plateau. SAGES has developed their MASTERS program to advance skill in practice from competency (chief resident/fellow level) to mastery. Beyond video and lecture content, the platform allows for surgical video assessment allowing peer review and feedback. Attaining mastery-level skills would push the surgeon to participate as a surgical coach for more junior participants [40]. This type of program has many beneficial aspects including access to high-quality educational materials and networking within one's specialty. On a similar regional level, the Wisconsin Surgical Coaching Program was developed to provide peer coaching for practicing surgeons to facilitate performance improvement [41]. While not universal across areas of expertise or regions, similar programs will continue to develop as performance improvement and quality metrics remain a focus at the hospital and governmental levels.

One's own performance and outcomes should be monitored on a continuous basis and compared to state or national benchmarks. The ACS Surgeon Specific Registry (SSR) serves as a repository for operative procedures and performance/quality metrics and permits the individual to be benchmarked against their peers. Ongoing improvement of the SSR has permitted mobile data input, delegation of account access, and addition of custom data fields. Future development would include the capacity to interface with electronic health records to prepopulate important data. The ACS goal is to create a unified platform quality improvement, whether it is the TQIP (trauma), MBSAQIP (bariatric), NABPC (breast), or any other database.

Beyond their own practice, a surgeon should contribute to quality improvement in their group and institution. At the departmental level, this may be accomplished through morbidity and mortality conferences or peer review. Within these endeavors, the "environment moves away from blame and shame while expecting all health care professionals to accept responsibility and accountability for their actions" [19]. The shared goal is to identify the basis of the error and work to prevent similar events in the future. The surgeon should take advantage of opportunities to become involved in institutional committees to feedback and shape their practice environment. This could include medical staff service to address the needs of the physician cadre or subcommittees focused on specific issues (e.g., infection control, purchasing, graduate medical education). Quality and performance improvement will remain a focal point in the modern hospital as reimbursements are tied to these metrics. The surgeon must maintain an up-to-date knowledge base and review their performance at a personal and institutional level.

Surgical Leadership Challenges: Diversity and Generational Issues

The modern surgeon understands the strengths of a diverse workforce and is prepared to lead a multi-generational team.

The American College of Surgeons' 2018 Statement on Diversity affirms a "strong commitment to multiculturalism and equal opportunity, respecting and nurturing the diversity of its membership. It recognizes that specific recruitment and development of Fellows from diverse and underrepresented groups is essential to enhancing the strength of the ACS" [42]. A recent survey of US physicians noted that surgeons and surgical trainees were less diverse both demographically and in self-acknowledgment than non-surgeons in terms of gender, prior work experience, and political and gender/sexual identity [43]. Thus diversity in the surgical workforce is a work in progress.

Despite women being equally proportioned to men in medical school matriculation and graduation, they are underrepresented at higher levels of faculty and leadership. Females represent approximately one-third of surgical residents, one-quarter of surgical faculty, and one-tenth of surgical chairs. Traditional gender roles, manifestation of sexism, and lack of effective mentors may contribute to the observed salary and advancement gaps [44]. Interestingly, Dr. Keith Lillemoe's 2017 Presidential Address for the American Surgical Association focused on improving surgical mentorship and leadership opportunities, specifically for women surgeons [45]. Efforts to increase recruitment of women and minorities may benefit from efforts similar to the Nth Dimensions Summer Internship Program which saw a greater than 70% match rate in procedural specialties for participants [7]. With increasing awareness of these shortcomings, the surgical community must strive to embrace workforce diversity and have zero tolerance for offensive and divisive behaviors. The modern surgical practice should be dedicated to "the principle of just, equitable and compassionate care, and surgeons should affirm their individual commitment to this principle through introspection and education" [46]. The modern surgeon strives for cultural competence – the appreciation of race, ethnicity, gender, culture, and religion that impact healthcare decision-making and delivery of care.

Challenging dynamics go beyond gender and diversity to the incorporation of multiple generations into the workforce. By 2020, Millennials (born approximately 1982–1999) will account for over half of the workforce and outnumber all other generations combined. Each generation has its own unique defining events and characteristics that influence their interface with technology and the surgical community. The millennial generation is viewed as technologically adept, accustomed to teamwork, structured learning environments, and driven by self-interest (Table 29.2). As Waljee et al. state "...the values, expectations, and ethos that define millennials are perceived as substantially different from their predecessors and have caught the attention, and concern, of older generations. This is particularly true in medicine where training, advancement, and mentorship are steeped in tradition and where change often comes slowly" [47].

Table 29.2 Characteristics of the Millennial generation

"Digital natives" – technologically savvy, competent, and connected
Facile with information gathering, need to be challenged with critical thinking
Comfortable with a collaborative, team-based approach
May struggle with the traditional hierarchy of surgical teams
Embrace mentorship and desire frequent performance feedback
Strong sense of purpose and socially conscious
Interconnected and less distinction between work and personal life

The modern surgeon will be forced to engage a multigenerational team and optimize performance from all members. "Teachers must avoid assuming that current learners will share the same learning style, goals, and interests they themselves had as learners a generation earlier" [48]. There may exist friction with leadership methods, time line of engagement, and purposing. The Millennial generation is comfortable with a team-based approach to problems and embraces a flat hierarchy. They may view the entire team as "surgeons" whether a third-year medical student, intern, fellow, or attending. Senior staff should anticipate being engaged by junior team members – a situation possibly unfamiliar in their personal experience. They must acknowledge differing perspectives and guide application of knowledge to facilitate effective learning. Both the Millennial and 2020 generations are considered "digital natives" having grown up with cellphones, digital learning tools, and near-continuous access to resources [49], as contrasted to older generations, "digital immigrants," that may be slower to adopt and less facile with technology. Within such a framework, this may translate into an expectation of 24/7 availability for guidance and education; thus it may be necessary to set limits on access.

This generation has a strong sense of interconnectedness, and the division of work and personal life is not as well-defined as in previous generations [48]. One prime example is the realm of social media. It is exciting to hear that *JAMA Surgery* reaches 60,000 individuals per week electronically with over 20,000 Twitter followers and 22,000 Facebook followers [50]. While social media platforms may allow the surgical community to connect and rapidly exchange information such as the International Hernia Collaborative on Facebook, there remains a real risk to the physician-patient relationship. Surgeons need to be cognizant of the pitfalls associated with social media and maintain the expected professional standards. Guidelines are available from multiple societies on what constitutes appropriate social media engagement, including protecting privacy, minimizing conflicts of interest, and avoiding defamatory or negative posting [51]. Concerns exist that, given the digital landscape, it is difficult for the younger generations to learn professional behavior. More than ever, modeling of appropriate physician-patient interaction, often through the apprenticeship model, is necessary to shape the next generation of surgeons. While this technique may lack the team dynamic the Millennial generation is comfortable with, it assuredly serves as a platform for mentoring/coaching to obtain clinical skills and knowledge [49]. The modern surgeon must create an effective team while overcoming these generational differences.

Disease-Based Management in a Multidisciplinary Team

The modern surgeon recognizes the poly-system impact of disease states and fosters the interaction of multiple team members to optimize care and outcomes.

"Working in teams does not come easily to physicians, who still often see themselves as heroic lone healers" [52]. The modern surgeon recognizes the limitations of physician autonomy and embraces a team approach to optimize disease management. In multiple conditions, a team approach is recognized to improve quality and outcomes. Team composition varies based upon the disease state and goals of care. For instance, a reduction of readmissions in chronic health conditions requires a team of allied health professionals. Geisinger Health System has had success in their efforts to reduce the number of readmissions through the use of care coordinators. These individuals create a therapeutic alliance between patients and their physicians to monitor post-discharge care. The physician's role in this team is to empower the care coordinators to reach out to patients, answer their questions, and forge a therapeutic alliance [52]. Similarly, oncology patients benefit from multidisciplinary tumor board-driven cancer care to ensure access to a range of specialists and enhance treatment decision-making. Recognize that the composition of this team will include more physician stakeholders (oncologic surgeons, radiation and medical oncologists). A recent study proposed a multifaceted instrument (ATLAS) to evaluate the leadership of a tumor board in major areas of care – case prioritization, establishing treatment plans, and conflict management [53]. Finally a multidisciplinary approach to trauma will incorporate therapists, case management, surgical specialists, and social service/outreach coordinators to optimize care and reduce recidivism. The modern surgeon must recognize the stakeholders in their unique multidisciplinary team and identify their common goals. They should be ready to engage and maximize the contribution of each and create an environment of collaboration.

Conclusion

The surgeon of the modern hospital will practice in an era of innovation, changing interpersonal dynamics and team-based care. As stated by Gloviczki, "Surgical innovations are essential to advance cost-effective care and shared decision making on adopting new therapies by an ethical surgeon, and a well informed patient is the cornerstone of ethical patient care" [38]. They will need to be adaptable as they pursue lifelong learning and professional development, reflecting on their weaknesses and seeking opportunities for improvement. The surgeon will encounter a patient population that is better informed and engaged in their care, requiring a collaborative approach. The modern surgeon will experience challenges but also great potential and opportunities.

References

1. American College of Surgeons comments on introduction of ensuring access to general surgery act. American College of Surgeons. 15 June 2017, www.facs.org/media/press-releases/2017/access061517.
2. Dill MJ. The state of the physician workforce. 4 Nov 2017, Presentation downloaded from www.aamc.org.
3. Ellison EC, Pawlik TM, Way DP, Satiani B, Williams TE. The impact of the aging population and incidence of cancer on future projections of general surgical workforce needs. Surgery. 2018;163:553–9.
4. Etzioni DA, Finlayson SR, Ricketts TC, Lynge DC, Dimick JB. Getting the science right on the surgeon workforce issue. Arch Surg. 2011;146(4):381–4.
5. Tierney J, Terhune K. Expanding the National Health Service Corps Scholarship Program to general surgery: a proposal to address the national shortage of general surgeons in the United States. JAMA Surg. 2017;152(4):315–6.
6. Grover K, Agarwal P, Agarwal N, Tabakin MD, Swan KG. Students to surgeons: increasing matriculation into surgical specialties. Surg Innov. 2016;23(6):623–34.
7. Mason BS, Ross W, Chambers MC, Grant R, Parks M. Pipeline program recruits and retains women and underrepresented minorities in procedure based specialties: a brief report. Am J Surg. 2017;213(4):662–5.
8. 2016 physician specialty data report. Association of American Medical Colleges. www.aamc.org/data/workforce/reports/457712/2016-specialty-databook.html. Accessed 1 Apr 2018.
9. Sirinek KR, Willis R, Stewart RM. Geographic maldistribution of general surgery PGY1 residents: another US surgical desert. Am J Surg. 2014;208(6):1023–8.
10. Khoushhal Z, Hussain MA, Greco E, Mamdani M, Verma S, Rotstein O, Tricco AC, Al-Omran M. Prevalence and causes of attrition among surgical residents. JAMA Surg. 2017;152(3):265–72.
11. Ableson JS, Sosa JA, Symer MM, Mao J, Michelassi F, Bell R, Sedrakyan A, Yeo HL. Association of expectations of training with attrition in general surgery residents. JAMA Surg. 2018;153:712; e-pub ahead of print.
12. Lynge DC, Larson EH, Thompson MJ, Rosenblatt RA, Hart LG. A longitudinal analysis of the general surgery workforce in the United States, 1981–2005. Arch Surg. 2008;143(4):345–50.
13. Khubchandani JA, Shen C, Ayturk D, Kiefe CI, Santry HP. Disparities in access to emergency general surgery care in the United States. Surgery. 2018;163:243–50.
14. Maykel JA. Leadership in surgery. Clin Colon Rectal Surg. 2013;26:254–8.
15. Statement on high-performance teams. American College of Surgeons. 1 Feb 2010, www.facs.org/about-acs/statements/66-high-performance-teams.
16. Ford K, Menchine M, Burner E, Arora S, Inaba K, Demetriades D, Yersin B. Leadership and teamwork in trauma and resuscitation. West J Emerg Med. 2016;17(5):549–56.
17. Stone JL, Aveling EL, Frean M, Shields MC, Wright C, Gino F, et al. Effective leadership of surgical teams: a mixed methods study of surgeon behaviors and functions. Ann Thorac Surg. 2017;104:530–7.
18. Jaffe GA, Pradarelli JC, Lemak CH, Mulholland MW, Dimick JB. Designing a leadership development program for surgeons. J Surg Res. 2016;200:53–8.
19. Hoyt DB, Ko CY. Optimal resources for surgical quality and safety. 1st ed. Chicago: American College of Surgeons; 2017.
20. Taylor K. Paternalism, participation and partnership – the evolution of patient centeredness in the consultation. Patient Educ Couns. 2009;74:150–5.
21. Holmström I, Röing M. The relation between patient-centeredness and patient empowerment: a discussion on concepts. Patient Educ Couns. 2010;79:167–72.
22. Kravitz RL, Melnikow J. Engaging patients in medical decision making. BMJ. 2001;323(7313):584–5.
23. Healy JM, Davis KA, Pei KY. Comparison of internal medicine and general surgery residents' assessments of risk of postsurgical complications in surgically complex patients. JAMA Surg. 2018;153(3):203–7.
24. Evers BM. The evolving role of the surgeon scientist. J Am Coll Surg. 2015;220(4):387–95.
25. Merani S, Switzer N, Kayssi A, Blitz M, Ahmed N, Shapiro AMJ. Research productivity of residents and surgeons with formal research training. J Surg Educ. 2014;71(6):865–70.
26. Brochu A, Aggarwal R. Research during general surgery residency: a Web-based review of opportunities, structure and outputs. J Surg Res. 2018;223:149–54.
27. Papasavas P, Filippa D, Reilly P, Chandawarkar R, Kirton O. Effect of a mandatory research requirement on categorical resident academic productivity in a university-based general surgery residency. J Surg Educ. 2013;70:715–9.
28. Hsieh H, Paquette F, Fraser SA, Feldman LS, Meterissian S, Fried GM, Bergman S. Formal research training during surgical residency: scaffolding for academic success. Am J Surg. 2014;207:141–5.
29. Grova MM, Yang AD, Humphries MD, Galante JM, Salcedo ES. Dedicated research time during

surgery residency leads to a significant decline in self-assessed clinical aptitude and surgical skills. J Surg Educ. 2017;74:980–5.
30. Suliburk JW, Kao LS, Kozar RA, Mercer DW. Training future surgical scientists. Ann Surg. 2008;247:741–9.
31. Valsangkar NP, Kays JK, Feliciano DV, Martin PJ, Parett JS, Joshi MM, et al. The impact of members of the Society of University Surgeons on the scholarship of American surgery. Surgery. 2016;160:47–53.
32. Valsangkar NP, Milgrom DP, Martin PJ, Parett JS, Joshi MM, Zimmers TA, Koniaris LG. The positive association of Association for Academic Surgery membership with academic productivity. J Surg Res. 2016;205:163–8.
33. Mansukhani NA, Patti MG, Kibbe MR. Rebranding "the lab years" as "professional development" in order to redefine the modern surgeon scientist. Ann Surg. 2017;266:937–8.
34. Riskin DJ, Longaker MT, Gertner M, Krummel TM. Innovation in surgery: a historical perspective. Ann Surg. 2006;244:686–93.
35. Buschemeyer WC, Cunningham DK, Edwards MJ. Surgical training and implementation of emerging surgical technologies. Am J Surg. 2005;190:166–72.
36. Pradarelli JC, Thornton JP, Dimick JB. Who is responsible for the safe introduction of new surgical technology? An important legal precedent from the da Vinci surgical system trials. JAMA Surg. 2017;152(8):717–8.
37. Stefanidis D, Fanelli RD, Price R, Richardson W. SAGES guidelines for the introduction of new technology and techniques. Surg Endosc. 2014;28:2257–71.
38. Gloviczki P. ESVS volodos lecture: innovations and the hippocratic oath. Eur J Vasc Endovasc Surg. 2018;55(5):605–13.
39. Exam pass rates. American Board of Surgery. www.absurgery.org/default.jsp?statgeneral. Accessed 1 Apr 2018.
40. Jones DB, Stefanidis D, Korndorffer JR, Dimick JB, Jacob BP, Schultz L, Scott DJ. SAGES University MASTERS Program: a structured curriculum for life-long learning. Surg Endosc. 2017;31:3061–71.
41. Greenberg CC, Ghousseini HN, Pavuluri Quamme SR, Beasley HL, Frasier LL, Brys NA, et al. A statewide surgical coaching program provides opportunity for continuous professional development. Ann Surg. 2018;267:868–73.
42. Statement on diversity. American College of Surgeons. 1 Jan 2018, www.facs.org/about-acs/statements/104-diversity.
43. French JC, O'Rourke C, Walsh RM. A current assessment of diversity characteristics and perceptions of their importance in the surgical workforce. J Gastrointest Surg. 2014;18:1936–43.
44. Zhuge Y, Kaufman J, Simeone DM, Chen H, Velazquez OC. Is there still a glass ceiling for women in academic surgery? Ann Surg. 2011;253:637–43.
45. Lillemoe KD. Surgical mentorship: a great tradition, but can we do better for the next generation. Ann Surg. 2017;266:401–10.
46. Walsh RM, Jeyarajah DR, Matthews JB, Telem D, Hawn MT, Michelassi F, Reid-Lomardo KM. White Paper: SSAT commitment to workforce diversity and healthcare disparities. J Gastrointest Surg. 2016;20:79–84.
47. Waljee JF, Chopra V, Saint S. Mentoring millennials. JAMA. 2018;319(15):1547–8.
48. Roberts DH, Newman LR, Schwartzstein RM. Twelve tips for facilitating Millennials' learning. Med Teach. 2012;34:274–8.
49. DiLullo C, McGee P, Kriebel RM. Demystifying the Millennial student: a reassessment in measure of character and engagement in professional education. Anat Sci Educ. 2011;4:214–26.
50. Kibbe MR. JAMA surgery – the year in review, 2017. JAMA Surg. 2018;153:405–6. e-published March 21, 2018.
51. Logghe HJ, Boeck MA, Gusani NJ, Hardaway JC, Hughes KA, Mouawad NJ, et al. Best practices for surgeons' social media use: statement of the Resident and Associate Society of the American College of Surgeons. J Am Coll Surg. 2018;226(3):317–27.
52. Lee TH. Turning doctors into leaders. Harv Bus Rev. 2010;88(4):50–8.
53. Jalil R, Soukup T, Akhter W, Sevdalis N, Green JSA. Quality of leadership in multidisciplinary cancer tumor boards: development and evaluation of a leadership assessment instrument (ATLAS). World J Urol. 2018;36(7):1031–8; E-pub ahead of print Mar 3, 2018.

30 The Solo Surgeon in the Modern Hospital

James A. Unti

The Changing Physician Practice Landscape

Recent decades have born witness to a dramatic transition in the practice patterns of physicians and surgeons in the United States [1, 2]. This transition has been significant, and one observer has described it as the "quiet revolution" in healthcare [3]. Not only have both medical doctors and surgical specialists been leaving their private practices to become employees of hospitals at an increasing rate, newly minted physicians are choosing the employed model of practice with greater and greater frequency [4].

Healthcare is undergoing many changes, and one of the most dominant themes is the consolidation and integration of delivery systems within the marketplace. The drivers behind these changes are definitely multifactorial. They include changes in healthcare policy, technological advancements, and the belief that patient care and overall safety are enhanced both by facilitated teamwork among providers and better coordination in the delivery processes themselves [5]. But at their core, the primary drivers are economic ones [6]. And despite the changes that have occurred so far, cost containment has been elusive, and current trends in healthcare delivery may still price the system as we know it out of existence [7].

The solo surgeon and small two-to-three surgeon private practice groups have been the bedrock of surgical practice since the late nineteenth century. Within the new world of health system consolidation, however, many questions about surgeons and their private practice situations increasingly arise. Smaller groups – and the solo surgeon in particular – are increasingly finding themselves in precarious situations. Changing payor reimbursement models are leaving them with little negotiating leverage, and with the passing of time, many are finding it difficult to survive [8].

One concern is the practice situation of the solo surgeon. Can the solo practicing surgeon survive in the evolving healthcare marketplace? Should the solo surgeon survive? What value does the solo surgeon bring to the hospital in the evolving "value-based" healthcare system? What particular value, if any, does the solo surgeon bring to the care of his or her patients? All of these questions are legitimate ones to ask, and similarly, they all deserve legitimate answers.

In 2010, The Physicians Foundation, with the assistance of Merritt Hawkins and an advisory panel of healthcare experts, published a white paper that examined the effects of the recently passed Patient Protection and Affordable Care Act (ACA) on physician practices [9]. The experts concluded that the legislation would "usher in substantive and lasting changes" and

J. A. Unti (✉)
Department of Surgery, Saint Joseph Hospital, Chicago, IL, USA

R. Latifi (ed.), *The Modern Hospital*, https://doi.org/10.1007/978-3-030-01394-3_30

that the "independent, private practice model will be largely, though not uniformly, replaced." They observed that individual practitioners and physicians in smaller groups would find it necessary either to consolidate, become hospital employees, or align with large hospitals and health systems in order to survive. They would need to do so for capital support, administrative assistance, and access to technical resources. Interestingly, the paper also concluded that healthcare reform would likely exacerbate physician shortages, not resolve the long-standing physician maldistribution problem, and because of increased reporting and tracking demands in an environment of high potential liability and problematic reimbursement, physicians would be placed under ever increasing stress.

In the early days of modern medicine, hospitals were places where people went to die. The predecessors of modern hospitals were almshouses and infirmaries. Likewise, the physician was typically a solo practitioner. To earn a living, he would travel to see patients in their homes. His office had the most basic equipment, his medical armamentarium was quite limited, and there were no third-party payors. He was paid in cash or would trade for his services. Unlike those early days, modern hospitals are complex, highly technical environments in which patients receive numerous types of sophisticated, life-saving care, and doctors' practices have become integrated into virtually all of their most important operations.

Initially, when the transition to the modern-day environment first began, physicians saw hospitals as an extension of their offices [10]. They formed useful associations with them but remained largely independent in their practice situations. Doctors were in possession of the essential scientific knowledge, and it was through their resultant cultural authority that they could do so. They admitted patients to hospitals and utilized their services, and as a result they helped hospitals generate their revenues. As time progressed and capabilities expanded, doctors began to share their authority with the hospitals within the community. Physicians were quite busy taking care of patients and overseeing clinical matters, and hospital administrators increasingly began to address external community healthcare needs. A relationship evolved in which hospitals would provide the places, technologies, and support staff for physicians to treat their patients, and in return, physicians would serve in non-paid (or minimally paid) medical staff governance positions and on various hospital oversight committees. This relationship, while generally harmonious, was also kept at arm's length because the hospital's and the medical staff's objectives were not always completely aligned [11]. The result was that in general, progress was made, but services were delivered in disorganized ways.

Another part of the problem was the financing system employed by third-party payors. The 1930s saw the rise of third-party payors, and the financing system set in motion at the time had far-reaching consequences that persist to this day. Hospitals and doctors were paid separately by insurers, and both were paid retrospectively for usual and customary charges without any cost-containment incentives. Medicare, which began in 1965, adopted the same reimbursement approach as the private insurers with its separate part A (hospital) and part B (physician) payment structure. By 1982, the majority – 54% – of all personal healthcare spending was paid for by private and public insurance means, and this financing system, together with scientific and technological advancements, fueled the exorbitant rise in healthcare costs [12]. Without any cost-containment incentives in place, the more services that doctors and hospitals provided, the more they billed, and the more they billed, the more they got paid. It isn't hard to see that left unchecked, one day overwhelming costs would threaten the sustainability of the entire system. Various attempts by policymakers to alter this trajectory, including Medicare's Prospective Payment System (PPS) with its diagnostic-related groups (DRGs), and the subsequent rate-setting resource-based relative value scale (RBRVS) mechanism failed to reign in healthcare spending.

The New Era of Healthcare Financing

Now let's turn to the current period, ushered in by the passage of the Patient Protection and Affordable Care Act. The Act, signed into law in 2010, expanded the Centers for Medicare and Medicaid Services' (CMS) authority to develop alternative payment models [13]. The framework it authorized was oriented around two goals: reduce costs and improve the quality of patient care. As "value-based" models of care delivery were being developed, they focused on advancing the triple aim of providing better care for individuals, improving population health management, and reducing healthcare costs [14, 15]. They centered on patient outcomes and how well providers could improve quality based on specific measures, such as reducing hospital readmissions, implementing the use of certified health information systems, and improving preventative care [16].

The ACA legislation included numerous provisions designed to transform the system away from the traditional, fragmented fee-for-service model toward one of more efficient, coordinated care. It provided grants to assess community-based Patient-Centered Medical Homes with the hope that a more team-based approach would improve care coordination, a hospital readmissions reduction program with reduced payments for various potentially preventable hospital readmissions, payment reductions for several potentially avoidable hospital-acquired conditions, and, importantly, the development of Accountable Care Organizations (ACOs). ACOs would require redesigning care processes, making them much more vertically integrated [17]. The hope was that with better coordination, clinical care processes would become much more efficient, much less redundant, and therefore much more cost-effective. Such improvements would lead to overall better healthcare delivery.

Most of the cost savings was expected to come from hospitals, but reimbursements would be restructured through a shared savings program that encompassed primary care physicians as well as specialists [18]. Importantly, viewing the traditional fee-for-service reimbursement framework as one of the main drivers of costs, bundled payment programs would be piloted and eventually put into place [19].

In 2011, the CMS Innovation Center introduced the Bundled Payments for Care Improvement (BPCI) initiative [20]. In its purest form, doctors and hospitals would receive bundled payments for selected services based on "episodes of care" with hopefully better aligned incentives covering the whole spectrum of care delivery [21]. A bundled episode of care payment would include all of the services provided to a patient during the acute hospitalization period as well as all related services for periods up to 90 days after hospital discharge. Providers would be collectively reimbursed for the expected costs to treat each specific condition. Both doctors and hospitals would need to reduce costs together in order to increase margins on their reimbursements. Implementation of the BPCI initiative increased pressure on both doctors and hospitals in two major ways. First, it increased the risks of financial loss by imposing financial penalties, and second, it increased the costs of compliance by requiring the reengineering of patient care processes.

In 2015, the Medicare Access and CHIP (Children's Health Insurance Program) Reauthorization Act (MACRA) was signed into law. This legislation resulted in CMS combining several distinct programs – the Physician Quality Reporting System (PQRS), the Value-Based Payment Modifier (VBM), and the electronic health record (EHR) incentive program into one single program called the Merit-Based Incentive Payment System, or "MIPS" [22]. Under this merit-based system, a composite performance score would be developed, and eligible providers would receive either a payment bonus, a payment penalty, or no payment adjustment at all depending on how well they succeeded in meeting certain "quality" metrics. The composite performance score would be based on four performance categories: quality, resource use, clinical practice improvement activities, and the meaningful use of certified electronic health records technology. By early 2017, the MIPS program was up and running, and eligible providers had to start providing annual reports on metrics in each of these four performance categories.

The major needs by hospitals today are to both increase (or at least maintain) their financial reimbursements and reduce their potential risks for financial loss. The primary strategy to do so is to capture as broad a patient base as possible and improve all patient care processes. They have no choice but to purchase and implement the health information systems with which to capture and report on all of the various performance and quality metrics mandated by the MIPS legislation. And they have no choice but to integrate, continually review, and optimize all of their patient care activities. To be highly successful, they need to control as many external facets of the care delivery process as possible, including practitioner services, outpatient care, and post-hospitalization patient management [23].

In this new environment, physician groups that have a larger patient base are more attractive to hospitals. Because of their larger size, they also have greater leverage and are in a better position to negotiate more favorable terms. Thus, the impetus for hospitals to buy physician practices and make doctors employees has blossomed.

Navigating Through the Process

For the time being, many physician groups, including smaller groups and specialists, have been able to navigate through the initial phases of these changes and maintain their independence by contracting with hospital systems as "in-network" providers. Physicians and hospitals in the 1990s formed Physician-Hospital Organizations (PHOs) and other networks in order to better contract with third-party payors, accepting decreased payments for services in exchange for guaranteed access to certain patient populations. As time passed many of these PHOs underwent a metamorphosis, becoming structures that are now recognizable as ACOs. During this process, shared control moved away from physicians and toward hospital administrators, but independent physicians and physician groups who were already part of the system could participate as long as they would meet all of the newly mandated performance metrics.

Here is where smaller physician groups, and especially solo practitioners, are encountering their greatest difficulties today. Clearly each physician practice is in its own unique situation, and by no means are they all uniform. Any individual practice may have circumstances that are different from others. But, by and large, many are finding it impossible to survive in the new environment because the burdens they face are increasingly overwhelming them. The major burdens physicians face today are twofold: financial and administrative. Both are substantial. They have little to do with the art and science of delivering good medical care. They have everything to do with achieving and maintaining compliance with all of the reporting requirements and with getting reimbursed fairly for the services provided. Physicians must be able to capture and report on a whole host of data points, and smaller practices and solo practitioners are finding that meeting these goals is becoming a financial and administrative nightmare [24].

Part of the financial burden stems from the considerable costs of implementing, maintaining, and upgrading EHR systems and other administrative information technologies. Unfortunately, many of the available systems are viewed as being quite suboptimal from the clinician's perspective. Other financial burdens arise from the increased costs of redesigning office-based patient care processes as well as the increased staffing costs associated with the time commitments and resources necessary to navigate through all of the ongoing changes. Often, outside consulting advice is necessary to ensure that compliance is proper and correct. Interestingly, despite all of the new policies and programs being put in place, the cost of healthcare continues to rise in America. According to a new (2018) survey by the West Health Institute in La Jolla, California, and the non-partisan and objective research organization NORC at the University of Chicago, 44% of Americans didn't go see a physician last year when they were sick or injured because of increased out-of-pocket costs [25]. Thus, not only are overall practice costs continuing to rise, higher patient out-of-pocket expenses are affecting physician practices financially in a negative way as well because patients are choosing not to seek the healthcare that they otherwise would.

Complicated administrative processes are causing major headaches too. A major concern pertains to the EHR itself. There are many benefits to the use of EHRs, but in truth, most of them don't function optimally for the practitioner [26]. On the front end, most of them appear to be designed for hospitals and hospital systems and how these systems are designed to capture data rather than for how doctors and other practitioners actually take care of patients. The quality of smaller systems designed with the practitioner's office in mind is variable, and determining which one is best for any given practitioner can be a costly and difficult task. Each system seems to have its positive and negative attributes, and changing from one to another is not always a straightforward, easy task. It is true that EHRs can facilitate information retrieval, but using them the way they are constructed can be more of a time-consuming burden for physicians than a facilitator of clinical patient care. A proper design would enhance practitioners' capabilities, making them more efficient. They would not be a time-consuming burden that detracts from patient care interactions.

Another administrative nightmare relates to third-party payors [27, 28]. Most working people receive health insurance coverage through their employers. While larger employers may self-insure their employees, most employers contract with any one of several commercial insurers, with or without benefit plan administrators. Although relatively small in number, third-party payors have many different types of plans with many different degrees of coverage. These plans have different premium, co-pay, and deductible amounts and may have benefits that are either unrestricted or restricted to "in-network" providers. The financing system has become so big and confusing that at times it seems to have taken on a life of its own. It is so confusing that often the consumer – and the provider as well – can't clearly decipher exactly what services are covered and how much will be paid under the plan they have chosen. If a consumer has insurance coverage that limits payments to a certain healthcare network and mistakenly receives care from an out-of-network provider, he or she could be faced with a very large bill despite the fact that all premiums have been properly paid. The same thing could happen if required authorization for certain services wasn't properly obtained ahead of time. These situations create a great deal of anxiety and tremendous amounts of paperwork for both consumers and providers, none of which is improving quality in healthcare delivery. Both hospitals and physician practices have had to employ full-time staff just to deal with this financing mess. Doctors, for the most part, have shielded themselves from directly dealing with these third-party payor issues by hiring personnel whose jobs are solely devoted to doing so. As a result, most of them don't even have a full appreciation for what it really takes to navigate through the system – making lengthy back and forth phone calls, forwarding clinical documents, obtaining authorizations for referrals and pre-authorizations for procedures, addressing and readdressing payment denials, submitting and resubmitting billing codes, etc. If doctors had to address these matters personally, they wouldn't have time to take care of their patients. It is the smaller groups – and especially the solo practitioner – that have suffered most from these administrative demands because they simply don't have the resources to deal with them.

So, the amount of time that a private practitioner spends each day actually taking care of patients is being squeezed by the amount of time required to address all of these administrative concerns. And day after day, the mandates and reporting requirements keep growing and growing. The unintended consequence is increasing physician dissatisfaction and burnout [29, 30]. Some physicians are retiring; others are seeking job opportunities outside of clinical medicine. Others are giving up their private practice situations completely to become hospital employees. Most solo physicians are finding it impossible to survive. Some surgical specialists have been able to survive independently so far, and several subspecialists in disciplines like orthopedic surgery, cardiothoracic surgery, urology, and others have banded together in different regions to form very large, market-dominating groups. These supergroups have been able to maintain a considerable amount of leverage.

General surgeons, because of the nature of their practices, have found it more difficult to do the same. Historically, any given hospital has had a relatively small number of general surgeons on its medical staff. The general surgeons would be in solo practice, or in one-, two-, or perhaps three- or four-surgeon groups. The surgeons would rotate emergency room call coverage, and each practice would have its own established primary care referral base. Surgeons could easily be on staff at more than one hospital, even if the hospitals were in different networks. Although these surgeons were collegial with each other and would readily support each other with call coverage, their small practices were in competition with each other as well, and banding together in business relationships was often more problematic.

Dedication, Pride, and Stress

The nature of the general surgeon's practice is such that in-hospital and emergency room consults are a frequent, daily occurrence. Attending to these consults in a timely manner is important because many of them are based on urgent or even emergent, potentially life-threatening conditions. Other surgical specialties function similarly, but to varying degrees depending on the particular specialty. Besides scheduled office and clinic visits and scheduled surgical cases, unscheduled hospital or emergency room consults and resultant unscheduled surgical procedures are the norm. More often than not, the workday of the general surgeon doesn't end up the way it originally was scheduled when the day began. Attending to urgent and emergent clinical cases on top of scheduled activities by itself is an inherent cause of stress in the life of the surgeon, and this stress is increased further if an unscheduled patient's case happens to be a life-threatening one.

Furthermore, disruptions in work schedules don't happen in a vacuum. They create all kinds of logistical disruptions on the operating room schedule that can permeate the entire system. These ramifications can impact completely unrelated patients and their families, other surgeons and ancillary personnel, and operating room staffing. All of these factors add up to relatively long workdays and workweeks and higher degrees of stress. This environment is the baseline norm in the general surgeon's line of work.

Admittedly, even with the stresses noted above, the typical surgeon will say that the rewards are substantial, both personally and professionally, and that they greatly outweigh any of the less desirable aspects of the job. There is something noble about the profession, and most surgeons don't mind the long, erratic hours or the added efforts needed to keep abreast of new technologies and developments. With the goal of doing one's best and helping each patient to the best of his or her ability, committing the time and participating in continuing medical education activities are part of the surgeon's life. Patients who allow surgeons to operate on them place their lives in the surgeon's hands, and all dedicated surgeons take this privilege seriously. The traditional culture instilled by the profession from its earliest days is that the surgeon does whatever it takes, irrespective of the time of the day or the day of the week, to provide the necessary care to the patient. Part of the culture has been that surgeons do not abandon their patients. Thus, in terms of putting in the required time, doing their jobs well, working toward optimal surgical outcomes, and maintaining an up-to-date knowledge base, dedicated surgeons take considerable pride in their work. However, when one adds to these professional demands, (1) the litany of financial and administrative burdens involved in reengineering ancillary delivery care processes, (2) the mandated reporting of all of the "quality" and performance metrics, and (3) the time-consuming interactions necessary to navigate through the dysfunctional third-party payor financing system, the general surgeon in private practice is increasingly being pushed toward the breaking point [31, 32].

A special mention must be made for solo surgeons who practice in a rural setting, especially if there is only one general surgeon available in any given geographic area. In such cases, it may be possible for a solo general surgeon to survive because the hospital may be so in need of his or her services that the hospital's administration may make an offer with very favorable practice conditions and support. But even in these situations, today hospital administrators are increasingly likely to offer an employed-physician status [33, 34].

Toward Hospital Employment

Let's look at some of the benefits of becoming a hospital-employed general surgeon vis-a-vis the advantages of this model over the solo practitioner one. The employed surgeon doesn't have to deal with the myriad of business elements of running an office practice. The surgeon in this situation doesn't have to hire and train office staff; negotiate wages and benefits; evaluate workers and either retain or replace them; hire an answering service; hire a billing service; pay office rent; pay for phone service; maintain office and other medical equipment; buy office supplies; submit billing codes and collect payments; appeal payment denials; interact with third-party payors; purchase, implement, and maintain certified EHR systems; track quality metrics; improve performance processes; collect data and report on them; or pay for professional liability insurance, not to mention the scheduling of patients, obtaining appropriate referrals, obtaining appropriate pre-authorizations, etc. All of these things (and more) are typical elements of running a private practice. Even though most practices have an office manager, the physician-owner is still ultimately responsible. For the employed physician, most (if not all) of these elements are handled by hospital personnel.

Other benefits include possible signing bonuses, salary guarantees, ensured vacations, time off for continuing medical education activities, and easier access to an immediate patient base. Surgeons are guaranteed to receive the same salary check every two-to-four weeks, which is perhaps the primary reason to be employed. The risk of revenue generation is assumed by the organization. In many cases, the salary exceeds what the surgeon can actually make, but the hospital accepts this loss in lieu of the overall revenue gain that they receive from the associated services that the surgeon generates. Younger surgeons entering the workforce are increasingly finding this employment model attractive, anticipating that their lifestyles will likely be better. The guaranteed salary offers an increased sense of security as well, especially if the new surgeon is starting out with a high level of education-related debt [35].

But like anything else, there are aspects of being hospital-employed that may be negative for the surgeon, and they may not be so readily discernable at first look [36, 37]. Hospitals and surgeons may not always agree on policy matters, for example, or on the way some patient care measures are implemented, or on capital expenditures regarding the purchases of instruments and supplies. To be fair, these kinds of issues are not unique to hospital-employed surgeons – they occur in all businesses in other sectors of the economy and even in physician group practices that utilize junior surgeons as salaried employees. For years there have been environments in which solo surgeons dominated the marketplaces, and they worked against each other as often as with each other, fighting change and grumbling about bureaucracy. The truth is that conditions can vary wildly depending on the personalities of the physicians and administrators involved and the particular culture of an institution.

Surgeons traditionally do not receive training in the business aspects of medicine, and care must be taken when signing employment contracts. Exact means of dispute resolution must be known, and termination and exit conditions must be clarified up front. Exit planning is perhaps the most important issue for the surgeon to address when thinking about becoming an employee. It is not uncommon for doctors, both surgeons and primary care physicians, to leave their first job after just a couple of years. An orthopedic and spine surgeon article published in 2012 noted that approximately 70–80% of young surgeons leave their first job within two years of practice [38]. Therefore, all areas of the employment contract need to be examined carefully by both the surgeon and his or her counsel.

There are other even more subtle aspects of becoming a hospital employee that can significantly impact the degree to which a surgeon may or may not find job satisfaction [39]. It is not uncommon to find that the individuals that execute the employment contract are not the same individuals that carry them out, and without proper documentation, surgeons may find themselves in compromised situations. Surgeons, by their training (and by their nature), tend to be proactive rather than passive individuals. They lean toward greater control of their environments. Shouldering immense responsibility for the successful execution of many fine-tuned surgical procedures, they have to be oriented this way. They are taught to gather information efficiently, make timely assessments, and act expeditiously if necessary. They strive for both accuracy and precision. The question is: Does the hospital-employer truly value these traits? The employed surgeon will likely lose some control in many day-to-day activities. Some real-world, significant questions are: Will the surgeons have viable decision-making capability in regard to what equipment can or cannot be used for their patients? Will they have a credible say in what technologies may or may not be used? Will they be able to determine where they can send their patients for therapy or other ancillary services? Perhaps the biggest negative for the employed surgeon – one that has caused the solo surgeon to remain in solo practice for as long as possible – is this loss of autonomy.

Paradoxically, some forms of administrative bureaucracy will likely be greater in the hospital-employed environment. Large institutions of all kinds tend to be filled with bureaucracies and inefficiencies that can be problematic for the surgeon. In large, integrated healthcare systems, real decision-makers are often removed from the local site, and they may be hard to reach in a timely manner. As part of a large organization, employed surgeons may find that what would be a simple process for the private practitioner can be a lengthy, complex one inside the system. A basic request, for example, may require the completion of multiple forms, the involvement of many people, and passage through multiple bureaucratic layers before any resolution is achieved. The process could take months instead of days.

Also, paradoxically, by becoming employed, surgeons may think that they are being freed up from the business management side of practice and that they will have more time to dedicate to patient care. But they may find that this circumstance is not necessarily the case. Many hospital administrators and managers lacking in clinical experience don't necessarily have a thorough understanding of what surgeons do and what their needs really are. They don't necessarily know the intricacies involved in optimal patient management, and they may be more likely to misallocate vital resources. An article in American Medical News in 2013 noted that out of all the hospitals rated for both economic efficiency and clinically effective care by the Centers for Medicare and Medicaid Services (using 12 measures of clinical care, patient satisfaction, and readmission rates), nine out of the ten best hospitals were physician-owned [40]. Employed surgeons may find themselves spending a great deal more time sitting on committees, advisory boards, and tasks forces than they initially had imagined, and they may not have as much time to focus on patient care as they had anticipated.

One of the real consequences of giving up a private practice and becoming an employed surgeon is the loss of authority over staff and other ancillary associates in the workplace. Independent surgeons have the ability to determine who they want to hire and who they want to let go. Choosing the right staff can lead to a positive, functional workplace environment, and working together with highly competent staff can be extremely rewarding. The true worth of working alongside dedicated, hardworking associates is immeasurable. It makes all the difference in the world and is one of those intangibles that greatly impacts the degree to which true job satisfaction is achieved. If employed surgeons have no control over their office management staff, their coworkers and their medical assistants, they may encounter any number of disheartening problems. The office personnel of the hospital-employed surgeon may not perform at levels desired by the surgeon.They may not be as dedicated or as willing to work as hard as the surgeon would like. They may not be motivated to "go that extra mile" or "stay a little later" to be certain that all clinical work is completed in the most timely, efficient manner. For the surgeon who takes pride in delivering the best care possible, these kinds of situations can be frustrating.

For the newly minted general surgeon who has never known a high degree of autonomy, however, the loss of this type of authority may not be an important issue. This younger surgeon may prefer a more balanced lifestyle with more regular working hours compared to those experienced by past generations [41]. Such an orientation actually may be healthier in the long run. Whether preferred or not, changes in training philosophy with mandated work hour restrictions are the norm today, fostered by the belief that fewer medical errors will be made if imposed limits are placed on the duration that residents can participate in clinical activities over any given period of time [42]. Younger physicians are training in a shiftwork environment and therefore they are more likely to embrace it [43]. The question is: Will the newer generation of surgeons be as prepared as they should be to meet the needs of their patients? Will they be willing to "go the extra mile" themselves for their patients when situations demand that they do so?

The Question of Survival

So, the question resurfaces: Does the solo surgeon bring value to the modern hospital? The answer is yes. A good solo surgeon who is a genuine professional – one who is collegial and truly dedicated to the care of his or her patients, has both an excellent bedside manner and highly developed technical skills, and is a team player interested in improving healthcare delivery – brings tremendous value to the modern hospital. The problem in the modern healthcare environment has nothing to with the capabilities of the solo surgeon; rather, it has everything to do with the overbearing demands of the new regulatory environment. They are becoming too costly and burdensome for the solo surgeon to survive.

In the end, if current trends continue, the solo surgeon will become extinct. But here is where attitude is important [44]. The profession of surgery is not being threatened, just the traditional platform upon which it is being practiced. For the foreseeable future, human beings will still need surgery, and an interest in the profession and in what surgeons are capable of doing will remain very much alive. There will always be opportunity for the capable surgeon who is interested in helping people.

Evolution is a continuous process, and there will always be something else that follows what is coming next. Change is the constant [45]. Although change can be difficult, it can be made easier by adjusting one's attitude. Although not all change is truly for the better, trying to make it better can be a very rewarding endeavor by itself. William Edwards Deming (1900–1993) was one of the world's most widely respected business advisors and management consultants. He was recognized as a distinguished author, engineer, statistician and teacher, and along with others he helped pioneer transformational advancements in production by applying innovative concepts in quality control and cost reduction. A popular quote often attributed to him may be fitting here: "It is not necessary to change. Survival is not mandatory"[46]. The truth is that more apropos words have never been spoken. Present-day solo surgeons don't have to change their practice situations. Some of them may survive. Many likely won't. But the choice is theirs.

References

1. Isaacs L, Jellinek PS, Walker R. The independent physician. Going, going.... N Engl J Med. 2009;360(7):655–7.
2. Japsen B. Feel like selling your practice? you're not alone. Chic Med. 2018;121(5):17–20. http://www.cmsdocs.org/news-publications/chicago-medicine-magazine/2018-issues/May2018Issue.pdf. Accessed 4 June 2018.
3. Harris G. More doctors giving up private practices. NY Times. 2010. https://nytimes.com/2010/03/26/health/policy/26docs.html. Accessed 21 May 2018.

4. Charles AG, et al. The employed surgeon. A changing paradigm. JAMA Surg. 2013;148(4):323–8.
5. Frenk J. Reinventing primary health care: the need for systems integration. Lancet. 2009;374:170–3.
6. Porter ME, Kaplan RS. How to pay for health care. Bundled payments will finally unleash the competition that patients want. Harv Bus Rev. 2016:88–100. https://hbr.org/2016/07/how-to-pay-for-health-care. Accessed 8 May 2018.
7. Centers for Medicare & Medicaid Services. CMS.gov. Historical. Retrieved from: https://www.cms.gov/Research-Statistics-Data-and-Systems/Statistics-Trends-and-Reports/NationalHealthExpendData/NationalHealthAccountsHistorical.html. Accessed 6 May 2018.
8. Ruggieri PA. The solo general surgeon is a dying breed. What is next? http://skepticalscalpel.blogspot.com/2014/08/the-solo-general-surgeon-dying-breed.html. Accessed 8 May 2018.
9. The Physicians Foundation. Health reform and the decline of physician private practice. 2010. https://physiciansfoundation.org/wp-content/uploads/2018/02/Health_Reform_and_the_Decline_of_Physician_Private_Practice.pdf. Accessed 8 May 2018.
10. Starr P. The social transformation of medicine. New York: Basic Books; 1982. p. 178.
11. Crosson F, Tollen L, editors. Partners in health – how physicians and hospitals can be accountable together, vol. 20. San Francisco: Jossey-Bass; 2010.
12. Crosson F, Tollen L, editors. Partners in health – how physicians and hospitals can be accountable together, vol. 73. San Francisco: Jossey-Bass; 2010.
13. Henry J Kaiser Family Foundation. Summary of the affordable care act. 2013. https://www.kff.org/health-reform/fact-sheet/summary-of-the-affordable-care-act/. Accessed 9 May 2018.
14. Centers for Medicare & Medicaid Services. CMS.gov. What are the value-based programs? Retrieved from: https://www.cms.gov/medicare/quality-initiatives-patient-assessment-instruments/value-based-programs/value-based-programs.html. Accessed 9 May 2018.
15. NEJM Catalyst. What is value-based healthcare? January 1st, 2017. Retrieved from: https://catalyst.nejm.org/what-is-value-based-healthcare/. Accessed 21 May 2018.
16. RevCycle Intelligence. What is value-based care, what it means for providers? Retrieved from: https://revcycleintelligence.com/features/what-is-value-based-care-what-it-means-for-providers. Accessed 23 May 2018.
17. Kocher R, Sahni NR. Physicians versus hospitals as leaders of accountable care organizations. N Engl J Med. 2010;363(27):2579–82.
18. Mehrotra A, Hussey P. Including physicians in bundled hospital care payments – time to revisit an old idea? JAMA. 2015;313(19):1907–8.
19. Hackbarth G, Reischauer R, Mutti A. Collective accountability for medical care – toward bundled medicare payments. N Engl J Med. 2008;359(1):3–5.
20. Press MJ, Rajkumar R, Conway PH. Medicare's new bundled payments: design, strategy and evolution. JAMA. 2016;315(2):131–2.
21. Hardin L, Kilian A, Murphy E. Bundled payments for care improvement – preparing for the medical diagnosis-related groups. J Nurs Adm. 2017;46(6):313–9.
22. American College of Physicians (ACP). MACRA and the quality payment program. Retrieved from: https://www.acponline.org/practice-resources/business-resources/payment/medicare/macra. Accessed 23 May 2018.
23. Brown B Crapo J. The key to transitioning from fee-for-service to value-based reimbursement. 2017. https://www.healthcatalyst.com/hospital-transitioning-fee-for-service-value-based-reimbursements. Accessed 26 May 2018.
24. McCaughey B. Death by paperwork. 2014. http://humanevents.com/2014/07/09/death-by-paperwork/. Accessed 3 May 2018.
25. Westhealth. New survey finds large number of people skipping necessary medical care because of cost. Retrieved from: https://www.westhealth.org/press-release/survey2018/. Accessed 3 June 2018.
26. Verghese A. How tech can turn doctors into clerical workers. The New York Times. May 16, 2018. Retrieved from: https://www.nytimes.com/interactive/2018/05/16/magazine/health-issue-what-we-lose-with-data-driven-medicine.html. Accessed 4 June 2018.
27. Robert Wood Johnson Foundation. What are the costs to physicians of administrative complexity in their interactions with payers? HCFO Find Brief. 2010;13(2):1–3.
28. Mazzolini C. Keeping payers, other third parties from interfering with patient care. Med Econ 2018. http://www.medicaleconomics.com/payers/keeping-payers-other-third-parties-interfering-patient-care. Accessed 5 May 2018.
29. Valentine RJ. The hidden cost of medicine. J Am Coll Surg. 2016;225(1):1–8.
30. Robb MJA. Fulfillment vs. burnout. J Am Phys Surg. 2017;22(4):101–4.
31. Squiers JJ, et al. Physician burnout: are we treating the symptoms instead of the disease? Ann Thorac Surg. 2017;104:1117–22.
32. DeCaporale-Ryan L, et al. The undiagnosed pandemic: burnout and depression within the surgical community. Curr Prob Surg. 2017;54:453–502.
33. Barr P. Looking for an oasis; large sections of rural America continue to suffer from a drought of general surgeons. Mod Healthc. 2012;42(13):28.
34. Jarman BT, et al. Factors correlated with surgery resident choice to practice general surgery in a rural area. J Surg Ed. 2009;66(6):319–24.

35. Leichtle SW, Hartin CW Jr. Physician leadership and the future of surgical practice. Bull Am Coll Surg. 2012;97(5):15–9.
36. Copeland EM III. Surgeons as employees: is the lining always golden? Bull Am Coll Surg. 2014;99(1): 48–50.
37. Napolitano LM. Surgeons as hospital employees. Good, bad or indifferent? JAMA Surg. 2013;148(4):329–30.
38. Miller L. 25 Key concepts for young orthopedic and spine surgeons to build a successful practice. Becker's Spine Rev. 2012. https://www.beckersspine.com/spine/item/11832-25-key-concepts-for-young-orthopedic-spine-surgeons-to-build-a-successful-practice.html. Accessed 12 May 2018.
39. Heiney JP. An examination and discussion of unintended consequences of being an employed physician. J Orthop Trauma. 2013;27(10 Suppl):S17–21.
40. Henry T. Physician-owned hospitals seize their moment. Am Med News. 2013;56:5–6.
41. Jackson T, et al. The physician attrition crisis: a cross-sectional survey of the risk factors for reduced job satisfaction among US surgeons. World J Surg. 2018;42:1285–92.
42. MacMullin G. Resident work hour restrictions: balancing resident education and patient safety. DMJ. 2013;40(1):32–6.
43. Brooks JV, Bosk CL. Remaking surgical socialization: work hour restrictions, rites of passage, and occupational identity. Soc Sci & Med. 2012;75:1625–32.
44. Finnegan J. Independent physician practice survival: a doctor's story. [Q&A] Fierce Healthcare 2016. https://www.fiercehealthcare.com/practices/how-one-independent-physician-Practice-survives-and-thrives-today-s-healthcare. Accessed 3 May 2018.
45. Klasko S. Change is gonna come. Are physicians ready? Athenainsight 2017. https://www.athenahealth.com/insight/change-gonna-come-are-physicians-ready. Accessed 23 May 2018.
46. Graban M. Don't threaten people with this famous Dr. Deming quote. Mark Graban's Lean Blog. February 19, 2013. Retrieved from: https://www.leanblog.org/2013/02/dont-threaten-people-with-this-deming-quote/. Accessed 22 May 2018.

The Role of Hospitalists in a New Hospital: Physician's Perspective

31

Christopher Nabors, Stephen J. Peterson, and William H. Frishman

History of the Hospitalist Movement

In this chapter, we discuss the rise of the hospitalist movement. In the most fundamental sense, this model of patient care arose as a solution to pressures being brought to bear on internal medicine generalists. Those pressures were of two sorts – the first relating to the finite capacity of the human mind to attain skill and knowledge and the other relating to efficiency.

The traditional model of internal medicine practice long consisted of the physician managing a group of patients in the outpatient setting and when one of these patients developed an acute illness admitting them to a nearby hospital, where he or she directed their care through discharge. This approach had the advantages of the patient being able to derive emotional support from a well-known provider at each step of the process and the potential for excellent care, since relevant health information would likely be known to the provider. And because the same provider cared for the patient regardless of setting, there was no need for patient handoff or risk of information loss at care transitions.

In the late 1980s, the financial underpinnings of this system began to erode. Managed care firms established a foothold in the private insurance industry, and the federal government began to reimburse for hospitalizations under diagnostic-related groups. As a result, the clinician was pressured to be more efficient. This significantly discouraged travel between clinic and hospital. At the same time, with improvements in care and increases in the average life span, the complexity of patient care was also increasing. Accordingly, the practitioner's burden to keep current with the latest inpatient and outpatient practices became ever more challenging. This pressure encouraged specialization and separated general internists into those who focused mainly on outpatient practice and those who emphasized inpatient care (Fig. 31.1). By the early 1990s, general internists spent less than 10% of their time performing hospital care [2].

The pace of change varied throughout the United States, but practices in many areas felt the force of the new medical landscape. One of those places was Valhalla, New York. There at Westchester Medical Center (WMC) in 1995, a small group of internists was establishing a new practice to cover the internal medicine service of a county-funded, medical school-affiliated hospital. The experience of this group will be used to illustrate the major concerns of the practitioner and how these concerns shaped adaptations on the

C. Nabors · W. H. Frishman (✉)
Department of Medicine, Westchester Medical Center, New York Medical College, Valhalla, NY, USA
e-mail: william.frishman@nymc.edu

S. J. Peterson
Department of Medicine, New York Presbyterian Brooklyn Methodist Hospital, Brooklyn, NY, USA

R. Latifi (ed.), *The Modern Hospital*, https://doi.org/10.1007/978-3-030-01394-3_31

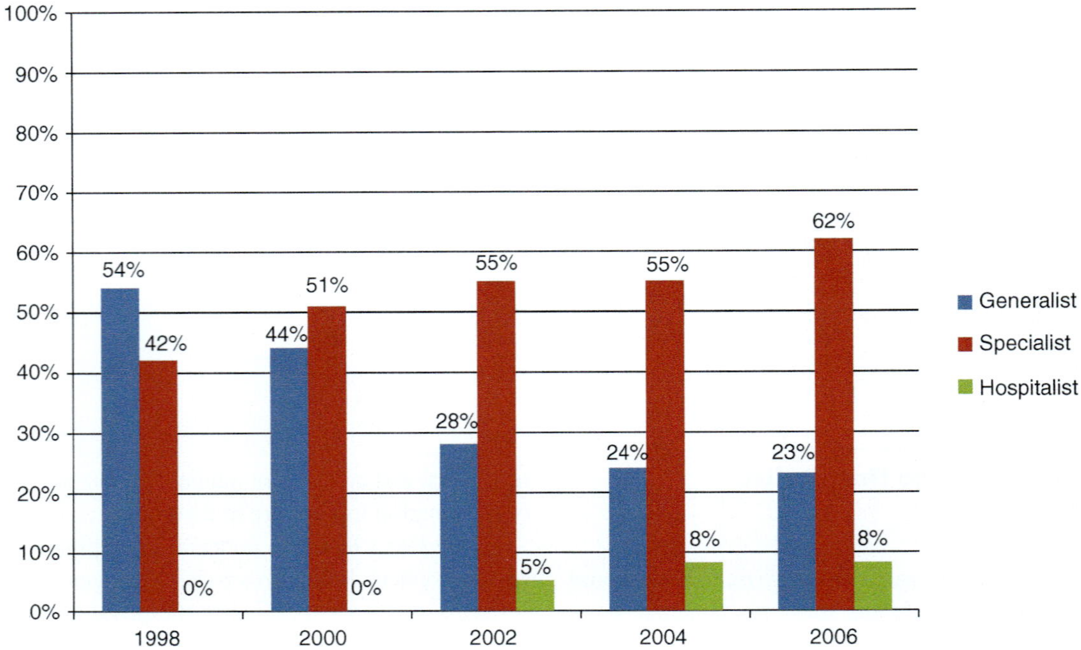

Fig. 31.1 Early Hospitalist Movement Internal Medicine Resident Career Choices, ACGME Internal Medicine In-Training Examination surveys. (Adapted from Okie [1]. With permission from Massachusetts Medical Society)

local scale which in turn reflected change happening on the national scale. In this location, the need was for internal medicine staffing in a private outpatient faculty practice, on a resident ambulatory clinic, on the general hospital wards and in a medical intensive care unit (MICU, with critical care backup), in a rehabilitation unit and on-campus skilled nursing facility, and within a prison primary care clinic and its associated inpatient prison ward. In addition, the group would serve as faculty (New York Medical College) for the internal medicine residency program, teaching residents and medical students.

From the outset, it was apparent that the provision of efficient and effective service in each of these settings required specialization and division of labor – much as envisioned by Wachter and Goldman [3]. The practice was a private one, though not for profit. This made financial considerations tangible with each pay cycle. For that reason, each area would be staffed by a small group of practitioners who offered to make their primary role patient care in that particular area, with adjustments as needed and some overlap to permit off-hour coverage. All providers also assumed variable levels of responsibility for teaching and scholarship activities (Fig. 31.2).

Elsewhere, other practices had been and were adapting to their local needs as well. In the early 1990s, inpatient managers had already been created on the West Coast to enhance inpatient care, and in the Midwest, the Park Nicollet group established an early hospitalist program [3–5]. Ultimately, enough physicians were emphasizing or solely practicing inpatient medicine to be recognized as "hospitalists" by the medical community [3] (Fig. 31.3).

A formal society for the field was established in 1997, and soon thereafter, investigators began to explore how the new care model was impacting patient care and other measures [7, 8]. Over the next two decades, the shape of hospital care evolved rapidly and included members of many other specialties. By 2006, the president of the Society for Hospital Medicine (SHM) explained, the "strength of hospital medicine and SHM is based on our 'big tent' that embraces physicians

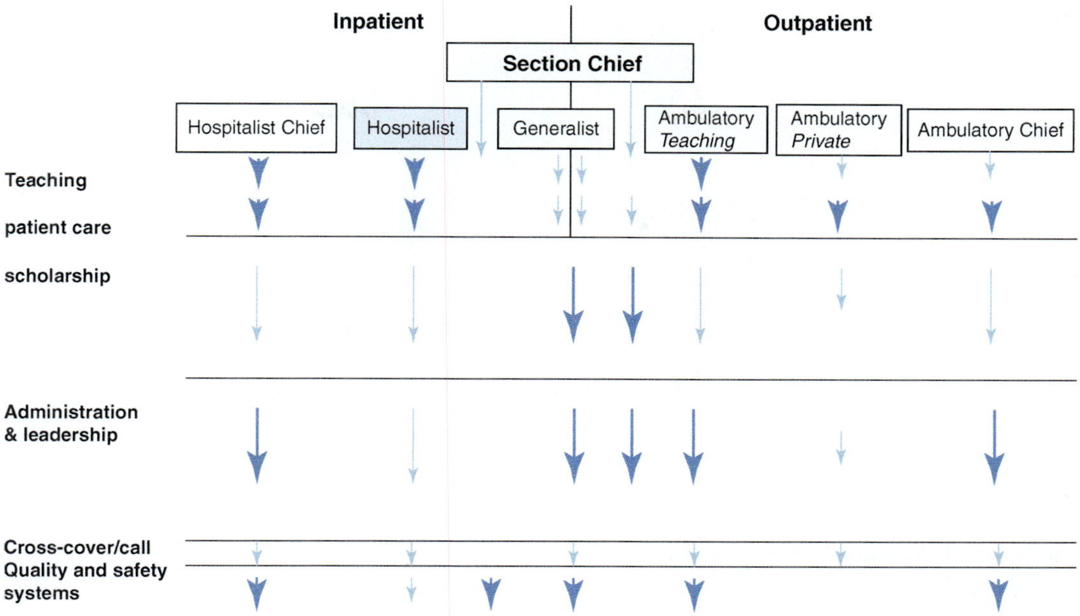

Fig. 31.2 Model of WMC General Internal Medicine Division Relative contributions to domain is identified by weight/length of arrows. (Courtesy of WMC Westchester Medical Center)

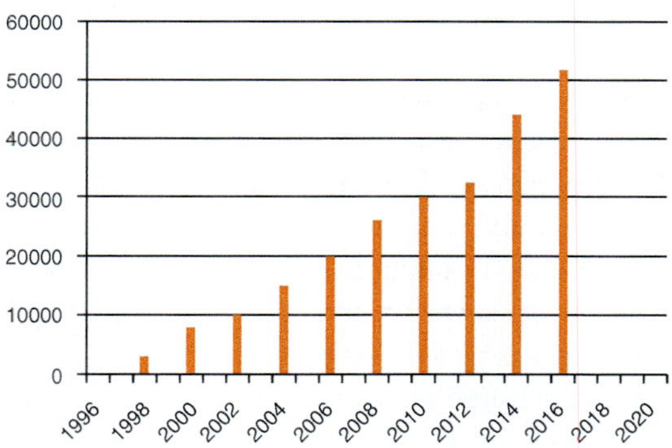

Fig. 31.3 Number of hospitalists 1995–2020. (Adapted from Wachter and Goldman [6]. With permission from Massachusetts Medical Society. (Data from American Hospital Association))

who work as hospitalists (internists, family physicians, and pediatricians) in all settings—community practice, academia, and industry" [9]. To accommodate the diverse needs of its members, the society established pediatrics and family medicine committees to address issues relating to hospitalists in these specialties. And a list of new names for these new subspecialists arrived: nocturnists, laborists, subacutists, transitionalists, and SNFists (skilled nursing facility practitioners). In 2017, most hospitalists worked in groups averaging 19 physician and 3 nonphysician providers. Local hospital groups averaged 13 physicians, hospital corporations 20 physicians, and university/medical school centers 26 physicians. Annual compensation ranged from 259,000 (Northeast) to 309,000 (Southwest). Those who worked for over 10 years earned 292,000 compared to 254,000 for those who worked 2 years or less. Mean annual pay for men was $291,000 and women $261,000. Fifty-five percent of hospitalist worked a block schedule with the remainder working a flexible schedule. Blocks were most commonly 5 days on/5 days off (5/5) or 7 days on/7 days off (7/7) in which hospitalists worked shifts of 12 hours (56%), 10 hours (20%), or over 13 hours (7%) (Fig. 31.4).

Sixty-five percent of providers completed 14–16 shifts per month with an average of 3–4 weekend shifts per month. Sixty-seven percent of primary shifts involved daytime or mostly daytime care, and nighttime coverage was provided by rotating hospitalists (30%), nocturnists (29%), or primarily nocturnists with some hospitalist rotations (25%) [10].

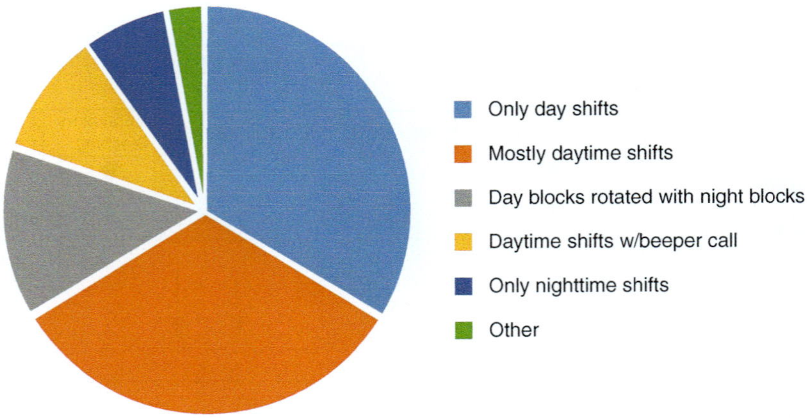

Fig. 31.4 Most common hospitalist schedules. (Based on data from Today's Hospitalist Survey 2017)

Patient Care

Early US Hospitalist Medicine Era (1990–2005)

The hospitalist model is credited with a number of benefits. In early reports published between 1998 and 2005, most found hospitalist care associated with reduced resource use [11, 12] or cost [12–14], length of stay [13–16], and need for consultation [15, 17] with some exceptions [4, 18–20]. Results regarding patient outcomes were inconsistent with some studies finding readmission rates and mortality unchanged [11, 17, 21–23]; others noting decreased readmissions with unchanged mortality [16]; or showing no change in mortality, but increased readmissions [24] and still others demonstrating decreased in-hospital mortality rate with no change in readmissions [13]. A limited amount of evidence suggested the model might improve inpatient teaching of house officers [25]. At WMC, end-of-rotation evaluations by residents indicated that the introduction of hospitalist teams improved rounding efficiency, communication, and supervision (unpublished results). And the introduction of nocturnists permitted round-the-clock supervision of house staff, as required by state regulations. With respect to management of particular conditions, hospitalist care of orthopedic surgery patients resulted in reduced time to surgery and length of stay [26]. Patients admitted for either heart failure or pneumonia had shorter length of stay when cared for by hospitalists and were more likely to have important clinical parameters documented [27].

Mid-Current Era Hospitalist Medicine (2006–Present)

As the movement matured, further studies confirmed the initial findings that hospitalist care improved efficiency. In a 2011 review, a shorter length of stay for patients managed by hospitalists was reported in 35/58 (60%) of articles. This was consistent across all hospitalist models. Thirteen reports (22%) identified no significant differences in length of stay between hospitalist and nonhospitalist providers, and seven (12%) reports found increased length of stay among hospitalists [28]. In a subsequent report, increasing hospitalist workload was associated with increased LOS and cost [29]. Analysis of overall quality of hospitalist care has been limited by the heterogeneity of study designs and methodological concerns. In general, evidence suggesting improvements in the effectiveness of care provision is limited. With respect to mortality, 7/35 studies (20%) reported reduced mortality rates among patients cared for by hospitalists. Of 43 studies examining readmissions, 34/43 (79%) found no differences, 6/43 (14%) reported reduced readmissions, and 3/43 (7%) reported higher rates of readmissions [28]. In a 2013 analysis of 2005–2008 Medicare data, compared to cardiologists, hospitalist care was associated with a small increase in mortality for patients admitted with heart failure but a decrease in length of stay [30]. In a 2017 study, patients who were cared for by their own primary care physician had a lower 30-day mortality than patients being cared for by hospitalists (OR 0.94) or by other generalists (OR, 1.09) [31]. Among surgical patients, there were lower rates of surgical complications among those cared for by hospitalists in two studies [32, 33]. One of these studies, however, involved patients with a lower anticipated length of stay being admitted to the hospitalist service. In another report, high-risk patients undergoing limb salvage or reconstructive surgery had higher complication rates when comanaged by hospitalists when compared to previous care only by the surgical team [34]. Of reports analyzing adverse events or hospital complications, five of eight reports described no significant differences between provider types. Financial data from the California's Office of Statewide Health Planning and Development indicated that for each increase in percentage of hospitalist coverage per daily census, there was a corresponding decrease in malpractice insurance premiums [35].

Trade-Offs and Innovations of the Hospitalist Model

Despite its advantages, the hospitalist model has inherent flaws. The trade-off of robust and specialized inpatient management is fragmented care which requires the involvement of multiple providers and care transitions fraught with potential for miscommunication. The patient in this model who faces potentially serious illness and who may be confused or uncertain about treatment options is unlikely to have any support from his or her primary physician. This could manifest later as low scores on a patient satisfaction survey but more fundamentally relates to a weakening of the traditional patient/provider bond and trust that was, prior to the hospitalist movement, held sacrosanct [36]. Participation of multiple providers could further erode this bond, as each might feel a lesser depth of involvement in the case.

At institutions where there is a clear delineation between inpatient/outpatient and on-/off-duty periods, a shift mentality could arise such that the physician's desire to guard against inefficiencies or gaps in care related to "gray areas" around shift changes or definitions of roles could weaken. Similarly, the off-duty clinician might be less inclined to devote nonclinical time to activities such as leadership in quality improvement or other scholarly works. As hospital physician staffs decline and fewer primary clinicians from the community are involved in hospital care, their stake in decision-making is likewise diminished. This could lead to a hospital-centric approach to care which ultimately might not be in the best interest of community's overall health. Finally, providers who exclusively manage only inpatient or outpatient care could tend to become less familiar with or adept at managing care in alternate settings. This could have a deleterious effect on overall care in that patient needs at care transitions might not be well anticipated. Or, the collective skill level of practitioners who work in only one rather than multiple settings could diminish over time.

Two final problems with the hospitalist movement relate to lack of depth training and experience. When starting practice, many hospitalists have just completed residency, and 41% of practicing hospitalists are age 40 or under [10]. Lack of experience has been linked to higher mortality rates [37], and absence of specialty training may tend to limit the clinician's ability to carry out substantive research or other scholarly activities. This in turn could hinder career development or satisfaction. Early on, studies by hospitalists tended to focus on quality measures such as length of stay, cost of hospitalization, and readmission rates. This led to calls for hospitalist groups to become more involved in research focused on the comparative effectiveness, bench-to-bedside, and bedside-to-community research agendas of the National Institutes of Health [38].

Innovations

In 1996, Robert Wachter described a potential blueprint for either the academic or nonacademic general medicine service which relied on subspecialization within the group.

At Westchester Medical Center, the general medicine division was established in almost complete accord with this model. How that structure facilitated the integration of a hospitalist component into a well-functioning division of general internal medicine is detailed here. First, having *some trained as generalists, others as specialists* permitted not only sharing of inpatient duties but freed up enough manpower to maintain one clinician to be the group's director of scholarly activity. This led to grant funding from the State of New York's Empire Clinical Research Investigator Program (ECRIP) and other sources which allowed us to engage in a variety of research and quality and safety initiatives [39–41]. As foreseen by Wachter, *not everyone in the group possess[ed] the skills to oversee the development of practice guidelines and to study the outcomes of care*; however, because the group always retained several clinicians expert in the area of research design and implementation, we were able to explore projects that were not only related to generalist-focused activities but to bench-to-bedside translational research as well as clinician outcome research [42–49].

Wachter also envisioned some portion of the group being able to *participate in developing and disseminating guidelines, as well as teaching clinical medicine*. The core teaching faculty for internal medicine residents and rotating medical students were the hospitalists and the clinicians assigned to the center's resident-based ambulatory clinic. Over the years, these faculty members were consistently recognized as among the best educators in the Department of Medicine.

In a well-integrated division, Wachter also believed that the division's members would *develop strong relationships with hospital staff, discharge planners, specialty consultants, and outpatient physicians. The outpatient physicians, in turn,* [would] *have more time in the office to see patients and less hospital duty. Potential problems with the transfer of care between the outpatient and inpatient settings are prevented by meticulous communication between office and hospital.* In this regard, our division was particularly active. As a matter of routine, the director of the ambulatory resident clinic also served as the chair of the ambulatory quality committee and oversaw the quality initiatives of all ambulatory care clinics, including those outside the medical specialties. Another generalist typically headed the Department of Medicine Quality committee. In 2005, the division became a part of the Accreditation Council for Internal Medicine's Educational Innovations Project (EIP) [50]. As part of the EIP, our division led or collaborated in a variety of scholarly ventures. Recognizing that residency training focused largely on inpatient medicine could promote a shift mentality during training, we devised a system-based practice curriculum (termed the "Administrative Internship") to permit residents to learn key aspects of the institution's legal/risk, pharmacy, case management, social, fiscal, and quality and safety operations. Nonphysicians from various hospital departments were appointed as instructors in medicine and collaborated on making this an enriching experience for the residents and shared in the publication of the work [51]. Their interactions during this initiative led to an enduring culture of patient safety and to further quality improvement initiatives. To help identify best practices in balancing inpatient versus outpatient medicine training, we collaborated with other programs to study how care/training models impacted on resident and patient satisfaction as well as clinical outcomes [52–54]. In anticipation of the Next Accreditation System, our division participated in an ABIM/ACGME pilot study of the milestones and implemented one of the earliest milestone-based evaluation processes [55]. Prior to the institution's acquisition of an event reporting system (MIDAS®), the division worked with the chief quality officer to develop a handoff software platform which incorporated a quality and safety event reporting module [56]. The platform also included an oversight module by which faculty reviewed and corrected resident sign-outs [57]. This, we believe, importantly taught residents the value of and how to generate high-quality handoffs but also allowed leadership to track and address deficiencies in handoff [58]. Over several years, hospitalists in our division worked with a team from Long Island Jewish Medical Center to develop a mobile version which further enhanced events reporting by house officers [41, 59]. The system permitted association of handoff quality with numbers of quality and safety reports and led to several quality awards (Figs. 31.5 and 31.6).

Metric	Performance of hospitalist comapred to other providers
Length of stay	↑↑
Cost of care	↑↑
Time to surgery	↑
Emergency room throughput	(---)
Mortality	↑ (---)
Readmission rate	↑ (---) (---) ↓
Complications	↑ (---) ↓
Outpatient follow up	↑ (---)
Emergency room visits	(---)
Satisfaction	↑ (---)
Malpractice premiums	↑

↑ Majority of studies favor hospitalist care

↑↑ Large proportion of studies favor hospitalist care

(---) Indicates no difference in performance between providers

↓ Majority of studies favor non-hospitalist care

↓↑ Some studies favor hospitalist and some favor non-hospitalist care

Fig. 31.5 Hospitalists versus nonhospitalist performance. (Based on data from systematic reviews [28, 60] supplemented by literatures search of "hospitalist" and "hospital-based medicine" related articles, PubMed, 2011 to April 2018)

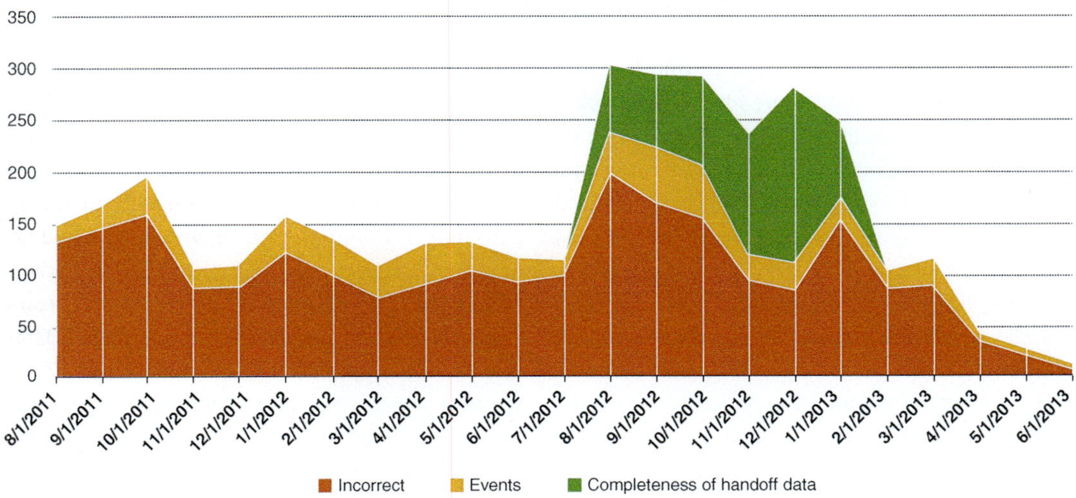

Fig. 31.6 Association between accuracy of handoff data and safety concerns

Innovations in handoff such as these and important initiatives at other institutions demonstrate the hospitalist's commitment to optimize patient care while mitigating against any negative effects of the hospitalist model [41, 57, 61–63].

Teaching and Supervision

Residency Training

Hospitalists now comprise the largest internal medicine subspecialty. The movement has undergone remarkable growth over the past 20 years. Yet as with any field, its value and durability will depend on new adaptations to the changing needs of the medical community. One of the most important considerations is how well the training of those who will practice hospital medicine prepares them for their career. Traditional internal medicine residency training has focused on preparing graduates to manage acutely ill adults admitted to the hospital. And despite a larger proportion of inpatient education by hospitalists, programs still may not adequately teach the skills needed for independent hospital practice at graduation [64]. Recognizing this, residency programs have increasingly incorporated hospitalist-specific rotations into their curricula. At Baylor College of Medicine, following a 1-month second year hospitalist rotation, resident confidence in managing hospitalized patients and leading a ward team increased significantly as did self-assessed knowledge deficits related to care transitions, cost-conscious care, hospital quality measure metrics, and billing/coding and hospital reimbursement. Interest in pursuing hospital medicine as a career also increased after the experience [65]. Similar rotations and internal medicine tracks are in place in many internal medicine programs. In a 2018 survey, the prevalence of hospitalist-focused rotations was 50% (41/82) with an additional nine programs (11%) planning to start one. Of these 85% were elective, and 15% were mandatory, typically involving clinical responsibilities as well as nonclinical activities such as teaching, research, and work on quality improvement and patient safety [66]. Programs are also exploring ways to adapt ward teaching methods to changing needs of learners, and many institutions now require completion of additional quality/safety education such as online modules offered by the Institute for Healthcare Improvement [67].

Fellowships in hospital medicine are now available at a number of centers for both internal and family medicine [68, 69]. At the University of Colorado, the Hospital Medicine Group developed a Health Innovations Scholars Program (HISP) to provide medical students with skills needed to function as quality and safety leaders and an Advanced Practice Fellowship (APF) in hospital medicine to provide intensive training to nurse practitioners (NPs) and physician assistants (PAs) entering a hospital-based career [70]. These programs illustrate how hospitalists are working to foster leadership and hospital-related skills even prior to residency as well as expanding hospitalist expertise to nonphysician providers who help form the inpatient team. And although there is currently not a separate certifying board under the American Board of Medical Specialties, the boards of internal medicine and family medicine have created a recertification pathway for hospitalists – called Recognition of Focused Practice in Hospital Medicine (RFPHM) [71]. This permits recertification in the clinician's area of practice and is likely a welcome avenue to hospitalists.

Career Satisfaction and Burnout (Fig. 31.7)

In general, hospitalists have reported fairly high levels of career satisfaction in recent surveys. In May 2017, of 624 hospitalists (94% of whom care only for adults), 55% reported being either extremely or very satisfied with their career as a hospitalist. Other levels of satisfaction (very or extremely) were opportunity for growth (72%) respect from specialists, administration (70%), specific job (88%), current duties (88%), autonomy (85%), patient load (73%), and pay structure (70%). Annual pay (40%) and amount of time on paperwork (46%) were the lowest rated item.

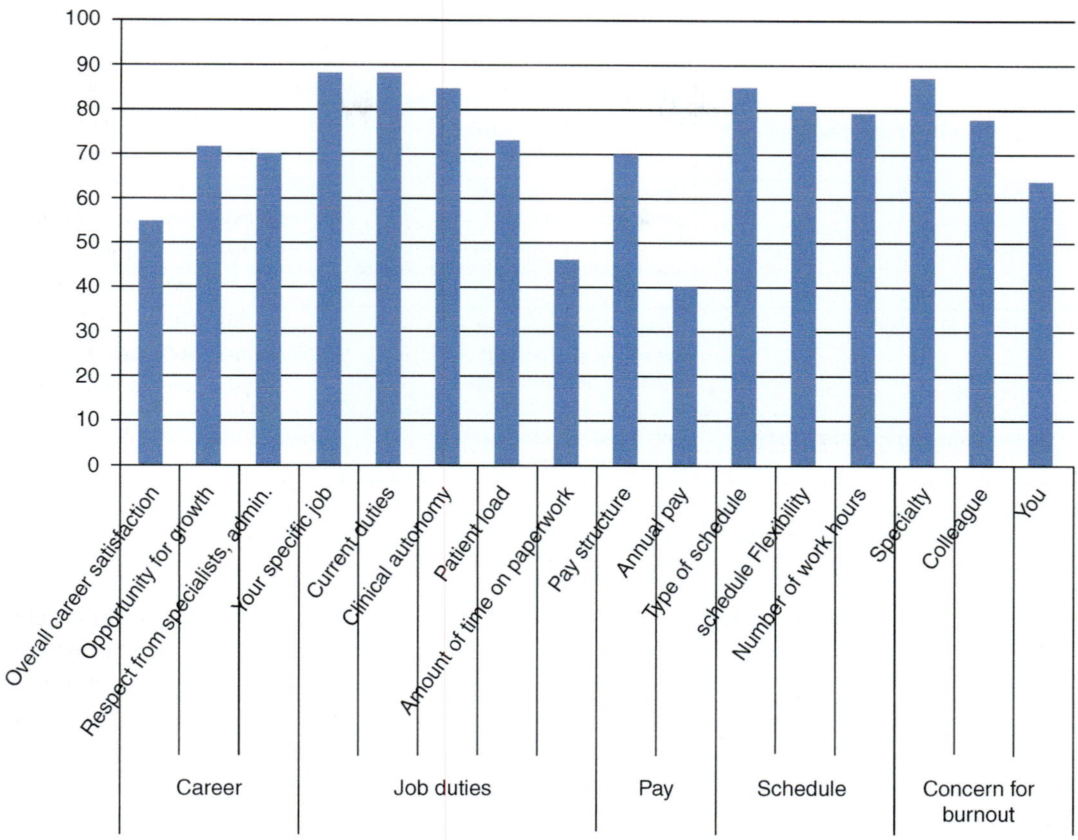

Fig. 31.7 Hospitalist satisfaction and burnout satisfaction rated as percentage responding either "extremely or very satisfied." Burnout rated as percentage agreeing that "burnout is a significant issue for...". (Based on data from Today's Hospitalist Survey 2017)

However, 87% agreed that burnout is a significant issue for the specialty overall, for colleagues (78%), and for the respondent (64%) [10] (Fig. 31.8).

Themes represented in another survey to be relatively important were excitement about daily work, being respected and recognized, and dissemination of work. Nevertheless, in the same survey, clinicians reported ambivalence toward the academic value of clinical work, scholarship, and promotion [73]. Burnout was found to be relatively common among both hospitalists and outpatient general internists with 43.8% of internal medicine hospitalists affected by emotional exhaustion [74]. These feelings could potentially arise from growing pressure to increase productivity to compensate for declining revenue or to meet new responsibilities [74]. One of the solutions to this may be peer mentoring. In one program, 86% of mentees and 67% of mentors reported increased job satisfaction after completing the program; 80% of mentees reported feeling more prepared to be a hospitalist and felt that mentorship positively affected their career management, knowledge, skills, and attitudes. Both mentors and mentees reported a stronger sense of connection and cohesion within their department after program completion. And the study author suggested that the program may have contributed to a low attrition rate of new hires (2 out of 26) after >1 year [75]. This was consistent with prior reports which have suggested that having a sense of calling in the provider's practice may promote career resilience [76]. In studies not specific to hospital practice, control over schedule and hours worked, total

Technology	Potential impact	Challenges
Electronic health records (EHRs)	Platform on which to build other innovations	Competing financial interests; cost
EHRs integration and interoperability	Permit big data analysis, enhance outcomes, value	Technological and security requirements; privacy laws
iOT-based devices	Permit round-the-clock, services/monitoring; enhance patient engagement and efficiency using mobile devices	Dissemination and integration of new technologies; Patient confidentiality, cyber security, and data governance.
Big data and analytics	Facilitate development of perdictive models and enhance decision support	Pace of software development and integration
Telemedicine, videoconferencing	Enhanced at home care for elderly and immobile	Training, implementation
Smart Health platforms; information architecture advances	Engage patients in their care; facilitate patient/provider collaboration	Relationship between IA and health outcomes

Fig. 31.8 Major technologies that may impact hospitalists. (Based on from data from Ref. [72], iOT (Internet of Things))

work hours, marital status, and having child dependents in the household were important factors in mediating the relationship between work–life balance and career satisfaction. Apart from these factors, the relationship between career satisfaction and work–life balance was weaker. In contrast to work–life balance, measures of burnout (emotional resilience and personal accomplishment) were strongly associated with career satisfaction [77]. Taken together, it appears that schedules which emphasize flexibility and predictability are most likely to improve career satisfaction and decrease work-related stress and burnout could – either for hospitalists or other providers.

A large-scale adjustment to hospitalist scheduling patterns may also be in order to improve career satisfaction and reduce burnout. The block schedule (e.g., "7-on, 7-off") or other variation favored early on and still common permits extended time off but is fairly rigid and requires multiple straight days of intensive patient management. It is now criticized as most suited to the 30-year-old who just graduated [78]. This has prompted many centers to increase scheduling flexibility and to emphasize weekday duty and shift work [79], but empiric data by which to determine how scheduling changes affect safety and quality outcomes and work–life balance are limited and require further study. One schedule which emphasizes patient continuity was implemented at Johns Hopkins. Called the CICLE (Creating Incentives and Continuity Leading to Efficiency) schedule, this was found to reduce length of stay and cost by promoting care continuity and effective discharge management while avoiding any incentives; other schedules might have generated to keep patients needlessly in the hospital [80]. Because the model was designed to address patient care measures as well as to promote highly professional behavior among physicians, the model also holds some potential to enhancing career satisfaction.

Other possible antidotes to burnout include measures external to the provider: institutional-level changes in scheduling and workload, development of support groups and/or designation of a wellness officer, web-based resources (AMA STEPS forward Preventing Physician Burnout website (https://www.stepsforward.org/, Stanford's WellMD Center at http://wellmd.stanford.edu/), and conferences (e.g., 2017 American Conference on Physician Health; Society of Hospital Medicine). Factors intrinsic to the provider include finding work-related interest outside of direct patient care, focus on mindfulness and self-compassion, and willingness and ability to cultivate meaningful social connections in and out of the workplace. To some extent the provider who is committed to wellness must become a student of his/her own internal psychological milieu and chart his/her own course toward fulfillment. However, in some circumstances, the provider must also be willing to seek help from a mental health professional.

Pediatric Hospitalists

On entering Pediatric Hospital Medicine (PHM), 70% of residents envision long-term PHM careers, with PHM career goals more frequently reported among residents entering community hospitalist positions [81]. Among pediatric hospitalists, those working in community hospitalists emphasized diversity of clinical responsibilities, resource availability, and work schedules as being important domains relating to career satisfaction, while tertiary care hospitalists gave priority to having diverse nonclinical responsibilities and career development [82]. Both groups found recognition, schedule, and work environment as well as nonclinical factors such as institutional support, involvement in program administration/leadership activities, and opportunities for career development to be relevant [81].

New Technologies

The advancement of health-care information technology (IT) will likely provide major benefits to hospitalist-based care and overall health care in the next decade. Transformation is proceeding in two overlapping major steps: the first relates to implementation of local EHRs which function as information nodes within the larger health information system and the second involves coordination and exchange of data among EHRs, web portals, and other sources such as the Internet of Everything (iOE) (i.e., smart devices, wearables, mHealth applications) backed by sophisticated analytics. Both stages are underway within the United States and globally. The Henry Ford Health System Health Data Exchange now connects with more than 1200 hospitals across 50 states and shares more than 14 million patient records using an EHR linked to a statewide health information network [83]. An EHR-based dashboard at Lehigh Valley Hospital collates key throughput indicators to facilitate flow through the overall hospital, emergency department, and operating rooms. At our health center, in 2015, telehealth program was developed to facilitate care across a 6200-square-mile service area including a 10-hospital network. The system permits critical care specialists to view and remotely guide intensive care unit interventions and has been shown to reduce mortality and length of stay [84]. While implementation of an EHR in a single institution can improve the quality, safety, and cost of care for the local patients, the integration of EHRs across institutions promises to facilitate big data analysis with potential for wide-ranging improvements in health-care quality and value. Realizing these benefits will require information unification and sharing through interoperable platforms. Innovation in the area of machine learning should facilitate the development of predictive models that can be more precise than current clinical scoring systems. Decision support and monitoring tools are expected to make possible improvements in many areas of clinical management and are already helping to identify deteriorating patients more quickly [85]. And telemedicine or videoconferencing offers at home care options to the elderly and to the mobility challenged. This technology has already been used in the post discharge follow-up of surgical patients [86] and might reduce medication errors, missed test results, and patient harms attributed to the hospital to home care transition [87].

The Future of Hospitalists

An emphasis on value-based care coupled with the need to diminish overall health-care spending as a percentage of US gross domestic product is likely to drive change in the health-care environment for the foreseeable future. Hospitalists are particularly well positioned to facilitate coming changes, owing to their skill in the collaborative management of the sickest patients and in leading efforts to improve quality in the complex health environment of the hospital. Continuing realignment of residency training with hospital and community needs will promote well-being of providers and the durability of hospital medicine. Following graduation, mentoring and hospital administrative support will be important in enabling the hospitalist to achieve career goals and long-term satisfaction. Just as the hospitalist movement arose rapidly in response to a changing financial and practice landscape, future adjustments in the movement should allow hospital medicine to endure in the long term.

Acknowledgments The authors graciously acknowledge the support received from Michael Israel, Chief Executive Officer, Westchester Medical Center, and the hospital administration, which made possible the initiatives described herein.

References

1. Okie S. Innovation in primary care–staying one step ahead of burnout. N Engl J Med. 2008;359(22):2305–9.
2. Wachter RM. Response to David meltzer's paper, "Hospitalists and the doctor patient relationship". J Legal Stud. 2001;30(2):615–23.
3. Wachter RM, Goldman L. The emerging role of "hospitalists" in the American health care system. N Engl J Med. 1996;335(7):514–7. https://doi.org/10.1056/NEJM199608153350713.
4. Craig DE, Hartka L, Likosky WH, Caplan WM, Litsky P, Smithey J. Implementation of a hospitalist system in a large health maintenance organization: the kaiser permanente experience. Ann Intern Med. 1999;130(4 Pt 2):355–9. doi: 199902161-00005 [pii].
5. Freese RB. The park Nicollet experience in establishing a hospitalist system. Ann Intern Med. 1999;130(4 Pt 2):350–4. doi: 199902161-00004 [pii].
6. Wachter RM, Goldman L. Zero to 50,000 – the 20th anniversary of the hospitalist. N Engl J Med. 2016;375(11):1009–11.
7. Timeline of SHM's history. Society of Hospital Medicine Web site. https://www.hospitalmedicine.org/about/history-mission/#Timeline_of_SHM's_History. March 17, 2018.
8. Lindenauer PK, Pantilat SZ, Katz PP, Wachter RM. Hospitalists and the practice of inpatient medicine: results of a survey of the national association of inpatient physicians. Ann Intern Med. 1999;130(4 Pt 2):343–9. doi: 199902161-00003 [pii].
9. Pantilat S. What is a hospitalist? Hospitalist. 2006(2) (February 2006). https://www.the-hospitalist.org/hospitalist/article/123072/what-hospitalist. Accessed 17 March 2018.
10. 2017 today's hospitalist career and compensation survey results. Today's Hospitalist Web site. https://www.todayshospitalist.com/survey/17_salary_survey/d01.php. Accessed 8 Apr 2018.
11. Halpert AP, Pearson SD, LeWine HE, Mckean SC. The impact of an inpatient physician program on quality, utilization, and satisfaction. Am J Manag Care. 2000;6(5):549–55. doi: 923 [pii].
12. Meltzer D, Manning WG, Morrison J, et al. Effects of physician experience on costs and outcomes on an academic general medicine service: results of a trial of hospitalists. Ann Intern Med. 2002;137(11):866–74. doi: 200212030-00007 [pii].
13. Auerbach AD, Wachter RM, Katz P, Showstack J, Baron RB, Goldman L. Implementation of a voluntary hospitalist service at a community teaching hospital: improved clinical efficiency and patient outcomes. Ann Intern Med. 2002;137(11):859–65. doi: 200212030-00006 [pii].
14. Halasyamani LK, Valenstein PN, Friedlander MP, Cowen ME. A comparison of two hospitalist models with traditional care in a community teaching hospital. Am J Med. 2005;118(5):536–43. doi: S0002-9343(05)00070-7 [pii].
15. Rifkin WD, Conner D, Silver A, Eichorn A. Comparison of processes and outcomes of pneumonia care between hospitalists and community-based primary care physicians. Mayo Clin Proc. 2002;77(10):1053–8. doi: S0025-6196(11)62526-3 [pii].
16. Diamond HS, Goldberg E, Janosky JE. The effect of full-time faculty hospitalists on the efficiency of care at a community teaching hospital. Ann Intern Med. 1998;129(3):197–203.
17. Hackner D, Tu G, Braunstein GD, Ault M, Weingarten S, Mohsenifar Z. The value of a hospitalist service: efficient care for the aging population? Chest. 2001;119(2):580–9. doi: S0012-3692(15)38240-4 [pii].
18. Tingle LE, Lambert CT. Comparison of a family practice teaching service and a hospitalist model: costs, charges, length of stay, and mortality. Fam Med. 2001;33(7):511–5.
19. Kearns PJ, Wang CC, Morris WJ, et al. Hospital care by hospital-based and clinic-based faculty: a prospective, controlled trial. Arch Intern Med. 2001;161(2):235–41. doi: ioi00064 [pii].
20. Kaboli PJ, Barnett MJ, Rosenthal GE. Associations with reduced length of stay and costs on an academic hospitalist service. Am J Manag Care. 2004;10(8):561–8. doi: 2658 [pii].
21. Wachter RM, Katz P, Showstack J, Bindman AB, Goldman L. Reorganizing an academic medical service: impact on cost, quality, patient satisfaction, and education. JAMA. 1998;279(19):1560–5. doi: jsc80075 [pii].

22. Stein MD, Hanson S, Tammaro D, Hanna L, Most AS. Economic effects of community versus hospital-based faculty pneumonia care. J Gen Intern Med. 1998;13(11):774–7.
23. Davis KM, Koch KE, Harvey JK, Wilson R, Englert J, Gerard PD. Effects of hospitalists on cost, outcomes, and patient satisfaction in a rural health system. Am J Med. 2000;108(8):621–6. doi: S0002-9343(00)00362-4 [pii].
24. Bellet PS, Whitaker RC. Evaluation of a pediatric hospitalist service: impact on length of stay and hospital charges. Pediatrics. 2000;105(3 Pt 1): 478–84.
25. Wachter RM, Goldman L. The hospitalist movement 5 years later. JAMA. 2002;287(4):487–94. doi: jrv10099 [pii].
26. Phy MP, Vanness DJ, Melton LJ 3rd, et al. Effects of a hospitalist model on elderly patients with hip fracture. Arch Intern Med. 2005;165(7):796–801. doi: 165/7/796 [pii].
27. Lindenauer PK, Chehabeddine R, Pekow P, Fitzgerald J, Benjamin EM. Quality of care for patients hospitalized with heart failure: assessing the impact of hospitalists. Arch Intern Med. 2002;162(11):1251–6. doi: ioi10299 [pii].
28. White HL, Glazier RH. Do hospitalist physicians improve the quality of inpatient care delivery? A systematic review of process, efficiency and outcome measures. BMC Med. 2011;9:58. https://doi.org/10.1186/1741-7015-9-58.
29. Elliott DJ, Young RS, Brice J, Aguiar R, Kolm P. Effect of hospitalist workload on the quality and efficiency of care. JAMA Intern Med. 2014;174(5):786–93. https://doi.org/10.1001/jamainternmed.2014.300.
30. Kociol RD, Hammill BG, Fonarow GC, et al. Associations between use of the hospitalist model and quality of care and outcomes of older patients hospitalized for heart failure. JACC Heart Fail. 2013;1(5):445–53. https://doi.org/10.1016/j.jchf.2013.07.001.
31. Stevens JP, Nyweide DJ, Maresh S, Hatfield LA, Howell MD, Landon BE. Comparison of hospital resource use and outcomes among hospitalists, primary care physicians, and other generalists. JAMA Intern Med. 2017;177(12):1781–7. https://doi.org/10.1001/jamainternmed.2017.5824.
32. Abenhaim HA, Kahn SR, Raffoul J, Becker MR. Program description: a hospitalist-run, medical short-stay unit in a teaching hospital. CMAJ. 2000;163(11):1477–80.
33. Huddleston JM, Long KH, Naessens JM, et al. Medical and surgical comanagement after elective hip and knee arthroplasty: a randomized, controlled trial. Ann Intern Med. 2004;141(1):28–38. doi: 141/1/28 [pii].
34. Pinzur MS, Gurza E, Kristopaitis T, et al. Hospitalist-orthopedic co-management of high-risk patients undergoing lower extremity reconstruction surgery. Orthopedics. 2009;32(7):495. https://doi.org/10.3928/01477447-20090527-14.
35. Lee J. Impact of hospitalist care on hospital malpractice premiums using California hospital data. Appl Econ Lett. 2017;24(11):742–52.
36. Conigliaro RL. A piece of my mind. satisfaction? JAMA. 2005;293(18):2193. doi: 293/18/2193 [pii].
37. Goodwin JS, Salameh H, Zhou J, Singh S, Kuo YF, Nattinger AB. Association of hospitalist years of experience with mortality in the hospitalized medicare population. JAMA Intern Med. 2018;178(2):196–203. https://doi.org/10.1001/jamainternmed.2017.7049.
38. McMahon LF Jr. The hospitalist movement–time to move on. N Engl J Med. 2007;357(25):2627–9. doi: 357/25/2627 [pii].
39. Gupta T, Mujib M, Agarwal P, et al. Association between opioid abuse/dependence and outcomes in hospitalized heart failure patients. Am J Ther. 2016;23(2):e350–6. https://doi.org/10.1097/MJT.0000000000000190.
40. Nabors C, Khera S, Forman L, et al. Electronic capture of written handoff information: what are the next steps? Am J Ther. 2016;23(3):e785–91. https://doi.org/10.1097/MJT.0000000000000052.
41. Nabors C, Patel D, Khera S, et al. Improving resident morning sign-out by use of daily events reports. J Patient Saf. 2015;11(1):36–41. https://doi.org/10.1097/PTS.0b013e31829e4f56.
42. Abraham NG, Li M, Vanella L, Peterson SJ, Ikehara S, Asprinio D. Bone marrow stem cell transplant into intra-bone cavity prevents type 2 diabetes: role of heme oxygenase-adiponectin. J Autoimmun. 2008;30(3):128–35. https://doi.org/10.1016/j.jaut.2007.12.005.
43. Barbagallo I, Vanella A, Peterson SJ, et al. Overexpression of heme oxygenase-1 increases human osteoblast stem cell differentiation. J Bone Miner Metab. 2010;28(3):276–88. https://doi.org/10.1007/s00774-009-0134-y.
44. Kannam HC, Satou G, Gandelman G, et al. Anomalous origin of the left main coronary artery from the right sinus of valsalva with an intramural course identified by transesophageal echocardiography in a 14 year old with acute myocardial infarction. Cardiol Rev. 2005;13(5):219–22. doi: 00045415-200509000-00001 [pii].
45. Yalamanchili K, Aronow WS, Kilaru R, et al. Coronary artery disease is more severe in older persons with rheumatoid arthritis than in older persons without rheumatoid arthritis. Cardiol Rev. 2006;14(2):55–6. https://doi.org/10.1097/01.crd.0000166172.07216.98.
46. Sukhija R, Aronow WS, Sorbera C, et al. Left ventricular ejection fraction and prevalence of new left ventricular wall motion abnormality at long-term follow-up in patients with automatic implantable cardioverter-defibrillators treated with dual-chamber rate-responsive pacing at a rate of 70/minute versus backup ventricular pacing at a rate of 40/minute. Am J Cardiol. 2005;96(3):412–3. doi: S0002-9149(05)00744-7 [pii].
47. Sule S, Aronow WS, Babu S. Prevalence of risk factors and of coronary artery disease, ischemic

stroke, carotid arterial disease and lower extremity peripheral arterial disease in 96 patients undergoing elective surgery for an abdominal aortic aneurysm. Int J Angiol. 2008;17(3):141–2.
48. Sule S, Aronow WS. Therapy of patients hospitalized for heart failure with abnormal versus normal left ventricular ejection fraction. Compr Ther. 2009;35(1):50–4.
49. Sule S, Palaniswamy C, Aronow WS, et al. Etiology of syncope in patients hospitalized with syncope and predictors of mortality and rehospitalization for syncope at 27-month follow-up. Clin Cardiol. 2011;34(1):35–8. https://doi.org/10.1002/clc.20872.
50. Accreditation Council for Graduate Medical Education. Educational innovation project. Available at http://www.acgme.org/acWebsite/RRC_140/140_EIPindex.asp. Accessed 22 Aug 2013.
51. Nabors C, Peterson SJ, Weems R, et al. A multidisciplinary approach for teaching systems-based practice to internal medicine residents. J Grad Med Educ. 2011;3(1):75–80. https://doi.org/10.4300/JGME-D-10-00037.1;10.4300/JGME-D-10-00037.1.
52. Francis MD, Julian KA, Wininger DA, et al. Continuity clinic model and diabetic outcomes in internal medicine residencies: findings of the educational innovations project ambulatory collaborative. J Grad Med Educ. 2016;8(1):27–32. https://doi.org/10.4300/JGME-D-15-00073.1.
53. Francis MD, Thomas K, Langan M, et al. Clinic design, key practice metrics, and resident satisfaction in internal medicine continuity clinics: findings of the educational innovations project ambulatory collaborative. J Grad Med Educ. 2014;6(2):249–55. https://doi.org/10.4300/JGME-D-13-00159.1.
54. Francis MD, Wieland ML, Drake S, et al. Clinic design and continuity in internal medicine resident clinics: findings of the educational innovations project ambulatory collaborative. J Grad Med Educ. 2015;7(1):36–41. https://doi.org/10.4300/JGME-D-14-00358.1.
55. Nabors C, Peterson SJ, Forman L, et al. Operationalizing the internal medicine milestones-an early status report. J Grad Med Educ. 2013;5(1):130–7. https://doi.org/10.4300/JGME-D-12-00130.1.
56. Nabors C, Peterson SJ, Aronow WS, et al. Physician reporting of clinically significant events through a computerized patient sign-out system. J Patient Saf. 2011;7(3):155–61. https://doi.org/10.1097/PTS.0b013e31822d7a66;10.1097/PTS.0b013e31822d7a66.
57. Nabors C, Peterson SJ, Lee WN, et al. Experience with faculty supervision of an electronic resident sign-out system. Am J Med. 2010;123(4):376–81. https://doi.org/10.1016/j.amjmed.2009.12.010.
58. Frishman WH, Nabors C, Peterson SJ. Faculty supervision of the house staff handoff process: the time has come. Am J Med. 2013;126(1):e1–2. https://doi.org/10.1016/j.amjmed.2012.07.014;10.1016/j.amjmed.2012.07.014.
59. Nabors C, Peterson SJ, Aronow WS, et al. Mobile physician reporting of clinically significant events-a novel way to improve handoff communication and supervision of resident on call activities. J Patient Saf. 2014;10(4):211–7. https://doi.org/10.1097/PTS.0b013e31829952ff.
60. Peterson MC. A systematic review of outcomes and quality measures in adult patients cared for by hospitalists vs nonhospitalists. Mayo Clin Proc. 2009;84(3):248–54.
61. Parent B, LaGrone LN, Albirair MT, et al. Effect of standardized handoff curriculum on improved clinician preparedness in the intensive care unit: a stepped-wedge cluster randomized clinical trial. JAMA Surg. 2018. https://doi.org/10.1001/jamasurg.2017.5440.
62. Starmer AJ, Spector ND, Srivastava R, et al. Changes in medical errors after implementation of a handoff program. N Engl J Med. 2014;371(19):1803–12. https://doi.org/10.1056/NEJMsa1405556.
63. Wohlauer MV, Arora VM, Horwitz LI, et al. The patient handoff: a comprehensive curricular blueprint for resident education to improve continuity of care. Acad Med. 2012;87(4):411–8. https://doi.org/10.1097/ACM.0b013e318248e766.
64. Glasheen JJ, Siegal EM, Epstein K, Kutner J, Prochazka AV. Fulfilling the promise of hospital medicine: tailoring internal medicine training to address hospitalists' needs. J Gen Intern Med. 2008;23(7):1110–5. https://doi.org/10.1007/s11606-008-0646-5.
65. Lin D, Shah C, Campbell S, Bates JT, Lescinskas E. Getting it RITE: impact of a dedicated hospital medicine curriculum for residents. South Med J. 2018;111(1):30–4. https://doi.org/10.14423/SMJ.0000000000000751.
66. Ludwin S, Harrison JD, Ranji S, Sharpe BA, Kneeland P. Training residents in hospital medicine: the hospitalist elective national survey. J Hosp Med. 2018. https://doi.org/10.12788/jhm.2952.
67. Institute for Health Care Improvement Open School. http://app.ihi.org/lms/onlinelearning.aspx?CatalogGUID=6cb1c614-884b-43ef-9abd-d90849f183d4. March 10, 2018.
68. Hospitalist fellowships. Society of Hospital Medicine. https://www.hospitalmedicine.org/membership/hospitalist-fellowships/?hkey=7faea954-15f1-4eef-aa6c-ca29674d0838. April 2, 2018.
69. Ranji SR, Rosenman DJ, Amin AN, Kripalani S. Hospital medicine fellowships: works in progress. Am J Med. 2006;119(1):72.e1–7. doi: S0002-9343(05)00673-X [pii].
70. University of Colorado Hospital Medicine Group. http://www.ucdenver.edu/academics/colleges/medicalschool/departments/medicine/GIM/ClinicalCare/HospitalMedicine/impact/Pages/Innovations.aspx. Updated 2017 March 20, 2018.
71. Ireland J. ABFM and ABIM to jointly participate in recognition of focused practice (rfp) in hospital medicine pilot approved by abms. Ann Fam Med. 2010;8(1):87. https://doi.org/10.1370/afm.1084.
72. Edelstein P. Top trends in health information & communications technology for 2017. https://

www.elsevier.com/connect/top-trends-in-health-information-and-communications-technology-for-2017. Accessed 8 Apr 2018.
73. Cumbler E, Yirdaw E, Kneeland P, et al. What is career success for academic hospitalists? A qualitative analysis of early-career faculty perspectives. J Hosp Med. 2018. https://doi.org/10.12788/jhm.2924.
74. Roberts DL, Shanafelt TD, Dyrbye LN, West CP. A national comparison of burnout and work-life balance among internal medicine hospitalists and outpatient general internists. J Hosp Med. 2014;9(3):176–81. https://doi.org/10.1002/jhm.2146.
75. Fredrickson M. Utilizing peer mentorship to improve job satisfaction and engagement in an academic community hospitalist group. [Hospital Medicine abstract 91]. J Hosp Med. 2018. https://www.shmabstracts.com/abstract/utilizing-peer-mentorship-to-improve-jobsatisfaction-and-engagement-in-an-academic-community-hospitalist-group/. Accessed 17 March 2018.
76. Yoon JD, Daley BM, Curlin FA. The association between a sense of calling and physician well-being: a national study of primary care physicians and psychiatrists. Acad Psychiatry. 2017;41(2):167–73. https://doi.org/10.1007/s40596-016-0487-1.
77. Keeton K, Fenner DE, Johnson TR, Hayward RA. Predictors of physician career satisfaction, work-life balance, and burnout. Obstet Gynecol. 2007;109(4):949–55. doi: 109/4/949 [pii].
78. Frellick M. Wachter: we got it wrong with 7 on, 7 off work schedules. Medscape Medical News; March 15, 2016. https://www.medscape.com/viewarticle/860409. Accessed 1 April 2018.
79. Ryan L. Flexibility is king. Hospitalist. 2011(3). https://www.the-hospitalist.org/hospitalist/article/124935/flexibility-king. Accessed 17 March 2018.
80. Chandra S, Wright SM, Howell EE. The creating incentives and continuity leading to efficiency staffing model: a quality improvement initiative in hospital medicine. Mayo Clin Proc. 2012;87(4):364–71. https://doi.org/10.1016/j.mayocp.2011.12.015.
81. Leyenaar JK, Frintner MP. Graduating pediatric residents entering the hospital medicine workforce, 2006–2015. Acad Pediatr. 2018;18(2):200–7. doi: S1876-2859(17)30317-0 [pii].
82. Leyenaar JK, Capra LA, O'Brien ER, Leslie LK, Mackie TI. Determinants of career satisfaction among pediatric hospitalists: a qualitative exploration. Acad Pediatr. 2014;14(4):361–8. https://doi.org/10.1016/j.acap.2014.03.015.
83. Hoppszallern S. Henry ford health system's health data exchange fuels next gen ACO data interoperability critical for value-based care. Hosp Health Netw. 2017;91(9):14. https://www.hhnmag.com/articles/8507-henry-ford-health-systems-health-data-exchange-fuels-next-gen-aco. Accessed 17 March 2018.
84. Becker C, Frishman WH, Scurlock C. Telemedicine and tele-ICU: the evolution and differentiation of a new medical field. Am J Med. 2016;129(12):e333–4. doi: S0002-9343(16)30839-7 [pii].
85. Escobar GJ, Turk BJ, Ragins A, et al. Piloting electronic medical record-based early detection of inpatient deterioration in community hospitals. J Hosp Med. 2016;11(Suppl 1):S18–24. https://doi.org/10.1002/jhm.2652.
86. Gunter RL, Chouinard S, Fernandes-Taylor S, et al. Current use of telemedicine for post-discharge surgical care: a systematic review. J Am Coll Surg. 2016;222(5):915–27. https://doi.org/10.1016/j.jamcollsurg.2016.01.062.
87. Kripalani S, LeFevre F, Phillips CO, Williams MV, Basaviah P, Baker DW. Deficits in communication and information transfer between hospital-based and primary care physicians: implications for patient safety and continuity of care. JAMA. 2007;297(8):831–41. https://doi.org/10.1001/jama.297.8.831.

The Nurse in the Modern Hospital 32

Jane C. Shivnan and Martha M. Kennedy

Nursing: Precious Resource

While never static, the profession of nursing has evolved rapidly in the last few decades to meet the needs of patients and families navigating complex health systems. Globally, nurses are seeking advanced certifications and education to prepare themselves as expert partners in care. This chapter focuses on nursing in the United States, but many of the themes discussed here are echoed or even amplified in other countries.

Nursing is defined by the American Nurses Association as "the protection, promotion, and optimization of health and abilities, prevention of illness and injury, facilitation of healing, alleviation of suffering through the diagnosis and treatment of human response, and advocacy in the care of individuals, families, groups, communities, and populations" [1]. The World Health Organization states that nursing "encompasses autonomous and collaborative care of individuals of all ages, families, groups and communities, sick or well and in all settings. It includes the promotion of health, the prevention of illness, and the care of ill, disabled and dying people" [2]. In the modern hospital, the nurse is an essential member of the healthcare team, collaborating to facilitate care and advocating for the patient and family. The nurse uses professional knowledge and skills to provide direct care, to protect the patient from harm, and to efficiently coordinate care.

The demands of efficiency and throughput in acute hospital settings may seem at odds with nurses' desire for personal connections with patients and families. Nursing time is often spent documenting care, managing machines, interacting with computers, and directing ancillary staff members. Nurses working in such complex and fast-paced settings may experience stress, job dissatisfaction, and even burnout. Time spent on valuable nursing activities such as patient education, psychological and spiritual support, advocacy, and caring at the bedside is often pressured by competing priorities and the need to meet regulatory requirements.

Professional nursing is a precious resource in the modern hospital. While assessments differ somewhat in numbers, there is widespread consensus that the twenty-first century will bring an increased need for nurses. Major contributing factors in the United States include an aging nursing workforce and aging population (Table 32.1: Factors influencing nursing workforce). By 2050 the number of Americans over the age of 65 is expected to double to almost 84 million. Some of those older Americans will be retired nurses – as of 2013 about 55% of the nursing workforce was age 50 or older. By 2024, over one million job openings for nurses will be

J. C. Shivnan (✉)
Health Care Consultant, Glen Burnie, MD, USA
e-mail: jshivna1@jhmi.edu

M. M. Kennedy
Department of Surgery, The Johns Hopkins Hospital, Baltimore, MD, USA

R. Latifi (ed.), *The Modern Hospital*, https://doi.org/10.1007/978-3-030-01394-3_32

Table 32.1 Factors influencing nursing workforce

Developed world	Developing world
Increased demand	Increased demand
Faculty shortages	Faculty shortages
Aging nurse population	Global migration
Alternative careers	Gender-based discrimination
Pay and benefits	Infectious diseases
Unacceptable work environments	Unacceptable work environments

created in the United States, reflecting the impact of nurses leaving the workforce and increased demand. Inequitable distribution of the workforce is expected to lead to significant local shortages [3].

The landmark 2010 Institute of Medicine report, *The Future of Nursing*, recommended that the number of nurses with baccalaureate degrees should be 80% of the workforce by 2020. Currently, only 55% of nurses are prepared at the baccalaureate or graduate level [3]. Schools of nursing have limited capacity due to shortages in faculty, clinical sites, classroom space, and clinical preceptors. Local and national nursing shortages are often mitigated by economic downturns as inactive and part-time nurses take on more hours of work to support families, and young people (and second-career job seekers) turn to nursing for secure employment. Nevertheless, the projections paint a grim picture of a potential future without enough appropriately educated RNs to care for older adults with complex healthcare needs and multiple comorbidities.

The modern hospital must therefore provide a supportive workplace environment for nurses to attract and retain this precious resource. The chief nursing officer (CNO) must be a transformational leader, form a strong partnership with other members of the executive team, and be an advocate for nursing to the board of directors. The CNO is accountable for the organizational nursing structure and standards of nursing practice. In collaboration with other departments and disciplines, the CNO establishes programs and policies that support and engage nurses and promote excellence in patient care. From servant leader to bedside, nurses help create an organizational culture of excellence.

Evolving Roles

Nurses are registered (RNs) or licensed (LPNs) in the United States, distinguished by their education, role, and autonomy in practice. LPNs typically receive training for a year beyond high school and become licensed after passing the NCLEX-PN exam. They provide a variety of direct care services under the direction of RNs, physicians, or other healthcare providers, with most working in residential facilities and home health. RNs most often have a bachelor's degree in nursing or a 2-year associate's degree in nursing and are licensed to practice after passing the NCLEX-RN. While there is overlap in the direct care activities provided by RNs and LPNs, the RN's work is more complex and analytical, and the RN has greater autonomy in practice.

Within a supportive healthcare organization, nurses are empowered to practice to the full extent of their professional license and educational preparation. The professional nurse acting at the point of care – the direct care or bedside nurse – is the foundation of the modern hospital's patient care system. At the core of nursing is the nursing process: assess, plan, implement, and evaluate. The direct care nurse coordinates the multidisciplinary plan of care and assures continuity of care across settings.

Nurses have also developed specialized roles to meet the needs of patients and families and provide optimal care within complex healthcare systems. Such roles provide advancement opportunities to individuals and keep expertise close to the bedside. Clinical ladders also provide opportunities to direct care nurses for recognition of expert practice. Specialized roles now frequently require advanced education and/or certifications and may be further regulated by licensing and other requirements (Table 32.2: US nursing roles and current requirements). The chief nursing officer, in collaboration with other members of the executive team, creates a nursing structure and

Table 32.2 US nursing roles and current requirements

Role	Focus	Education requirement	Certification	Notes
Registered nurse, direct care nurse, clinical nurse	Direct care	BSN or associate degree	Specialty certifications available	
Clinical nurse leader	Coordination and direct care for a cohort	MSN	CNL certification available	
Clinical nurse specialist	Clinical care, consultation and education, and research	MSN or DNP	CNS certification required	States vary in independent practice and prescriptive authority
Nurse practitioner	Direct care including medical diagnosis and interventions	MSN[a] or DNP	NP Certification required[b]	States vary in independent practice and prescriptive authority
Certified registered nurse anesthetist	Anesthesia and pain management services	MSN[c] with nurse anesthesia	CRNA certification required	States vary in independent practice and prescriptive authority
Certified nurse-midwife	Women's health, labor, and delivery	MSN	CNM certification required	States vary in independent practice and prescriptive authority
Nurse educator	Orientation and continuing education for staff	BSN or MSN	Certifications available	
Nurse case manager	Transitions of care for high-risk patients and populations	BSN or MSN	Certifications available	
Nurse navigator	Assisting individual patients with complex healthcare needs	BSN or associate degree	Certification available	
Clinical research nurse	Direct care and study coordination	BSN or associate degree	Certifications in clinical research available	

[a]Graduate education not required for NP in Indiana
[b]Specialties include family, acute care, emergency, women's health, psychiatric, neonatal, pediatric, adult gerontology
[c]Graduate education not required for CRNA in South Dakota

organization that leverages the expertise of nurses to meet patient care needs.

Clinical Nurse Leader

The clinical nurse leader (CNL) role is designed to enhance patient safety and care by placing master's prepared generalist nurses as clinical leaders at the point of care. Key components of the role include care coordination and management of transitions of care, outcomes measurement, risk assessment, interprofessional communication and team leadership, implementation of evidence-based best practices, and quality improvement. The CNL works with a distinct group of patients and interdisciplinary team – a cohort, rather than a population. This microsystem focus is a fundamental characteristic of the CNL role and helps distinguish it from the clinical nurse specialist.

The CNL role is relatively new. It was first introduced in 2003 through the American Association of Colleges of Nursing (AACN) as a strategy to improve patient outcomes [4]. Diffusion and implementation of this role have been slow, however. A 2016 study noted that CNLs represented only 0.1% of the RN workforce and 1.3% of RNs with a master's degree [5]. The survey reached out to the 3375 certified CNLs via email and 601 (19%) responded. Of the study participants, just 347 (58%) were practicing in a formal CNL role, although 480 (80%) were involved in a CNL initiative. The majority of study participants worked in urban acute care hospitals in the South.

Evidence for the impact of the CNL role consists mostly of case reports, with just seven qualitative and/or survey studies and three quantitative studies found in a 2014 narrative review of the CNL literature [6]. Many of the case reports describe CNL pilots and quality improvement activities with a broad array of positive outcomes: increased patient satisfaction, improved team communication and collaboration, improved Joint Commission core measures, and reductions in healthcare-associated infections, use of resources, and length of stay. None of the research studies measured the CNL impact on patient outcomes. These studies demonstrated a positive impact of the CNL role on the individual's own job satisfaction, less anticipated turnover and greater happiness among nurses working on CNL units, and improved patient satisfaction.

Advanced Practice Nursing

The term advanced practice registered nurse (APRN) is used most often to represent four nursing specialty roles: clinical nurse specialist (CNS), nurse practitioner (NP), certified registered nurse anesthetist (CRNA), and certified nurse-midwife (CNM). APRNs have completed additional specialty training and/or graduate course work and clinical hours to supplement their foundation as registered nurses. While the focus of each role is different, common to all are essential competencies in both clinical (e.g., patient care, critical thinking) and nonclinical (e.g., leadership, academic, research, outcome evaluation) skills. Over 267,000 APRNs are practicing in the United States. Each state determines the level of independent practice and prescriptive authority for APRN roles. Not all states recognize the four roles, and there is considerable variation in APRN scope of practice across states [7].

Clinical Nurse Specialist

CNSs deliver care to patients, families, and groups of patients, provide direct mentorship and coaching of clinical staff, and improve care through establishment of standards of care and quality improvement initiatives at the local and institutional level. The CNS may identify and research common clinical problems in order to improve care delivery and outcomes, focusing on patient populations and healthcare systems. Through their work with both staff and patients, CNS integration into practice has been found to positively impact prevention of hospital-acquired conditions and readmissions and length of stay [8]. CNSs often specialize in practice areas such as oncology, critical care, and women's health.

Nurse Practitioner

In the 1960s, a shortage of primary care physicians available to provide care in rural areas of the United States led to the introduction of the NP role. Over time, the role has expanded to include acute as well as primary care. Depending on the setting and state or institutional regulations, NP care may be provided independently, under the supervision of physician colleagues, or as a member of a collaborative team of providers. With increasing specialization has come more specific education and certification requirements that address the patient acuity level, chronicity or acuteness of the disease process, and age-specific competencies required to provide safe and expert care [9]. NPs may now be certified in primary and/or acute care and in specialties such as neonatology, pediatrics, adult, psychiatric/mental health, oncology, women's health, and gerontology.

While there are few randomized controlled trials comparing physician and NP outcomes, two systematic reviews found comparable clinical outcomes and patient satisfaction, adherence to guidelines, and more thorough patient education [10, 11]. A review by Stanik-Hutt et al. [12] did not find differences in health status outcomes and physical function across settings (ambulatory, home, and inpatient settings) linked to patient oversight by a NP or physician. Landsperger et al. [13] conducted a large cohort study of MICU patients in an academic medical center. Patients were cared for consistently by either NP or resident teams and had similar outcomes at hospital discharge and at 90-day post-discharge. In many institutions, especially academic settings with increasing limitations on house staff work hours, the NP role is also valued for its impact on improving workflow and throughput. Patients, staff, and faculty alike value the continuity of care provided by a NP who may manage patients' care throughout their hospital stay and then coordinate their transition to the next level of care. Nurse practitioners can be valuable partners to physician faculty as they strive to meet both clinical and academic goals as well as provide training and mentorship to the next generation of physicians in training.

Certified Registered Nurse Anesthetists

CRNAs are registered nurses who have completed a graduate nurse anesthesia education program. Working in collaboration with anesthesiologists, surgeons, and other healthcare professionals, CRNAs attend to patients of all ages in a variety of settings. They provide anesthesia services, pain management, airway management, and invasive monitoring as required and may support emergency response and resuscitation teams. Each state determines the extent to which CRNAs can work independently and the rate of reimbursement for their care. Additionally, the federal government, through Medicare and Medicaid regulations, also determines some reimbursement rates. Reviews of the literature comparing morbidity and mortality outcomes of CRNAs are challenged to find significant differences in CRNA care when compared to anesthesiologists [14, 15]. Both sides cite concerns related to study designs, measurement choices, and interpretation of results [16].

Certified Nurse-Midwives

CNMs are registered nurses educated and certified to provide reproductive care and primary care and to attend births. Their scope of practice includes gynecologic and family planning services, antepartum and postpartum care, nutrition counseling, parenting and patient education, and attending childbirth. As of 2010, all entry-level CNMs are required to have a graduate degree from an accredited graduate educational program to enter midwifery practice.

A Cochrane systematic review of studies comparing midwife-led vs other models of care was completed in 2013 and updated in 2016. The review included studies conducted in the public health systems in Australia, Canada, Ireland, and the United Kingdom. The authors found that women in midwife-led care models had fewer epidurals, instrumented vaginal births, and preterm births than their counterparts and more spontaneous vaginal births [17]. It is important to note that this review excluded women with significant maternal disease and substance abuse, hindering the generalizability of these findings.

Nurse Educator

The modern hospital must assure its nurses are competent and safe providers of care. Traditionally, those in the nurse educator role partnered with the manager to evaluate staff performance and develop plans for addressing identified needs. Often those needs were met with practical training at the bedside or through classroom instruction. Educator practice has evolved due to graduate programs in education and the availability of new learning technology and strategies based on adult learning principles. Academic and clinical educators have been moving from a "teaching/instruction" paradigm to a "learning" paradigm. In the modern hospital, the nurse educator identifies the desired learning outcomes, creates a collaborative and supportive environment with learning activities where the learner can discover and construct knowledge, and facilitates its application [18, 19]. Ideally, learning principles are integrated in orientation programs and by preceptors as the new graduate nurse is supported to move from theoretical and classroom learning to practical and applied learning, with the expectation of repeated assessment of competencies over time. Many institutions have recognized that the new graduate nurse requires proactive support to transition from student to care provider. This has led the development of evidence-based "transition to practice" programs. In these programs, new nurses are supported over their first year to increase their personal confidence, competency, and comfort in their role [19–21].

Increasingly, institutions are now requiring nurse educators to obtain certification in education or nursing professional development or to have a graduate degree with an emphasis in education. To enable workforce training and education, hospitals may provide simulation laboratories with experts in simulation practice, learning resource centers to support development of learning materials and strategies, and research support for quality and performance initiatives.

The nurse educator facilitates new learning experiences, and the evaluation of the need for revision of existing learning activities over time. Additionally, nurse educators partner with other nurse leaders and disciplines to identify ongoing developmental needs for more experienced staff. When integrated fully, the nurse educator is a valuable member of the leadership team, who partners in education, research, quality, and performance improvement initiatives.

Case Manager

The modern hospital does not exist in isolation – its capacity for horizontal and vertical integration reduces structural barriers to transitions of care and may help reduce length of stay, cost of care, and readmission rates. Managing these transitions of care remains a significant challenge for most organizations. Contemporary case management expanded in the 1970s to help contain costs while assuring quality outcomes in an increasingly complex American health system. Case managers are widely used in multiple settings, but there is no universal set of standards and expectations of the role. Nurse case managers apply skills in assessment, planning, and patient education to the case management role. They frequently work with a specific patient population within an interdisciplinary team. The opportunity for role ambiguity and confusion has only increased with the development and implementation of facility-specific roles such as admission or discharge coordinators.

Nurse Navigator

The nurse navigator role has emerged as a unique partnership between the professional nurse, patient, and healthcare system. Nurse navigation has been best defined and studied in oncology, but there are many examples of its successful application to other high-risk clinical scenarios including emergency departments, heart failure management, and obstetric and neonatal care. Pederson and Hack (2010) identified five critical patient navigator attributes in their concept analysis: the nurse navigator facilitates access to care, is a skilled communicator and listener, is knowledgeable of the system and resources in which they work, acts as an empathic patient advocate, and provides information and education [22]. The role's focus on the relationship with an individual patient provides the nurse navigator with the opportunity to remove barriers to care, improve patient outcomes, and enhance the overall quality of healthcare delivery.

Dr. Harold Freeman and his colleagues at Harlem Hospital in New York are generally credited with implementing the first oncology patient navigation program in the 1990s, designed to address health disparities for marginalized communities [22]. Federal funding for patient navigation projects was provided in 2005 under the Patient Navigator Outreach and Chronic Disease Act. In cancer care, expectations for navigation processes have been built into accreditation standards from the American College of Surgeons (ACS) and the National Accreditation Program for Breast Centers (NAPBC). Patient navigation programs do not require nurse navigators, however the specialized knowledge and skills of professional nurses make them uniquely suited to facilitate timely access to care and reduce barriers to treatment. In 2013 (and updated in 2016) the Oncology Nursing Society (ONS) established a definition and core competencies for the Oncology Nurse Navigator (ONN) [23].

Clinical Research Nurse

Clinical research in hospital settings is highly regulated to protect the rights of human subjects and ensure robust, replicable outcomes. The principal investigator often engages a multidisciplinary team of providers, pharmacists, nurses, clinical trial coordinators, and data analysts to conduct a clinical trial. Such research teams work in all settings where complex clinical trials are conducted – oncology, cardiology, pediatrics, nephrology, and infectious disease. Clinical research nurse (CRN) roles are multidimensional. An oncology role delineation study confirmed that CRNs provide direct patient care, generally related to the goals of the study, e.g., educating patients and families, monitoring for adverse events, and collecting study data [24]. CRNs support the study with activities such as subject recruitment, eligibility screening, informed consent, and coordination of study visits. They use their expertise to help develop and implement the research protocol and may create and provide educational materials for research participants as well as educating staff about the study. CRNs often help administer and lead the study, managing budgets and teams and data and producing regulatory reports.

The Nurse and the Team

Nursing Practice

Nurses use the nursing process to guide holistic, patient-centered care. Multidimensional *assessment* collects and analyzes patient data: physiologic, psychologic, sociocultural, and spiritual. The nurse uses these data and makes a clinical judgment about the patient's response to actual or potential healthcare problems and needs, the nursing *diagnosis*. In collaboration with the patient and family, the nurse creates measurable goals and uses evidence-based interventions to design the *plan of care* for the patient. Nursing care is provided and documented based on the nursing plan of care and in collaboration with other disciplines, the *implementation* phase. Ongoing and systematic *evaluation* of the patient's response to the plan of care is used to modify the care plan.

In the United States, each state has enacted a nurse practice act and established a Board of Nursing (BON) with the authority to provide licenses to nurses and issue administrative rules and regulations. For example, BONs issue regulations and guidance defining the nursing role in practice areas such as delegation to unlicensed assistive personnel, procedural sedation, telephone triage, use of complementary therapies, and bolusing epidural anesthesia. BON activities establish the legal basis for nursing in each state. The scope of nursing practice includes activities that nurses pursue independently and activities that are interdependent with other disciplines such as the medication process. At a national level, professional and specialty nursing organizations publish nursing practice standards and scope documents, providing guidance to nurses working in clinical specialties and specialty roles. Examples include the Hospice and Palliative Nurses Association 2014 position statement on the use of medical marijuana and the Association of periOperative Registered Nurses' position statement delineating the scope of practice and qualifications for the Registered Nurse First Assist (RNFA) role.

Communication

With the patient and family at the center, the nurse provides and coordinates care in collaboration with the many disciplines and departments that create the modern hospital. Effective interpersonal communication is crucial in this complex system. Electronic medical records, orders, rounds, handoffs, and patient education all require timely, accurate, and useful communication. The link between poor communication and poor patient outcomes has been well documented by the Joint Commission, the Institute of Medicine, and others. Ineffective communication in healthcare results in sentinel events, misdiagnosis, delayed treatment, medication errors, and patient injury. Ineffective communication also results in frustration, stress, job dissatisfaction, and attrition.

Studies of interprofessional communication in healthcare have demonstrated clear themes that provide a framework for understanding and improving communication [25, 26]. Barriers to effective communication include lack of confidence, lack of experience, complexity of healthcare, professional jargon, distractions and interruptions, physician dominance in decision-making, and lack of structure and standardization. Many studies have demonstrated differences in communication styles between physicians and nurses, ascribed to differences in training and socialization as well as gender. Nurses are trained to be descriptive and supportive in communication, whereas physicians are trained to be succinct and provide opinions. It is worth remembering that these styles are not right or wrong and that these differences can and should be embraced to enhance communication and ultimately benefit the patient.

Research has demonstrated that interprofessional communication skills can be significantly improved with training, including use of simulation exercises and standardized communication tools [25]. These findings have important implications for academic education of physicians, nurses, and other disciplines. They also imply that the modern hospital must establish communication standards and expectations, provide standardized communication tools, and invest in interprofessional training. Supportive practice environments that empower nurse participation in hospital operations and interprofessional activities also improve nurses' perceptions of nurse-physician communication. Nurses can be catalysts for change in workplace climate and organizational culture, promoting respectful communication and trust.

Standardized communication tools provide a framework for concise and organized information transfer. They can guide reports and handoffs between individuals or between settings. They can convey critical information, for example, in requesting a rapid response team intervention, or check accuracy, for example, with the read-back technique. Standardized communication tools can also be used to structure team meetings such as rounds and huddles. One example, the situation-background-assessment-recommendation (SBAR) framework, is relatively simple to teach and use, can be implemented in multiple situations and settings, and can be used within or between professions. It also has the advantage of streamlining information, eliminating assumptions, and flattening the hierarchy among caregivers [25].

Collaboration

Teamwork and collaboration are terms often used interchangeably in healthcare, but there are subtle differences. Teamwork represents the combined actions of a group of people toward goals and objectives, for example, the successful implementation of a weaning protocol for a patient in a MICU or the pain management and mobilization of a postoperative patient. Collaboration is one of several activities that characterize effective teamwork. It implies a high level of professional accountability and engagement within the healthcare team – sharing knowledge and skills to establish and achieve an objective. Effective communication and collaboration are essential competencies for healthcare professions and prerequisites for highly performing teams.

Interprofessional training focused on improving communication and collaboration can use a variety of approaches – workshops, online modules, case studies, and simulation. TeamSTEPPS™ (Team Strategies and Tools to Enhance Performance and Patient Safety) instruction was developed by the Department of Defense (DoD) and the Agency for Healthcare Quality and Research (AHRQ) to provide training, tools, and strategies to improve team performance in healthcare. Its goal is to improve patient safety by improving teamwork. Released in 2006, the program addresses core competencies of leadership, situation monitoring (mutual performance monitoring), mutual support (backup behavior), and communication [27].

The Comprehensive Unit-Based Safety Program (CUSP) was developed and initially implemented in ICUs at the Johns Hopkins Hospital in Baltimore, Maryland. It includes training and quality improvement strategies to engage clinicians and support change at the unit level. AHRQ provides the CUSP toolkit to healthcare organizations, funding a national effort to reduce healthcare-associated infections such as central line-associated bloodstream infections (CLABSI) and catheter-associated urinary tract infections (CAUTI) [28].

A recent literature review investigating interprofessional interventions designed to promote patient safety included 89 studies published between 2005 and 2015 [29]. The majority of the studies were conducted in North America (76%) and in acute clinical organizations (82%). Most studies (68%) employed educational interventions to improve collaboration, sometimes adding practice interventions such as team checklists, team briefings, or patient safety rounds. Although most studies measured interim outcomes such as perceptions of patient safety culture, several reported improvements in patient outcomes such as rates of morbidity, reduction of adverse events, and timely delivery of patient medications. The authors conclude that interprofessional education should be combined with changes in practice and organizational activities to promote collaboration and patient safety.

Patient- and Family-Centered Care

Various organizations have defined and endorsed patient-centered care (PCC) including the Institute of Medicine, the Agency for Healthcare Research and Quality, the Planetree Initiative, the Picker Institute, and the National Cancer Institute [30]. PCC is care that respects the patient's beliefs and values, includes patients' personal and social support systems, and is provided and coordinated in the context of a caring and therapeutic relationship. This relationship between clinician and patient includes open (and two-way) communication of knowledge, personal expertise, and clinical expertise. PCC also requires patient engagement in care, enabled by providing the education, information, evidence, and resources needed to allow patients to be involved in managing their own care [30]. The expanded concept of patient- and family-centered care appropriately recognizes the important role of family (as defined by the patient) and is particularly meaningful in settings such as ICUs, pediatrics, and neonatology.

The nurse is uniquely placed in the healthcare system to identify and promote opportunities for patient- and family-centered care. Patients expect nurses to act in their best interests and to respect their dignity. The therapeutic nurse-patient relationship protects the patient's autonomy and gives the nurse the insights and information needed to individualize the plan of care and advocate for the patient. The modern hospital supports PCC with policies, structures, and processes that facilitate the engagement of patients and families in care. Examples include open visitation, bedside rounds, bedside hand-offs, patient-/family-activated rapid response teams, shared care plans, and daily goals sheets. Patients and family members may be engaged in care by tracking medications, assisting with or providing care, and accessing information including medical records. Patient and family advisory councils and other committees provide opportunities for patients and family members to influence hospital policies and procedures and support PCC initiatives. Healing environments such as those described by the Planetree Initiative, single rooms, amenities for families, and strategies for noise reduction are examples of environmental changes that support PCC and should be considered in hospital renovations and design.

Family-centered care in ICUs has been described in an updated set of 2016 evidence-based guidelines from the American College of Critical Care Medicine and endorsed by multiple professional organizations [31]. The authors did not find strong evidence for any of their recommendations and noted the importance of further high-quality research studies. The evidence supports offering open or flexible family presence at the bedside, including during resuscitation efforts, family education programs, routine interdisciplinary family conferences and structured approaches to communication with families, and reducing noise and providing families with an opportunity to sleep. The implementation of PCC has resulted in positive measurable outcomes in numerous research studies [30, 31]. Reported benefits include increased patient and family satisfaction, decreased costs, decreased lengths of stay in ICUs and in the hospital, fewer diagnostic tests and referrals, fewer symptoms of depression and anxiety, and greater self-efficacy. Changes in organizational structures, policies, and processes are doomed to fail without a sustained cultural change and commitment to viewing the patient as an engaged partner in care. PCC is based on relationships – individual professional relationships with patients and families and organizational relationships. Its successful implementation can be readily measured with patient and family satisfaction measurement tools.

Patient and Family Education

Adoption of PCC requires an even greater emphasis on patient and family education. Patients need knowledge and understanding of their illness and the actions they must take to mitigate its effects and achieve their health goals. Effective patient education improves outcomes by increasing adherence to medications and treatment plans, enhancing self-care, and promoting appropriate healthcare utilization [32].

The modern hospital uses evidence-based strategies and a formal system for patient and family education. Approaches to patient and family education must account for learning needs, health literacy, and learning styles. An organization-wide interprofessional committee can establish standards, support the development of enduring materials and mixed media, and help train staff in patient education methods. For example, written materials should be assessed for readability using a tool such as Flesch reading ease score. The Suitability Assessment of Materials (SAM) instrument or a similar tool can assess the presentation of information, including graphics, layout, learning stimulation and motivation, and cultural appropriateness. Ideally, patient and family representatives should also provide feedback in iterative consumer testing. Healthcare professionals benefit from learning structured methods of patient education, including "teach-back" and motivational interviewing.

While all healthcare providers have responsibilities for patient and family education, nurses play a key role in assuring that patients and families have the knowledge and skills needed for safe transitions of care. The nurse partners with an individual patient to identify learning needs and develop a teaching-learning plan based on an assessment of willingness and readiness to learn, barriers to learning, and preferred methods for learning. In educational sessions nurses complement spoken instruction with enduring materials such as printed, individualized instructions. Sessions are focused and often brief, using plain language and allowing the patient to control the flow of information. The nurse checks frequently with patient for understanding. Effective nurse teachers eliminate excessive details, use graphics and pictures, and ensure all parts of the message are coherent. Proven methods such as "teach-back" give the nurse the opportunity to assess the patient's understanding.

Measuring the Impact

Nurse-Sensitive Quality Indicators

Quality indicators that measure the structures, processes, and outcomes most influenced by nurses are referred to as nurse-sensitive indicators (NSIs). A wide range of possible NSIs have been proposed over time, but many of these indicators are not regularly collected due to measurement challenges (Table 32.3: Nurse-sensitive quality indicators). As a result, organizations such as the American Nurses Association (ANA), National Quality Forum, and the Joint Commission provide a limited set of structure and outcome NSIs.

The most widely reported NSIs in the United States are derived from the National Database for Nursing Quality Indicators (NDNQI®). Originally developed by ANA and managed by The University of Kansas School of Nursing, the NDNQI program was acquired in 2014 by Press Ganey. More than 2000 hospitals participate in NDNQI, with the opportunity to benchmark nursing quality at the unit, service, and organizational level. Continued work is needed to develop and test NSIs and to further expand their use in specialty and ambulatory settings.

Table 32.3 Nurse-sensitive quality indicators

Structural indicators	Process indicators	Outcome indicators
RN education level	*Nursing interventions*	Fall rate
Hours of nursing care per patient day	*Nursing documentation*	Fall with injury rate
Workload intensity	*Nursing care plans*	Hospital-acquired pressure injury (HAPI) rate
Skill mix	*Compliance with protocols*	Central line-associated bloodstream infection (CLABSI) rate
Support for bedside nurses	*Pediatric pain assessment, intervention, reassessment (AIR) cycle*	Catheter-associated urinary tract infection (CAUTI) rate
Quality of professional relationships	*Fall risk assessment*	Ventilator-associated pneumonia and events (VAP, VAE)
Voluntary nurse turnover	*Smoking cessation counseling*	Patient/family satisfaction
Nurse vacancy rate	*Delirium screening*	Length of stay
RN years of experience		Readmissions
		Nurse job satisfaction
		Medication errors
		Failure to rescue
		Pediatric peripheral intravenous infiltration rate
		Restraint and seclusion
		Mortality

NSIs in italics are not regularly collected and reported due to measurement challenges

Nursing Research- and Evidence-Based Practice

The complex body of knowledge and skills that defines a profession grows through investigation, research, and dissemination. Nursing research uses qualitative and quantitative systematic approaches to study and improve patient care and care systems. A nursing research program is an important addition to the modern hospital's department of nursing. Ideally, nurse leaders develop a strategic plan for nursing research and allocate resources to support research. Expertise can be engaged through partnerships with doctorally prepared faculty at Schools of Nursing or by recruiting a Director of Nursing Research. A committee structure – either nursing or interdisciplinary – can develop research competencies through education and mentorship, peer review for research proposals, and assistance with presentations and publications. Hospital and IRB policies and procedures should support nurses as principal investigators (PIs). Limiting PIs to individuals with advanced degrees or faculty members creates a barrier for many nurses. Appropriate training to ensure adequate protection of human subjects and compliance with research regulations can help prepare clinical nurses to participate in, and lead, nursing research.

Dissemination of nursing research is a professional responsibility – to internal and external audiences, with presentations and publications. Translating research findings into practice is as critical as generating new knowledge through investigation. Many organizations adopt a formal evidence-based practice (EBP) model, for example, the Johns Hopkins Nursing Evidence-Based Practice Model [33] or the Iowa Model [34]. EBP competencies have been defined for RNs and APRNs, but most nurses lack the knowledge and skills needed to achieve those competencies [35]. The nursing research program structure can be expanded to include EBP activities, or EBP can be embedded within the structure used for policies and procedures.

Magnet® Recognition Program

The American Nurses Credentialing Center's Magnet® Recognition Program is based on a 1983 research study that identified 14 "Forces of Magnetism" characterizing work environments most likely to attract and retain well-qualified nurses. From the first ANCC Magnet-designated organization in 1994, the program has grown to recognize over 430 healthcare organizations around the world [36]. Rigorous analyses have clustered the original Forces of Magnetism into a conceptual model with five key components: transformational leadership; structural empowerment; exemplary professional practice; new knowledge, innovations, and improvements; and empirical outcomes. A major revision of the Magnet Recognition standards in 2008 shifted the focus from descriptive measures to empirical outcomes. The release of the 2019 Magnet Application Manual continues to raise the bar for achieving this mark of organizational nursing excellence, emphasizing benchmarked empirical outcomes, generation of new knowledge through nursing research, and expanded requirements for ambulatory settings. While there are many organizations that have improved the practice of nursing and delivery of patient care, the robust research-based standards of this important program has undoubtedly been one of the most significant. Its importance is reflected in its inclusion in other measures of excellence, including the Leapfrog Group and the US News and World Report's annual ranking of best hospitals.

The process of Magnet application (and redesignation, required every 4 years) consists of application, submission of written documentation, and site visit. At least three independent expert nurse appraisers review the written documentation and conduct the site visit to determine whether the organization meets a threshold of excellence. Their written report is provided to the 12-member Commission on Magnet Recognition who make the decision [36].

Many recent research studies have demonstrated the positive impact of Magnet Recognition and the standards it establishes for excellence in nursing. Friese and his colleagues studied outcomes for Medicare patients undergoing coronary artery bypass surgery, colectomy, or lower extremity bypass surgery between 1998 and 2010 at US Magnet hospitals as compared to matched control non-Magnet hospitals [37]. Thirty-day mortality rates and failure to rescue complication rates were significantly lower in Magnet hospitals, independent of nurse staffing levels. Another study demonstrated 20% reduction in mortality for patients admitted between 2009 and 2011 to Magnet adult trauma centers in Pennsylvania, as compared to non-Magnet adult trauma centers [38]. A companion study of patients with ischemic stroke admitted to New York hospitals between 2009 and 2013 found that Magnet hospitals were associated with lower mortality, decreased length of stay, and decreased rate of discharge to a facility [39]. Magnet hospitals have recently been shown to be associated with lower CLABSI rates [40], lower HAPU rates [41], and higher scores in the Centers for Medicare and Medicaid Services Hospital Value-Based Purchasing (VBP) Program [42].

Some research studies have not found differences in outcomes between Magnet and non-Magnet hospitals or, rarely, have found better outcomes at non-Magnet hospitals. A 2015 systematic review considered ten quantitative studies and concluded that the evidence remains mixed and inconclusive for the impact of Magnet on nurse and patient outcomes. Seven of the ten studies showed statistically significant but general small effects, and three showed no effect [43]. A large study comparing pediatric critical care outcomes in Magnet and non-Magnet freestanding children's hospitals between 2004 and 2015 did not find any differences in mortality overall or when stratified by subgroups [44].

Preparing for the Future

Technology

In the modern hospital, technology transforms all aspects of operations and care delivery – from communication to supply management to decisions about patient care. Innovations in patient technology and monitoring have the potential to improve the quality and safety of care, resource utilization, coordination of care across settings and organizations, and accountability. As technology advances, nurses must acquire new competencies in data management and utilization and additional skills in the use of computer-based medical equipment and interfaces.

Nurses are primary end-users of many new technologies. Examples include point-of-care testing, automated dispensing systems and bar coding of medications and supplies, computerized provider order entry, and smart infusion pumps. Each of these significant innovations has the potential for positive and negative impact. While many technologies enhance patient safety, nurses (and other disciplines) express concerns about the amount of time added to the performance of activities such as medication administration and the potential loss of independent professional critical thinking when decisions and care are circumscribed by the technology.

The newest technologies have yet to reach most bedside nurses. Schools of nursing and healthcare organizations need to prepare nurses for widespread application of genomics and personalized precision medicine, clinical decision-making support software, and further dissemination of mobile technology and its implications for telehealth. A number of research studies have identified barriers and facilitators to technology adoption and use among nurses [45]. Best practices in demonstrating organizational commitment, high-quality training, support from peers, and perceived usability and usefulness will contribute to successful implementation of new technology.

Education

Nurse education in the United States is conducted by university-based schools of nursing (baccalaureate and graduate degrees), community colleges (associate degrees), and historically with diploma programs based in hospitals. The landmark 2010 Institute of Medicine report, *The Future of Nursing*, included strong recommendations for baccalaureate preparation of nurses based on the proven link between educational preparation and positive patient outcomes and for increasing the number of nurses with advanced degrees. Recent trends in nursing education include expanded availability of online programs, entry-level master's programs, and the Doctor of Nursing Practice (DNP) clinical doctorate program designed to prepare advanced practice nurses and nurse leaders (Table 32.4: Nurse education).

Lifelong Learning

As a professional, the nurse is accountable to maintain current knowledge, skills, and competencies. Continuing nursing education (CNE) provides systematic learning activities that augment the nurse's education and experience. Accredited CNE providers follow evidence-based standards for developing, providing, and

Table 32.4 Nurse education

Educational program	Offered by	Prepares student for	Length (full-time)	Other options
Associate degree in nursing (ADN, ASN)	Community colleges	NCLEX exam and RN licensure	2–3 years	
Bachelor's degree in nursing (BSN)	Colleges and universities with schools of nursing	NCLEX exam and RN licensure	4 years	RN to BSN programs for RN students with ADN or diploma (2–3 years) Accelerated BSN program for students with BA or BS (12–18 months)
Master's degree in nursing (MSN) Most curricula offer specialty role focus	Colleges and universities with graduate schools of nursing	Advanced practice nurse roles, nurse leader roles, nurse educator, nursing faculty	2 years	Entry-level MSN for students with BA or BS (15–24 months)
PhD in nursing	Colleges and universities with graduate schools of nursing	Nursing faculty, nurse researchers, nurse executives	4–6 years	BS to PhD MS to PhD
Doctor of Nursing Practice (DNP)	Colleges and universities with graduate schools of nursing	Advanced practice nurse roles, nurse leader roles, nursing faculty	18 months – 4 years	BS or BSN to DNP MS to DNP

evaluating educational activities. CNE can be provided in more traditional in-person settings, through simulation and through synchronous and asynchronous online activities.

Most states require continuing education as a condition of licensure. Nurses are also required to participate in CNE to obtain or renew specialty certifications, and many healthcare organizations require CNE for clinical ladder advancement and promotions. Increasingly, interprofessional education (IPE) activities are used by organizations to ensure that disciplines learn together. Brandt and colleagues found that most IPE research has focused on the assessment of its short-term impact on individual knowledge, skills, and attitudes, changes in practice-based processes, and organizational policy changes [46]. They argued for the pressing need to conduct well-designed research studies exploring the impact of IPE (and interprofessional collaborative practice) on the Triple Aim: the mandate to simultaneously improve patient experiences of care, population health, and per capita cost.

Conclusion

Nursing is the single largest profession in the healthcare workforce and a precious resource for the modern hospital. Nursing is creative and flexible, adapting to changes in healthcare delivery, technology, and patient care needs with evolving roles and focused evidence-based practice. Nursing is a trusted profession, with a strong commitment to ethical practice and patient advocacy. Structures and processes that allow nurses to practice to the full extent of their professional knowledge and skills will benefit patients, families, and the healthcare organization. As a profession, nursing continues to face challenges, for example, preparing and retaining sufficient well-educated new nurses, standardizing APRN roles and competencies across states, agreeing on entry-level education, demonstrating its impact through research, and increasing diversity in the workforce. Nevertheless, it is well worth taking on these challenges in order to assure the continued important contributions of nursing to healthcare and the modern hospital.

References

1. American Nurses Association [Internet]. Silver Spring, MD: American Nurses Association; c2018 [cited 2018 Jan 29]. What is nursing; [about 1 screen]. Available from: http://www.nursingworld.org/EspeciallyForYou/What-is-Nursing.
2. World Health Organization [Internet]. Geneva, Switzerland: World Health Organization; c2018 [cited 2018 Jan 29]. Nursing; [about 1 screen]. Available from: http://www.who.int/topics/nursing/en/.
3. American Association of Colleges of Nursing [Internet]. Washington, DC: American Association of Colleges of Nursing; c2017 [cited 2018 Jan 29]. Nursing shortage fact sheet; [about 1 screen]. Available from: http://www.aacnnursing.org/News-Information/Fact-Sheets/Nursing-Shortage.
4. American Association of Colleges of Nursing [Internet]. Washington, DC: American Association of Colleges of Nursing; c2017 [cited 2018 Jan 29]. Clinical Nurse Leader; [about 5 screens]. Available from: http://www.aacnnursing.org/CNL.
5. Bender M, Williams M, Su W. Diffusion of a nurse-led healthcare innovation: describing certified clinical nurse leader integration into care delivery. JONA. 2016;46(7–8):400–7.
6. Bender M. The current evidence base for the clinical nurse leader: a narrative review of the literature. J Prof Nurs. 2014;30(2):110–23.
7. National Council of State Boards of Nursing [Internet]. Chicago, IL. National Council of State Boards of Nursing. c2018 [cited 2018 Jan 29] APRN consensus model; [about 1 screen] Available from: https://www.ncsbn.org/aprn-consensus.htm.
8. National Association of Clinical Nurse Specialists. Impact of the clinical nurse specialist role on the costs and quality of healthcare. Policy briefing paper. 2013. Clin Nurse Spec. 2014;28(5):300–3.
9. National Organization of Nurse Practitioner Faculties [Internet]. c 2016[cited 2017 Dec 12]. Washington D.C: National Organization of nurse practitioner faculties; adult-Gerentology acute care and primary care NP competencies. Available from: http://www.nonpf.org/?page=14.
10. Moore J, McQuestion M. The clinical nurse specialist in chronic disease. Clin Nurse Spec. 2012;26(3):149–63.
11. Swan M, Ferguson S, Chang A, Larson E, Smaldone A. Quality of primary care by advanced practice nurse: a systematic review. Int J Qual Health Care. 2015;27(5):396–404.
12. Stanik-Hutt J, Newhouse R, White K, Johantgen M, Bass E, Zangaro G, et al. The quality and effectiveness of care provided by nurse practitioners. J Nurse Pract. 2013;9(8):492–500.
13. Landsperger J, Semler M, Wang L, Byrne M, Wheeler A. Outcomes of nurse practitioner-delivered critical care: a prospective cohort study. Chest. 2015;149(5):1146–54.
14. Pine M, Holt K, Lou Y. Surgical mortality and type of anesthesia provider. AANA J. 2003;71(2):109–16.
15. Simonson DC, Ahern MM, Hendryx MS. Anesthesia staffing and anesthetic complications during cesarean delivery. Nurs Res. 2007;56(1):9–17.
16. American Association of Nurse Anesthetists. [Internet]. c2009 [cited 2018 Feb 10]. Park Ridge, IL. American Association of Nurse Anesthetists; Quality of care in anesthesia. Available from: https://www.aana.com/news/news-detail/2017/06/05/quality-of-care-in-anesthesia.
17. Sandall J, Soltani H, Gates S, Shennan A, Devane D. Midwife-led continuity models versus other models of care for childbearing women (Review). Cochrane Database Syst Rev. 2015;15(9):CD004667.
18. Barr RB, Tagg J. From teaching to learning—a new paradigm for undergraduate education. Change: The Magazine of Higher Learning. 1995;27(6):12–26.
19. Chappy S, Jambunathan J, Marnocha S. Evidence-based curricular strategies to enhance BSN graduates' transition into practice. Nurse Educ. 2010;35(1):20–4.
20. Dyess SM, Sherman RO. The first year of practice: new graduate nurses' transition and learning needs. J Contin Educ Nurs. 2009;40(9):403–10.
21. Hofler L, Thomas K. Transition of new graduate nurses to the workforce: challenges and solutions in the changing health care environment. N C Med J. 2016;77(2):133–6.
22. Pederson A, Hack TF. Pilots of oncology health care: a concept analysis of the patient navigator role. ONF. 2010;37(1):55–60.
23. Lubejko BG, Bellfield S, Kahn E, Lee C, Peterson N, Rose T, et al. Oncology navigation: results of the 2016 role delineation study. CJON. 2017;21(1):43–50.
24. Purdom MA, Peterson S, Haas BK. Results of an oncology clinical trial nurse role delineation study. ONF. 2017;44(5):589–95.
25. Foronda C, MacWilliams B, McArthur E. Interprofessional communication in healthcare: an integrative review. Nurse Educ Pract. 2016;19:36–40.
26. Tan TC, Zhou H, Kelly M. Nurse-physician communication – an integrated review. J Clin Nurs. 2017;26(23-24):3974–3989.
27. King HB, Battles J, Baker DP, Alonso A, Salas E, Webster J, et al. TeamSTEPPS™: team strategies and tools to enhance performance and patient safety. In: Henriksen K, Battles JB, Keyes MA, Grady ML, editors. Advances in patient safety: new directions and alternative approaches (Vol. 3: Performance and tools). Rockville (MD): Agency for Healthcare Research and Quality (US); 2008. Available from: https://www-ncbi-nlm-nih-gov.ezp.welch.jhmi.edu/books/NBK43686/.
28. Agency for Healthcare Research and Quality [Internet]. c2018. [cited 2018 Feb 11]. Agency for Healthcare Research and Quality Rockville, MD. CUSP Toolkit; [about 1 screen]. Available from: http://www.ahrq.gov/professionals/education/curriculum-tools/cusptoolkit/index.html.

29. Reeves S, Clark E, Lawton S, Ream M, Ross F. Examining the nature of interprofessional interventions designed to promote patient safety: a narrative review. Int J Qual Health Care. 2017;29(2):144–50.
30. Pelletier LR, Stichler JF. Patient-centered care and engagement: nurse leaders' imperative for health reform. JONA. 2014;44(9):473–80.
31. Davidson JE, Aslakson RA, Long AC, Puntillo KA, Kross EK, Hart J, et al. Guidelines for family-centered care in the neonatal, pediatric, and adult ICU. Crit Care Med. 2017;45:103–28.
32. Miller TA. Health literacy and adherence to medical treatment in chronic and acute illness: a meta-analysis. Patient Educ Couns. 2016;99:1079–86.
33. Dang D, Dearholt SL. Johns Hopkins nursing evidence-based practice: model and guidelines. 3rd ed. Indianapolis: Sigma Theta Tau International; 2017.
34. Buckwalter KC, Cullen L, Hanrahan K, Kleiber C, McCarthy AM, Rakel B, et al. On behalf of the Iowa Model Collaborative. Iowa Model of evidence-based practice: revisions and validation. Worldviews Evid-Based Nurs. 2017;14(3):175–82.
35. Melnyk BM, Gallagher-Ford L, Zellefrow C, Tucker S, Thomas B, Sinnott LT, et al. The first US study on nurses' evidence-based practice competencies indicates major deficits that threaten healthcare quality, safety, and patient outcomes. Worldviews Evid-Based Nurs. 2017; https://doi.org/10.1111/wvn.12269. [Epub ahead of print].
36. American Nurses Credentialing Center [Internet]. Silver Spring, MD: American Nurses Credentialing Center; c2017 [cited 2018 Jan 29]. Magnet Program overview, history, and growth; [about 4 screens]. Available from: http://www.nursecredentialing.org/Magnet/ProgramOverview.
37. Friese CR, Xia R, Ghaferi A, Birkmeyer JD, Banerjee M. Hospitals in 'Magnet' program show better patient outcomes on mortality measures compared to non-'Magnet' hospitals. Health Aff. 2015;34(6):986–92.
38. Evans T, Rittenhouse K, Horst M, Osler T, Rogers A, Miller JA, et al. Magnet hospitals are a magnet for higher survival rates at adult trauma centers. J Trauma Acute Care Surg. 2014;77(1):89–94.
39. Bekelis K, Missios S, MacKenzie TA. Association of Magnet status with hospitalization outcomes for ischemic stroke patients. J Am Heart Assoc. 2017;6:1–9.
40. Barnes H, Rearden J, McHugh MD. Magnet® hospital recognition linked to lower central line-associated bloodstream infection rates. Res Nurs Health. 2016;39:96–104.
41. Ma C, Park SH. Hospital magnet status, unit work environment, and pressure ulcers. J Nurs Schol. 2015;47(6):565–73.
42. Lasater KB, Germack HD, Small DS, McHugh MD. Hospitals known for nursing excellence perform better on value based purchasing measures. Policy Polit Nurs Pract. 2016;17(4):177–86.
43. Petit dit Dariel O, Regnaux JP. Do Magnet®-accredited hospitals show improvements in nurse and patient outcomes compared to non-Magnet hospitals: a systematic review. JBI Database System Rev Implement Rep. 2015;13(6):168–219.
44. Rettiganti M, Shah KM, Gossett JM, Daily JA, Seib PM, Gupta P. Is Magnet® recognition associated with improved outcomes among critically ill children treated at freestanding children's hospitals? J Crit Care. 2018;43:207–13.
45. Kaye SP. Nurses' attitudes toward meaningful use technologies: an integrative review. Comput Inform Nurs. 2017;35(5):237–46.
46. Brandt B, Lutfiyya MN, King JA, Chioreso C. A scoping review of interprofessional collaborative practice and education using the lens of the Triple Aim. J Interprof Care. 2014;28(5):393–9.

33 Wound Healing: Proof-of-Principle Model for the Modern Hospital: Patient Stratification, Prediction, Prevention and Personalisation of Treatment

Olga Golubnitschaja, Lara Stolzenburg Veeser, Eden Avishai, and Vincenzo Costigliola

Why Is Changing the Current Paradigm of Reactive Medicine Crucial for Healthcare?

Examples of the failures of the current paradigm of reactive medicine are readily available: (1) it is estimated there are nearly 0.5 billion diabetic individuals worldwide – truly an epidemic chronic pathology [1]. (2) Breast cancer has reached similar epidemic proportions: almost 2 million new cases and 0.5 million disease-related deaths annually [2].

Until recently, both pathologies were considered to be diseases primarily of the elderly: 60+-year-old patients with diabetes mellitus (DM) type 2 and postmenopausal type of breast cancer patients. However, highly alarming statistics demonstrate an increasing number of young people affected by both pathologies. Regarding DM, in some populations one-third of new cases present in teenagers [3]. The incidence of a particularly aggressive pregnancy-associated breast cancer (PABC) has increased from 1:10,000 at the beginning of the millennium to the currently registered 1:3000 of all pregnancies

O. Golubnitschaja (✉)
Radiological Clinic, Rheinische Friedrich-Wilhelms-Universität Bonn, Bonn, Germany

Breast Cancer Research Centre, Rheinische Friedrich-Wilhelms-Universität Bonn, Bonn, Germany

Centre for Integrated Oncology, Cologne-Bonn, Rheinische Friedrich-Wilhelms-Universität Bonn, Bonn, Germany

European Association for Predictive, Preventive and Personalised Medicine, EPMA, Brussels, Belgium
e-mail: olga.golubnitschaja@ukbonn.de

L. S. Veeser
Department of Business Administration, Carlos III University, Getafe, Madrid, Spain

E. Avishai
Department of Immunology, Department of Neuroscience, The Ruth and Bruce Rappaport Faculty of Medicine, Technion-Israel Institute of Technology, Haifa, Israel

V. Costigliola
European Association for Predictive, Preventive and Personalised Medicine, EPMA, Brussels, Belgium

R. Latifi (ed.), *The Modern Hospital*, https://doi.org/10.1007/978-3-030-01394-3_33

(about 100.000 new cases annually) [4]. Since a large portion of PABC demonstrates the characteristics specific for the triple-negative breast cancer (TNBC) subtype, the situation is particularly dramatic: 50% of patients affected by the TNBC subtype die within the first 6 months of the metastatic BC diagnosis [5].

The brain is one of the predominant sites of the breast cancer metastatic disease; the phenomenon has been well addressed in a recently published article [6]. Prognosis for brain malignancies is generally one of the poorest in oncology. The standard treatment protocol is temozolomide combined with radiation therapy – at a cost of about 50.000 € per capita for 2–4 months prolonged overall survival. With regard to DM, by the year 2025, it is estimated that the annual DM-related costs for the USA alone will be $595 billion US [1].

Considering the above evidence, if the current "reactive medicine" model is allowed to persist, economic collapse of healthcare systems on a global scale will be the result. Moreover, ethical issues make the current "reactive medicine" model unacceptable when alternatives are being developed that can greatly reduce the healthcare burden on society as a whole.

In contrast, modern healthcare promotes the paradigm change from delayed interventional to predictive medicine tailored to the person, from reactive to preventive medicine and from disease to wellness. The innovative predictive, preventive and personalised medicine (PPPM) paradigm is emerging as the focal point of efforts in healthcare aimed at curbing the prevalence of both communicable and non-communicable diseases such as diabetes, cardiovascular diseases, chronic respiratory diseases, cancer and dental pathologies. The cost-effective management of diseases and the critical role of PPPM in modernisation of healthcare have been acknowledged as priorities by global and regional organisations and health-related institutions such as the United Nations, the European Union and the National Institutes of Health. The integrative approach by PPPM can be considered the healthcare model for the future. Being at the forefront of the global efforts, the European Association for Predictive, Preventive and Personalised Medicine (EPMA) promotes the integrative concept of PPPM among healthcare stakeholders, governmental institutions, educators, funding bodies, patient organisations and in the public domain [7].

Why Has Been Wound Healing Chosen to Demonstrate the Principles of Predictive, Preventive and Personalised Medicine (PPPM) as the Medicine of the Future?

The economics of wound healing (WH) is not a minor issue for healthcare at large: in the USA alone, over $25 billion US are spent annually for the treatment of chronic wounds affecting 6.5 million patients [8]. Problematic WH and chronic wounds may result from a broad spectrum of suboptimal health conditions [9], severe pathologies, and comorbidities predisposing the affected individuals and corresponding patient cohorts to hindered WH and consequent pathologic developments such as chronic inflammation, persistent infections, "open wounds", cancerous wound transformation, etc. [10]. The quality of WH is highly individual resulting from both non-modifiable (genetic predisposition, age) and modifiable (nutrition, lifestyle, preventable collateral pathologies such as DM type 2) risk factors. The quality of WH is considered an essential parameter of individualised patient profiling and the subject for advanced approaches by systems medicine, predictive diagnostics, targeted preventive measures and treatments tailored to the person – altogether the innovative approaches of PPPM as the Medicine of the Future. To achieve this goal, multilevel diagnostics utilising comprehensive biomarker panels are proposed. The potential application is multi-faceted: early diagnostics of related pathologies and disease predisposition, effective prevention and treatment of collateral pathologies, prediction and prognosis of post-surgical complications, improved individual outcomes in plastic surgery etc. [11].

Complexity of the Wound Healing, Main Players and Health Conditions Characteristic for Compromised Healing Quality: Potential Indicators for PPPM Approach

Wound healing is a highly complex process that aims to restore tissue integrity and function after an injury. The process is composed of a well-controlled sequence of four overlapping phases: haemostasis, inflammation, proliferation and tissue remodelling – as demonstrated in Fig. 33.1. Every phase is characterised by highly specific cellular and molecular makeup, the regulation of which is of great clinical utility as a biomarker panel. Systemic factors regulating the molecular makeup play a crucial role in the overall WH quality as discussed below.

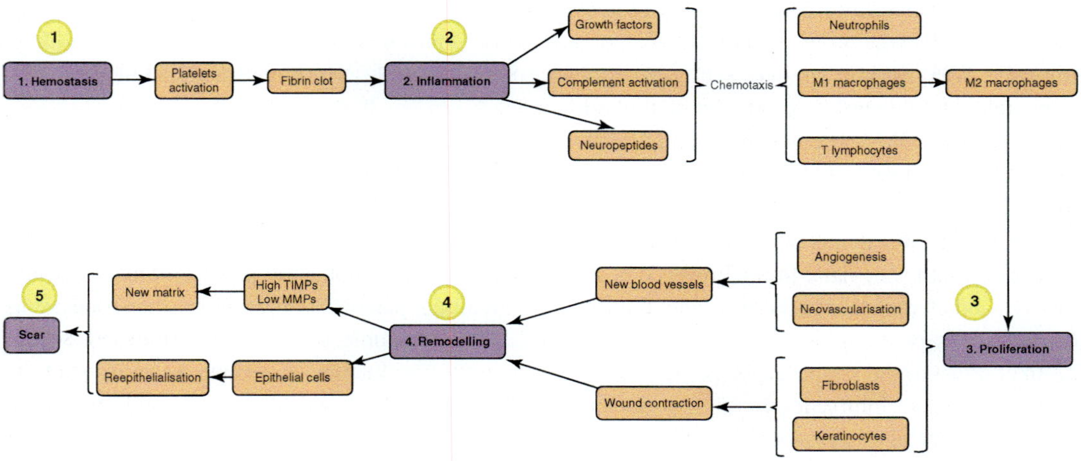

Fig. 33.1 The "roadmap" of physiologic wound healing; After an acute injury, the first phase of the wound healing is *haemostasis* (1), when platelets and the coagulation cascade get activated together leading to formation of the fibrin clot (composed of fibrin, fibronectin, vitronectin and thrombospondin). On the other hand, there is a temporary hypoxia in the early wound that contributes to the release of growth factors and cytokines by the activation of HIF-1. The release of growth factors (mainly PDGF, TGF, FGF, VEGF, EGF, and IGF) by platelets and the fibrin clot starts in the second phase of healing – *inflammation* (2), where several factors act as chemoattractants for inflammatory cells. These include growth factors, the activated components of the complement cascade (especially C3a and C5a) and neuropeptides produced by peripheral neurons, such as SP, NPY, CGRP and NGF. Further, also DETCs, as well as epigenetics, play a role in inflammation. This results in recruitment of inflammatory cells (neutrophils, macrophages and T lymphocytes). Neutrophils arrive at the place by 24–36 h after injury performing phagocytosis of bacteria in the wound area, as well as recruiting further immune cells by releasing pro-inflammatory cytokines (IL-1, IL-6 and TNF- α). It is important to note that neutrophils release MMPs, which play a critical role in many steps of wound healing. Macrophages arrive later on (by 48–72 h after injury) demonstrating the M1 (pro-inflammatory) phenotype and releasing pro-inflammatory cytokines (IL-1, IL-6, IL-12 and TNF-α) and MMPs. Afterwards the transition to M2 macrophages occurs with pro-healing phenotype releasing anti-inflammatory cytokines (e.g. IL-10), growth factors that contribute to the formation of new blood vessels through angiogenesis (TGF-β, β-FGF and VEGF) and TIMPs, which are critical for balancing the MMP activity for physiologic tissue remodelling; thereby, growth factors released by M2 macrophages interact with reorganised extracellular matrix. By 72 h after injury, T lymphocytes arrive promoting recruitment of fibroblasts and triggering the *proliferative* (3) phase; active M2 macrophages are the prerequisite for switching from inflammation to proliferation. Effective angiogenesis and neovascularisation are critical for this phase: angiogenesis extends the formation of blood vessels based on pre-existing vasculature, whereas by neovascularisation new blood vessels are created based on bone marrow-derived stem cells. The phase is characterised by the migration and proliferation of fibroblasts producing the main components of the ECM (collagen, glycosaminoglycans and proteoglycans) and substituting the original fibrin clot by granulation tissue. Myofibroblasts synergistically with keratinocytes promote the wound contraction. *Tissue remodelling* (4) is characterised by several regulatory events such as downregulation of MMPs versus upregulation of TIMPs leading to the matrix accumulation. New epithelium is formed by migration and proliferation of epithelial cells accompanied by well-controlled apoptosis of excessive fibroblasts and macrophages, decreasing number of inflammatory cells, normalised vascular functioning and cross-linking of collagen in the extracellular matrix. All the events lead to *scar formation* (5), the quality of which depends on specific molecular setup (e.g. TGF-β, CTGF, IL-4, IL-13). Tissue remodelling and scar formation are the longest phase of healing and may last up to 1–2 years depending on an individual patient profile

Hypoxic Environment

The early wound is characterised by a *temporary hypoxic environment* resulting from the vascular disruption and high oxygen consumption by metabolically active cells in the wound [12–14]. The hypoxic environment specifically upregulates production of the hypoxia-inducible factor-1 (HIF-1), which is essential for the physiologic healing processing at the stage of inflammation, angiogenesis, neovasculogenesis, fibroplasia and tissue remodelling. HIF-1 dysregulation is characteristic of an impaired WH, fibrotic wounds and hypertrophic scars related frequently to vascular pathologies, stress, obesity, DM and other metabolic disorders [12–17]. Therefore, HIF-1 expression level could serve as a reliable biomarker for physiologic versus pathologic WH that is of great clinical utility – indicative on the one hand for an impaired healing process and on the other hand for a potential cause of the pathology.

In contrast to the temporary hypoxic condition created by acute injury, a *chronic hypoxic environment* is typical of a systemic vascular dysregulation resulting in chronic wounds [10]. Chronic wounds lead to onset of (pre)cancerous lesions; therefore, delayed healing is strongly indicative for predisposition to severe pathologies such as cancer that is of great importance for a predictive medical approach [10]. Although of different origin, a systemic vascular dysregulation is characteristic of both diabetic angiopathy in ageing and Flammer syndrome in adolescence. The latter cohort is less investigated to date regarding the healing quality. However, Flammer syndrome phenotype has been demonstrated to be highly relevant for cancer development and aggressive metastatic disease [18, 19]. Contextually, the Flammer syndrome phenotype is of particular importance for innovative screening programmes, predictive diagnostics, targeted prevention and personalised treatment algorithms created specifically for needs of young populations [10], [20].

Matrix metalloproteinases (MMPs) – the central processors of tissue remodelling and overall healing (reacting to hypoxia, cellular damage and apoptosis) – have been demonstrated to play a role in both DM comorbidities [21] and pathologies related to Flammer syndrome [19, 22]. Consequently, MMPs represent an important biomarker panel that can be used to predict severity of pathologies linked to the compromised healing quality [23]. Further, the quality of tissue remodelling and scar formation is crucial for individual outcome in plastic surgery and aesthetic medicine, where – due to underdeveloped predictive diagnostics – the quality of individual outcomes is still uncertain for all three parties involved, namely, the treating doctor, the affected patient and their insurance. Innovative PPPM approaches can address this uncertainty. Syndromes and pathologies leading to chronic hypoxia as well as MMPs (MMP-1, MMP-2, MMP-3, MMP-7, MMP-8, MMP-9, MMP-10, MMP-11, MMP-13) and HIF-1 patterns are strongly indicative of tissue remodelling and quality of scar formation, which therefore might be the first choice biomarker panel for predictive individualised patient profiles in aesthetic medicine [23]. For example, senescent fibroblasts and keratinocytes are known to secrete proteins such as MMP-2, MMP-3 and MMP-9 (antifibrotic effect) or maspin (antiangiogenic effect) – leading to an overall reduction of healing quality [24]. Finally, specific miRNAs are involved in regulating the quality of scarring: downregulation of miRNA-196a correlates with an increased production of type I and type III collagens and consequent overproduction of collagens in keloid scar formation. On the other hand, fibrosis and hypertrophic scarring may be caused by excessive migration of keratinocytes to the centre of the wound. The miRNA-200 family and miRNA-205 are known to regulate this process through epithelial–mesenchymal transition (EMT): downregulation of both miRNAs induces the process and therefore could lead to the formation of hypertrophic scars. There is also a set of lncRNAs that appears to be involved in scar formation such as lncRNA8975–1, AC097662.2 and RP11-586K2 – having a role in collagen synthesis and matrix degradation [25]. Liquid biopsy is useful for the biomarker detection such as blood plasma and wound liquid [26].

Advanced and accelerated ageing is a risk factor for ageing-related pathologies (cancer, DM type 2, etc.) and important systemic factors that affect healing quality, chronic wounds, wound dehiscence and persistent wound infections [27–29]. Hypoxic wounds are characteristic of this patient cohort [30] where the essential switch between inflammation and proliferation WH phases does not occur; therefore non-healing wounds are more prone to remain in the inflammatory stage. Disturbed microcirculation further contributes to the impaired WH. Consequently, individualised patient profiles demonstrating premature ageing are predictive for both diminished healing quality and severe pathologies such as cancer [13, 31].

Malnutrition is a factor negatively affecting the healing quality. Strict diets and starvation are generally not recommended to individuals predisposed to compromised WH [32].

Psychological stress and depression both negatively impact healing process through chronically elevated cortisol levels, which prolong WH due to their immunosuppressive effects and increased susceptibility to infections [33, 34].

Hormonal dysregulation directly affects the quality of healing, since several hormones play a role in tissue restoration. For example, the sex hormone oestrogen has positive effects as an anti-inflammatory regulator, whereas androgen has been shown to negatively impact WH [35].

Chronic systemic inflammation is critical for developing chronic wounds. Permanent stress, accelerated ageing, hormonal dysregulation, chronic infections, metabolic syndrome, compromised nutrition and immune response are the factors supporting chronic inflammatory processes. Excessive inflammation causes chronic wounds [36], which in turn fail to complete the initial microbial decontamination inside the wound and to perform the switch between the inflammatory and proliferative phases in the healing process [28, 37]. Elevated MMP activity and defective extracellular matrix are the characteristic attributes of chronic inflammation [19, 38].

Metabolic syndrome is the classical example of a strongly impaired WH linked to chronic wounds and lower extremity amputations [39]. DM patients are at high risk of developing a cascade of secondary pathologies: systemic angiopathy, chronic inflammation, susceptibility to infections, stroke, cancer and metastatic disease. Deficient healing process in DM patients is characterised by a strongly hypoxic and pro-inflammatory environment, non-healing wounds, delayed activation of neutrophils and macrophages, dysfunction of phagocytosis, excessive production of reactive oxygen species, poor collagen accumulation etc. [19, 30, 40]. The biomarker panel proposed above including systemic hypoxia and specific patterns of HIF-1 and MMPs are of great clinical utility to predict the impaired healing and strong predisposition to cancer and aggressive metastatic disease typical of this patient cohort [41].

Cancer and metastatic disease have been demonstrated to be pathologies of systemic origin. Impaired WH, cancer and metastatic progression share several key pathways and molecular repertoires. Characteristics are an accelerated cell proliferation and migration, greater turnover of the extracellular matrix (ECM) and enhanced neovascularisation – as well as abnormal growth factor profiles and elevated MMP levels [29, 38]. Moreover, there is accumulating evidence that wounding stimulates hair follicle stem cells to promote the growth of basal cell carcinoma [19, 42]. Specific cellular repertoires are similar for both an impaired healing process and cancer progression [42, 43]. Consequently, individuals demonstrating deficient healing process should be further considered as strongly predisposed to cancer; individualised patient profiles should be thoroughly analysed predicting outcomes and implementing targeted preventive measures [23].

Deficient Wound Healing Reflects Pathological Processes and Predicts Severe Diseases Before Their Clinical Manifestation: Proposed PPPM Approach

The facts summarised above clearly demonstrate that deficient WH reflects ongoing pathological processes and may be strongly indicative of a number of diseases before their clinical manifestation. Consequently, the quality of WH is considered a powerful predictor for individuals in suboptimal health condition and argues in favour of developing innovative diagnostic approaches and targeted preventive measures applied according to the individual patient profile. Both non-modifiable (of genetic origin) and modifiable risk factors synergistically predispose to deficient healing processes [10], [44] .

Modifiable Risk Factors as the First Choice for Individualised Prevention

Preventable modifiable risks include durable stress conditions of any origin, toxic environment, inappropriate lifestyle (harmful habits such as smoking and abnormal alcohol consumption), imbalanced diet and/or malnutrition, vascular dysregulation of non-genetic origin etc. as described above. Modifiable risk analysis serves as the first choice of measures for targeted prevention [45–48].

Each risk factor is associated with its unique fingerprint of alterations in the WH process that can be used to assess the degree of WH impairment and to evaluate the specific effect that risk factor has on an individual [10, 23].

Questionnaires as a Tool to Create Individualised Patient Profiles

Despite the accumulating knowledge regarding WH risk factors and associated pathological processes, to date quality-based prediction and prevention measures have not been efficiently implemented. Currently, when a person visits the family doctor practice, nobody questions whether the patient may observe delayed healing, e.g. from a finger cut while working in the garden or preparing a meal. A simple, practical and extremely efficient solution would be introduction of questionnaires in daily practice by general practitioners. These questionnaires would help primary caregivers to assess the predisposition of an individual to deficient healing processes – even in adolescence and at early stages of impairment. Puberty would be an optimal age to start the assessment of suboptimal health conditions such as Flammer syndrome that can give a clue to individual predispositions early enough to protect the affected individuals against severe pathologies later on in life [18, 49, 50]. At this young age, educational measures are well-accepted and individual habits are not yet fixed. Thus habits can still be fairly easily changed with the correct guidance and support in order to keep control over modifiable risk factors.

The questionnaires can be introduced in the form of a diagnostic tree by "yes" versus "no" answers and corresponding measure linked to either a positive or a negative answer.

The relevant questionnaire should include the following aspects:

- Family history – disorders recorded for the family which might provide a genetic predisposition to impaired healing processes and/or pathologies linked to dysregulated pathways
- Lifestyle – to evaluate an option to optimise habits such as sedentary lifestyle, imbalanced nutrition, level of stress, smoking and abnormal alcohol consumption
- Quality of the healing process – to evaluate the level of impairments, if any
- Pre-existing medical/suboptimal conditions linked to potentially deficient healing such as abnormal weight (both overweight and underweight), signs and symptoms of Flammer syndrome, depression, hormonal dysregulation etc., as described above

The questionnaire would help the responsible family doctor to stratify the patient, to estimate potential risks, to identify individuals at high risk, to suggest follow-up laboratory tests and medical examinations as well as to recommend individualised preventive measures.

Predictive Liquid Biopsy Analysis

The questionnaires described above provide valuable information to estimate the necessity of follow-up analysis and to specify molecular profiling to be performed in case of an increased risk. Corresponding predictive biomarker panels can be evaluated utilising body fluids (blood, saliva, urine, tear fluid etc.). Multiomic analysis is strongly recommended for predictive diagnosis as demonstrated by the most recent scientific literature [11, 51]. Based on the results of multilevel diagnostics, the responsible general practitioner can recommend follow-up preventive measures using personalised treatment algorithms. The overall procedure is demonstrated by the patient case below.

General Diagnostic and Treatment Scheme: An Example

An example is illustrated in Fig. 33.2.

Patient description by the responsible family doctor:

- A 15-year-old female with BMI = 28 kg/m^2 has not been treated for any medical condition.
- Additional information received: the patient (1) is physically inactive, (2) suffers frequently from cold hands/feet, (3) has mood disorders, (4) due to being overweight is subjected to unfriendly attitude by other pupils in school and (5) has irregular menstrual cycles, i.e. hormonal dysregulation.
- The questionnaire revealed potentially deficient healing process in the adolescent patient.

Family history:

- Diabetic family history
- Grandmother died of metastatic breast cancer

Laboratory analysis:

- Laboratory tests included glucose, cytokines, endothelin-1, activity of both MMP-2 and MMP-9 in blood and "comet assay" analysis of peripheral leucocytes.
- Results revealed normal glucose level, increased plasma cytokine and endothelin-1 levels, high metalloproteinase activities and DNA fragmentation demonstrated by "comet assay" analysis.

Conclusions: a deficient healing process indicative for risks linked to cancer development. Supportive findings include risk profile of persisting inflammation, hormonal and vascular dysregulation and increased stress reactions.

Recommendations: (1) magnesium therapy to improve the vasodilatation; (2) nailfold capillary microscopy monitoring to evaluate the therapy efficacy; (3) consultations by physiotherapist and endocrinologist for individual optimisation of physical activities, weight, stress response and hormonal regulation that synergistically may positively impact the quality of healing and related processes; (4) regular blood tests for glucose; (5) repeated tests for metalloproteinase activity and "comet assay" analysis; and (6) evaluation of specific miRNA [25], HIF-1 [17] and hypoxia-responsive long

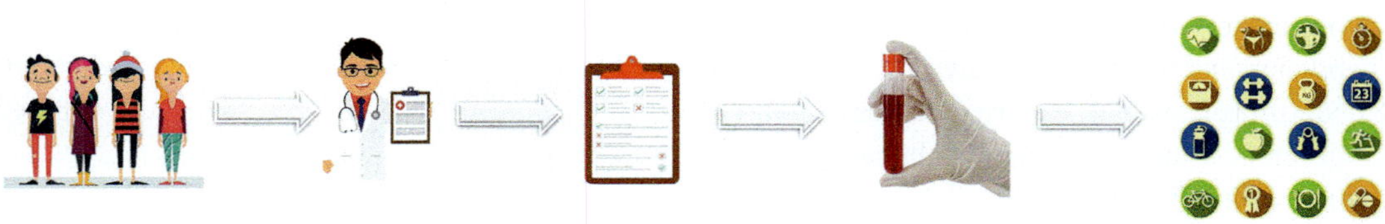

Fig. 33.2 General scheme for PPPM action in adolescence; responsible family doctor (general practitioner) performs the first consultation with the teenager identifying a specific character of potential suboptimal health condition, modifiable risk factors and family history (non-modifiable risk factors); application of pathology-specific questionnaires are strongly recommended; depending on the output, laboratory tests will be ordered and the results analysed for the follow-up preventive measures and personalised treatment algorithms as proposed in subchapter "General diagnostic and treatment scheme – an example"

non-coding RNA patterns in blood that correlate with healing quality and reflect cancer predisposition [52].

Concluding Remarks: Requirements for the Modern Hospital

The concepts for the modern hospital described above should follow the requirements listed below:

1. To increase the overall quality of medical services and improve socio-economic aspects, the paradigm should be shifted from the present "reactive" to a predictive, preventive and personalised medical approach in healthcare.
2. Primary caregivers (family doctors/general practitioners) should be more actively involved in innovative screening programmes focused on identification of suboptimal health conditions before the clinical onset of severe pathologies.
3. Signs and symptoms of suboptimal health conditions – such as deficient healing processes discussed above – can alert well-educated caregivers to predictive diagnostic and targeted preventive measures based on individualised patient profiling. Questionnaires linked to corresponding lab tests and multilevel diagnostics are mandatory.
4. Adolescent patients in suboptimal health are the central target group for an effective implementation of PPPM approaches. Many severe pathologies known to result from modifiable risk factors synergistically developed early in life have been overlooked and underestimated at the level of primary and secondary prevention.
5. Multi-professional expertise is essential to develop a cost-effective healthcare system based on PPPM principles.
6. PPPM educational programmes are essential at the levels of both the general population (e.g. school programmes) and caregivers.
7. A tight collaboration with policymakers is required for effective implementation of PPPM in healthcare systems and society at large. Realisation of modern healthcare based on the principles of PPPM saves human and financial resources by improving the quality of life for the entire population. Innovative PPPM programmes should be supported administratively and economically at all stages of their development and implementation. Long-term legislation is required to guarantee continuous support for PPPM. The healthcare of society as a whole deserves modern PPPM.

References

1. Duarte AA, Mohsin S, Golubnitschaja O. Diabetes care in figures: current pitfalls and future scenario. EPMA J. 2018;9(2). 10.1007/s13167-018-0133-y.
2. Golubnitschaja O, Debald M, Yeghiazaryan K, Kuhn W, Pešta M, Costigliola V, Grech G. Breast cancer epidemic in the early 21st century: evaluation of risk factors, cumulative questionnaires and recommendations for preventive measures. Tumor Biol. 2016;37(10):12941–57. https://doi.org/10.1007/s13277-016-5168-x.
3. Golubnitschaja O. Three levels of prediction, prevention and individualised treatment algorithms to advance diabetes care: integrative approach. In: Mozaffari M, editor. The book "new strategies to advance pre/diabetes care: integrative approach by PPPM". Dordrecht/Heidelberg/New York/London: Springer; 2013. p. 15–28. ISBN 978-94-007-5970-1.
4. Polivka J Jr, Altun I, Golubnitschaja O. Pregnancy associated breast cancer: the risky status quo and new concepts of predictive medicine. EPMA J. 2018;9(1):1–13. https://doi.org/10.1007/s13167-018-0129-7.
5. Vaz-Luis I, Lin NU, Keating NL, Barry WT, Winer EP, Freedman RA. Factors associated with early mortality among patients with de novo metastatic breast cancer: a population-based study. Oncologist. 2017;22:386. https://doi.org/10.1634/theoncologist.2016-0369.
6. Polivka J, Kralickova M, Polivka J, Kaiser C, Kuhn W, Golubnitschaja O. Mystery of the brain metastatic disease in breast cancer patients: improved patient stratification, disease prediction and targeted prevention on the horizon? EPMA J. 2017;8(2):119–27. https://doi.org/10.1007/s13167-017-0087-5.
7. Golubnitschaja O. Foreword, book series "advances in predictive, preventive and personalised medicine". Dordrecht/Heidelberg/New York/London: Springer. http://www.springer.com/series/10051.
8. Sen CK, Gordillo GM, Roy S, Kirsner R, Lambert L, Hunt TK, et al. Human skin wounds: a major and snowballing threat to public health and economy. Wound Repair Regen. 2009;17(6):763–71.
9. Kunin A, Polivka J Jr, Moiseeva N, Golubnitschaja O. "Dry Mouth" and "Flammer" Syndromes - Neglected Risks in Adolescents and New Concepts by Predictive, Preventive and Personalised Approach.

EPMA J. 2018;9(3):307–317. https://doi:10.1007/s13167-018-0145-7.
10. Avishai E, Yeghiazaryan K, Golubnitschaja O. Impaired wound healing: facts and hypotheses for multi-professional considerations in predictive, preventive and personalised medicine. EPMA J. 2017;8(1):23–33. https://doi.org/10.1007/s13167-017-0081-y.
11. Golubnitschaja O, Costigliola V, Grech G. EPMA World Congress: traditional forum in predictive, preventive and personalised medicine for multi-professional consideration and consolidation. EPMA J. 2017;8(Suppl):1–54. https://doi.org/10.1007/s13167-017-0108-4.
12. Bayat A, McGrouther DA, Ferguson MW. Skin scarring. BMJ. 2003;326(7380):88–92.
13. Bentov I, Reed MJ. Anesthesia, microcirculation, and wound repair in aging. Anesthesiology. 2014;120(3):760–72. https://doi.org/10.1097/ALN.0000000000000036.
14. Bhargava M, Viken KJ, Dey S, Steinbach MS, Wu B, Jagtap PD, Higgins L, Panoskaltsis-Mortari A, Weisdorf DJ, Kumar V, Arora M, Bitterman PB, Ingbar DH, Wendt CH. Proteome profiling in lung injury after hematopoietic stem cell transplantation. Biol Blood Marrow Transplant. 2016;22(8):1383–90. https://doi.org/10.1016/j.bbmt.2016.04.021.
15. Al-Shaqsi S, Al-Bulushi T. Cutaneous scar prevention and management: overview of current therapies. Sultan Qaboos Univ Med J. 2016;16(1):e3–8. https://doi.org/10.18295/squmj.2016.16.01.002.
16. Bhattacharya S, Aggarwal R, Singh VP, Ramachandran S, Datta M. Downregulation of miRNAs during delayed wound healing in diabetes: role of dicer. Mol Med. 2015;21(1):847–60. https://doi.org/10.2119/molmed.2014.00186.
17. Brady NJ, Chuntova P, Schwertfeger KL. Macrophages: regulators of the inflammatory microenvironment during mammary gland development and breast cancer. Mediat Inflamm. 2016;2016:4549676. https://doi.org/10.1155/2016/4549676.
18. Zubor P, Gondova A, Polivka J Jr, Kasajova P, Konieczka K, Danko J, Golubnitschaja O. Breast cancer and Flammer syndrome: any symptoms in common for prediction, prevention and personalised medical approach? EPMA J. 2017;8(2):129–40. https://doi.org/10.1007/s13167-017-0089-3.
19. Bubnov R, Polivka J Jr, Zubor P, Koniczka K, Golubnitschaja O. Pre-metastatic niches in breast cancer: are they created by or prior to the tumour onset? Flammer Syndrome relevance to address the question. EPMA J. 2017;8(2):141–57. https://doi.org/10.1007/s13167-017-0092-8.
20. Kunin A, Polivka J Jr, Moiseeva N, Golubnitschaja O. "Dry Mouth" and "Flammer" Syndromes - Neglected Risks in Adolescents and New Concepts by Predictive, Preventive and Personalised Approach. EPMA J. 2018;9(3):307–317. https://doi:10.1007/s13167-018-0145-7].
21. Golubnitschaja O, Jaksche A, Moenkemann H, Yeghiazaryan K, Karl SE, Schild HH, Löffler KU. Molecular imaging system for possible prediction of active retinopathy in patients with Diabetes mellitus. Amino Acids. 2005;28:229–37.
22. Yeghiazaryan K, Flammer J, Orgül S, Wunderlich K, Golubnitschaja O. Vasospastic individuals demonstrate significant similarity to glaucoma patients as revealed by gene expression profiling in circulating leukocytes. Mol Vis. 2009;15:2339–48.
23. Stolzenburg-Veeser L and Golubnitschaja O. Mini-encyclopaedia of the wound healing - Opportunities for integrating multi-omic approaches into medical practice. Journal of Proteomics. 2018;188:71-84. https://doi:10.1016/j.jprot.2017.07.017.
24. Eming SA, Martin P, Tomic-Canic M. Wound repair and regeneration: mechanisms, signaling, and translation. Sci Transl Med. 2014;6(265):265sr6. https://doi.org/10.1126/scitranslmed.3009337.
25. Luan A, Hu MS, Leavitt T, Brett EA, Wang KC, Longaker MT, Wan DC. Noncoding RNAs in wound healing: a new and vast frontier. Adv Wound Care (New Rochelle). 2018;7(1):19–27. https://doi.org/10.1089/wound.2017.0765.
26. Lindley LE, Stojadinovic O, Pastar I, Tomic-Canic M. Biology and biomarkers for wound healing. Plast Reconstr Surg. 2016;138(3 Suppl):18S–28S. https://doi.org/10.1097/PRS.0000000000002682.
27. Csősz É, Deák E, Kalló G, Csutak A, Tőzsér J. Diabetic retinopathy: proteomic approaches to help the differential diagnosis and to understand the underlying molecular mechanisms. J Proteome. 2017;150:351–8. https://doi.org/10.1016/j.jprot.2016.06.034.
28. Darby IA, Laverdet B, Bonté F, Desmoulière A. Fibroblasts and myofibroblasts in wound healing. Clin Cosmet Investig Dermatol. 2014;7:301–11. https://doi.org/10.2147/CCID.S50046.
29. MacLeod AS, Mansbridge JN. The innate immune system in acute and chronic wounds. Adv Wound Care. 2016;5(2):65–78. https://doi.org/10.1089/wound.2014.0608.
30. Martin P, Nunan R. Cellular and molecular mechanisms of repair in acute and chronic wound healing. Br J Dermatol. 2015;173(2):370–8. https://doi.org/10.1111/bjd.13954.
31. Leonardi GC, Accardi G, Monastero R, Nicoletti F, Libra M. Ageing: from inflammation to cancer. Immun Ageing. 2018;15(1):1. https://doi.org/10.1186/s12979-017-0112-5.
32. Mikesh LM, Aramadhaka LR, Moskaluk C, Zigrino P, Mauch C, Fox JW. Proteomic anatomy of human skin. J Proteome. 2013;84:190–200. https://doi.org/10.1016/j.jprot.2013.03.019.
33. Golubnitschaja O, Yeghiazaryan K, Stricker H, Trog D, Schild HH, Berliner L. Patients with hepatic breast cancer metastases demonstrate highly specific profiles of matrix metalloproteinases MMP-2 and MMP-9 after SIRT treatment as compared to other primary and secondary liver tumours. BMC Cancer. 2016;16:357. https://doi.org/10.1186/s12885-016-2382-2.
34. Molnar JA, Underdown MJ, Clark WA. Nutrition and chronic wounds. Adv Wound Care. 2014;3(11):663–81. https://doi.org/10.1089/wound.2014.0530.

35. Nauta TD, van Hinsbergh VW, Koolwijk P. Hypoxic signaling during tissue repair and regenerative medicine. Int J Mol Sci. 2014;15(11):19791–815. https://doi.org/10.3390/ijms151119791.
36. Cazander G, Jukema GN, Nibbering PH. Complement activation and inhibition in wound healing. Clin Dev Immunol. 2012;2012:534291. https://doi.org/10.1155/2012/534291.
37. George AL, Bangalore-Prakash P, Rajoria S, et al. Endothelial progenitor cell biology in disease and tissue regeneration. J Hematol Oncol. 2011;4:24. https://doi.org/10.1186/1756-8722-4-24.
38. Falanga V. Wound healing and its impairment in the diabetic foot. Lancet. 2005;366(9498):1736–43.
39. Ren Y, Gu G, Yao M, Driver VR. Role of matrix metalloproteinases in chronic wound healing: diagnostic and therapeutic implications. Chin Med J. 2014;127(8):1572–81.
40. Franco C, Hess S. Recent proteomic advances in developmental, regeneration, and cancer governing signaling pathways. Proteomics. 2015;15(5–6):1014–25. https://doi.org/10.1002/pmic.201400368.
41. Cebioglu M, Schild HH, Golubnitschaja O. Cancer predisposition in diabetics: risk factors considered for predictive diagnostics and targeted preventive measures. EPMA J. 2010;1(1):130–7. https://doi.org/10.1007/s13167-010-0015-4.
42. Rieger S, Zhao H, Martin P, Abe K, Lisse TS. The role of nuclear hormone receptors in cutaneous wound repair. Cell Biochem Funct. 2015;33(1):1–13. https://doi.org/10.1002/cbf.3086.
43. Jiang M, Qiu J, Zhang L, et al. Changes in tension regulates proliferation and migration of fibroblasts by remodeling expression of ECM proteins. Exp Ther Med. 2016;12(3):1542–50. https://doi.org/10.3892/etm.2016.3497.
44. Kunin A, Polivka J Jr, Moiseeva N, Golubnitschaja O. "Dry Mouth" and "Flammer" Syndromes - Neglected Risks in Adolescents and New Concepts by Predictive, Preventive and Personalised Approach. EPMA J. 2018;9(3):307–317. https://doi:10.1007/s13167-018-0145-7].
45. Ahn C, Mulligan P, Salcido RS. Smoking-the bane of wound healing: biomedical interventions and social influences. Adv Skin Wound Care. 2008;21(5):227–36. quiz 237–8.
46. Szabo G, Mandrekar P. A recent perspective on alcohol, immunity, and host defense. Alcohol Clin Exp Res. 2009;33(2):220–32.
47. Kiecolt-Glaser JK, Marucha PT, Mercado AM, Malarkey WB, Glaser R. Slowing of wound healing by psychological stress. Lancet. 1995;346(8984):1194–6.
48. Demling RH. Nutrition, anabolism, and the wound healing process: an overview. Eplasty. 2009;9:e9.
49. Konieczka K, Ritch R, Traverso CE, Kim DM, Kook MS, Gallino A, Golubnitschaja O, Erb C, Reitsamer HA, Kida T, Kurysheva N, Yao K. Flammer syndrome. EPMA J. 2014;5(1):11. https://doi.org/10.1186/1878-5085-5-11.
50. Golubnitschaja O. Feeling cold and other underestimated symptoms in breast cancer: anecdotes or individual profiles for advanced patient stratification? EPMA J. 2017;8(1):17–22. https://doi.org/10.1007/s13167-017-0086-6.
51. Golubnitschaja O, Filep N, Yeghiazaryan K, Blom HJ, Hofmann-Apitius M, Kuhn W. Multi-omic approach decodes paradoxes of the triple-negative breast cancer: lessons for predictive, preventive and personalised medicine. Amino Acids. 2018;50:383. https://doi.org/10.1007/s00726-017-2524-0.
52. Kapinova A, Kubatka P, Zubor P, Golubnitschaja O, Dankova Z, Uramova S, Pilchova I, Caprnde M, Opatrilova R, Richnavsky J, Kruzliak P, Danko J. The hypoxia-responsive long non-coding RNAs may impact on the tumor biology and subsequent management of breast cancer. Biomed Pharmacother. 2018;99:51–8. https://doi.org/10.1016/j.biopha.2017.12.104.

34 Home Healthcare Services as an Extension of Intensive Care Unit

Priya Goyal and Rifat Latifi

Introduction

More than 5.7 million patients are admitted annually to intensive care units (ICUs) in the USA because of acute or life-threatening surgical and medical problems. Approximately 20% of acute care admissions in the hospital are to an ICU [1]. The annual cost of ICU hospitalization due to prolonged hospital length of stay is estimated to be 33 billion dollars [2]. This cost is bound to further increase the cost of healthcare. Prolonged ICU stay has proven medical disadvantages in terms of poor patient outcomes as it increases risk of nosocomial infections, bed sores, and psychological issues such as delirium and psychosis. The Society of Critical Care Medicine in their consensus paper on admission and discharge criteria from ICU admits that there is limited amount of high-quality evidence related to ICU admission, discharge, and triage [3]. Transition to home healthcare offers a cost-effective alternative to the ICU for the management of patients in need. We have observed that there are two types of patient population who will benefit from transitioning ICU care at home: patients who are not acutely ill but are not fully ready for discharge from ICU and patients who are at the end stage of their lives and need life support as a continuum of care at home. There are numerous advantages of extending intensive care services at home as they promise a friendly environment with reduced disturbance favoring the return to more physiological status [4]. Transition of care from ICU to home involves a multidisciplinary team effort involving ICU medical and nursing staff, families, social worker, equipment supply offices, insurance offices, and discharge planning coordinators. This chapter is an effort to explain the importance of extending home healthcare services after ICU discharge as an effective means of assuring safer and better outcomes in terms of health and financial benefits.

Home Healthcare Model: The Rising and Importance

National Research Council (NRC) in its report on home care in 2011 declared that "Health care is coming home." Home healthcare brings down the costs of care and promotes healthy living and well-being [5]. Dr. John Burton from Johns Hopkins School of Medicine and Dr. Donna Regenstreif from John A. Hartford Foundation conceived the idea of extending home healthcare in 1995 to provide safe and effective hospital-level care in the home [6]. In 1999 a 17-patient pilot trial conducted by Leff showed that home

P. Goyal
Department of Surgery, Westchester Medical Center, Valhalla, NY, USA

R. Latifi (✉)
New York Medical College, School of Medicine, Department of Surgery and Westchester Medical Center, Valhalla, NY, USA
e-mail: rifat_latifi@nymc.edu; rifat.latifi@wmchealth.org

R. Latifi (ed.), *The Modern Hospital*, https://doi.org/10.1007/978-3-030-01394-3_34

healthcare is a feasible, safe, and cost-effective method of healthcare [7].

A public/private partnership in 2010 tested a modified model of Hospital at Home, in which home-based care is provided by nurses, with physician consult via two-way telemedicine video. This is considered a big leap in a way that technological advances were incorporated for homebound patients' still needing attention and rather closer monitoring. The senior author of this chapter being an authority figure in telemedicine firmly believes that telemedicine is and will be the pillar of transition of ICU care at home model.

Briefly, home healthcare model works as follows: After informed consent and ensuring family participation, the patient was transported home by an ambulance. The hospital-at-home nurse examines the patient on his arrival at home. The patient gets one-on-one nursing supervision for an initial period for a few days. When direct nursing supervision was no longer required, the patient gets intermittent nursing visits at least daily. The hospital-at-home physician made at least daily home visits and is available 24 h a day for urgent or emergent visits. Apart from nursing, other care components, such as medical equipment, oxygen therapy, and skilled and pharmacy support, were provided by a partner Medicare-certified home health agency. Diagnostic studies, such as electrocardiography and radiography; intravenous fluids, intravenous antimicrobial agents, and other medications; and oxygen and other respiratory therapies are also provided at home. The patient was followed by the same hospital-at-home physician until his or her condition was stable enough for discharge. Patient's care after discharge is resumed by a primary care physician [8].

Designing an ICU-Driven Home Healthcare Model

We all have been to a modern hospital ICUs as healthcare provider, family, or friend. We all are familiar with the sight of people waiting outside, eyes piercing through the glass windows waiting for news about their loved ones. Now imagine an ICU where a family member can sit beside the patient and hold the patient's hand at their home. There are existing home ICU care models in many countries like the UK, New Zealand, France, and Australia. These health systems deploy multidisciplinary home healthcare teams which include physicians, ICU nurses, and home health suppliers at the patient's home rather than a hospital after emergency department evaluation and diagnosis or after a short hospital stay in acute care settings. The basic requirements for transition from hospital ICU to home ICU care are illustrated in Fig. 34.1.

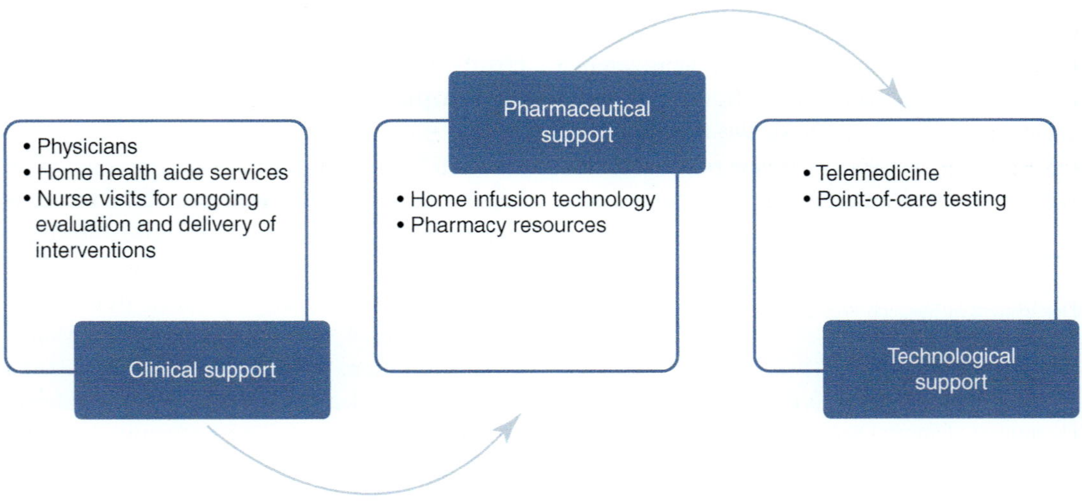

Fig. 34.1 Essential interdependent components of intensive home healthcare model

ICU care at home is different than ICU settings in the hospitals. Physicians working or interested in this arena have a little different role and some extra responsibilities. Physicians are not available around the clock in an ICU-driven home healthcare model. The communication between physicians and nurses becomes imperative. The senior author (RL) being in the field of trauma and critical care surgery for years cannot emphasize enough the importance of incorporating telemedicine in day-to-day clinical practice of physicians and critical care specialist treating the patient from their homes while driving a car, attending the conference, or doing their daily chores. Telemedicine and advanced technologies that ensure telepresence have become a common practice and are an effective way of providing healthcare services [9]. The essence is that telemedicine is telepresence of healthcare providers into the home of patients in need of critical care. Telemedicine will help physicians to do more virtual home visits with a video; it is a very efficient way of collecting vital sign remotely. Telemedicine will improve medication compliance and promote patient and family education. Clinical conditions that are suitable for ICU-based home care are exacerbations of heart failure or chronic obstructive pulmonary disease (COPD), stable pulmonary embolism (PE), deep-vein thrombosis (DVT), pneumonia, and skin or soft tissue infections such as cellulitis [10]. We believe that this list can be extended to many other conditions including trauma patients who recover from acute life-threatening phase but still need ICU level of care as they gradually resume their functionality. Adding home physical therapy will greatly enhance their outcome. Ventilator-dependent patients are another group of patients being treated at home settings. This intervention has shown to reduce the rate of emergency readmissions [11]. We propose outcome indicators of this model in Table 34.1. They can be used to gauge the effectiveness of the program.

Extending ICUs to home offers numerous advantages. Home is a familiar place; it offers sense of peace and safety and offers a comfort zone. Patients who need critical care but are dischargeable when found themselves at a familiar place such as home, along with effective and robust clinical care, have shown improved health clinically as well as physically. A meta-analysis conducted by Sheppered et al. in 2009 showed that shifting acute hospital care at home increased the patient satisfaction, reduced use of antipsychotic drugs in patients with dementia, reduced lower urinary tract and bowel complications, reduced costs, and resulted in a significant difference in 6-month mortality (hazard ratio, 0.62; 95% confidence interval [CI], 0.45–0.87; $P = 0.005$) [12]. On a more personal level, there is reduced disturbance in sleep and easier access to personal belongings, such as books, computers, TV, etc. There is greater interaction with family, relatives, and friends.

Table 34.1 Outcome indicators of intensive home healthcare model

Mortality
Readmissions
Disease-specific health status
Functional status
Psychological well-being
Complications
Patient and family satisfaction
Cost

Current Status in the USA and Limitations

At present established intensive home healthcare services are being offered by Presbyterian Healthcare at Home in Albuquerque, New Mexico, Cedars–Sinai Medical Center in Los Angeles, and the Kaiser Permanente Riverside Medical Center in Riverside, California [13]. Presbyterian Healthcare published a favorable report on its outcome. Costs of care for patients in the Healthcare at Home program were 19% lower than those for a matched cohort, and although 30-day post-episode hospital utilization rates were similar, patient satisfaction scores were higher in intensive home healthcare program [14]. Lack of financial support and encouragement in the system is an important hurdle that we need to remove, hospitals tend to lose revenue, and outpatient care providers have no incentive to work collaboratively with home care providers. To encourage outpatient ambulatory services, Centers for Medicare and Medicaid Services (CMS) awarded a grant to New York's Icahn School of Medicine at Mount Sinai to test Mobile Acute Care Team (MACT) Services, which studied the expertise of multiple providers to address acute care needs in an outpatient setting. Such initiatives will definitely bring change in payment system and encourage tertiary care centers to adopt this program.

Patient selection and eligibility criteria for intensive home healthcare need to be established for effective allocation of resources. But we understand that this is a gradual process and this field offers a potential area of research and more literature is warranted. Nonetheless, the idea of extending ICU care in home settings is being embraced gradually and is going to be the new world order.

Summary

The focus of patient care now is integrating cure with comfort. There is a shortage of beds for incoming critically ill patients; healthcare providers are pressed toward early discharges or shifting patients to regular floor. This in a way promotes readmissions, increasing cost of care and artificially increasing ICU morbidity and mortality. This is an era of "innovations," and healthcare technology is at a boom. Extending ICU care in home settings is a bold but possible move. This program is being offered by few hospitals in the country, and many other institutions are beginning to accept it. This is a multidisciplinary effort involving physicians, nurses, allied healthcare providers, pharmaceutical companies, and home service providers. CMS and Medicaid have been more positive toward this unique step. There are numerous benefits to the patients in terms of more comfort, familiar surroundings, and more interaction with their loved ones. Hospitals have more space to accommodate the rising number of patients in critical shape. Extending ICU care at home will reduce readmissions and decrease morbidity in terms of less delirium and low urinary and respiratory complications. There is a growing evidence of literature supporting ICU at home healthcare model. We can say with confidence that extending "ICU to home healthcare" model is here to stay.

References

1. Society of Critical Care Medicine. Critical care statistics. http://www.sccm.org/Communications/Pages/CriticalCareStats.aspx. Accessed 30 Apr 2018.
2. Beaulieu RA, McCarthy MC, Markert RJ, Parikh PJ, Ekeh AP, Parikh PP. Predictive factors and models for trauma patient disposition. J Surg Res. 2014;190(1):264–9.
3. Guidelines for intensive care unit admission, discharge, and triage. Task Force of the American College of Critical Care Medicine, Society of Critical Care Medicine. Crit Care Med. 1999;27:633–8.
4. Razavi SS, Fathi M, Hajiesmaeili M. Intensive care at home: an opportunity or threat. Anesthesiol Pain Med. 2016;6(2):e32902.
5. NRC (National Research Council). Health care comes home: the human factors. Washington, DC: The National Academies Press; 2011.
6. Hospital at Home. History. Retrieved from: http://www.hospitalathome.org/about-us/history.php.
7. Leff B, Burton L, Guido S, Greenough WB, Steinwachs D, Burton JR. Home hospital program (a pilot study). J Am Geriatr Soc. 1999;47:697–702.
8. Leff B, Burton L, Mader SL, Naughton B, Burl J, Inouye SK, et al. Hospital at home: feasibility and outcomes of a program to provide hospital-level Care at Home for acutely ill older patients. Ann Intern Med. 2005;143:798–808.
9. Latifi R, Tilley EH. Telemedicine for disaster management: can it transform chaos into an organized, structured care from the distance? Am J Disaster Med. 2014;9(1):25–37.
10. Ticona L, Schulman KA. Extreme home makeover – the role of intensive home health care. N Engl J Med. 2016;75(18):1707–9.
11. Kastrup M, Tittmann B, Sawatzki T, et al. Transition from in-hospital ventilation to home ventilation: process description and quality indicators. GMS German Med Sci. 2017;15:Doc18.

12. Shepperd S, Doll H, Angus RM, et al. Hospital at home admission avoidance. Cochrane Database Syst Rev. 2008;(4):CD007491. https://doi.org/10.1002/14651858.CD007491.
13. Klein S, Hostetter M, McCarthy D. The hospital at home model: bringing hospital-level care to the patient. 2016. Retrieved from http://www.commonwealthfund.org/publications/case-studies/2016/aug/hospital-at-home.
14. Cryer L, Shannon SB, Van Amsterdam M, Leff B. Costs for 'hospital at home' patients were 19 percent lower, with equal or better outcomes compared to similar inpatients. Health Aff (Millwood). 2012;31:1237–43.

Part IV

The Future of Modern Hospital

The Hospital of the Future: Evidence-Based, Data-Driven

35

John A. Savino and Rifat Latifi

Introduction

Predicting the future modern hospital may be difficult and should be based on current technological advances. In the future, hospitals will have command centers that equip decision-makers with real-time support tools to help them make quicker clinical and operational decisions similar to an airport's air traffic control system. Digital data are the foundation of such centers, and many hospitals have already adopted such digital technologies, and it is expected that this trend grows tremendously. In 2016 the national health expenditures [1] were estimated at $3.4 trillion with a projected increase from 17.8% to 19.9% of the GDP between 2015 and 2025. The estimate of the artificial intelligence (AI) market is poised to reach $6.6 billion by 2021 [2] and by 2026 will annually save the US healthcare $150 billion [3]. Other emerging digital technologies help hospitals move from episodic to collaborative and longitudinal care which creates ways to continually monitor patients and integrate the data to manage individual patients and operational units. Such technologies will include wearable and microfluidic sensors and artificial intelligence that constantly will monitor the data to alert hospital operators and caregivers, which can enable more efficient care and improve outcomes. Through big data analytics, machine learning, and AI, patient medical errors can be predicted before they occur, and suggested interventions can be fed to caregivers. Such clinical command centers exist at Johns Hopkins Hospital and the Cleveland Clinic [4, 5].

Clinical Command Centers

Newly established clinical command centers (CCC) manage a variety of clinical, operational, and administrative processes and can span from data on admissions, inter-facility transfers, and predictive analytics on possible days for discharge. Command center analysts can help staff manage patient flow and improve care delivery, better manage lengths of stay, and enhance the discharge process. More importantly, it is expected that such CCC will assist in elimination altogether or reducing substantially errors on medications and many other man-made errors. In other words, they will help with providing precision medicine. These command centers also can track social media for open feedback and identify any patterns in comments to generate alerts for rapid response from appropriate leaders [4]. Newer technology advancements, including 3D printing, robotics, nanotechnology, genetic

J. A. Savino (✉)
Westchester Medical Center Health Network, New York Medical College, Valhalla, NY, USA
e-mail: John.savino@wmchealth.org

R. Latifi
New York Medical College, School of Medicine, Department of Surgery and Westchester Medical Center, Valhalla, NY, USA

R. Latifi (ed.), *The Modern Hospital*, https://doi.org/10.1007/978-3-030-01394-3_35

coding based on genomic mapping, and therapeutic options, will permit more personalized and accessible patient care (see Chaps. 13 and 14), which is expected to become more portable with treatments that will become more targeted and precise. Subsequently, clinicians will be able to quickly find the best treatment option rather than try multiple interventions. Based on a patient's genetic profile and precision medicine, medications will become more personalized and biology based (see Chap. 28). Designs for 3D-printed prostheses will be based largely on a patient's specific anatomy [4].

As medical equipment and sensors become smaller and more portable, clinicians may be able to perform various tests and procedures at the patient's bedside rather than transporting the patient to different areas of the hospital. Patient rooms will be built to include more equipment options and robotic equipment to deliver medications to patients. Additionally, medical interventions will continue to become less invasive which will result in better outcomes and more rapid recoveries. The long-elusive goal of electronic health records (EHR) populated by interoperable data from different sources beyond a network will likely be a reality in the hospital of the future. EHR coupled with AI will create process efficiencies and improve decision-making necessary to boost quality. Moreover, data can be better integrated into daily care, and patients can play a role in collecting their own data [4].

Real-Time Data

Important real-time patient data at the point of care can affect the treatment and improve patient outcomes [6]. The data can include genetic, biologic, social, and behavioral patient information, as well as financial, clinical, and administrative records. Securing and ability to access such data in real time will become a challenge, however. Many hospitals will need cognitive analytics to sort through and find the most important personalized data points and trends. This information can be presented to clinicians, patients, and caregivers in a comprehensible format that fits into their daily activities. Patients can own their own data, add to and edit their health records, and proactively communicate with their caregivers. The data can easily be de-identified which will be ideal for research purposes [7]. Will data fatigue and how to sort through and select only what really matters become an issue with massive data present and stored become the next challenge?

Digital Technology and Bedside Patient Experience

Digital technology may improve the patient experience by providing real-time access to medical knowledge. Although, there will always be a need for clinical providers at the bedside, an AI-powered bedside virtual care assistant can answer or direct patient queries to the most appropriate person at the hospital. The virtual assistant can answer questions about diagnoses, expected recovery times and experiences, and daily medication schedules and also can act on a data repository for patients' medical history, test results, consultation times, and appointment schedules [4]. Patients often complain about filling out multiple forms that ask for similar data or receiving conflicting discharge instructions. As hospital processes convert to digital, staff can use AI to improve them by eliminating the patient registration process. When the patient's physician recommends admission, the patient will receive an application on their own or on a hospital device that helps direct their experience. Clinical, financial, and demographic information can be prepopulated from the patients' records. These stored records should be easily accessible to key stakeholders. AI incorporated into the application can help physicians, medical staff, and patients converge on decisions such as modulating staffing needs, selecting room type, stocking required medications, determining diagnostic choices, and meeting nonmedical support based on the patient's sociodemographic profile [4].

Eventually AI algorithms approach may be integrated into the discharge workflow by creating customized discharge guidelines and integrated into the virtual care assistant and delivered to the patient at discharge and throughout recovery. Patients can take as long as they need to understand the instructions and can also ask questions. Nurses and medical staff are available if needed. Post-discharge patients can use a personal device to schedule appointments with various caregivers such as nutritionists, eye specialists, and pharmacists. The EHR can automatically capture results of these visits [4].

Ensuring Financial Viability of Modern Hospital

Hospitals traditionally were constructed with the anticipation that there would be predictable price growth, continuous demand for its services with minimal competition, and regulatory protections. Unfortunately, Medicare reimbursement has progressively decreased with projections in the future of a steady decline. Hospital occupancy across the country on the average is 60% which will probably continue in the future based on the focus on patient-centered care and initiatives dedicated to management of multiple conditions at home. Additionally, many hospitals have placed greater focus to ambulatory sites [8]. Acute care substitutes have emerged as competition in the acute care delivery system at lower costs. In 2018 Walmart and Humana were negotiating a potential deal that would provide inexpensive healthcare competitive options to the hospital industry. CVS Health's $70 billion bid for Aetna [9] and Cigna's $ 54 billion offer for Express Scripts potentially could mean a shift toward cheaper care provided at clinics and prescription drugs with reduced spending on hospital services which are less efficient and more costly. Clearly, Walmart's massive retail presence would expand its outpatient capabilities as a low-cost offering. Walmart's negotiating power for employee health benefits would be a threat to hospitals especially with Humana's data and infrastructure that could position a combined entity to offer competitive health plans [10]. Humana will reimburse hospitals based on quality improvement and performance metrics under a new program that it revealed April 25, 2018. The insurer's National Hospital Incentive Program pertains to hospitals treating its commercial members. The program will compensate hospitals based on three key areas: patient experience, patient safety, and patient outcomes. It will also use other measures including healthcare-associated infection rates, care coordination, palliative care, and other performance parameters. Earned annual rate increases in participating hospitals will be based on the continuous improvement of the three performance measures [10].

In order to survive in a new financial and competitive environment, hospitals have pursued mergers, acquisitions, and expansion. This complex process has not yielded the expected effects in these transactions, and most systems aggregate without consolidation and decreasing costs. Many of the institutions within a network compete with each other by providing a duplication of services without adequate volume. A fully integrated strategy that has a clear perception of the actual market availability of prospective patients will benefit the system by reducing overhead and operational costs. The smaller hospitals have fixed costs and attempt to consolidate redundant services to maintain financial viability. However, low occupancy rates inevitably threaten survivability leading to a reduction in bed count and conversion to a more ambulatory facility [8].

Tertiary Medical Institution of the Future

The institutions that provide care for patients with complex conditions, specifically tertiary care hospitals of the future, will emulate the University of Pennsylvania's new $ 1.5 billion 17-story hospital, the Pavilion, which is designed to deliver the best care to patients based on current standards but also will have the ability to adapt to any advancements that occur over the next few decades [11]. The hospital will have 500 private rooms and 47 operating and interventional rooms. The hospital is broken down into smaller neighborhoods meant to provide a sense of community. Patients, families, and employees will have access to daylight and landscaped views of outdoor green space with foliage.

Each of the hospital's rooms will be designed to be converted to a higher level of care such as a critical care unit room, and the nursing staff in that circumstance will be changed to nurses specialized in critical care. Consequently, unnecessary transfers to different units can be avoided. Technology in the rooms will strengthen communication between patients, families, and care teams and will provide educational programming. Rooms are typically 300–400 square feet in size to accommodate electrical outlets, medical gases, observation window, and data ports found in the ICU. The rooms are divided into three zones for the patient, family, and care team. Older institutions have the option to renovate individual units by decreasing the number of beds but increasing room size to accommodate family members. The extra space allows for larger mattresses and equipment bed lifts which will accommodate elderly and disabled patients [11]. In other words, the future tertiary medical centers will be technologically driven, "smart hospitals" and compatible to provide the best possible care. They will be in fact intensive care units for the most part.

Outpatient Services and Skilled Nursing Facilities (SNF)

Technology has advanced to a level of sophistication that allows many procedures to be performed on an outpatient basis. To adapt to this environment, institutions have converted to the hospital without beds which has all the services available at a typical inpatient hospital including primary care, specialties, imaging, laboratories, pharmacy, and ambulatory surgery center. These institutions do not provide care in the emergency department, inpatient beds, and an ICU [12].

Other sites prefer to accommodate patients requiring acute care that do not require a full-service hospital but more specifically supervision or short-term recovery from a procedure. Medicare payment reform has allowed medical patients in these sites. These institutions use the 3-day skilled nursing facility waiver to decrease hospital length of stay [13]. Currently, in traditional fee-for-service Medicare, beneficiaries are eligible for Medicare-covered skilled nursing facility services when a beneficiary is admitted within 30 days of either an inpatient hospital stay of 3 consecutive days or more (i.e., qualifying hospital stay, starting with the day the hospital admits the beneficiary as an inpatient, but not including the day they leave the hospital) or a previous SNF stay. The time the beneficiary is in the hospital being observed or in an emergency room before they are admitted does not count toward the 3-day qualifying inpatient hospital stay. However, the next-generation ACO waiver allows an aligned beneficiary to be eligible for Medicare-covered SNF services when admitted to a SNF without a 3-day qualifying inpatient hospital stay or previous SNF stay, including beneficiaries who are in the hospital for fewer than 3 days or admitted directly from a physician's office. The waiver relieves the system to send the patient directly to a cost appropriate site of care. Even for organizations currently without the 3-day waiver, a preferred post-acute care network is crucial to managing acute care costs. These preferred partner networks are relatively common, but others have established joint ventures with post-acute care providers and exclusive partnerships with single providers for high-frequency services for a limited set of clinical conditions, or they can use them as low-cost site for low-acuity medical needs [13].

There are alternatives for ailing Medicare patients for whom the hospital may not be the ideal locations of their care. Hospitals can be an unsafe environment for these patients because of possible infections, medical errors, or falls. Advances in smartphone and sensor technologies have digitized a range of medically relevant biometric data. Certain conditions such as chronic obstructive pulmonary disease (COPD), cellulitis, dehydration, congestive heart failure, and pneumonia would be amenable to manage at home. Creative innovations have the potential to provide post-discharge monitoring capabilities; provide observation that the patient is living in a healthy manner at home; detect disease patterns, risk of falls, and mood assessment; and provide a window for caregivers to diagnosis and tailor treatments remotely.

Medical Homes of The Future

Medical homes of the future can have installation of floor mat pressure sensors, cameras, infrared, visual motion sensors, and pulse-Doppler radar [14]. All of these have been shown to be useful for fall detection and gate analysis in specially equipped senior living apartments. Integrated data streams from these sensors, communicated in real-time with caregivers, and could improve safety oversight by providing alerts on the detection of an in-home emergency and a longitudinal evaluation of a person's mobility trend. In addition, future medication adherence could be assessed by smart pill boxes, as well as radio-frequency-labeled medications, facial recognition, and swallowing monitored by smartphone video, TVs, or video-equipped mirrors in the home. Dietary patterns could be assessed using information from smart fridges and online food ordering requests, and mobile device spectrometers are in development to capture and analyze food intake. By combining such dietary information with passively collected weights taken by scales in the floor of the bathroom or toilet seats, individualized eating plans could be recommended. Body-worn devices such as wrist-worn accelerometers could be useful in detecting position changes (seated to standing), falls, activity, and health status. Wearable devices in chairs and beds could monitor heart rate and rhythm, blood pressure, respiratory rate, or blood oxygen concentration. Point-of-care diagnosis using breath, urine, saliva, or finger stick of blood can predict early stages of disease and clearly could preemptively provoke the initiation of treatments remotely. Emergency services could be notified in an automated fashion along with the patient's location, family, and care providers [14].

Patient Empowerment

Recently, journalist Laura Landro reported in The Wall Street Journal a review of the changes that are occurring in the US healthcare system but most importantly the variety of healthcare outpatient institutions that exist [15]. Traditional hospital care is overly expensive and inefficient for many medical conditions. In an era of consumerism, the patients have become empowered to select the venues where they prefer to be treated. There is greater focus today and in the future to prevent diseases. Amazon Inc., Berkshire Hathaway, Inc., and JPMorgan Chase formed a company with the intention to provide less expensive healthcare for their employees [16]. Mount Sinai Hospital developed a hospital at home program, HaH-Plus, for patients who are evaluated for an acute situation [17]. If they are eligible for care in a Mobile Acute Care Team (MACT) program, as well as sick enough to require hospitalization and meet previously validated medical eligibility criteria, they are considered for the program. These patients must live in a stable residence that meets the needs for safety, shelter, and basic utilities and reside within Manhattan. If MACT concludes that the patient qualifies for admission, the HaH is designated. The provider must receive written consent from the patient or a family member, must write an admission note and specific orders for infusions and medications, and must arrange for the patient's transportation home. The patient subsequently receives hospital-level care from a team of doctors, nurses, and other healthcare professionals. The care includes daily visits or more frequently if appropriate from a medical doctor or nurse practitioner or home care nurses to monitor vital signs regularly and administer certain medications, e.g., infusions, laboratory services, I.V. medications, and other equipment or therapy as needed. Additionally, 24/7 coverage is available to address any urgent or immediate concerns or needs, and social worker coordination of care, and follow-up plans. The patient is eventually discharged, and the MACT continues to be available to patients for 24/7 for 30 days to deal with any emergencies or concerns. Many patients who require subacute rehabilitation prefer to return home immediately after an illness or a surgical procedure with the proper support and services in place. Rehab at Home (RaH) is an alternative service provided by Mount Sinai [17].

Providing Care from The Bunker

Cleveland Clinic has in a nondescript part of Cleveland in a bunker a doctor, nurses, and medical technicians that monitor over 150 patients in special care units and intensive care beds. These patients are scattered around the region in clinics that have no specialist covering the night shift. They track their vital signs and they can zoom in with a camera at the foot of the bed. High-speed Internet remote monitoring technology and analysis of enormous amounts of data have diminished the need for a hospital with sophisticated monitoring units. A hospital would resemble an air traffic control tower from which medical teams would monitor patients near and far to standards only possible in ICUs [4, 15].

Banner Health, a large nonprofit health system, operates 28 hospitals and several specialized facilities across 6 states [18]. It is Tele-ICU program for which Philips, a Dutch health technology firm, provides equipment, programming, and software support. It manages care for critically ill patients who may be thousands of miles away. Patients are assisted to leave the hospital earlier than anticipated for their heath condition. The patients remain under constant monitoring and care in their homes with an ability to contact their doctor or nurse by audio-visual methods. Johns Hopkins University in Baltimore, MD, has built a NASA-inspired command center to manage its patient's flow [19]. Surrounded by 22 beeping flat-screens, live video streams, and innumerable phones, staff members wearing head sets orchestrate the 1100 bed institution around the clock. In the future, a command center could watch over patients not only in hospitals but also at home. Wearable devices that track vital signs, contact lenses that monitor blood-sugar levels, and smart stitches that measure the pH level of fluid in wounds would diminish the number of patients requiring hospitalizations.

In the hospitals that manage the complex patients confined in critical care units, the importance of predictive analytics and big data is critically important. The volume of data in the Electronic Health Record (EHR) creates a staggering challenge in complex environments such as intensive care units and emergency medicine departments. Individual physicians have to scrutinize thousands of data points to find key information. Relying only on EHR data greatly limits the insights derived from artificial intelligence algorithms or big data analytics. The investigators and researchers at the Mayo Clinic in Rochester, Minnesota, decided to combat the data deluge with ambient intelligence which is a set of decision-making tools powered by data on insights into clinician's goals, work environments, and strengths and performance constraints [20]. When layered on top of existing information infrastructure, ambient intelligence applications can cut through the clutter and deliver the right information in a form that clinicians can use, quickly and effectively, at the patient's bedside. The researchers needed to deliver the information at the point of care by building an EHR interface for the clinician's in the ICU called Ambient Warning and Response Evaluation (AWARE) [20]. AWARE filters out the meaningless data and deliver context-specific, high-value information in real time and improve cognitive performance, efficiency, and reliability of human decision-makers. The AWARE saves 3–5 min on chart review per patient, per day. With an average ICU clinician workload of 15 patients per day, that savings cumulatively provides 1 h of additional clinician time that can be devoted to the patient bedside. Additionally, implementation of AWARE has improved patient outcome and reduced costs in the ICU. AWARE delivers results that clearly suggest the importance of human insights and creatively in developing information technology for clinicians [21].

As of 2016 the Westchester Medical Center Health Network has instituted a state of the art telehealth program where intensivists (doctors and nurses) manage 114 ICU beds across the network as a supplementary support to the ICU team members. The eICU monitors best practice performance indicators including stress ulcer prophylaxis, venous thromboembolism prophylaxis, ventilator days, oxygen ratio based on tidal volume level, blood transfusion report based on hemoglobin level, and average daily glucose levels. The eICU utilizes APACHE IV which employs a risk stratification and outcome prediction tool to assist in the evaluation of critical care performance. It employs the Acute Physiology Score (APS) in conjunction with the admission diagnosis, chronic health factors, and admission source details to generate risk-stratified mortality and length of stay predictors that can be employed for comparative purposes.

Telemedicine Connects the Hospital to the Home

The US Congress passed legislation in February 2018 that includes healthcare provisions affecting telehealth. The law signaled a broader use of telehealth which allows private Medicare reimbursement for telestroke services and allows patients receiving home dialysis to have the required monthly physician visits conducted by the telehealth technology. The program impacts specifically patients and beneficiaries who receive care through Accountable Care Organizations (ACO) and Medicare Advantage's private health plans beginning in 2020 [22]. Technological advances including high-resolution video cameras and stable broadband Internet have made real-time telemedicine an increasingly common mode of healthcare delivery in such diverse fields as dermatology, neurology, intensive care, and psychiatry. The American Hospital Association encouraged the Senate Finance Committee on Rural Health Care to strengthen the Rural Health Care Program in order to provide more support for rural telemedicine services to improve access to healthcare services [23]. A quarter of the US population lives in rural communities. However, approximately only 10% of physicians practice in these areas. Broadband enables telehealth services to connect patients and providers in a variety of ways that include videoconferencing, remote monitoring, electronic consults, and wireless communications, while electronic health records enable efficient exchange of patients' treatment information improving the continuity of care, reducing redundant treatment, and improving outcomes. Currently, telemedicine budgets are modest, and the academic medical centers anticipate more growth than community hospitals. Security of data and HIPPA compliance are the most significant requirements for successful deployment. For telehealth to continue evolving and expanding, clinicians need to reassure regulators and patients that critical data is properly secured yet accessible for patients. Independent accreditation of telehealth programs can help assure that organizations meet rigorous standards [24].

The regulatory landscape for telehealth provided care remains fragmented and complex, especially when the doctor patient relationships cross state lines. Certain medications, specifically opioids, present prescribing issues using telehealth technology because of a strict regulatory environment. The Interstate Medical Licensure Compact [25] which was developed by the Federation of State Medical Boards has developed an expedited and improved pathway for physicians to seek licenses in different states. Many are on board while others are debating legislation to join by reducing regulatory hurdles and aligning processes. For the healthcare industry to be successful, patients will need opportunities to assess the quality of care that is provided. One advantage is that the physicians have more time to engage with their patients with reduced overhead. From a reimbursement perspective, government financial remuneration by Medicare and Medicaid, as well as private insurers, has inconsistent policies, and individual states have independent laws. However, CMS has expanded in 2018 the list of telehealth services that are reimbursed as Medicare services and decreased the burdens for physicians in billing the government as well. CMS added new categories of Telehealth services including psychotherapy services, counseling services, interactive complexity, administration of health risk assessments, and assessments for patients requiring chronic care management services [26].

There are opportunities to ameliorate the current challenge of progressively rising healthcare costs by utilizing telehealth. The cumulative anticipated positive effect includes a reduction in readmissions to the hospital, preemptive outreach potentially prevents hospitalizations, and there is better utilization of staff. Telehealth technology permits accumulation of data which allows clinicians to analyze the information more effectively. The concept of patient-centered care is not a clinic appointment in which patients see their physicians in their clinic environment, but rather a house call. When viewed from that perspective, the benefits, limitations, and tradeoffs in telehealth and traditional care are more apparent. Providing smartphones to persons in need will be essential to ensure that current disparities in care are not amplified by differential access to the next generation of care delivery [27].

Because of the potential of technology to transform healthcare, venture capital funding in digital health has nearly quadrupled from $ 1.1 billion in 2011 to $ 4 billion in 2015. In the near future, many advances will be connected to smartphones, which 90% of the world will have by 2020. The increasingly sophisticated sensors, wearables, and growing number of peripheral assessments may enable smartphones to monitor a person's health passively, facilitate diagnosis, and connect patients to clinicians when needed. The ability to exchange patient-generated real-world data, including data from sensors, laboratories, and imaging, with the doctor during or in advance of a telehealth visit, may enhance the value of such interactions [28].

Telemedicine involved in the care of cardiovascular disease patients has revolutionized healthcare in terms of modality and quality attributes. The attributes for these patients include reduced hospitalizations and readmissions, improved mortality rates, increased cost effectiveness, improved outcomes, improved quality of life, and increase in self-management. More than 85 million Americans, approximately 26% of the US population, suffer from cardiovascular disease, and nearly 7 million (2.2%) are stroke survivors [29]. Significant reduction in hospitalizations and increased self-management by patients epitomize the economic perceptive of telemedicine, since it has helped reduce the monetary side of readmissions. The American Heart Association [29] has endorsed the use of telemedicine in the care of cardiovascular disease and stroke patients which are significant public health burdens. Care becomes more accessible and affordable while reducing many of the widespread disparities in access to care, particularly those attributable to geography or provider shortages. Effective telehealth interventions exist in many diseases such as diabetes mellitus, in-pain management, and medication adherence, in ambulatory patients in heart failure, and in those with implanted cardiac devices with remote monitoring. Barriers to the effective implementation of telehealth across broad populations of patients and providers can be broken down into three areas of legal/regulatory, technological, and financial.

Emerging Technologies in Future Hospital Care

Artificial intelligence can be defined as the ability of a digital computer or computer-controlled robot to perform tasks commonly associated with intelligent beings. The term is frequently applied to the project of developing systems endowed with intellectual processes characteristic of humans, such as the ability to reason, discover meaning, generalize, or learn from past experience [30].

A source of clinician assistance lies in the domain of artificial intelligence which focuses on spoken language and machine learning. Machine learning [31] entails building knowledge from patterns in data rather than being specified by human programmers. Computer vision allows machines to see and understand the visual world. When applied to computer vision, tasks such as discernment of people, objects, and their motion, cameras, and imaging sensors supply data for learning. Computer vision is poised to gain a foothold in screening medical images for clinician analysis. The use of computer vision to continuously monitor bedside behavior could off-load low-value work better suited to machines, augmenting rather than replacing clinicians. If successfully developed, ambient computer vision carries the potential to discern diverse bedside clinician and patient behaviors at superhuman performance levels and send user-designed prompts in real time. Such systems could remind a doctor or a nurse to perform hand hygiene if they begin to enter a patient room without doing so, alert a surgeon that an important step has been missed during a complex procedure, or notify a nurse that an agitated patient is dangerously close to pulling out an endotracheal tube [32].

Given its rapid pace of improvement in accuracy and affordability in other industries, computer vision may bring us closer to resolving an intractable mismatch between the growing complexity of intended clinician behaviors and human vulnerability to error. Cognitive computing [32] is a specialized area of AI that attempts to mimic or stimulate human thought processes. Statistic and analytic, symbolic reasoning and bioinspired systems are three high-level approaches that make up cognitive computing. Each approach brings different strengths and capabilities to AI challenges, allowing cognitive computing approaches to address a wide variety of tasks. It is important to note that AI works best when paired with humans, as systems may not perform predictably when faced with parameters outside of their normal range of experience. There is the development of an AI-based operating system combined with cognitive capabilities to enable organizations to seamlessly manage massive quantities and complexity of data. All medical information including clinical data, images, omics, or wearables can be integrated into intelligent systems that provide insight and decision support based on this data [33].

Researchers have developed deep-learning neural networks that can identify pathologies in radiological images such as bone fractures and potentially cancerous lesions, in some cases more reliable than the average radiologist [34]. Deep learning is rapidly advancing, and it is superior to previous approaches to medical image analysis. Radiologists do more than read and interpret images. The deep-learning models are trained for specific image recognition tasks such as nodule detection on chest CT or hemorrhage on brain MRI. Thousands of such narrow detection tasks are necessary to fully identify all potential findings in medical images, and only a few of these can be done by AI today. The job of image interpretation encompasses only one set of tasks that radiologists perform. They also consult with other physicians on diagnosis and treatment, treat diseases with ablative therapy, perform image-guided medical interventions (interventional radiology), define the technical parameters of imaging examinations to be performed, relate findings from images to other medical records and test results, discuss procedures and results with patients, and many other activities. Even in the unlikely event that AI took over image reading and interpretation, most radiologists could redirect their focus to these other essential activities [34].

There are substantial medical and productivity benefits to be gained from integrating AI with radiological practice. The productivity improvements may even mean that radiologists can spend more time doing what many of them find most fulfilling: consulting with other physicians about diagnoses and treatment strategies. If predicted improvements in deep-learning image analysis are realized, then providers, patients, and payers will gravitate toward the radiologists who have figured out how to work effectively alongside AI [34].

One of the most dominant conditions confronting healthcare providers is the challenge of chronic disease. In the United States, chronic disease accounts for $3 of every $4 spent on healthcare or $7900 for every American with chronic disease causing seven out of every ten deaths. Chronic disease is both predictable and preventable, and AI can play a pivotal role in addressing solutions that can provide personalized medicine and interventions. AI has already started revolutionizing the healthcare by leveraging big data analysis to optimize healthcare services. A perfect example is Google's DeepMind Health Project [35]. IBM Watson for Oncology [36] has advanced ability to analyze a patient's data and provide personalized treatment plans that combine the attributes from the patient's file, clinical expertise, external research, and data. These techniques can also be leveraged to detect cancer or vascular diseases in their very early stage.

Identifying patterns in huge data sets of genetic information and medical records (Precision Medicine and Deep Genomics), looking for mutations and linkages in diseases, and personalizing the treatment and process protocols for a patient will play a key role in increasing the efficacy to address chronic disease. Atomwise [37] has launched a virtual search for safe, existing medicines that could be redesigned to treat the Ebola virus. Similarly, nearly 50% of the population of the United States, and almost 90% of people 65 years and older, which amounts to 36 million patients, take at least one prescription drug and more than 10% of the US population, and almost 40% of people 65 years and over (approximately 16 million patients), take five or more prescription drugs. By understanding patient's diseases precisely and providing personalized patient-centric care, the outcomes will dramatically be optimal.

Problems around medical imaging seem ideally suited for this computer support. Case studies have highlighted the potential of deep learning. Pathologists face the task of identifying and quantifying cancerous regions by investigating tissue samples on microscopy slides, and in a recent study an AI-based algorithm [38] achieved a detection rate surpassing that of a trained pathologist. In the case of skin cancer detection, a team of researchers have successfully trained a computer to identify melanoma from images as accurately as a human dermatologist [39]. In the case of radiotherapy treatment, planning the aim is to kill cancer cells while avoiding damaging healthy tissue within the patient's body. The task is therefore to distinguish precisely between regions targeted by the X-ray beam and those areas that must be spared. This can require many hours of outlining both pathological regions and healthy organs, in a process labeled as segmentation, to ensure successful and safe treatment. The radiation therapy workflow could be streamlined if AI was used to automate the segmentation. All the doctor would need to perform is a relatively fast review of the results produced by the computer [40].

Precision medicine is an emerging approach for disease treatment and prevention that takes into account individual variability in genes, environment, and lifestyle for each person. This approach will allow doctors and researchers to predict more accurately which treatment and prevention strategies for a particular disease will work in which groups of people [41]. It is in contrast to a one size fits all approach, in which disease treatment and prevention strategies are developed for the average person, with less consideration for differences between individuals. Pharmacogenomics is a part of precision medicine and is the study of how genes affect a person's response to particular drugs. This relatively new field combines pharmacology and genomics (the study of genes and their functions) to develop effective and safe medications and doses that are tailored to variations in a person's genes. The Precision Medicine Initiative intends to increase the knowledge of the genetics and biology of cancer to find new and more effective treatments for various forms of disease. The NIH plans to study (All of Us Research Program) [42] one million volunteers who will provide genetic data, biological samples, and other information about their health. Participants will be able to access their health information, as well as research that uses their data, during the study. Researchers will use these data to study a large range of diseases, with goals of better predicting disease risk, understanding how diseases occur, and finding improved diagnosis and treatment strategies.

One of the benefits of the precision medicine will be to find new approaches for protecting research participants, particularly patient's privacy and confidentiality of their data. It will provide new tools for building, analyzing, and sharing large sets of medical data. Additionally, there will be improvement of FDA oversight of tests, drugs, and other technologies to support innovation while ensuring that these products are safe and effective. In the long term, physicians will use patient's genetic and other molecular information as part of routine medical care and will have improved ability to predict which treatments will be most effective for specific patients. Inevitably, there will be a better understanding of the underlying mechanisms by which various diseases occur, as well as improved approaches to preventing, diagnosing, and treating a wide range of diseases. If decision medicine approaches are to become part of routine healthcare, physicians and other providers will need to become more knowledgeable about molecular genetics and biochemistry in order to interpret the results of tests, understand how the information is relevant to treatment or prevention approaches, and convey this knowledge to patients [42].

Another technology, 3D printing, that has potential to streamline manufacturing allows healthcare organizations to design and produce new products cheaply, expeditiously, and efficiently. 3D printing is a process that lays down successive layers of material to build three-dimensional objects [43]. It can produce objects using a wide range of materials, including polymers (plastics, rubber, resins), powdered metals and alloys (aluminum, steel, titanium), ceramics, wax, sand, organic materials (stem cells, wood), and other composites. Initially, in the 3D printing process, a digital model is created which is done with computer-aided design software but may also involve a 3D object scanner or medical imaging. Within the software workflow, users can adjust the printing process to match their needs regarding segmentation (e.g., outlining and coloring the structure of a heart model), functionality (e.g., the need for an object to include a movable hinge), or structural complexity (e.g., shape, texture, layer thickness). The design is then imported into a slicer program that determines how the printer will build each layer before it is converted into a file format that can be read by the printer. Once the print process begins, the machine works autonomously, following the rules of the digital file with little or no need for human involvement. After the printing is complete, there is often a post-processing phase which can include coloring, sanding, sterilization, polishing, or removing structures that were needed to support printed overhangs on the 3D object [44].

There are many medical applications in the healthcare industry already with anticipated future developments. In surgical planning providers can 3D print patient-specific models of organs, nerves, tumors, and other tissues from CT and MRI scans [44]. These models are used for educational purposes, to help diagnose illness, or for surgeons to plan for an upcoming surgery. 3D-printed limb prosthetics are cheaper and faster to produce than traditional prostheses especially for amputees. 3D printing is also used to develop exoskeletons [44], which can help patients learn to walk again after injuries. Most of the in-ear hearing aids are made using 3D printing to custom fit for each patient's ear canal. 3D printing is used for Hip and knee joints, spinal disks, and bone replacements for the sternum and craniofacial reconstruction. In the field of "Bioprinting," researchers are testing new ways to use 3D printers and stem cells to print blood vessels, muscles, bones, cartilages, and functional organs [45]. 3D-printed tissues and organs may be used for testing pharmaceuticals or cosmetics, modeling the effects of different diseases, and reducing problems with organ rejection. Patient satisfaction increases and outcomes improve when patient-specific custom-made devices such as implants, anatomical models, and surgical tools are readily available in health systems and hospitals.

In an article published in Forbes magazine in 2014, Vinod Khosla, founder of Sun Microsystems, speculated that entrepreneurs are trying to use machine learning technologies to replace human judgment in many areas including farm workers, warehouse workers, hamburger flippers, legal researchers, financial investment intermediaries, and in healthcare including cardiologists, psychiatrists, ear-nose-throat specialists, and the previously mentioned radiologists, pathologists, and others [46]. He continued to predict that the future is promising and this technology revolution may result in dramatically increasing productivity and abundance, yet the process of arriving there raises all sorts of questions about the changing nature of work and likely increases in income disparity [46]. With less need for human labor and judgment, labor will be devalued relative to capital and even more so relative to ideas and machine learning technology. He stated that in an era of abundance and increasing income disparity, there may be a need for a version of capitalism that is focused on more than just efficient production and also places greater prioritization on the less desirable side effects of capitalism [46]. Historically, technology augmented and amplified human capability, which increased the productivity of human labor. Education was one method for humans to leverage technology as it evolved and improved. However, if machine learning technologies become superior in both intelligence and knowledge relevant to a particular job, human employees may be rendered unnecessary or in the very least, they will be in far less demand and command lower pay [46].

References

1. Centers for Medicare and Medicaid Services. National Health Expenditure Data Fact Sheet. 2018, April 17. Retrieved from: https://www.cms.gov/research-statistics-data-and-systems/statistics-trends-and-reports/nationalhealthexpenddata/nhe-fact-sheet.html.
2. Frost & Sullivan. From $600 M to $6 billion, artificial intelligence systems poised for dramatic market expansion in healthcare [press release]. 2016, January 5. Retrieved from: https://ww2.frost.com/news/press-releases/600-m-6-billion-artificial-intelligence-systems-poised-dramatic-market-expansion-healthcare.
3. Collier M, Fu R, Yin L. Artificial intelligence in healthcare. Accenture. 2018. Retrieved from: https://www.accenture.com/us-en/insight-artificial-intelligence-healthcare.
4. Gordon R., Perlman M, Shukla M. The hospital of the future how digital technologies can change hospitals globally. Deloitte. 2017. Retrieved from: https://www2.deloitte.com/content/dam/Deloitte/global/Documents/Life-Sciences-Health-Care/us-lshc-hospital-of-the-future.pdf.
5. Sweeney E. The digitalized hospital of the future will include clinical command centers and interoperable EHRs. 2017, October 05. Retrieved from: https://www.fiercehealthcare.com/analytics/digitized-hospital-clinical-command-center-ehr-interoperability-cloud.
6. Toussaint JS, Mannon M. Hospitals are finally starting to put real-time data to use. Harv Bus Rev. 2014. Retrieved from: https://hbr.org/2014/11/hospitals-are-finally-starting-to-put-real-time-data-to-use.
7. MyChart. The Ohio State University: Wexner Medical Center. Retrieved from: https://wexnermedica.osu.edu/features/osumychart.
8. Dowling MJ. Michael Dowling: are hospitals obsolete? No, they are evolving. Becker's Hospital review. 2018, April 2. Retrieved from: https://www.beckershospitalreview.com/hospital-management-administration/michael-dowling-are-hospitals-obsolete-no-they-are-evolving.html.
9. Humer C, O'Donnell C. CVS health to acquire Aetna for $69 billion in year's largest acquisition. Reuters. 2017, December 3. Retrieved from: https://www.reuters.com/article/us-aetna-m-a-cvs-health/cvs-health-to-acquire-aetna-for-69-billion-in-years-largest-acquisition-idUSKBN1DX0NC.
10. Haefner M. Humana launches national value-based hospital incentive program. Becker's Hospital review. 2018, April 26. Retrieved from: https://www.beckershospitalreview.com/payer-issues/humana-launches-national-value-based-hospital-incentive-program.html.
11. Penn: Facilities & Real Estate Services. University of Pennsylvania. 2018. Retrieved from: https://www.facilities.upenn.edu/maps/locations/pavillion.
12. Barth B. "A hospital without beds." American Builders Quarterly. Retrieved from: https://americanbuildersquarterly.com/2015/06/15/montefiore-medical-center/.
13. Next Generation ACO Model: skilled nursing facility (SNF) three-day rule waiver. 2018, January. Retrieved from: https://innovation.cms.goc/files/x/pioneeraco-snfwaiver.pdf.
14. Muse ED, Barrett FM, Steinhubls SR, Topol EJ. Toward a smart medical home. Lancet. 2017;389(10067):358. https://doi.org/10.10116/S0140-6736(17)30154-x.
15. Landro L. What the hospitals of the future look like. Wall Street J. 2018.; Retrieved from: https://www.wsj.com/articles/what-the-hospitals-of-the-future-look-like-1519614660.
16. Chappell B, Dwyer C. Amazon, Berkshire Hathaway and JPMorgan chase launch new health care company. 2018, January 30. Retrieved from: https://www.npr.org/sections/thetwo-way/2018/01/30/581804474/amazon-berkshire-hathaway-and-jpmorgan-chase-launch-new-healthcare-company.
17. Mobile Acute Care Team (MACT). Icahn School of Medical at Mount Sinai. Retrieved from: https://www.mountsinai.org/patient-care/service-areas/geriatrics-and-aging/mobile-acute-care-team.
18. Erikson J. Banner health eICU shortens hospital stays, improves patient care. 2014, May 21. Retrieved from: https://telemedicine.arizona.edu/blog/banner-health-eicu-shortens-hospital-stays-improves-patient-care.
19. Slabodkin G. Johns Hopkins Hospital Command Center is first of its kind. Health data management. 2017, January 24. Retrieved from: https://www.healthdatamanagement.com/news/johns-hopkins-hospital-command-center-is-first-of-its-kind.
20. Gajic O, Herasevich V, Pickering B. How Mayo Clinic is combatting information overload in critical care units. Harv Bus Rev. Retrieved from: https://hbr.org/2018/03/how-mayo-clinic-is-combating-information-overload-in-critical-care-units.
21. PHILIPS News Center. Philips debuts new cloud-based clinical analytics dashboard to enhance patient care and staff efficiency in critical care. 2016, March 1. Retrieved from: https://www.usa.philips.com/a-w/about/news/archive/standard/news/press/2016/20160301-Philips-debuts-new-cloud-based-clinical-analytics-dashboard-to-enhance-patient-care-and-staff-efficiency-in-critical-care.html.
22. Spitzer J. Congress OKs telehealth measures in temporary funding bill. Becker's Hospital review. 2018,

February 9. Retrieved from: https://www.beckershospitalreview.com/telehealth/congress-oks-telehealth-measures-in-temporary-funding-bill.html.
23. AHA Statement before Senate Finance Committee on Rural Health Care in America: challenges and opportunities. https://www.aha.org/testimony/2018-05-24-aha-statement-senate-finance-committee-rural-health-care-america-challenges.
24. Adler-Milstein J, Kvedar J, Bates DW. Telehealth among US hospitals: several factors including state reimbursement and licensing policies, influence adoption. Health Aff (Millwood). 2014;33(2):207–15. Retrieved from: https://www.ncbi.nlm.nih.gov/pubmed/24493762.
25. American Medical Association: Advocacy Resource Center. Issue brief: interstate medical licensure compact. 2017. Retrieved from: https://www.ama-assn.org/sites/default/files/media-browser/specialty%20group/arc/fsmb-interstate-medical-licensure-compact-issue-brief.pdf.
26. Daniel JG, Uppaluru. New reimbursement for remote patient monitoring and telemedicine. C&M Health Law, November 3, 2017. Retrieved from: https://www.cmhealthlaw.com/2017/11/new-reimbursement-for-remote-patientmonitoring-and-telemedicine/.
27. Principi B. How hospitals are reducing medical costs with telehealth. American Well Blog. 2015, November 3. Retrieved from: https://www.americanwell.com/how-hospitals-are-reducing-medical-costs-with-telehealth/.
28. Dorsey RE, Topol EJ. State of telehealth. N Engl J Med. 2016;375:154–61. https://doi.org/10.1056/NEJMra1601705. Retrieved from: https://www.nejm.org/doi/full/10.1056/NEJMra1601705.
29. Schwamm LH, Chumbler N, Brown E. Recommendations for the implementation of telehealth in cardiovascular and stroke care: a policy statement from the American Heart Association. Circulation. 2017;135(7):e24–44. https://doi.org/10.1161/CIR.0000000000000475. Retrieved from: https://www.ncbi.nlm.nih.gov/pubmed/27998940.
30. Van Duin S, Bakhshi N. Part 1: artificial intelligence defined: the most used terminology around AI. Deloitte. 2017, March 28. Retrieved from: https://www2.deloitte.com/nl/nl/pages/data-analytics/articles/part-1-artificial-intelligence-defined.html.
31. Mastanduno M. Machine learning 101: 5 easy steps for using it in healthcare. HealthCatalyst. Retrieved from: https://www.healthcatalyst.com/learn-the-basics-of-machine-learning-in-healthcare.
32. Gao J, Lin P, Park DS, Yang Y. Computer vision in healthcare. J Healthcare Eng. 2018;2018: Article ID 5157020, 4 pages. Retrieved from: https://www.hindawi.com/journals/jhe/2018/5157020/.
33. Faggella D. Machine learning healthcare applications – 2018 and beyond. TechEmergence. Retrieved from: https://www.techemergence.com/machine-learning-healthcare-applications.
34. Davenport TH, Dreyer KJ. AI will change radiology, but it won't replace radiologists. Harvard Business Review. 2018, March 27. Retrieved from: https://hbr.org/2018/03/ai-will-change-radiology-but-it-wont-replace-radiologists.
35. DeepMind Health. Helping clinicians get patients from test to treatment, faster. 2017, February 27. Retrieved from: https://deepmind.com/applied/deepmind-health/.
36. IBM. Oncology and genomics. Retrieved from: https://www.ibm.com/watson/health/oncology-and-genomics/.
37. Atomwise. Artificial Intelligence for drug discovery. Retrieved from https://www.atomwise.com.
38. Carter A, Sharma G. Artificial intelligence and the pathologist: future frenemies? PubMed. 2017;141(5):622–3. https://doi.org/10.5858/arpa.2016-0593-ED. Retrieved from: https://www.ncbi.nlm.nih.gov/pubmed/28447905.
39. Welch A. AI better than dermatologists at detecting skin cancer, study finds. CBS News. 2018, May 29. Retrieved from: https://www.cbsnews.com/news/ai-better-than-dermatologists-at-detecting-skin-cancer-study-finds/.
40. The Medical Futurist. Top artificial intelligence companies in healthcare to keep an eye on. 2017, January 31. Retrieved from: https://medicalfuturist.com/top-artificial-intelligence-companies-in-healthcare/.
41. NIH: US National Library of Medicine. What is precision medicine? 2018, July 10. Retrieved from: https://ghr.nlm.nih.gov/primer/precisionmedicine/definition.
42. NIH: National Institutes of Health. About the All of Us research program. Retrieved from: https://allofus.nih.gov/about/about-all-us-research-program.
43. The Medical Futurist. The ultimate list of what we can 3D print in medicine and healthcare! 2017, April 11. Retrieved from: https://medicalfuturist.com/3d-printing-in-medicine-and-healthcare/.
44. Durben Hirsch M. Mayo Clinic uses imaging to expand point-of-care 3D printing. 2018, March 22. Retrieved from: https://www.healthdatamanagement.com/news/mayo-clinic-expands-use-of-point-of-care-3d-printing.
45. Center for Regenerative Medicine: Mayo Clinic. Renaissance in medicine. 2017, April 6. Retrieved from: https://regenerativemedicineblog.mayoclinic.org/2017/04/06/renaissance-in-medicine/.
46. Khosla V. The next technology revolution will drive abundance and income disparity. Forbes.com. 2014, November 6. Retrieved from: https://www.forbes.com/sites/valleyvoices/2014/11/06/the-next-technology-revolution-will-drive-abundance-and-income-dis parity/#3f845d271882.

Embracing the New Transformation Through Team Approach

36

Rachel Cyrus and Kevin J. O'Leary

Teamwork Is More Important than Ever

As we continue to navigate the move into the era of value-based care, high-functioning teams have become critical to provide well-coordinated care for complex patients. Over the last two decades, we have seen a shift from payment based on volume to payment models designed to improve health outcomes and lower costs. This shift has resulted in a focus on efficiency across the continuum of care. Specific changes for the inpatient setting include a trend toward fewer patients being admitted to the hospital, shorter lengths of stay, and financial pressures to improve outcomes such as 30-day readmissions, hospital-acquired infections, and patient experience [1, 2].

These changes have escalated the complexity of hospitalized patients and their care needs. Hospitalized patients often have multiple active medical problems. Though we are fortunate to have an increasing number of new options for testing and treatment, new options require close coordination with other team members and often carry new risks for patient safety [3, 4]. Once improving, patients are typically discharged prior to full recovery to complete convalescence in a lower acuity setting, leaving only the sickest patients in the hospital. Overall, taking care of these increasingly complex patient populations in today's environment, which challenges us to provide more efficient, high-quality, cost-effective, and safe care, has highlighted the need for optimally performing healthcare teams.

R. Cyrus (✉) · K. J. O'Leary
Department of Internal Medicine, Northwestern Feinberg School of Medicine, Chicago, IL, USA
e-mail: rcyrus@nm.org

Why Is Taking a Team Approach So Critical?

A large and growing body of evidence shows a clear association between teamwork and important outcomes related to patient safety, patient experience, and professional engagement.

Patient Safety Despite recent improvements since the publication of the Institute of Medicine's *To Err is Human* report [5], we are still a long way from consistently delivering safe care to hospitalized patients [6]. A recent estimate reported the number of deaths due to medical error to be approximately 251,000 each year, making it the 3rd most common cause of death in the USA [7].

Well established as a contributor to adverse events, communication, a key part of teamwork, is tightly linked to patient safety. For example, The Joint Commission has reported communication failure as a root cause in approximately 2/3 of reported sentinel events (i.e., adverse events

R. Latifi (ed.), *The Modern Hospital*, https://doi.org/10.1007/978-3-030-01394-3_36

that result in serious injury) [8] (see Fig. 36.1). Similarly, the Department of Veterans Affairs National Center for Patient Safety Root Cause Analysis database reported that communication failures contributed to 77% of all adverse events evaluated using root cause analyses between 2010 and 2013 [9]. In a study of 70 "mishaps" reported by residents in medicine, surgery, and obstetrics and gynecology, Sutcliffe and colleagues found communication failures were a contributing factor in 91% of instances [10]. Another study of surgical errors in three hospitals attributed 43% of incidents to communication breakdown [11]. Despite undoubtedly good intentions, consistently effective communication is lacking among healthcare professionals across a range of specialties within hospitals and contributes to adverse events.

Patient Experience Outcomes related to patient experience and overall satisfaction with care have also been shown to correlate with teamwork. A retrospective cohort study of 7872 patients in an academic urban emergency department (ED) setting in the USA over 4 years showed that better perceptions of provider-provider communication among doctors, nurses, and other staff were associated with higher patient satisfaction [12]. Another cross-sectional ED study of over 1000 patients showed patients with a very positive perception of ED teamwork were more likely to be satisfied with their overall care experience [13]. In inpatient populations, a large VA study looking at staff members' perception of teamwork culture at 125 hospitals showed a significant positive relationship between hospitals with high staff perception of teamwork culture and patient satisfaction [14] (see Fig. 36.2).

Professional Engagement A marker of high-performing healthcare systems, high levels of teamwork have been associated with stronger professional engagement as well. In a study of nurses in acute care patient units, higher perceptions of teamwork correlated with higher levels of satisfaction with current position and occupation [15]. Another study of nurses in obstetrics found that hospitals which scored higher in nurses' ratings of teamwork communication had higher job commitment and satisfaction and lower unanticipated turnover [16]. Additionally, Chang et al. found that higher perceptions of collaborative relationships were a predictor of higher job satisfaction for physicians, nurses, and other healthcare professionals [17]. There may be other positive downstream effects of a teamwork approach and

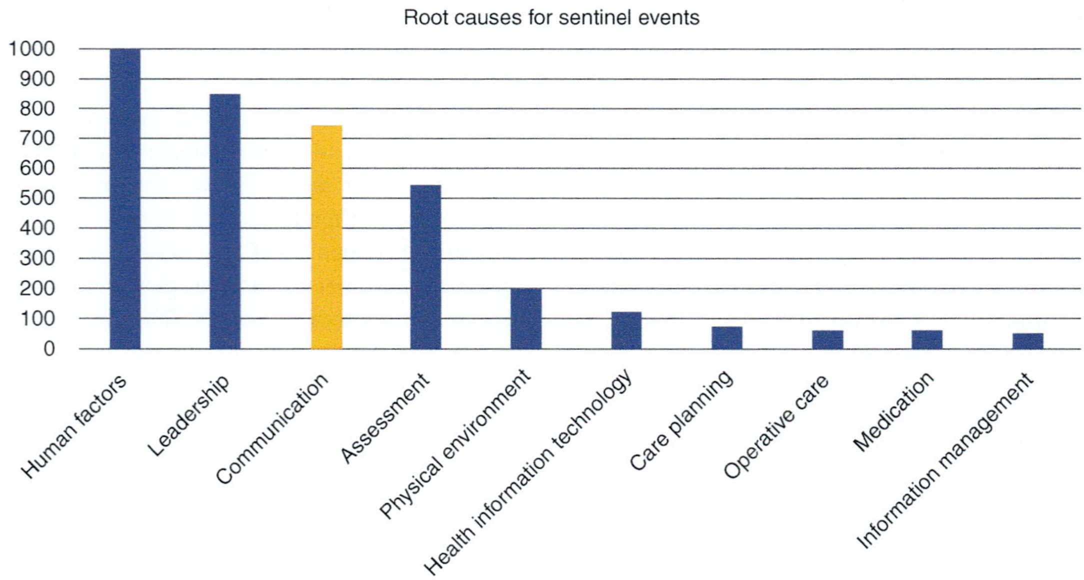

Fig. 36.1 The Joint Commission lists communication as the 3rd highest root cause of sentinel events

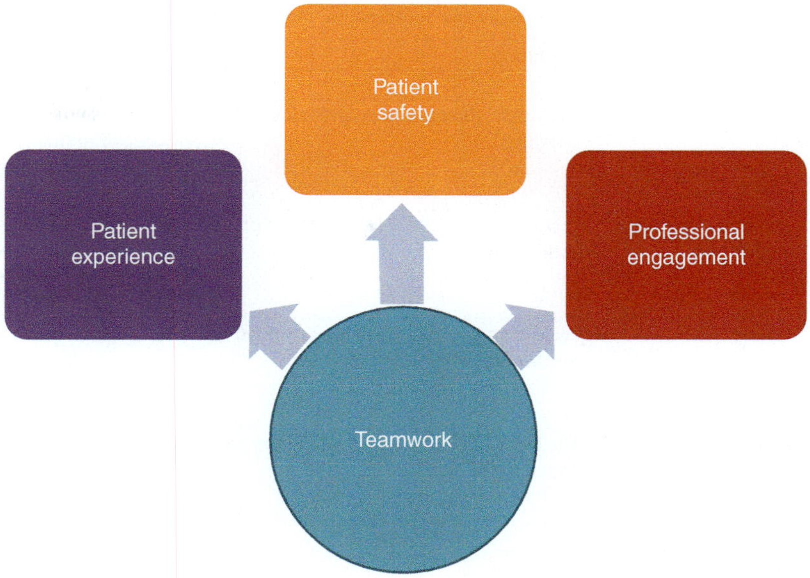

Fig. 36.2 Teamwork is a key factor in improving patient safety and experience as well as professional engagement

improved engagement, as well, with a study of 61 US hospitals finding there was a significant association between hospital culture and degree of reported quality improvement implementation. Hospitals with cultures that emphasized teamwork and a willingness to undertake some degree of risk reported a higher degree of quality improvement implementation [18].

Principles of a Team Approach

Definitions

> Team: Two or more individuals with specified roles interacting adaptively, interdependently, and dynamically toward a common and valued goal.
> Teamwork: A set of interrelated thoughts, actions, and feelings of each team member that are needed to function as a team and that combine to facilitate coordinated, adaptive performance and task objectives resulting in value-added outcomes [19].

Framework Several frameworks have been proposed to describe elements of teamwork and the relationships among those elements. After extensive study of teams across a range of industries, Salas and colleagues developed a useful framework which identifies the core components of teamwork as leadership, mutual performance modeling, backup behavior, adaptability, and team orientation (see Table 36.1). These core components are facilitated by coordinating mechanisms, namely, the development of shared mental models, achievement of mutual trust, and engagement in closed-loop communication [19]. Salas points out that merely assembling a team does not ensure that it will be successful and effective. Furthermore, teamwork differs from task work, depending not only on knowledge and skill of the team members but their ability to anticipate the needs of others, adjust to a changing environment, and have a shared understanding of how a procedure or plan should be completed [21].

Challenges to Effective Teamwork

The hospital presents unique challenges to forming effective teams, including those related to team composition, system factors, psychological factors, and education of healthcare professionals.

Team Composition Patient care teams in hospital settings are large, and team membership continuously evolves, because of the need to provide care 24 h a day, 7 days a week. Moreover, a patient's "team" may consist of several different subunits of professionals (e.g., primary service, specialist clinicians, nurses), each of which has a

Table 36.1 Teamwork components and coordinating mechanisms

Teamwork	Definition	Behavioral examples
Component		
Team leadership	The leader directs and coordinates team member activities	Facilitate team problem-solving Provide performance expectations Clarify team member roles Assist in conflict resolution
Mutual performance monitoring	Team members are able to monitor one another's performance	Identify mistakes and lapses in other team member actions Provide feedback to fellow team members to facilitate self-correction
Backup behavior	Team members anticipate and respond to one another's needs	Recognize workload distribution problems Shift work responsibilities to underutilized members
Adaptability	The team adjusts strategies based on new information	Identify cues that change has occurred and develop a plan to deal with changes Remain vigilant to change in the internal and external environment
Team orientation	Team members prioritize team goals above individual goals	Take into account alternate solutions by teammates Increased task involvement, information sharing, and participatory goal setting
Coordinating mechanism		
Shared mental model	An organizing knowledge of the task of the team and how members will interact to achieve their goal	Anticipate and predict each other's needs Identify changes in team, task, or teammates
Closed-loop communication	Acknowledgment and confirmation of information received	Follow-up with team members to ensure that the message was received Acknowledge that the message was received Clarify the information received
Mutual trust	Shared belief that team members will perform their roles	Share information Willingly admit mistakes and accept feedback

Adapted from Baker et al. [20]. With permission from Elsevier

different group of patients for which they provide care. Therefore, each patient's team looks different from all others, and each professional is a member of multiple patients' teams.

System/Organizational Challenges Hospital team members, especially physicians, often care for patients spread across many units. The dispersion of patients makes it difficult for team members to be in the same place at the same time. One consequence of this dispersion is the relatively low frequency of face-to-face communication between nurses and physicians. Studies have found that a given patient's nurse and physician report having face-to-face communication with one another only 50–60% of the time and often disagree about key elements of the plan of care [22]. That is, the low frequency of communication among team members results in a lack of a shared mental model. High workloads and stress also impede communication [19]. Brindley and colleagues found that physicians often fail to communicate during crises and when they do it is often with other physicians, rather than the team. Nurses tend to delay bringing up problems under high workloads and increased stress [23].

Technology is also not designed well to support teamwork. While pagers allow for immediate communication, the unidirectional nature of most paging systems does not allow for confirmation nor the ability of the recipient to reply or forward the message. Despite their limitations, pagers are still the most common technology used for patient care-related communication [24]. Although secure mobile messaging applications ensure security of protected health information and more functionality (i.e., ability to respond, forward, handle message differently based on designated urgency), a minority of health systems have yet to implement them [24].

Psychological Challenges Traditional hierarchies can impede effective teamwork as well. Social identity theory details how individuals identify within their own group as compared to others, creating intrinsic tension between individuals from different professional backgrounds (i.e., us vs. them mentality) [25]. Studies of critical care physician-nurse communication reveal differing attitudes about teamwork, with 33% of nurses rating the quality of collaboration as high or very high compared with 73% of physicians. Nurses noted difficulty speaking up and poor resolution of disagreements, desiring more input into decision-making and positive response for speaking up [26]. Similar results were seen in the operating room [27]. Hierarchies within disciplines (e.g., between an intern and an attending physician) can also prohibit team members from offering important information such as alternative diagnoses or anticipated problems with planned treatments [25].

Educational Challenges Education of healthcare professionals is frequently discipline-specific, with relatively few opportunities to interact with and learn alongside learners from other disciplines. The lack of interprofessional education results in decreased understanding of others' roles, responsibilities, and priorities [25]. Finally, few healthcare professionals have received specific training to improve teamwork skills [28].

Measurement of Teamwork

Measuring teamwork can be challenging. Methods of measuring teamwork can be grouped into self-assessment, peer assessment, direct observation, and surveys on teamwork climate [29].

Self-Assessment Though common and efficient, self-assessment is too weak to be helpful as individuals tend to overestimate their own performance [30].

Peer Assessment Peer assessment including 360° or multisource feedback is typically used to provide robust, formative feedback to individuals on their performance related to collaboration and communication [31]. However, peer assessment can be challenging to administer, and adequate sample sizes for each individual may be difficult to achieve.

Direct Observation The direct observation of a team allows for better assessment of team function by conducting real-time assessment using behavior-based team scoring assessment tools. Trained observers evaluate performance using checklists or behaviorally anchored rating scales (BARS), the latter which were first developed in the aviation industry and soon incorporated into other workplaces which require advanced individual and team performance [29, 32, 33]. Direct observation using a scoring system may be useful in assessing teamwork skills across a range of domains, including communication, coordination, leadership, monitoring, and cooperation. A number of instruments have been developed to assess teamwork using direct observation [34–39]. Drawbacks are that direct observation is resource intensive and may affect behavior during assessment [38, 40]. Direct observation is also not well suited to capture infrequent behaviors, and measurements are dependent upon observer skill [32]. Direct observation can be used to assess team performance during simulation exercises, and scenarios can be created to represent situations which are high risk yet occur infrequently in clinical settings. Assessments during simulation training are often formative and coupled with deliberate practice of skills [41, 42].

Surveys Survey instruments may be especially useful in settings where team members are seldom in the same place at the same time. Instruments assessing attitudes and teamwork climate are easy to administer but lack contextual information about specific behaviors and challenges [43–45].

So How Do We Optimize Teamwork?

Successful teamwork involves implementing strategies that foster and facilitate high-quality communication and interdisciplinary input. Interventions address the challenges previously described. The best approach is to use a combination of complementary interventions, tailored for the needs and goals of the specific setting (see Table 36.2).

Interventions Addressing Challenges Related to Team Composition Given that team membership is constantly evolving because of the need to provide care 24 h a day, 7 days a week, high-quality handoffs are critical. Many tools have been developed to aid in handoffs and have shown improved outcomes used in conjunction with other interventions. Tools such as IPASS (illness severity, patient summary, action items, situation awareness and contingency planning, synthesis by receiver), developed by Starmer et al. in 2012, have been shown to reduce rates of medical errors and preventable adverse events [46–48]. Assessment of handoffs, using a tool such as the handoff clinical examination exercise (CEX), can be used to provide formative feedback to improve handoff communication [33].

Interventions Addressing System/Organizational Challenges To address the dispersion of team members, some hospitals have localized physicians geographically so that a physician has all of her patients on just 1–2 units (see Fig. 36.3). Olson et al. localized internal medicine house staff and found that physicians felt a sense of greater collaboration and teamwork with nursing after localization. Nurses in the study also scored significantly higher in their perceptions of physician-nurse collaboration [49]. Another study localizing medicine hospitalists to a geographic unit resulted in improved ability of nurses and physicians to correctly identify each other by name and increased frequency of physician-nurse communication [50].

Though localization helps facilitate communication through proximity, it is not alone sufficient to ensure effective communication. One way to facilitate quality and consistency of communication is through the use of structured communication tools and checklists. These tools help ensure a shared mental model among team members. Studies in operating rooms have implemented checklists to make sure that surgeons, anesthesiologist, nurses, and other team members have an opportunity to share essential information with one another [51]. A literature review of surgical checklist use was conducted by Russ et al. and found that checklists were beneficial for operating room teamwork and communication and were associated with improved clinical outcomes. Observed mechanisms were through establishing open dialogue between interdisciplinary team members. Interestingly, nurses were shown to perceive maximum benefit [52], potentially due to having lower perceptions of teamwork and communication between physicians and nurses at baseline. Similarly, daily goals of care forms have been used in intensive care units in an effort to achieve a shared mental model among team members and have shown effectiveness in improving communication and team members' understanding of patient care goals [53–55].

Interdisciplinary rounds (IDR) have also shown to be effective in improving collaboration and teamwork. IDR consist of gathering the professionals involved in a patient's care to meet in a daily meeting. Team members attending IDR typically include the patient's nurse and physician but also may include pharmacists, social workers, case managers, physical and occupational therapists, nutritionists, respiratory care practitioners, unit nurse managers, and medical directors. When conducted at the bedside, IDR can help to inform and engage patients and family members. Similar to other settings, a checklist

Table 36.2 Interventions to optimize teamwork

Intervention	Description	Benefits	Implementation keys
Handoff tools	A standardized method of passing information between providers	Improves quality of communication Reduces adverse events	Consider combining with an evaluation tool to ensure quality of handoff
Localization of physicians	A structure in which physicians are localized to a minimal number of units, ideally 1–2	Improves physician-nurse collaboration Improves team members' efficiency	Helps increase quantity of communication and team member familiarity but does not address quality of communication
Checklists	Using a checklist to standardize communication and make sure key components are always communicated	Establishes dialogue between team members Allows for input from multiple team members Helps team members be on the same page about patient care goals Improves patient outcomes	Needs to be done in a conscientious way and needs to be updated on a routine basis to account for changes in care plan
Interdisciplinary rounds	Gathering of professionals involved in a patient's care in a daily meeting	Stronger interprofessional collaboration Improves patient and team satisfaction Reduces adverse events	Requires leadership to facilitate the conversation and ensure closed-loop communication. Requires a checklist to ensure all important aspects are covered. Participation of care team members is essential
Unit co-leadership	Nurse-physician shared responsibility for the quality delivered on a patient care unit	Facilitates interprofessional support and respect May improve patient safety outcomes	Synergy obtained through sharing a set of mutual core values, willingness to work together toward goals, and mutual respect
Teamwork training	Training aimed at improving skills and behaviors related to teamwork	Improves team performance May translate to improved patient outcomes	The effect of team work training likely depends on the duration of training and amount of practice of new skills
Interprofessional education	Combined training of students from different healthcare professions	May lead to better respect and understanding of others' roles	This may be challenging to incorporate but well worth the effort

should be used to ensure essential aspects of the patient plan and goals, quality metrics, and transitional needs are discussed. IDR has been shown in some studies to improve collaboration between nurses and physicians, improve patient and team satisfaction, and reduce adverse events [56–62] (see Table 36.3).

Interventions Addressing Psychological Challenges Hospitals can make organizational changes to address tension between different professional groups and foster a culture of better interprofessional collaboration. One such intervention is unit nurse-physician co-leadership, which is a collaborative model in which a nurse leader and physician leader share responsibility for quality on their unit [63–66]. Similar interprofessional leadership structures at all levels throughout an organization can support better relationships and respect. Though not rigorously evaluated, this interprofessional model may also improve patient outcomes and has been associated

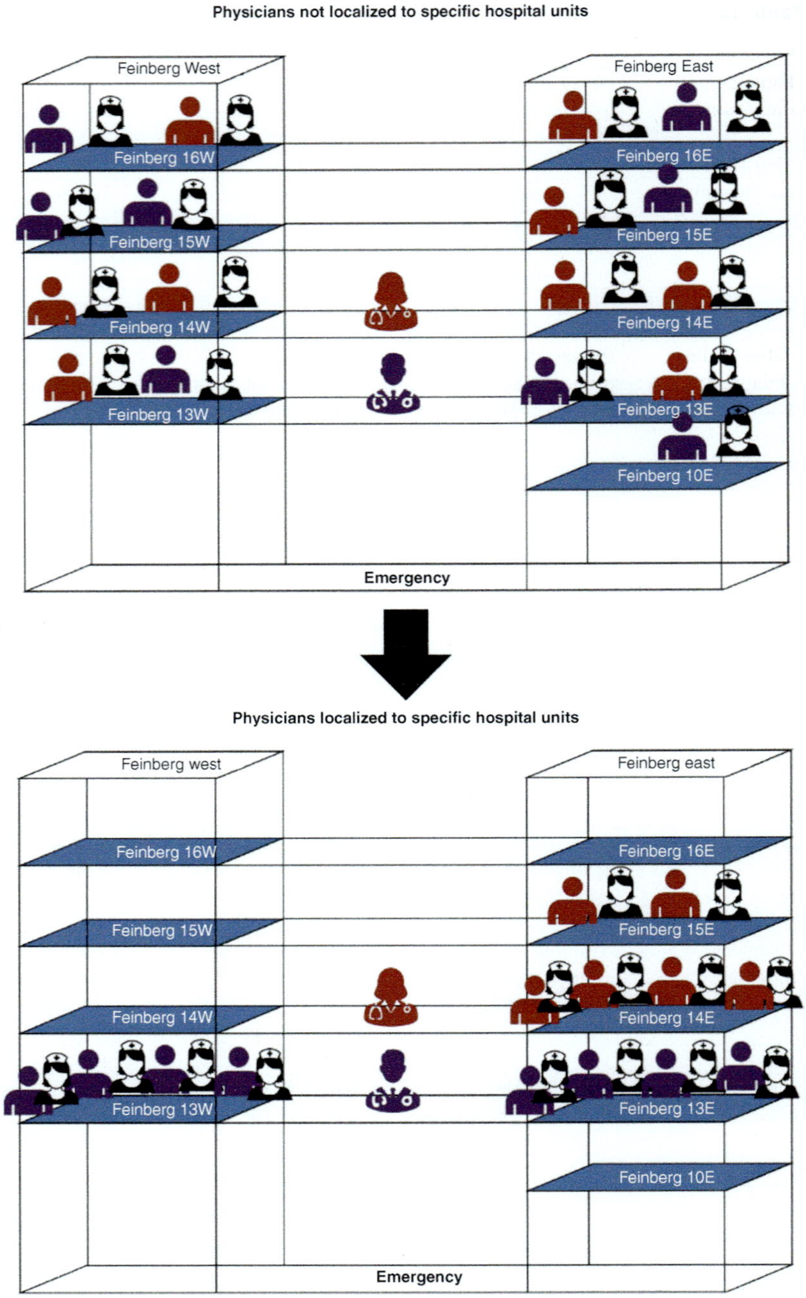

Fig. 36.3 Localizing physicians can help communication and teamwork by consolidating the professionals on a patient's care team

with reductions in central line-associated bloodstream infections, catheter-associated urinary tract infections, and pressure ulcers [67]. Key factors for successful co-leadership include common core value(s), willingness to work together toward a common vision and mission, clear and transparent communication with each other and the organization, mutual respect, and complementary leadership competencies [68].

Interventions Addressing Educational Challenges Teamwork training aims to improve behaviors and skills related to teamwork. Cockpit resource management (CRM) training in teamwork, developed from aviation, has been used in multiple clinical settings and focuses on nontechnical human factors such as group dynamics, leadership, interpersonal communication, and decision-making

Table 36.3 Example of IDR checklist. Each team member is responsible for certain items with some overlap

Category	Care team member	Items to discuss
Patient information	Physician	Room number Patient last name Primary nurse
Plan of care	Physician	Diagnosis Patient status (e.g., "doing well," "rough night") Tests/procedures today Medical milestones for patient to achieve before discharge (including consulting services, as needed) Medication – changes or issues Other items for discussion?

Patient safety and quality
Each item to be discussed ONLY if applicable to the patient
	Primary RN/CC (if primary RN unavailable)	VTE prophylaxis – *is patient on it/does patient need it*
		Central lines – *can central lines (including PICCs) be discontinued*
		Foley – *can Foley catheter be discontinued*
		Pressure ulcer risk – *does the patient have one and what can we do to reduce patient risk*
		Mobility assessment
		  Fall/injury risk
		  PT/OT needs
		Sitter – *does patient have/need one*
		Restraints – *does patient have/need them*
		Telemetry – *is patient on it/does patient need it*
		Delirium concerns
		Patient education – *what does patient need and who will do it*
		  Injection or insulin teaching
		  Wound care
		  Warfarin video
		  Inhaler teaching
		  Anything else
		Other items for discussion?

Discharge plans
Each item to be discussed ONLY if applicable to the patient
	Social worker	Readmission risk – *is patient at risk of readmission*
		Anticipated discharge date/time – *will patient be discharged by 2 pm that day or the next day*
		Discharge needs/barriers
		  Placement – *where is the patient going/what needs to be done*
		  Home health needs?
		    Oxygen
		    Other equipment
		  Transportation
		Other items for discussion?

Additional information	Pharmacist PT/OT Dietary	Medication – *changes or issues* PT/OT – *needs or issues* Dietary – *changes or issues* Are there any other questions, concerns, or issues?

CC Clinical Coordinator, *PP* Physical Therapy and *OT* occupational therapy

[69]. Using CRM principles, the Agency for Healthcare Research and Quality (AHRQ) and the Department of Defense partnered in developing the Team Strategies and Tools to Enhance Performance and Patient Safety (TeamSTEPPS®) program, which offers a number of online resources and training opportunities. TeamSTEPPS® and other CRM-based training programs have been used in multiple inpatient settings from the emergency room to surgery and medicine [70–72] and have been endorsed by The Joint Commission and the Institute for Healthcare Improvement (IHI). A recent systematic review and meta-analysis of 51 controlled studies of teamwork training found positive and significant medium-sized effects of training on teamwork and team performance [73]. Another systematic review sought to discover whether training resulted in improved teamwork in clinical settings and

improved outcomes and found evidence for both [69]. The impact of teamwork training appears to be dependent upon the duration of teamwork training and the degree of emphasis on deliberate practice of new skills (e.g., with the use of simulation-based training).

Interprofessional education is the systematic design of opportunities in which students from two or more healthcare professions learn together during all or part of their professional training. Though strong evidence for impact is not yet available, interprofessional education may help to address learners to better understand the roles and priorities of other professions and foster greater respect [74].

Assessment of Efficacy

While multiple studies have shown that the perception of teamwork improves with interventions [57, 75–77], studies vary significantly in rigor and quality of evidence, and many are qualitative in nature. Few studies evaluate how improvements in teamwork translate to improved management decisions or clinical outcomes [30, 62, 78–80]. One of the limitations is that available studies often evaluate the impact of a single intervention. In light of multiple challenges impeding teamwork in hospital settings, a more productive approach is to use complementary interventions which address the range of challenges to team performance.

Conclusion

Hospitals need to continue to strive toward providing consistently safe and patient-centered care. Achieving these goals requires coordinated teams of individuals performing at the highest levels. The hospital setting presents important challenges to teamwork, yet these challenges also represent opportunities. We recommend a combination of complementary of interventions with adaptations to fit unique clinical settings and local culture.

References

1. Kalra AD, Fisher RS, Axelrod P. Decreased length of stay and cumulative hospitalized days despite increased patient admissions and readmissions in an area of urban poverty. J Gen Intern Med. 2010;25(9):930–5.
2. American College of Physicians. Achieving a high-performance health care system with universal access: what the United States can learn from other countries. Ann Intern Med. 2008;148(1):55–75.
3. Zilberberg MD. The clinical research enterprise: time to change course? JAMA. 2011;305(6):604–5.
4. Epner PL, Gans JE, Graber ML. When diagnostic testing leads to harm: a new outcomes-based approach for laboratory medicine. BMJ Qual Saf. 2013;22(Suppl 2):ii6–ii10.
5. Institute of Medicine Committee on Quality of Health Care in A. In: Kohn LT, Corrigan JM, Donaldson MS, editors. To err is human: building a safer health system. Washington (DC): National Academies Press (US) Copyright 2000 by the National Academy of Sciences. All rights reserved; 2000.
6. Quality AfHRa. Saving lives and saving money: Hospital-Acquired Conditions Update. Rockville, MD; 2015. Available from: https://www.ahrq.gov/professionals/quality-patient-safety/pfp/interim-hacrate2014.html.
7. Makary MA, Daniel M. Medical error-the third leading cause of death in the US. BMJ. 2016;353:i2139.
8. Commission TJ. Sentinel Event Statistics Released for 2015. 2015 Available from: http://info.jcrinc.com/rs/494-MTZ-066/images/Sentinel39.pdf.
9. Sculli GL, Fore AM, Sine DM, Paull DE, Tschannen D, Aebersold M, et al. Effective followership: a standardized algorithm to resolve clinical conflicts and improve teamwork. J Healthcare Risk Manag. 2015;35(1):21–30.
10. Sutcliffe KM, Lewton E, Rosenthal MM. Communication failures: an insidious contributor to medical mishaps. Acad Med. 2004;79(2):186–94.
11. Gawande AA, Zinner MJ, Studdert DM, Brennan TA. Analysis of errors reported by surgeons at three teaching hospitals. Surgery. 2003;133(6):614–21.
12. Aaronson EL, Mort E, Sonis JD, Chang Y, White BA. Overall emergency department rating: identifying the factors that matter most to patient experience. J Healthc Qual. 2018:1.
13. Kipnis A, Rhodes KV, Burchill CN, Datner E. The relationship between patients' perceptions of team effectiveness and their care experience in the emergency department. J Emerg Med. 2013;45(5):731–8.
14. Meterko M, Mohr DC, Young GJ. Teamwork culture and patient satisfaction in hospitals. Med Care. 2004;42:492–8.
15. Kalisch BJ, Lee H, Rochman M. Nursing staff teamwork and job satisfaction. J Nurs Manag. 2010;18(8):938–47.

16. Gifford BD, Zammuto RF, Goodman EA. The relationship between hospital unit culture and nurses' quality of work life. J Healthc Manag. 2002;47(1):13–25. discussion -6.
17. Chang WY, Ma JC, Chiu HT, Lin KC, Lee PH. Job satisfaction and perceptions of quality of patient care, collaboration and teamwork in acute care hospitals. J Adv Nurs. 2009;65(9):1946–55.
18. Shortell SM, O'Brien JL, Carman JM, Foster RW, Hughes EF, Boerstler H, et al. Assessing the impact of continuous quality improvement/total quality management: concept versus implementation. Health Serv Res. 1995;30(2):377–401.
19. Salas E, Sims DE, Burke CS. Is there a “big five” in teamwork? Small Group Res. 2005;36(5):555–99.
20. Baker DP, Salas E, King H, Battles J, Barach P. The role of teamwork in the professional education of physicians: current status and assessment recommendations. Jt Comm J Qual Patient Saf. 2005;31(4):185–202.
21. Agency for Healthcare Research and Quality. Team Strategies and Tools to Enhance Performance and Patient Safety. 2017, April. Available from: https://www.ahrq.gov/teamstepps/about-teamstepps/index.html.
22. O'Leary KJ, Thompson JA, Landler MP, Kulkarni N, Haviley C, Hahn K, et al. Patterns of nurse-physician communication and agreement on the plan of care. Qual Saf Health Care. 2010;19(3):195–9.
23. Brindley PG, Reynolds SF. Improving verbal communication in critical care medicine. J Crit Care. 2011;26(2):155–9.
24. O'Leary KJ, Liebovitz DM, Wu RC, Ravi K, Knoten CA, Sun M, et al. Hospital-Based Clinicians' Use of Technology for Patient Care-Related Communication: a National Survey. J Hosp Med. 2017;12(7):530–5.
25. Weller J, Boyd M, Cumin D. Teams, tribes and patient safety: overcoming barriers to effective teamwork in healthcare. Postgrad Med J. 2014;90(1061):149–54.
26. Thomas EJ, Sexton JB, Helmreich RL. Discrepant attitudes about teamwork among critical care nurses and physicians. Crit Care Med. 2003;31(3):956–9.
27. Sexton JB, Thomas EJ, Helmreich RL. Error, stress, and teamwork in medicine and aviation: cross sectional surveys. BMJ. 2000;320(7237):745–9.
28. Medicine Io. Health professions education: a bridge to quality. Washington (DC): National Academies Press (US); 2003.
29. O'Leary KJ, Sehgal NL, Terrell G, Williams MV. Interdisciplinary teamwork in hospitals: a review and practical recommendations for improvement. J Hosp Med. 2012;7(1):48–54.
30. Marlow SL, Hughes AM, Sonesh SC, Gregory ME, Lacerenza CN, Benishek LE, et al. A systematic review of team training in health care: ten questions. Jt Comm J Qual Patient Saf. 2017;43(4):197–204.
31. Dominick PG, Reilly RR, McGourty JW. The effects of peer feedback on team member behavior. Group Organ Stud. 1997;22(4):508.
32. Klampfer B, Flin R, Helmreich RL, et al. Enhancing performance in high risk environments: recommendations for the use of behavioural markers. Swissair Training Centre, Zurich; July 5–6, 2001. Retrieved from: http://www.raes-hfg.com/reports/notechs-swiss.pdf.
33. Arora VM, Berhie S, Horwitz LI, Saathoff M, Staisiunas P, Farnan JM. Using standardized videos to validate a measure of handoff quality: the handoff mini-clinical examination exercise. J Hosp Med. 2014;9(7):441–6.
34. Fletcher G, Flin R, McGeorge P, Glavin R, Maran N, Patey R. Anaesthetists' Non-Technical Skills (ANTS): evaluation of a behavioural marker system. Br J Anaesth. 2003;90(5):580–8.
35. Frankel A, Gardner R, Maynard L, Kelly A. Using the communication and teamwork skills (CATS) assessment to measure health care team performance. Jt Comm J Qual Patient Saf. 2007;33(9):549–58.
36. Malec JF, Torsher LC, Dunn WF, Wiegmann DA, Arnold JJ, Brown DA, et al. The mayo high performance teamwork scale: reliability and validity for evaluating key crew resource management skills. Simul Healthc. 2007;2(1):4–10.
37. Sevdalis N, Davis R, Koutantji M, Undre S, Darzi A, Vincent CA. Reliability of a revised NOTECHS scale for use in surgical teams. Am J Surg. 2008;196(2):184–90.
38. Sevdalis N, Lyons M, Healey AN, Undre S, Darzi A, Vincent CA. Observational teamwork assessment for surgery: construct validation with expert versus novice raters. Ann Surg. 2009;249(6):1047–51.
39. Lineberry M, Bryan E, Brush T, Carolan TF, Holness D, Salas E, et al. Measurement and training of TeamSTEPPS dimensions using the medical team performance assessment tool. Jt Comm J Qual Patient Saf. 2013;39(2):89–95.
40. Hays RB, Davies HA, Beard JD, Caldon LJ, Farmer EA, Finucane PM, et al. Selecting performance assessment methods for experienced physicians. Med Educ. 2002;36(10):910–7.
41. Yang LY, Yang YY, Huang CC, Liang JF, Lee FY, Cheng HM, et al. Simulation-based inter-professional education to improve attitudes towards collaborative practice: a prospective comparative pilot study in a Chinese medical centre. BMJ Open. 2017;7(11):e015105.
42. Schmidt E, Goldhaber-Fiebert SN, Ho LA, McDonald KM. Simulation exercises as a patient safety strategy: a systematic review. Ann Intern Med. 2013;158(5_Part_2):426–32.
43. Sexton JB, Helmreich RL, Neilands TB, Rowan K, Vella K, Boyden J, et al. The safety attitudes questionnaire: psychometric properties, benchmarking data, and emerging research. BMC Health Serv Res. 2006;6:44.
44. Baggs JG. Development of an instrument to measure collaboration and satisfaction about care decisions. J Adv Nurs. 1994;20(1):176–82.

45. Hojat M, Fields SK, Veloski JJ, Griffiths M, Cohen MJ, Plumb JD. Psychometric properties of an attitude scale measuring physician-nurse collaboration. Eval Health Prof. 1999;22(2):208–20.
46. Starmer AJ, Sectish TC, Simon DW, Keohane C, McSweeney ME, Chung EY, et al. Rates of medical errors and preventable adverse events among hospitalized children following implementation of a resident handoff bundle. JAMA. 2013;310(21):2262–70.
47. Starmer AJ, Spector ND, Srivastava R, Allen AD, Landrigan CP, Sectish TC. I-pass, a mnemonic to standardize verbal handoffs. Pediatrics. 2012;129(2):201–4.
48. Starmer AJ, Spector ND, Srivastava R, West DC, Rosenbluth G, Allen AD, et al. Changes in medical errors after implementation of a handoff program. N Engl J Med. 2014;371(19):1803–12.
49. Olson DP, Fields BG, Windish DM. Geographic localization of housestaff inpatients improves patient-provider communication, satisfaction, and culture of safety. J Healthc Qual. 2015;37(6):363–73.
50. O'Leary KJ, Wayne DB, Landler MP, Kulkarni N, Haviley C, Hahn KJ, et al. Impact of localizing physicians to hospital units on nurse-physician communication and agreement on the plan of care. J Gen Intern Med. 2009;24(11):1223–7.
51. Haynes AB, Weiser TG, Berry WR, Lipsitz SR, Breizat AH, Dellinger EP, et al. A surgical safety checklist to reduce morbidity and mortality in a global population. N Engl J Med. 2009;360(5):491–9.
52. Russ S, Rout S, Sevdalis N, Moorthy K, Darzi A, Vincent C. Do safety checklists improve teamwork and communication in the operating room? A systematic review. Ann Surg. 2013;258(6):856–71.
53. Agarwal S, Frankel L, Tourner S, McMillan A, Sharek PJ. Improving communication in a pediatric intensive care unit using daily patient goal sheets. J Crit Care. 2008;23(2):227–35.
54. Narasimhan M, Eisen LA, Mahoney CD, Acerra FL, Rosen MJ. Improving nurse-physician communication and satisfaction in the intensive care unit with a daily goals worksheet. Am J Crit Care. 2006;15(2):217–22.
55. Pronovost P, Berenholtz S, Dorman T, Lipsett PA, Simmonds T, Haraden C. Improving communication in the ICU using daily goals. J Crit Care. 2003;18(2):71–5.
56. Gausvik C, Lautar A, Miller L, Pallerla H, Schlaudecker J. Structured nursing communication on interdisciplinary acute care teams improves perceptions of safety, efficiency, understanding of care plan and teamwork as well as job satisfaction. J Multidiscip Healthc. 2015;8:33–7.
57. Cao V, Tan LD, Horn F, Bland D, Giri P, Maken K, et al. Patient-centered structured interdisciplinary bedside rounds in the medical ICU. Crit Care Med. 2018;46(1):85–92.
58. Mudge A, Laracy S, Richter K, Denaro C. Controlled trial of multidisciplinary care teams for acutely ill medical inpatients: enhanced multidisciplinary care. Intern Med J. 2006;36(9):558–63.
59. Boyko WL Jr, Yurkowski PJ, Ivey MF, Armitstead JA, Roberts BL. Pharmacist influence on economic and morbidity outcomes in a tertiary care teaching hospital. Am J Health Syst Pharm. 1997;54(14):1591–5.
60. Curley C, McEachern JE, Speroff T. A firm trial of interdisciplinary rounds on the inpatient medical wards: an intervention designed using continuous quality improvement. Med Care. 1998;36(8 Suppl):As4–12.
61. Pannick S, Beveridge I, Wachter RM, Sevdalis N. Improving the quality and safety of care on the medical ward: a review and synthesis of the evidence base. Eur J Intern Med. 2014;25(10):874–87.
62. Bhamidipati VS, Elliott DJ, Justice EM, Belleh E, Sonnad SS, Robinson EJ. Structure and outcomes of interdisciplinary rounds in hospitalized medicine patients: a systematic review and suggested taxonomy. J Hosp Med. 2016;11(7):513–23.
63. Clark RC, Greenawald M. Nurse-physician leadership: insights into interprofessional collaboration. J Nurs Adm. 2013;43(12):653–9.
64. Kim CS, Calarco M, Jacobs T, Loik C, Rohde J, McClish D, et al. Leadership at the front line: a clinical partnership model on general care inpatient units. Am J Med Qual. 2012;27(2):106–11.
65. Kim CS, King E, Stein J, Robinson E, Salameh M, O'Leary KJ. Unit-based interprofessional leadership models in six US hospitals. J Hosp Med. 2014;9(8):545–50.
66. Rich VL, Brennan PJ, May L. Unit clinical leadership: a successful partnership between frontline clinicians, quality and senior leaders. 21st Annual National Forum on Quality Improvement in Health Care. Orlando; 2009; Found at https://pdfs.semanticscholar.org/presentation/f851/93b38c420b1969da2aac47d0d3c7290ec676.pdf.
67. Rich VL, Brennan PJ. Improvement projects led by unit-based teams of nurse, physician, and quality leaders reduce infections, lower costs, improve patient satisfaction, and nurse–physician communication. (AHRQ Health Care Innovations Exchange. Apr 14, 2010. (Updated: Jul 16, 2014.); https://innovations.ahrq.gov/profiles/improvement-projects-led-unit-based-teams-nurse-physician-and-quality-leaders-reduce.
68. Cortese DA, Smoldt RK. 5 success factors for physician-administrator partnerships: Medical Group Management Association; Available from: https://www.mgma.com/practice-resources/mgma-connection-plus/online-only/2015/september/5-success-factors-for-physician-administrator-partnerships.
69. Zeltser MV, Nash DB. Approaching the evidence basis for aviation-derived teamwork training in medicine. Am J Med Qual. 2010;25(1):13–23.
70. Morey JC, Simon R, Jay GD, Wears RL, Salisbury M, Dukes KA, et al. Error reduction and performance improvement in the emergency department through formal teamwork training: evaluation results of the MedTeams project. Health Serv Res. 2002;37(6):1553–81.

71. Hansen KS, Uggen PE, Brattebo G, Wisborg T. Training operating room teams in damage control surgery for trauma: a followup study of the Norwegian model. J Am Coll Surg. 2007;205(5):712–6.
72. Rudy SJ, Polomano R, Murray WB, Henry J, Marine R. Team management training using crisis resource management results in perceived benefits by healthcare workers. J Contin Educ Nurs. 2007;38(5):219–26.
73. McEwan D, Ruissen GR, Eys MA, Zumbo BD, Beauchamp MR. The effectiveness of teamwork training on teamwork behaviors and team performance: a systematic review and meta-analysis of controlled interventions. PLoS One. 2017;12(1):e0169604.
74. Reeves S, Perrier L, Goldman J, Freeth D, Zwarenstein M. Interprofessional education: effects on professional practice and healthcare outcomes (update). The Cochrane database of systematic reviews. 2013(3):Cd002213.
75. Kuy S, Romero RAL. Improving staff perception of a safety climate with crew resource management training. J Surg Res. 2017;213:177–83.
76. Buljac-Samardzic M, Dekker-van Doorn CM, van Wijngaarden JD, van Wijk KP. Interventions to improve team effectiveness: a systematic review. Health policy (Amsterdam, Netherlands). 2010;94(3):183–95.
77. Hughes KM, Benenson RS, Krichten AE, Clancy KD, Ryan JP, Hammond C. A crew resource management program tailored to trauma resuscitation improves team behavior and communication. J Am Coll Surg. 2014;219(3):545–51.
78. Lemieux-Charles L, McGuire WL. What do we know about health care team effectiveness? A review of the literature. Med Care Res Rev. 2006;63(3):263–300.
79. Manser T. Teamwork and patient safety in dynamic domains of healthcare: a review of the literature. Acta Anaesthesiol Scand. 2009;53(2):143–51.
80. Weaver SJ, Lyons R, DiazGranados D, Rosen MA, Salas E, Oglesby J, et al. The anatomy of health care team training and the state of practice: a critical review. Acad Med. 2010;85(11):1746–60.

37 Patient-Centered Care: Making the Modern Hospital Truly Modern

Olga Golubnitschaja and Russell J. Andrews

Medicine has evolved from ideologically guided treatments administered by shamans to evidence-based interventions directed by (hopefully well-informed) healthcare professionals. The hospital – the point where the most advanced and invasive treatments typically occur – must similarly evolve. In this chapter we consider some themes guiding the evolution of the modern hospital in the twenty-first century.

Economics Dictates that Healthcare Cannot Remain Reactive

In 2010, under the rubric "Intelligent Investing," *Forbes* published an article by Hilary Kramer entitled "Diabetes Is Killing Our Economy" [1]. Diabetes may be the best example of the urgent necessity for the paradigm shift from the current reactive medical services to the more cost-effective – not to mention more ethical – approach of predictive, preventive, and personalized medicine as the cornerstone for the modern hospital [2].

The diabetes epidemic is a snowballing threat to public health, healthcare systems, and the economy – due to the cascade of pathologies triggered in a long-term manner after diabetes become manifest. The total diabetes-related cost in the United States, including medical expenses and lost productivity, was about US $300 billion in 2010 [3]. If the current reactive approach to diabetes care is allowed to persist, the annual diabetes-related cost is estimated to increase to over US $510 billion by 2025 [3]. Similarly, it is estimated that by 2040, the annual diabetes-related cost in the United States will be over US $770 billion. Worldwide by 2040, it is estimated there will be 650 million diabetic patients and an annual diabetes-related cost of US $8.5 trillion [2].

Similar economic alarms are raised by the rapidly increasing numbers of patients diagnosed with cardiovascular disease, cancer, and neurological/neurodegenerative disorders [4]. Breast cancer, for example, has about 2 million new cases and 500,000 disease-related deaths annually [5]. Glaucoma – the second leading cause of blindness after diabetic retinopathy – affects about 70 million people worldwide [6]. If the currently practiced paradigm of reactive medical services persists, the implosion of healthcare systems predicted by economic experts will become a global reality.

O. Golubnitschaja (✉)
Radiological Clinic, Rheinische Friedrich-Wilhelms-Universität Bonn, Bonn, Germany

Breast Cancer Research Centre, Rheinische Friedrich-Wilhelms-Universität Bonn, Bonn, Germany

Centre for Integrated Oncology, Cologne-Bonn, Rheinische Friedrich-Wilhelms-Universität Bonn, Bonn, Germany

European Association for Predictive, Preventive and Personalised Medicine, EPMA, Brussels, Belgium
e-mail: olga.golubnitschaja@ukbonn.de

R. J. Andrews
Department of Nanotechnology & Smart System, NASA Ames Research Centre, Moffett Field, CA, USA

R. Latifi (ed.), *The Modern Hospital*, https://doi.org/10.1007/978-3-030-01394-3_37

PPPM: The Paradigm for the Modern Hospital

An optimistic scenario of the modern hospital is based on implementation of the innovative medical concepts of predictive, preventive, and personalized medicine (PPPM) (see Fig. 37.1) [7].

The new paradigm clearly discriminates between "disease care" and "healthcare." PPPM dramatically impacts both the ethical and economical aspects of medical services, affording both improved quality of life and cost-effective medicine. Predictive diagnostics are followed by targeted preventive measures triggered well in time; individualized treatment algorithms are tailored to the person, not "one size fits all." PPPM is a holistic approach comprised of preventive, curative, and rehabilitative medical care. Multidimensional interactions of internal and external risk factors are clearly recognized: genetic background, age, gender, environmental risk factors, lifestyle, culture and beliefs, as well as social status. The overall predisposition of individuals to specific diseases, the disease development, the natural course of the disease, and its response to therapeutic intervention all are incorporated into individualized patient profiling [7].

Furthermore, the individual plays an active role in the entire healthcare process: enhanced understanding of health versus illness and emphasized personalization of all medical services. The result is strong patient empowerment and the essential responsibility of every person for healthcare, at individual and community levels. Consequently, PPPM goes hand in hand with innovative educational programs provided to both the population and professional groups [7].

PPPM implementation into daily practice involves strategic and technological development of innovative medical fields: multilevel diagnostics instead of fragmented medical examinations, risk assessment by predictive technologies identifying an individual predisposition before clinical manifestation of pathologies, information/communication technology-based devices for

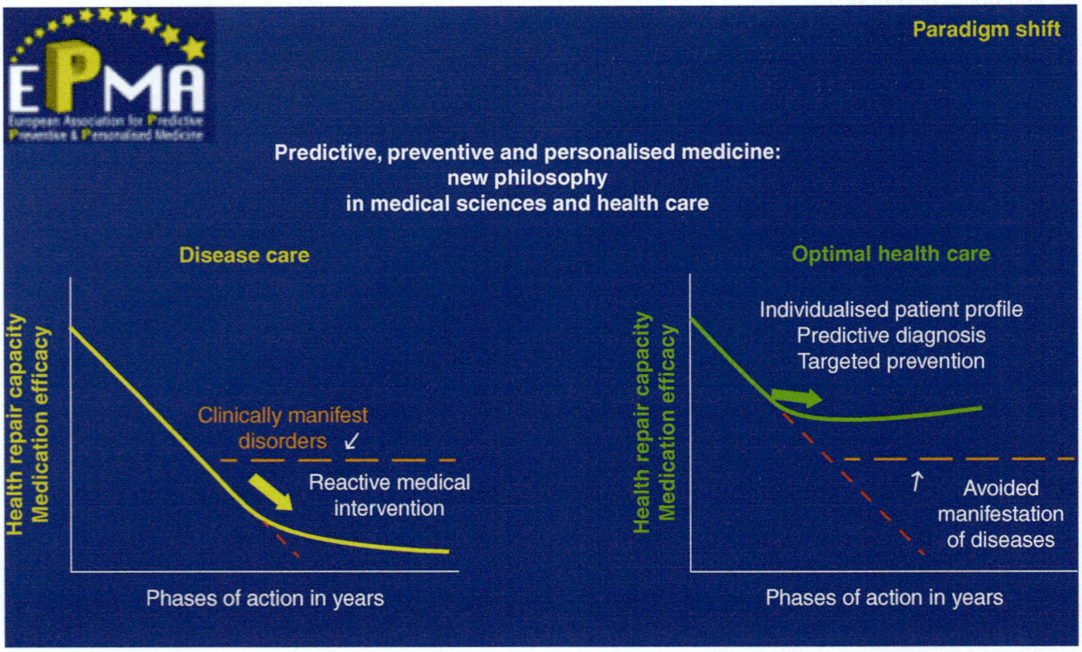

Fig. 37.1 PPPM implementation is based on the paradigm shift from delayed services to innovative medical approaches by individualized patient profiling, predictive diagnostics, and targeted preventive measures and treatments tailored to the individual (Reprinted from Golubnitschaja et al. [7]. With permission from Creative Commons License 4.0: https://creativecommons.org/licenses/by/4.0/)

telemedical services provided to chronically diseased people [7, 8] etc.

Setup of the "modern hospital" is, on the one hand, a process of healthcare transformation thoroughly designed for the long-term and, on the other hand, daily efforts in performing clinically relevant biomedical research and applying new programs focused on stratified patients. Examples include individuals in suboptimal health condition such as those affected by "Flammer syndrome" [9–12] as well as subpopulations needing much more investment into primary healthcare than is currently practiced (first of all-children, adolescents, and young adults) [13].

Below we provide clear examples for both emerging research branches and innovative screening programs.

Emerging Research Branches

- INTERNATIONAL BIOBANKING for long-term retrospective analyses in combating widespread, epidemic diseases – both communicable and noncommunicable. For this, well-organized global professional collaborations are essential.
- MULTIOMICS utilize all the collective advantages of biomedical knowledge and demonstrate a potential to advance medical services to the level of multilevel diagnostics.
- BIG DATA as an approach supports a comprehensive patient data analysis – data analysis that is essential for the prediction, prevention, and treatment of multifactorial diseases.
- MACHINE LEARNING maximizes the efficacy of the learning process, enabling ever-evolving disease modeling, innovative predictive screening approaches, and optimized treatment algorithms.

Innovative Screening Programs

Premenopausal breast cancer (PMBC) – with its notoriously poor prognosis – is an excellent example of the urgent necessity to incorporate innovative e-screening programs in the modern hospital [14].

Perhaps the best example to demonstrate an urgent necessity of innovative screening programs as the essential part of the overall concepts of a modern hospital is an increasing incidence of premenopausal breast cancer (PMBC) with poor outcomes, which we are currently fully unskilled to screen for in the population [15]. The situation is especially dramatic for specific subtypes such as triple-negative breast cancer – more than 50% of patients die within 6 months of being diagnosed with metastatic disease [16]. Equally dramatic is the increasing incidence of pregnancy-associated breast cancer (PABC): from 1:10,000 of all pregnancies in 2000 to 1:3000 presently [15]. In some populations, the incidence of PABC reaches 20% of all breast cancer patients [17]. For PABC there are presently no population screen programs, no generally accepted risk factors, no standardized diagnostic approaches, and no targeted preventive measures [15]. Given the devastating consequences of PABC to the affected women, their babies, their families, and the society at large, it is difficult to imagine a modern hospital without innovative programs targeting adolescent and young women, in order to reduce the burden of PMBC in general and PABC in particular.

What Are the Appropriate Steps to Create Such Innovative Programs?

- RELIABLE BIOMARKER PANELS – both pathology- and stage-specific – are essential to identify persons at high risk for targeted prevention by working on modifiable risk factors. Additionally, patients who already manifest a disorder can avoid a cascade of secondary pathologies and/or unnecessary therapies – clearly a cost-effective and ethically desirable approach.
- INDIVIDUALIZED PATIENT PROFILING is a powerful instrument to estimate an individual's risks and to create treatment algorithms tailored to that individual.
- MULTI-PROFESSIONAL EXPERTISE (medical doctors, technologists, educators, administrators) is essential to design cost-effective and treatment-effective programs.

- REGULATIONS by policy-makers are needed to motivate the stakeholders (in the healthcare, diagnostic, and pharmaceutical industries, as well as the general population) to implement the programs successfully.

Organizational Factors to Implement PPPM

From the discussion above, it is clear that healthcare in the modern hospital must evolve from "reactive" to "proactive" – to care that is predictive, preventive, and personalized to the individual member of society. Some themes that underpin the change in organizational structure of the modern hospital are now considered.

Several themes guide the modern medicine and the modern hospital:

- Proactive rather than reactive care (preventive rather than therapeutic interventions).
- Patient-specific rather than system-general interventions.
- Patients as partners in their healthcare rather than subjects of the healthcare system.
- Hospital management as innovative "big picture" leaders rather than administrators focused on short-term financial gain (dynamic rather than static leadership).
- Information technology to enable continuous updating and integrating
- Using technologies such as the cloud and fuzzy logic to optimize the benefit from "big data."
- Humanitarian healthcare is likely to be the most cost-effective healthcare in the long run.

What makes for an evolutionary – perhaps at times even revolutionary – modern hospital? Clues can be found in various studies, including the Lancet Commission on Education of Health Professionals for the 21st Century: A Global Independent Commission [18]. That study describes three types of healthcare management:

1. Experts – who impart a knowledge base (information or skills), usually identified by their academic qualifications and training. In surgery, for example, this is the technically gifted senior surgeon/instructor.
2. Professionals – who in addition to knowledge impart a value system; they can be considered those experts who by example give medicine its humanitarian and ethical aspect. In surgery, this is the mentor who imparts the ability for the in-training surgeon "to know when not to cut."
3. Leaders – who by their example impart transformation both in the healthcare system and in those being trained. In surgery, the neurosurgeon Harvey Cushing comes to mind. Not only did he contribute advances in surgical technique, but he also had mortality rates for craniotomy that were decades ahead of his time. He created the anesthetic record – having the anesthesiologist monitor the patient's pulse and blood pressure during surgery – to predict when retraction of the brain must be discontinued to avoid catastrophic infarction. Cushing nurtured collaboration with William Bovie, a young biophysics professor at Harvard, who developed what eventually became an essential surgical technique for hemostasis – electrocautery. The mutual respect between Cushing and Bovie is obvious: Cushing, "I shall hope to see you over here often [in the Operating Room]…I only wish you were here so that we could tap your ventricles and get some of your ideas more often." Bovie: "[I was] watching operations on the one hand and studying electrical currents on the other… [thus I] managed to learn a little bit of both ends of the problem" [19, 20].

The description by Swain and colleagues [19] of the three "ingredients" at Brigham and Women's Hospital (part of the Harvard Medical Center System in Boston) that fostered surgical innovation over the past century is instructive for the modern hospital:

1. "Multidisciplinary collaboration among surgical innovators and individuals outside of surgery who offered complementary skills and expertise"

2. "A rich institutional environment that sustained a diverse complement of innovators working in close proximity"
3. "Department Chairmen who facilitated the work of innovators and promoted their contributions, rather than seeking personal prestige or financial gain"

One might substitute "managerial innovators" and "individuals outside of management" for "surgical" and "surgery" in (1) and "hospital leadership" for "Department Chairmen" in (3) to describe what is required for the modern hospital to be transformative rather than constraining.

Another point raised in the previous paragraph is the concept of medicine guided by "personal prestige or financial gain." These are short-term notions or perceived personal benefits – not long-term investments in the health of the community as a whole. Even studies where financial benefit of the healthcare provider is tied to healthcare outcome measures ("pay for performance") show only modest if any benefit in low- and middle-income countries (LMICs) [21]. The difference between healthcare as a for-profit industry and healthcare as a for-society benefit is captured in the difference between healthcare "administration" and healthcare "management." Administrators enforce a system of rules; managers optimize the resources available. Administrating characterizes the structure of healthcare delivery in the United States; managing characterizes the structure of healthcare delivery in most other developed countries (where universal nonprofit healthcare is the norm) [22]. The difference in cost of healthcare delivery and the quality of the healthcare outcomes (e.g., life expectancy, infant mortality) between, for example, the United States and the United Kingdom, is quite striking – the United States spends 50% more per capita than the United Kingdom, but with shorter life expectancy and higher infant mortality.

Information technology (IT) is essential for the modern hospital. Obvious applications are electronic healthcare records (EHRs) and telemedicine. Clinicians recognize immediately an EHR developed without input from clinicians at every step – and rebel at the wasted time resulting from counterintuitive IT. Less obvious but equally important is input from the clinical side on all aspects of healthcare IT [23]:

> While nonclinical personnel can successfully implement and maintain technical systems, innovation and adaptation of such systems in a way that results in meaningful improvement in care requires a strong partnership between dedicated clinical… leadership and technical support personnel. Information systems cannot simply be viewed as a technical support activity.

These authors argue that IT must have a clinician as the "systems architect." In turn, the clinician/systems architect must engage IT professionals to create an integrated IT team. This echoes the three conditions noted above at Brigham and Women's Hospital that have been necessary for continuously innovative leadership.

Thanks to the "computer revolution" and "Internet connectivity," the challenge now is not data collection but rather data analysis. How to separate the wheat from the chaff? Medical data are often messy and not easily compartmentalized. Techniques such as fuzzy logic allow such data to be combined, compared, and analyzed in meaningful ways.

Another challenge is data extensibility, i.e., the ability to share and compare data from different laboratories or clinical settings [24]. The goal is a universally web-viewable laboratory shared across medical researchers (basic and clinical). Kiar and colleagues have described the components of such a platform, which they call "science in the cloud" (SIC – Latin for "thus was it written") [24]. The key aspects are cloud-based (universal access) data storage and open-source code/software. Such a system allows for continuous updating and modification – qualities essential for the modern hospital. Not only medical research IT but also hospital infrastructure and function IT needs to be continuously evolving and integrating across clinical "islands," hospital (and hospital system) "islands," and – eventually – national healthcare delivery system "islands."

The digital age may bring universality to healthcare data and progress. However, it also raises the specter of a new form of pandemic – a "digital Ebola virus." Breaches of digital information – from credit bureau and bank records to government agencies and healthcare files – are increasingly commonplace. Perhaps the most blatant breach of medical data occurred on May 12, 2017, when computer hackers violated the UK National Health Service (NHS) computer system with the ransomware worm "WannaCry" [25]. In the authors' terms, the NHS went into "electronic lockdown." Unfortunately, the health of a country's citizens does not go into lockdown in lockstep with an electronic virus. Indeed, it is conceivable that an "evil empire" – be it a group of rogue actors or a rogue state – could unleash both an electronic and an organic virus on a society simultaneously. The lethality of the organic virus (or, perhaps more likely, a chemical agent) would be all the more widespread with the paralysis of a healthcare system (including emergency response) dependent on "0's" and "1's" in a numberless (i.e., computerless) environment. Clarke and Youngstein argue for funding to keep the NHS IT a step ahead of the "bad guys."

With global mobility, global trade, and global medical/environmental issues (e.g., HIV, Ebola, pollution, and contamination) gaining importance at logarithmic acceleration, a universal "IT in the cloud" is imperative for the modern hospital. The modern hospital may be embarking on a cloud-based electronic medical arms race. Let us hope – in that "cloudy day" – the healthcare professionals of the modern hospital follow Shakespeare's inspiration [26]:

> And as the sun breaks through the darkest clouds,
> So honor peereth in the meanest habit.

References

1. Kramer H. Diabetes is killing our economy. Forbes.com. 13 Jan 2010. http://www.forbes.com/2010/01/13/kramer-obesity-nutrition-intelligent-investing-diabetes.html.
2. Duarte AA, Mohsin S, Golubnitschaja O. Diabetes care in figures: current pitfalls and future scenario. EPMA J. 2018;9(2):125–31. https://doi.org/10.1007/s13167-018-0133-y.
3. Institute for Alternative Futures. United States' diabetes crisis: today and future trends. Diabetes 2025 Forecasts; 2011. www.altfutures.org/diabetes2025.
4. Golubnitschaja O, Costigliola V, EPMA. General report & recommendations in predictive, preventive and personalised medicine 2012: white paper of the European association for predictive, preventive and personalised medicine. EPMA J. 2012;3(1):14. https://doi.org/10.1186/1878-5085-3-14.
5. Golubnitschaja O, Debald M, Yeghiazaryan K, Kuhn W, Pešta M, Costigliola V, Grech G. Breast cancer epidemic in the early 21st century: evaluation of risk factors, cumulative questionnaires and recommendations for preventive measures. Tumor Biol. 2016;37(10):12941–57. https://doi.org/10.1007/s13277-016-5168-x.
6. Golubnitschaja O. The key role of multiomics in the predictive, preventive and personalised medical approach towards Glaucoma management. Klin Monatsbl Augenheilkd. 2018;235(2):146–50. https://doi.org/10.1055/s-0044-101164.
7. Golubnitschaja O, Baban B, Boniolo G, Wang W, Bubnov R, Kapalla M, Krapfenbauer K, Mozaffari M, Costigliola V. Medicine in the early twenty-first century: paradigm and anticipation – EPMA position paper 2016. EPMA J. 2016;7:23. https://doi.org/10.1186/s13167-016-0072-4.
8. Brunner-La Rocca HP, Fleischhacker L, Golubnitschaja O, Heemskerk F, Helms T, Hoedemakers T, Allianses SH, Jaarsma T, Kinkorova J, Ramaekers J, Ruff P, Schnur I, Vanoli E, Verdu J, Zippel-Schultz B. Challenges in personalised management of chronic diseases-heart failure as prominent example to advance the care process. EPMA J. 2016;7:2. https://doi.org/10.1186/s13167-016-0051-9.
9. Konieczka K, Ritch R, Traverso CE, Kim DM, Kook MS, Gallino A, Golubnitschaja O, Erb C, Reitsamer HA, Kida T, Kurysheva N, Yao K. Flammer syndrome. EPMA J. 2014;5(1):11. https://doi.org/10.1186/1878-5085-5-11.
10. Avishai E, Yeghiazaryan K, Golubnitschaja O. Impaired wound healing: facts and hypotheses for multi-professional considerations in predictive, preventive and personalised medicine. EPMA J. 2017;8(1):23–33. https://doi.org/10.1007/s13167-017-0081-y.
11. Golubnitschaja O. Feeling cold and other underestimated symptoms in breast cancer: anecdotes or individual profiles for advanced patient stratification? EPMA J. 2017;8(1):17–22. https://doi.org/10.1007/s13167-017-0086-6.
12. Golubnitschaja O, Flammer J. Individualised patient profile: clinical utility of Flammer syndrome phenotype and general lessons for predictive, preventive and personalised medicine. EPMA J. 2018;9(1):15–20. https://doi.org/10.1007/s13167-018-0127-9.
13. Golubnitschaja O, Stolzenburg-Veeser L, Avishai E, Costigliola V. Wound healing quality: patient stratification, prediction, prevention and personalisation of treatment algorithms as the proof-of-principle model for advanced medical services. In: Latifi R, editor. The modern hospital: patients centered, disease

based, research oriented, technology driven. Springer Dordrecht Heidelberg: New York London; 2018.
14. Fröhlich H, Patjoshi S, Kuhn W, Golubnitschaja O. Premenopausal breast cancer: potential clinical utility of the multi-omic based machine learning approach for patient stratification. EPMA J. 2018;9(2). https://doi.org/10.1007/s13167-018-0131-0.
15. Polivka J Jr, Altun I, Golubnitschaja O. Pregnancy associated breast cancer: the risky status quo and new concepts of predictive medicine. EPMA J. 2018;9(1):1–13. https://doi.org/10.1007/s13167-018-0129-7.
16. Vaz-Luis I, Lin NU, Keating NL, Barry WT, Winer EP, Freedman RA. Factors associated with early mortality among patients with de novo metastatic breast cancer: a population-based study. Oncologist. 2017; https://doi.org/10.1634/theoncologist.2016-0369.
17. Hou N, Ogundiran T, Ojengbede O, Morhason-Bello I, Zheng Y, Fackenthal J, et al. Risk factors for pregnancy-associated breast cancer: a report from the Nigerian Breast Cancer Study. Ann Epidemiol. 2013;23(9):551–7. https://doi.org/10.1016/j.annepidem.2013.06.008.
18. Frenk J, Chen L, Bhutta ZA, et al. Health professionals for a new century: transforming education to strengthen health systems in an interdependent world. Lancet. 2010;376:1923–58.
19. Swain JD, Sharma G, Rumma RT, Fisichella PM, Whang E. A century of innovation at a Boston Hospital. J Laparoendosc Adv Surg Tech A. 2017;27:156–61.
20. Voorhees JR, Cohen-Gadol AA, Laws ER, et al. Battling blood loss in neurosurgery: Harvey Cushing's embrace of electrosurgery. J Neurosurg. 2005;45:990–1001.
21. Blacklock C, MacPepple E, Kunutsor S, Witter S. Paying for performance to improve the delivery and uptake of family planning in low and middle income countries: a systematic review. Stud Fam Plan. 2016;47:309–24.
22. Andrews RJ, Crisp N. The healthcare landscape: are doctors agents of change or impediments to change? World Neurosurg. 2017;105:997–1000.
23. Towbin A, Perry LA, Larson DB. Improving efficiency in the radiology department. Pediatr Radiol. 2017;47:783–92.
24. Kiar GK, Gorgolewski KJ, Kleissas D, et al. Science in the Cloud (SIC): a use case in MRI connectomics. Giga Science. 2017;6:1–10.
25. Clarke R, Youngstein T. Cyberattack on Britain's National Health Service – a wake-up call for modern medicine. N Engl J Med. 2017;377:409–11.
26. Shakespeare W. The Taming of the Shrew IV, iii, 173; 1594.

The Architecture of New Hospitals: Complex yet Simple and Beautiful

38

Collin L. Beers

Introduction

Each of us has a personal description of beauty, an ideology that combines elements resulting in something satisfying, that resonates and leaves us feeling fortunate for experiencing the sight or sound or experience of passing through. Rather than analyze what would only be a scant handful of projects, let us follow a train of thought that moves us from an understanding of why hospitals are so complex and what can be done to simplify the experience of working in, visiting, or needing a hospital for care. Can the result be beautiful? The answer should be yes, and more and more often we find it is.

The complexity of the modern hospital has crept up on us emerging slowly as community hospitals became regional institutions and healthcare networks and systems – as a result the hospital as a building type physically, conceptually, and organizationally grew. Once complexity creeps in, it takes persistence to push it back out. Complexity cannot be merely covered over – it needs to be addressed head-on through resolution and intervention.

It should certainly be expected that any book approaching the topic of the modern hospital would dwell on the physical aspects of the facilities that embody tertiary inpatient healthcare delivery. While hospitals are fundamentally complex operational and physical entities, there is an ever-present goal for architects to wrap that inherent complexity with a simple and beautiful outward expression.

As an architect, it is tempting to reflect on the evolution of the hospital as a building type culminating in the recent examples we see around us today and to anoint one or another as an exemplar for setting the standards of best practice to be modeled by others. While many fine examples exist and can be found in every country, it should be cautioned that any of these facilities having opened recently was necessarily [due to documentation schedule and construction durations] designed approximately 4–5 years ago based on prevailing information and the trends at that time. With that understanding, rather than reflect on the most recent examples and their evident features, it is much more beneficial to consider the trajectory of change and to envision what can be anticipated as future built configurations for hospitals – arguably the most complicated building type that the public regularly experiences as a visitor, patient, or employee/clinician practitioner.

Rather than incremental and iterative, the current pace of change in the healthcare industry itself and, therefore, in the facilities we call hospitals, has been accelerating. There has never been a greater transformation of the hospital facility paradigm than has been seen over the

C. L. Beers (✉)
Stantec Architecture, Philadelphia, PA, USA
e-mail: Collin.beers@stantec.com

R. Latifi (ed.), *The Modern Hospital*, https://doi.org/10.1007/978-3-030-01394-3_38

recent 20 years. This is true around the globe and will be equally true in less than 20 years from now as the momentum only quickens. The evolution of knowledge regarding disease, genetics, infection transmission and prevention, intervention alternatives, and the application/adoption of emerging technology, precision tools [robotics], and the "Internet of things" [IoT] has been exponential. The buildings that house the conglomeration of services available in today's healthcare delivery systems have been no less transformed and evolved with that infusion of knowledge and influencers.

The word evolution is also quite appropriate in describing hospitals. The facilities we encounter today had their genesis beginning years ago followed by a succession of encrusting additions and expansions, both horizontal and vertical, making most hospitals we may encounter today literal "complexes". Considering the progression of facility responses moving forward when the opportunity presents itself for starting with a clean slate we arrive at the "greenfield" hospital. These are the places where "complex yet simple and beautiful" have the best chance for expressions not constrained by the generative influence of encrustation around core aging assets. Unlike a pearl, smoothed to a beautiful luster in layers around an irritant, hospital facilities crafted around encapsulating an historic iconic "original" facility are often encumbered by the constraints of the previous generations and limited in their potential to evolve.

Opportunities for projects that can be characterized as "greenfield" are fortunately still occurring. There is a trend for replacement of aging facilities and a fresh proliferation of new hospitals being built to support the migration of population densities to new communities or to fill gaps in emerging hospital network development. Also, it would be best to consider the dialogue referring to these as examples of "whole" facility solutions rather than the forms and organization of major additions to existing facilities. While many additions embody partial expressions of formative ideas, a comprehensive stand-alone facility can evolve as a form without the constraints of attachment to existing systems, structures, and baked-in inefficiencies.

Of course, any specific discussion of architecture needs to address the context, culture, and climate to define parameters of built form and constructability. The term architecture in a more abstract sense can be useful in describing the characteristics of building components and the interconnections that become form, mass, and visual expression.

Hospitals, by virtue of their reflection of strategic purpose and community needs, range in size from the smallest critical access hospitals most often found in rural settings where distance to a significant facility is excessive, through modest community hospitals, to larger specialty facilities, culminating in the largest configuration, a unified academic medical center layering education on top of the highest levels of care for the acutely ill.

While many of the design principles described on the following pages could naturally be applied to various healthcare spaces such as ambulatory care centers, medical office buildings, or wellness centers, the thoughts articulated most accurately reflect the challenges and opportunities for true inpatient hospitals.

Building Blocks

Conceptually, a hospital consists of four broad clusters of places:

- Places for respite, observation, and restoration [healing] – the bed units
- Places for surgery, procedures, and imaging – diagnostic and intervents
- Places for materials, food preperation, equipment storage, repairs, and storing provisions – ancillary support
- A place for management, education, financial accountability, and organization – administration

These clusters are often formed by one or more departments of similar components and drive horizontal and vertical placement in an overarching organizational configuration that supports ideal adjacency needs. Often these are characterized by short physical distances for "walking" connectivity of staff and patient journey experiences reflecting care pathways traveled from admission to discharge. Many new hospital configurations make strong and successful efforts to enable lean efficiency to be realized in staff work patterns by creating fluid departmental boundaries that support flexibility of space allocation and the development of "care platforms" or "service lines" that bridge departmental definitions.

The modern hospital has an archetypal form that has evolved over generations of selective evolutionary variations [mutations]. Looking to the four main clusters of space, [the hotel, the factory, the warehouse, and the office], these often result in massing outcomes that resemble a wedding cake. Big layers of building at the base form a platform that usually contains all the elements of outpatient access at ground level as well as emergency services and heavy departments that like to sit on solid ground [e.g., MRI]. Smaller layers sit on top or side by side for the floors of inpatient bed units and for administrative space that can be a bit more distant from the nucleus of the facility infrastructure and vertical circulation nodes. Variations of this shape have become the prototype.

Complexity: Moving Toward Simplicity

In addition to size adding complexity to the built forms of modern hospitals, the technology and tools supporting delivery of modern healthcare and the interactions and interventions with patients are becoming increasingly complex. The pace of change among these aspects is accelerating. In the past, imaging equipment would be replaced once every 10 years due mainly to wear from repetitive use. In today's radiology suite, it is not unusual to see major equipment replacements happening on a 5-year cycle due to vendor's device redesigns delivering significant decreases in image acquisition time, enabling increased utilization and rapid delivery of diagnostic support, and the advancements in image resolution and precision. The need to anticipate smooth removal and replacement of large, fixed, sensitive equipment in an 24/7 operational building has required architects to develop ingenious solutions that enable change. A few of the gymnastics employed include removable building exterior panels and structurally reinforced pathways from delivery points for trucks and cranes to the imaging suite with width and height clearances.

This pace of inevitable change is leading architects to propose that instead of a building needing to be a specific complicated "thing," the building should rather be the "vehicle" for the thing. Adopting that perspective, the hospital building should become increasingly more simple, with a flexible framework that focuses not on the elements that require the most specificity for integrating devices but on the most human elements that can support the fragile state of illness and supportive caregiving. A way to think of this would be to envision that any given piece of artwork can be extremely complex and intricate, while the gallery where it is housed should be generous and supportive with a neutral background.

Since the 1960s, architects for healthcare have taken extreme pride in our ability to adapt modern built forms that accept emerging technology and result in precision-crafted bespoke spaces and facilities – bespoke not to support a person or a condition but for a *thing*! The current shift of perspective strives to reposition the patient as the central focus is helping to restore hospital design to being first about the people that inhabit these buildings. A machine is just a machine. It plugs in, as an invention it has become a constantly dynamic element, and it is not a static basis of design. Technology potentially takes us even farther from the point of human interaction, and our truest goal should be to support human interaction and allow for that to happen in places that are much more humane than are actually designed in many hospitals today – a return to simplicity. This mind-set follows a well-known axiom, thought to be coined by Louis Sullivan, that "form follows function," which was taught in every architectural class from the first year of college. Unfortunately, in healthcare the focus on function was misinterpreted to be referring to the complex tools not the function of the healing arts practiced by compassionate people for the benefit of people. Buildings became more mechanistic following the expression of the devices held within.

The other quote often repeated is from Winston Churchill – "We shape our buildings, thereafter they shape us." It reminds us that most elements of buildings are quite immutable, and although they may have been conceived to support a specific function and flow, they often become the obstacles to an evolving work practice pattern leading to frustration for progress. Interestingly, the quote above is only a fragment of a larger speech Churchill was giving following the bombing of the House of Commons and it reads:

> On the night of May 10, 1941, with one of the last bombs of the last serious raid, our House of Commons was destroyed by the violence of the enemy, and we have now to consider whether we should build it up again, and how, and when. *We shape our buildings*, and afterwards our buildings shape us. Having dwelt and served for more than forty years in the late Chamber, and having derived very great pleasure and advantage therefrom, I, naturally, should like to see it restored in all essentials to its old form, convenience and dignity. – October 18, 1943

Revealing in this quote is a striking attitude that there are those who, if given a fresh start, would "like to see it restored in all essentials to its old form, convenience and dignity." So often, given the opportunity to start fresh, we find architects following their user groups to the same conclusion – building a new version of the old facility to replicate the same work flow and create the same pattern for users and patients, unimproved apart from fresh construction materials and techniques. When we have a blank slate before us, we should use the idealized operational pathways as guidelines and detach from the physical spaces in which those operations are currently practiced, so we can discover opportunities to have the building become shaped by the "new us," exploring the freedoms in configuration that can become infused with lean future state pathways and enabling technology to facilitate new configurations and innovative physical embodiments.

In the new modern hospital, we see the ability to transition from an organization of bespoke spaces focused on functionality and adaptation to specific equipment requirements to one fostering a loose assemblage of activities that seamlessly and synergistically interface, through which patients and staff move toward health improvement and ultimately a return to home.

Simplicity

Simple. Not encumbered with extraneous or superfluous. That is a logical goal for buildings where the construction cost is a premium compared to a majority of other building types. Maintaining an attitude of responsible use of space is the balancing act of modern healthcare designers – creating a sense of place and an experience without using the traditional means associated with civic buildings where grandeur and volume are the indicators of significance and vitality of purpose.

Simple. Clear and direct without distractions – understandable. This is another goal for a facility where visitors are often mind-fogged with the concerns of pain or failing health or sudden situations demanding resolution. This aspect is most often associated with wayfinding or the ability to navigate the facility with visual cues and the potential lack of guidance or succinct signage. Often the placement of public circulation and elevators are driven by the opportunity to use views to the outside to aid instinctive navigation and a natural sense of orientation by associating interior building locations with persistent views to the landscape, other buildings, or site features in urban areas. Consistent location of elements of visitor users of a building, like public washrooms or information desks or vertical circulation [elevators, public stairs] and feature amenities of resource centers, lounges, waiting areas, cafés, etc., become the landmarks to anxiety-free navigation in a strange landscape.

Simple. Repetition promotes comprehension. It is an easily understood element that is repeatable and, therefore, comprehended with increasingly less exploration or explanation. For the staff in a hospital the predominant application of typical rooms becomes a strategy for design. Typical patient rooms, exam rooms, operating rooms, recovery positions, nursing/team stations, utility rooms, medication rooms, supply rooms, etc., are all examples of spaces that have become the willing targets for standardization and simplification. Internal configuration and appointments along with placement on a floor plan are the hallmarks of rigorous application of this strategy. It employs purposeful replication as an enabling effort to provide intuitive usability and limit the need for caregivers to "hunt" for items of patient care or another aspect of their duties.

Simple. Modularity and application of mass production. The modern hospital evolving from a greenfield opportunity is potentially a candidate for introduction of elements of construction technique applied to every other industry – mass production. There are many modern examples of taking a specific element of a hospital facility, like the patient's bedroom and washroom or the headwall of the patient's unit which houses all the essential complicated elements of piping for medical gases, power outlets, data jacks, monitor mounting brackets, lighting, nurse call, bed control, etc., and finding an approach to build these elements in a controlled factory environment for consistency. This approach is beneficial when quantity thresholds are attained, when the speed of construction is a priority driver, or when environmental control of the construction site [weather, labor force skills, etc.] is unfavorable.

Simple. Unadorned. In a hospital setting, there are overarching concerns beyond aesthetics to simplify the details of construction. Infection prevention is of utmost importance as the rampant examples of hospital-acquired disease or infection have emerged as the secondary epidemic to the initial causes of patient admission. Maintaining an environment of care that is easily cleaned and naturally constructed to limit dirt, deterioration, and heavy wear from continuous use challenges architects to layer the visual, acoustic, and textural appeal of hospitality facility role models onto the spaces where bleach and heavy moving equipment and urgency of movement are stressing the nature of fine attention to detail and craft.

Simple. Easily Comprehendible. As buildings of a single purpose are often wont to do, they become iconic physical objects in and of themselves. Can a person reasonably understand the purpose of the built form of a hospital and intuit on arrival the location of the main entry, the emergency department entry, the ambulatory destinations from the more serious inpatient spaces, etc.? Today we find that there is an opportunity to craft buildings as an aggregate of components that speak to the individual driving functionality of the program of spaces. The patient tower can become of a proportion and scale that evoke the efficiency of a hospitality building type – a hotel, a high-rise apartment building, etc. The ancillary support spaces can reflect the utility of a warehouse. The administrative areas become a reflection of an office building, and the diagnostic and interventional spaces can follow the design parameters of high-performance, infrastructure-intensive research and production facilities for high-technology industries. We are growing accustomed to these structures and the expressions proffered by modern design solutions. As you encounter buildings for the first time, it is becoming easier, following repeated exposure, to infer their purpose based upon similar encounters and recognition of the occupancies associated with materiality, proportion, and fenestration.

Simple. Generic elements become acuity adaptable - servicing both stable and emergent acute needs. We often see this aspect of simplicity expressed in the application of a design attitude of "universal rooms," whereby patient bedrooms are designed following a prototypical set of spaces each appointed with a consistent set of supportive infrastructure such as monitors, medical gases, electric outlets, space clearances, lighting, etc., thereby enabling the use of these rooms to support a wider range of patient needs and acuities. A predominant patient type with a similar acuity, medical fragility, or disease can be accommodated in the same room environment as another population with significantly better or worse disease status and progression. These universal rooms are set to accommodate the highest level of care but can also easily support a patient with significantly less physical distress. Changes in acuity are accommodated by modulating the equipment brought to support the patient and by the level of technical training of the staff in attendance on the unit. This approach is often challenged by the requirement to include the elements of the most critical use imagined, while most likely only being deployed at a less than critical daily use profile. There is debate that by designing spaces to follow the same dimension and proportions, there could be easy reconfiguration to support a shift in predominant use over time that represents a less costly first expense that preserves the option to incrementally supplement the base support elements bringing the acuity profile to higher levels in the future. This strategy allows for the most significant components of construction to remain constant while pushing the premium cost elements to later dates when true needs are more persistently observable and thus demonstrated for feasible capital allocations.

Divisions and Departments Soften and Dissolve into Service Lines

With physical proximity and face-to-face encounters to facilitate the sharing of information and collaboration on proposed actions, diagnosis, or courses of treatment available, departments were the preferred configuration for technically complex work to be performed with mutual support, relevant education and training, and technician familiarity with the specifics of complex equipment.

Traditional departmental siloes are being successfully eroded as the elements and tools of specialization are becoming increasingly pervasive and omnipresent as essential. Imaging is among the first from the technologic palette to seep into emergency departments and cardiology, catheterization, interventional, and surgical environments. The development of the "interventional platform" places imaging, interventional cardiology [cath], interventional radiology/angiography, and surgery in a horizontally continuous environment blending the tools with flexible uses. With the opportunity of co-location of all the specialties that utilize anesthesia and invasive procedures, these discrete elements, which formerly belonged to the siloed departments of imaging, cardiology, and perioperative services become a new cohesive conglomerate, sharing the physical attributes of restricted access, sterility for infection prevention, high levels of purified air supply and exhaust with a narrow range of temperature and humidity, support from anesthesiologists for sedation, and a "scrubbed-in" sterile field for the practitioners. The adoption of the concept bringing these elements into a common platform has been a fundamental shift away from siloes and the firm hierarchical patterns of subspecialties to a more modern, simple, and beautiful assemblage of spaces for the benefit of patient safety and clinical efficiency with vital support of anesthesiology as a locus of multifaceted practitioners.

Imaging as a department is also moving away from the traditional isolated cluster of fixed modalities to move more pervasively into any patient care area where imaging is frequently employed in determination of the progression of cure or to confirm patient stability. There is increased availability of smaller mobile devices that can go to the patient location versus the patient moving to and from the fixed devices. We even see the continued movement of imaging modalities [CT scanners and MRI units] inside the surgical suite, including the operating room itself, as image-guided interventions are increasingly commonplace. For the benefit of the patient and care team, pathways are evolving from engaging a series of destinations away from the bedroom to something more linear and colocated forming "service platforms" where all aspects of an avenue of care can be encountered in a more fluid manner with the patient in the center of the value stream.

Another strategy to achieve simplicity in modern hospital architecture is to eliminate the perception of complexity by moving it into the background. Complexity is out of sight. You may be familiar with the implication of "The Internet of things [IoT]." It is the reality that individual elements of technology are all undergoing the transition to allow them to interface seamlessly with each other without setups or arduous interventions. Cell phones connect via Bluetooth to car audio and navigation systems, ear buds pair to smartphones, and ventilators pair with CT scanners to pause inhalation when acquiring lung images. Well the last example is perhaps some years away; however, the notion that devices will share information to facilitate ease of use and automate actions will become increasingly prevalent. The complex will become simple by being unseen or directly encountered.

Simplicity in Automation

The more aspects of the daily activities that occur within the hospital that can be automated will simplify the logistics and limit background activity buzz and hum. Some of us have cars with temperature control that is based on setting the desired temperature and hitting a button that says "auto." After that we don't think about how fast the fan is blowing or whether the air needs heating or cooling to achieve the preferred stasis. Buildings are also getting into this with BAS [building automation systems] with sensors and programming to automate elements of heating and cooling, putting window shades up on the dark side of the building and shades down on the sunny side, and sun tracking sensors that cycle which rooms are programmed for cooling moving around the floorplan in total passive automatic response to keep the hospital temperature setting on "auto." The next generation of this concept is taking a complex environmental challenge and disguising the complexity as a "simple" response – self-darkening building glazing. These are windows that darken automatically to limit the amount of direct light penetrating the building which in turn generates heat which may or may not be valued depending on the season, climate, and occupant's desires for comfort. The next step is the linking of building automation system sensors to track an individual user [e.g., anesthesiologist or pharmacist] by the use of an RTLS [real-time location system] badge that can automatically adjust the room settings of their work environment to suit their predefined preferences. Light levels and temperature are attributes that can easily be controlled at a room by room level by occupants today, but the interoperability of automatic preference tracking will simplify the need for the user to actively facilitate their ideal environmental conditions as they move from area to area of the building.

The expansion of the use of RFID [radio-frequency identification] and RTLS [real-time location systems] will unlock traditional needs for a visual connection between object, equipment, patients, and staff colleagues when challenged with facility scale and magnitude to know "where" people and things are at any given moment. The true unlocking of common aggregate waiting areas to ensure medical assistants know where to look for the next patient or to find the lone ultrasound unit in a building of multiple levels and hundreds of patient encounter locations will be transformative to the design of future facilities. This technology essentially allows the building to be "aware" of your presence, location, movement, purpose [ID tied to itinerary of appointments and locations], destinations, time constraints, and authority [security to enter, exit, access] and even articulate and augment record keeping for medically significant events [unmanned] into a unique patient medical record for documentation and confirmation. One space and adjacency impact of RTLS is the ability to leverage this technology to break down the traditional "waiting room" into a system where the patient/family can chose to go anywhere in the facility and still be "found" and assisted to interface with staff when appointments are imminent.

With the prevalence of technology layered into every conceivable location creating instant connections between people and information, the necessity for direct physical proximity is eroding. It is no surprise that with access to images, data, voice, and live-streaming video, the emergence of tele-present applications is unfolding in the modern hospital setting. Access to colleagues, patient history, lab results, diagnostic images, voice recordings of consultations and oral patient history, and exhaustive data are banked in the "cloud"; the needs for side-by-side or face-to-face encounters can be diminished for many activities.

We see an increasing use of tug-enabled delivery or autonomous robots to supplant the footsteps and effort required to receive and distribute materials, equipment, meals, trash, medications, etc., well beyond the pneumatic tube which paved the way to enabling remote locations to rapidly shuttle small objects through interstitial spaces from point to point.

Onstage, offstage. The adoption of the language of theater and performance arts emerged in the healthcare design vocabulary with a realization that the complexities and messiness of many aspects of healthcare delivery could be hidden from casual observation of patients and families thus heightening their sense of calm and order, evoking the parallel expectations of hospitality destinations. To create this simplified patient/family experience often required a great deal of complexity in developing alternative support circulation routes to parallel the public pathways. Service elevators distinct from public elevators. Double-sided rooms that had a patient entry from one side and staff entry from another – meeting in the middle. Today a formative dialogue among design professionals and clinical users evolves around the ongoing desire or need to continue the illusion that the public/patient should not engage or visualize the inner workings of the complex healthcare delivery mechanisms animating the constituent functions of ancillary activities. A new attitude of increased transparency is emerging that celebrates the visibility of the care team to benefit the patient's experience, to witness the power of the team dynamic in support of their health improvement decisions and network of interrelated knowledge experts, and to ensure the patient is engaged at a human level beyond their disease, condition, or focused challenge.

Beautiful

Finally, we must address the claim that the modern hospital can be the blend of complexity and simplicity but, most significantly be a building type that engenders beauty. Beauty is in many ways the description of the perfect unity of form and function draped in an outward visible veil of culturally contextual materiality, color, pattern, and embellishment. Today we have come to anticipate that high-technology buildings [a category that includes hospitals] are best wrapped in sleek, precision-crafted glass and metal to exemplify those qualities anticipated in the practice of medicine.

More than a simple palette of building materials that have become associated with hospitals, we must consider the impact of regionality or cultural predisposition on form and scale [civic or residential], adornment [vernacular building materials, climate, and ornament], and customer expectations [read patient experience and expectations for caregiver participation].

Often, beauty can be defined as the resultant outcome of simplicity, but it is clear that aspects of personal preference influence our receptiveness to various artistic compositions which make a narrow absolute definition of beauty impossible to conceive with reliability.

Beauty can be evident in the underlying "bones" of a facility – the rigorous application of visible structural elements and the rhythm created, the repeatability. Successful integration with the landscape and surrounding context like other buildings and natural features like views, landscape, topography, etc. create a refinement of planning and contextual sensitivity that speaks of beauty. Beauty can also be discovered in the ingenuity of the structural system – heroics to judiciously use long spans and infrequent column placement to craft floorplates with freedom from fixed obstructions; this is most beneficial in designing for interoperative platforms [described earlier] to enable ultimate reconfiguration for a future that is tentative or unimagined in support of new procedures with space-hungry equipment [e.g, neurosurgical operating rooms with sliding MRI technology to enable image-guided surgery].

Beauty can also be readily visible in the outward "skin" of the facility – its facade. The surface materiality is visible at upper levels and tangible at lower levels. Healthcare facilities have long prized durable monumental materials to exemplify their stoic longevity and iconic presence in the community. Bricks from the past generations have been surpassed by floating terracotta panels or metal and resin composites. Granite and other noble materials are most often associated with buildings of civic importance. The goal is to produce a sense of stability and durability and in some cases evoke the monument or museum. Key attributes are also emulating the character of hospitality/hotel and high technology to demonstrate vision and embrace of the new, sleek, and glossy glass or metal to raise the notion of cleanliness and precision.

A hospital, like any civic building, should be comfortable in the architectural fabric of the community it serves. Architects use the term vernacular. The building materials, forms, and patterns should resonate with the predominant materials of the region and evoke and reflect the values of the residents in a geographic region. It should be familiar and commonplace while simultaneously speaking of a larger purpose and physical order of magnitude. Hospitals are often the largest contiguous buildings in a city or town, with exceptions of high-rise corporate towers or industrial manufacturing plants and warehouses. These large buildings set the civic vocabulary and make a dramatic impact among the town fabric.

The building sits in the landscape, and many of the most beautiful building expressions we find are those that meld seamlessly the inside and outside to become a harmonious composition of enclosed and exposed. Vital to health and healing is the beneficial exposure of the ill to the natural climate, light, vegetation, and views to stimulate cognitive participation in the healing process. The debate regarding living plants inside health facilities and the potential for exposure of fragile patients to contaminants, microbes, spores, etc., is ongoing. A beautiful solution often employed to mitigate these concerns is the use of the solarium, orangeries, greenhouses, etc., where patients can visually access these spaces from alongside or above overlooking. Family and staff and more stable patients can physically enter the green spaces. All patient rooms require outside windows for daylight and views; however, not all staff spaces have the same mandate, and this should be the next challenge we overcome as hospital designers.

In addition to outward visible beauty, we should explore the inner beauty potential for healthcare buildings. As was noted at the outset, we need to cease focusing our design efforts predominantly on the aspects of the bespoke needs of the technology and reclaim our obligation to design for the human condition that is supported within the walls. One step toward this compassion is the ongoing acceptance of the needs of the family/friend caregiver that fills the space between the patient and the physician as well as the space between the hospital [dependent and unstable] and the home life [independent and stable].

The embrace of "care partners" is a second patient focus for staff/physicians. The patient is not the only customer in the hospital. We have encouraged, rightly, for the patient to enjoin whomever they can in sharing responsibility for care both while in the hospital and most especially when they return to home. The family and designated care partners become secondary customers that have expectations and draw attention from the clinicians and core care team, their phones need charging, food is desired, they inquire if there is a place to nap or talk to the physician about concerns of genetic predispositions and their own health prognosis, etc. The modern hospital will continue to be challenged by the layers of customer expectations and finding the balance of satisfying each.

Substantive Innovations

The challenge is to design brick-and-mortar facilities that need a level of changeability to endure the ebb and flow of technologic advancement and breakthrough treatment options that radically modify the type, size, and quantity of spaces that support patient care today. Take as one small example the potential future impact of the development of oral medications to replace infusions for delivery of chemotherapeutic agents in the battle with cancer. What currently takes an environment of patient recliners and IV poles and 3–4 h per patient per treatment over days and weeks requiring space to achieve utilization and accommodation of the volumes may soon be extraneous as a pill or liquid medication that can be self-administered by the patient in their own home for convenience. Disruptive innovations will continue to influence the transition from complex and space needy to simple and lean.

Next

If we agree to some extent that complexity was born of hospitals getting bigger, then perhaps our search for simplicity is best first pursued by looking at hospitals that have chosen to get smaller – enter the age of micro-hospitals. A topic of ongoing debate is the rationale for health system organizations to move away from facilities that aggregate hundreds of beds in one super-center and focus instead on facilities that have a bed count in the low teens! While the scale of a facility and the composition of services offered will be a direct reflection of the strategic goals and community needs, it is a frequent occurrence that facilities are often modest in scale with a vision for growth or repeatability to support evolution and shifting population needs. These smaller facilities are helping to fill a much-needed gap between the scale and location of traditional community hospitals and specialty/teaching hospitals. Holding a smaller total compilation of clinical components, these facilities have an inherently more compact configuration and an approachable scale more easily comprehensible to the community.

Challenge

If you are involved in the medical profession in any capacity, are a healthcare architect or designer, or become part of a process to undertake work in existing or future hospital development, look around you and see the spaces and layers of infrastructure and the considerations that went into crafting those environments. Discover their failings or places where old drivers have been erased or replaced by new concerns or adaptations. Look for the complexity that still exists and that cannot be easily masked or moved into the "offstage" areas behind the scenes. Look for the simplicity of detail, of pathways and logistics, of access to information and supplies and interaction/interface, and of repeatable elements giving cues to intentional simplification in support of future flexibility. Look for beauty in the connectivity of the hospital to its community and of the physical facility to its contextual vernacular architecture and the landscape or site, be it urban or rural and evocative of the climate, cultures, and expectations, and in the aesthetic features that resonate with personal preferences or the ability to augment the experience with choice or adaptability of color, pattern, vibrancy, etc.

Patient's Perception is the New Reality: The Intersection of Multiple Stakeholders and Their Experience and Perception of Your Organization, and Why It Matters

39

Kara Bennorth and Jake Poore

Introduction

Growing up in a large family in the 1970s, our colleague didn't get to go out to a nice restaurant very often, but when he did, he remembers his mother was always on a mission to find the very best place for her money. Mom would pile seven kids into the Ford station wagon and drive from one restaurant to another. Many times, Mom put the car in park, left the car running, and told the kids to stay in the car while she checked the place out, only to emerge a few minutes later where one of two things would happen. Either she would drive to the next restaurant or, much to the kids' hungry relief, she would tell them to hop out of the car and go in and find a seat. Our colleague always wondered what she was doing—how did Mom decide the winners from the losers in restaurants? Was she looking at the menu selection? Checking the prices? The room décor? Years later, as an adult, our colleague kiddingly asked Mom one day what she was doing when they went out to eat. She said since the wait staff wouldn't let her into the kitchen, she took it upon herself to check out the restrooms. In her mind, if the restrooms were clean, that meant the restaurant was a good choice for her family. But if they were dirty? Forget it. It didn't matter how good the food may have been or how lovely the restaurant may have been decorated—if the restrooms were dirty and unkept, there was no way she was going to let her family eat there. Because dirty restrooms meant dirty kitchens. Dirty kitchens meant dirty food. Dirty food meant sick kids and sick kids meant a wasted weekly paycheck and a day off of work. To Mom, perception was reality.

This cliché is often said, but rarely understood by most caregivers seeing patients, and yet it has become one of the key drivers that separate the winners from losers in healthcare today. Patients' perceptions are shaped by many factors including television, social media, advertising, word of mouth from family and friends, and, of course, their own personal experiences. And with the advent of government-mandated national patient satisfaction surveys like HCAHPS (Hospital Consumer Assessment of Healthcare Providers and Systems), patients' perceptions are being captured and linked to hospital financial reimbursement. Simply put, a patient's perception is healthcare's new reality.

Hospital. To patients, what images does the word conjure up? Nurses in pressed uniforms and caps? Bustling emergency rooms? Bland food? Odd smells? Sounds of beeping and whirling machines? Life-saving teamwork in action? Grouchy attendants? Kind volunteers? Saying final goodbyes? Welcoming in new life? Not surprisingly, they are all true…and not.

K. Bennorth (✉)
Department of Administration, WMCHealth, Valhalla, NY, USA
e-mail: kara.bennorth@wmchealth.org

J. Poore
Integrated Loyalty Systems, Orlando, FL, USA

R. Latifi (ed.), *The Modern Hospital*, https://doi.org/10.1007/978-3-030-01394-3_39

So, what do your stakeholders think about your hospital? And does it really matter when their perceptions are the new reality?

A hundred or so years ago, most people never even saw the inside of a hospital. In fact, Jimmy Carter was the first US president born in a hospital. Hospitals were for the poor, the infirm, the abandoned, and the insane. Many hospitals were founded by religious orders as part of their mission and later by governments as part of theirs. Many private hospitals were initially organized by groups of doctors. As science and technology advanced and more and more progressive clinical care became available, hospitals became the vessels of and necessary controlled environments for this work, and inpatient care became more popular and eventually the mainstay of the US healthcare system.

Along the way, the growing popular medium of television portrayed doctors and nurses (*Marcus Welby, M.D.*, *House*) and emergency responders (*Emergency, Chicago Fire*) as glorified heroic figures and later serialized storylines (*ER, Grey's Anatomy*).

So, our perception of hospitals is a mixture of fiction and reality, our own experiences or what we've heard from someone else (advertising, social media posts, blogs, celebrity endorsements, or doctors who are celebrities), or reviewing hospital ratings and rankings from sources as varied as the federal government to national and local magazines to Yelp. Even how we define high quality differs (Fig. 39.1).

Even though hospitals in the United States have continued to modernize clinically over the past 200 years, they have not modernized culturally. Culture is defined as a system of shared assumptions, values, and beliefs, which governs how people behave and dictates how they dress, act, and perform their jobs. Yet, we continue to mandate that patients and their families adapt to our culture, our dress, and our processes and learn our hospital language as a "quid pro quo" to get the care they need, when they need it. Think about

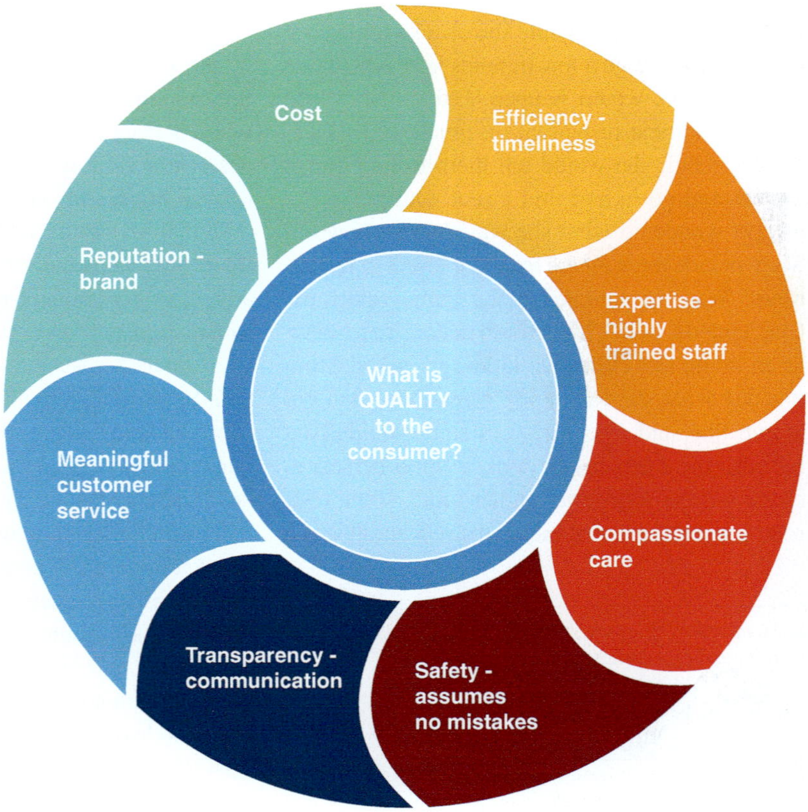

Fig. 39.1 What is quality to the consumer. (Courtesy of WMCHealth)

it, patients can only wear what we give them (and they still hate "the Johnny" gown), and we act as if the room they are assigned is not their room, it's ours. We leave the door open, and we don't always knock to enter. They eat when we tell them to eat and what we give them to eat. They are not allowed to use the toilet until we are able to get there and help them. Worst of all, we are still confusing them and their family with all the healthcare lingo, jargon, and acronyms (Fig. 39.2).

From the very first impression in the hospital emergency room, we confuse the patient by telling them, "We'll need to ***triage*** you first." Triage is an old word and patients still don't know what it means! Watch the elderly woman's face when the surgeon on evening rounds says, "Okay Mrs. Jones, I like what I see here. I think tomorrow we're going to want to ***discharge***." To an elderly woman, who has not been in the hospital in decades, the word *discharge* is personal, private, and feminine; it does not mean go home.

It is perception, then, where culture meets the patient.

Why This Matters

Improving the patient experience is more than just the right thing to do. It's just good business. The perception of your organization, true or not, deserved or not, among your patients, their families, your workforce, and the community at large, is important. How people think and feel about your organization, your brand (the picture they have painted in their minds), leads them in one of two directions: either toward or away from your organization, with their feet, their voice, or their pocketbook. Creating affinity and even loyalty to an organization is good business and directly related to volume and financial performance. But in healthcare, it is an incredibly complicated soup of people, processes, outcomes, ratings and rankings, customer service, and the experience that people have across thousands of employees and interactions.

Patients and referring physicians have many choices. So why would patients, referring physicians, and even prospective new employees

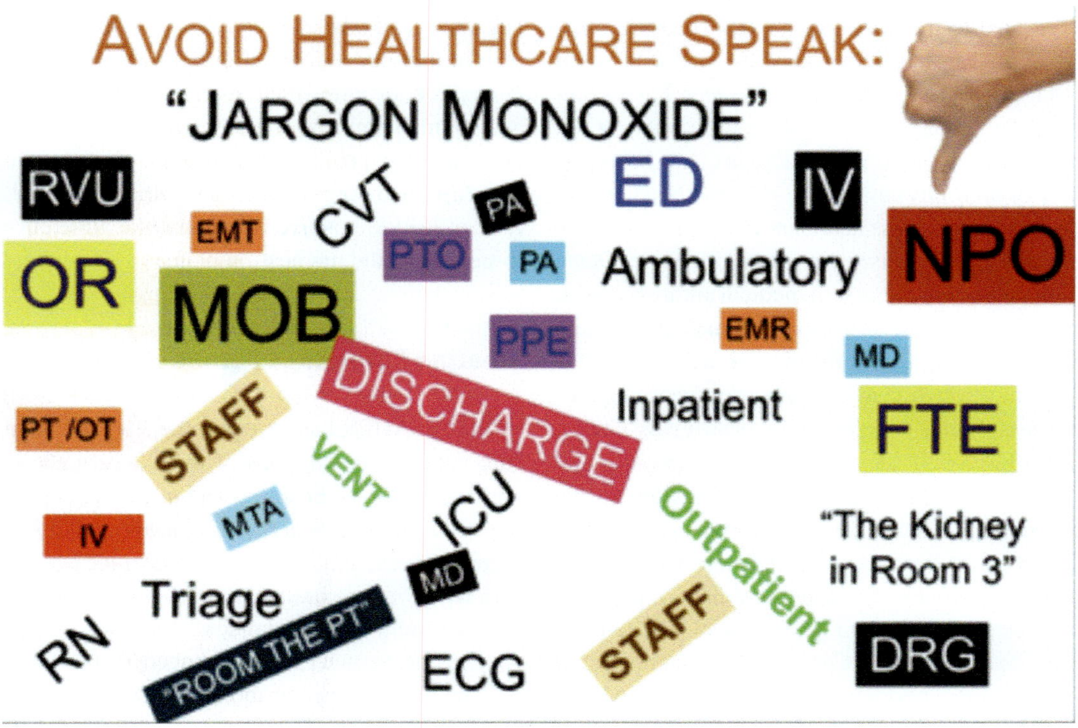

Fig. 39.2 Healthcare speak. (Courtesy of Integrated Loyalty Systems)

choose you and your organization as a place to work or as a place to be cared for? And, more importantly, after experiencing your organization and care for the first time—whether as a patient, referring physician, or new employee—why would they come back and give you their loyalty? This is especially relevant when considering that it costs less to retain existing patients and employees, than to acquire new ones.

There are also financial implications to consider, including the potential loss of patients and customers to the competition; a decline in patient loyalty and intent to return, refer, or give back; and the loss of reimbursement dollars. But, the picture you paint of your organization in the minds of your stakeholders is an important yet only a small step in the larger effort that is required today in securing your organization's economic future.

Patient Perception Measurement

For much of hospitals' short history in the United States, the "patient experience" of healthcare was relegated to the doctor or nurse's "bedside manner," a term that didn't arrive on the scene until 1848, according to Merriam-Webster. Early competition among hospitals, if there was any at all, was focused on clinical outcomes and the expertise of their physicians.

Enter Drs. Press and Ganey.

In the 1980s, two professors at Notre Dame University, Irwin Press, a medical anthropologist, and Rod Ganey, a sociologist and statistician, began looking at healthcare and the voice of the patient through statistical measurement and surveys and later founded their firm, Press Ganey, and developed an entirely new approach and industry for tracking patient satisfaction. At the beginning of the twenty-first century, the federal government began to take an interest in this statistical approach to and measurement of patients' experiences in United States' hospitals, launching the Hospital Consumer Assessment of Healthcare Providers and Systems (HCAHPS) survey in 2005, with hospitals receiving financial incentive for participation beginning in 2007, public reporting quickly following in 2008, and eventually Medicaid reimbursements for all participating hospitals were put on the line.

Hospital Consumer Healthcare Providers and Systems (HCAHPS) Controversy

It should be noted that the implementation of HCAHPS has not been without controversy. Recently, the federal Centers for Medicaid and Medicare changed the survey questions on pain management in response to potential pressures that clinicians felt to prescribe medications.

In 2017, the United States Government Accountability Office issued a report on the federal value-based purchasing program that pointed to disparities between safety-net hospitals and small urban and rural hospitals, a formula that provided bonuses to hospitals with lower quality outcomes as well as those with missing domain scores [1].

That being said, there is no doubt that HCAHPS and other surveys can provide valuable insight into our individual organization's patient perception of care, their interaction with staff, and their overall experience. There is certainly evidence that positive patient experiences, relationships, and communications with care providers can lead to positive behaviors like adherence to treatment and medication plans.

Treating Patients as People

While HCAHPS has changed the way we measure patients' perceptions of their experience in our organizations, hospitals and others remain on the front line of continuing developments in human interaction. Cultural competency is an area where many continue to struggle. Traditional rules of thumb like "treat someone the way you want to be treated" have morphed to the more holistic "treat someone the way they want to be treated."

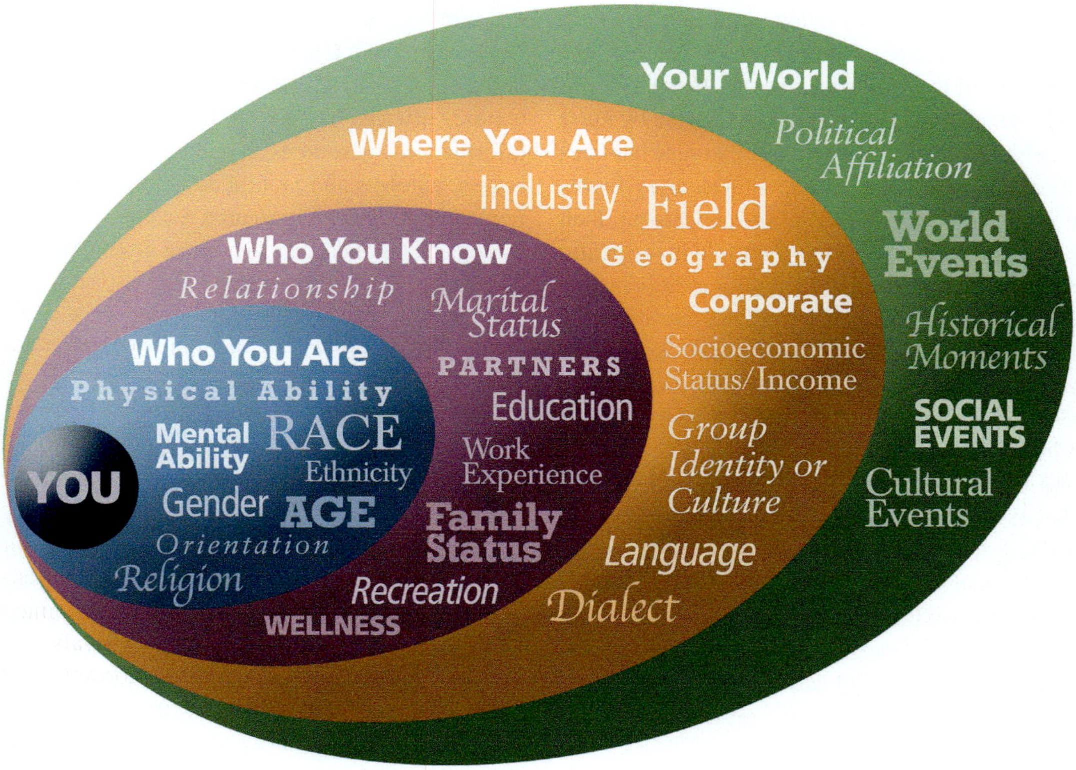

Fig. 39.3 Your universe. (Courtesy of WMCHealth)

We all bring a unique set of experiences and influences to bear in our interactions with others. Whether it is a lifetime of events, or something that happened just 15 min ago, how we see the world or approach a situation can be very different (Fig. 39.3). In fact, the one thing that we all have in common is that we are all different.

Compassion and the Patient Experience: The Impact of Injury and Illness on Patients, Families, and Caregivers

The Centers for Disease Control and Prevention define trauma as "an event, or series of events, that causes moderate to severe stress reactions… characterized by a sense of horror, helplessness, serious injury, or the threat of serious injury or death" [2].

For anyone who has ever worked in a healthcare setting, we can attest to the fact that many of our patients are feeling the impact of a traumatic event. From the more classic concept of trauma (those who were involved in an unexpected accident or incident that resulted in a serious injury or death) to those who are facing the helplessness of a newly diagnosed disease or disorder, many of our patients are "victims" of circumstances beyond their doing or control. They are normal people facing abnormal situations.

Most recently, trauma-informed care has emerged as another element of understanding and treating the "whole person," with empathy and understanding about the entirety of their life experiences, what brought them to our organization, and their current state, harkening back to our earlier discussion on cultural competence (Fig. 39.3).

Finally, healthcare organizations and their workforce members are in the unique position of regularly dealing with dying and death and have developed practices and programs to address both the needs of the patient and the workforce. No One Dies Alone (NODA) is a program started by nurse Sandra Clark in Oregon in 2001 that now has been adopted around the world. NODA uses highly trained volunteers to comfort patients in their dying hours. This service is multifold in that it also provides peace of mind to family members who may be unable to be at their loved one's bedside for one reason or another, and to staff, as well as a profound sense of service for volunteers. Patriot's Colony is a life care facility in Williamsburg, Virginia. In reviewing their end-of-life practices and working with leadership, staff, and residents, they developed The Final Farewell ceremony and reading to help family and workforce recognize the loss and its impact. Interestingly, both of these practices were developed by individual workforce members to address a gap in service, then recognized by superiors, and later adopted or hardwired as a formal practice for their organization (more about that later in this chapter.)

Often Ignored Part of the Patient Experience: Caring for the Caregiver

For a large part, much of the current focus on the patient experience ignores an entire segment of the provision of patient care, and that's the patient's caregivers—the friends and loved ones who are with them before, during and after their experiences in our healthcare organizations. Certainly, it has long been recognized that caregivers of chronically ill or dying family members often require care or respite themselves so that they can support and strengthen their own ability to provide care, similar to the airline industry's admonition to put on your own oxygen mask before helping others. No industry has limitless resources, so, in healthcare, like the No One Dies Alone program, we look to highly skilled and trained volunteers to work with caregivers. At Westchester Medical Center, in Valhalla, New York, a 1,800-square-foot enclave on the academic medical center's main concourse is dedicated to providing a retreat for family and friends, as well as staff, with emotional and physical support on hand for all who need it. The Caregiver Center (Fig. 39.4) is a space that incorporates the healing elements of art, design, and texture, offering access to the most up-to-date information resources, including computer access, wireless and mobile device charging stations, and information on area resources, as well as yoga, reiki and other therapies, aromatherapy, showers, and private rest stations [3].

Donors

Most healthcare organizations rely on philanthropy to support their programs and services in one way or another. Traditionally, about 80% of philanthropic giving comes from individuals. In healthcare, giving is most commonly from someone who has had an experience with the organization, either a patient, family member, or loved one. The Gobel Group, a leading healthcare philanthropy consulting group, connects philanthropy with healing by focusing on research on human relationships and happiness. According to the whitepaper, *Understanding Gratitude: The Connection Between Healing and Gratitude*, "The connection between clinicians and gratitude becomes more plausible when considering the true definition of philanthropy and the healing power that giving back can have for grateful patients and families" [4] (Fig. 39.5). So, if giving back to an organization actually makes patients and others feel better, why wouldn't they donate their time, energy, or even dollars? The flip side of the equation points directly to their experience with the organization, and, by no mere coincidence, patient gratitude drivers are very similar to the HCAHPS domains considered to influence patient satisfaction, such as how well the patient felt doctors communicated with them.

Perhaps more valuable than donor dollars are the donor's sphere of influence. Word-of-mouth and peer-to-peer marketing are commonly considered more powerful, more valuable, and lower-cost forms of marketing and advertising. Donors, grateful patients, and their friends and family members are a powerful force to be reckoned with for your organization. There is no

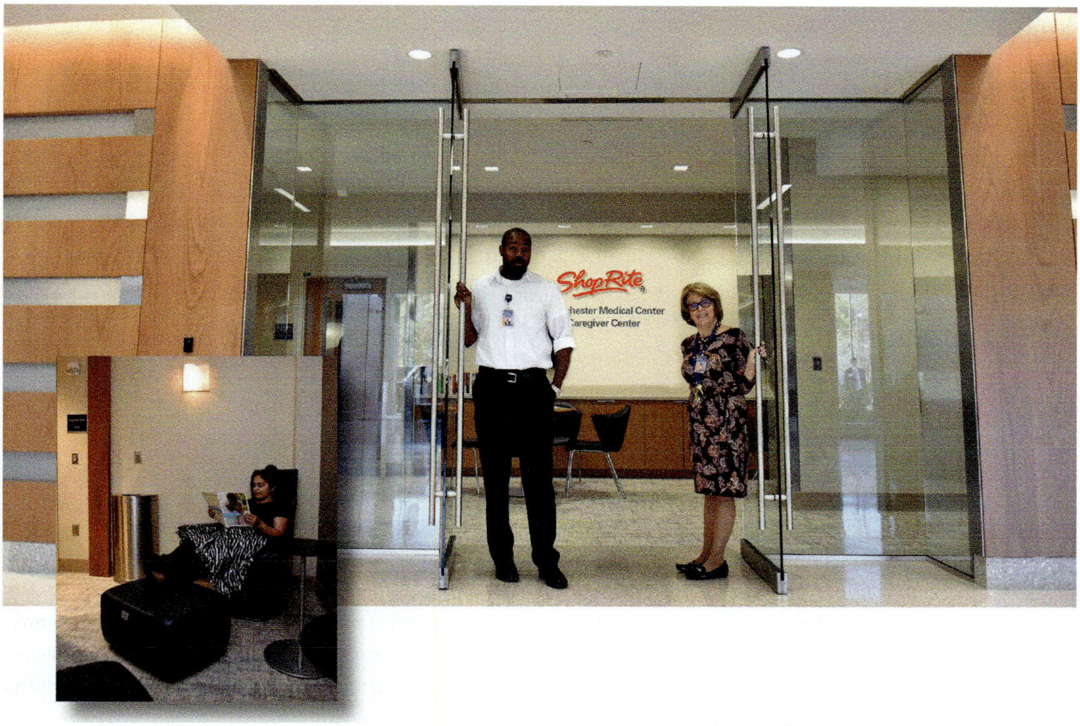

Fig. 39.4 The Caregiver Center. (Courtesy of WMCHealth)

Fig. 39.5 Continuum to care from healing. (Courtesy of the Gobel Group)

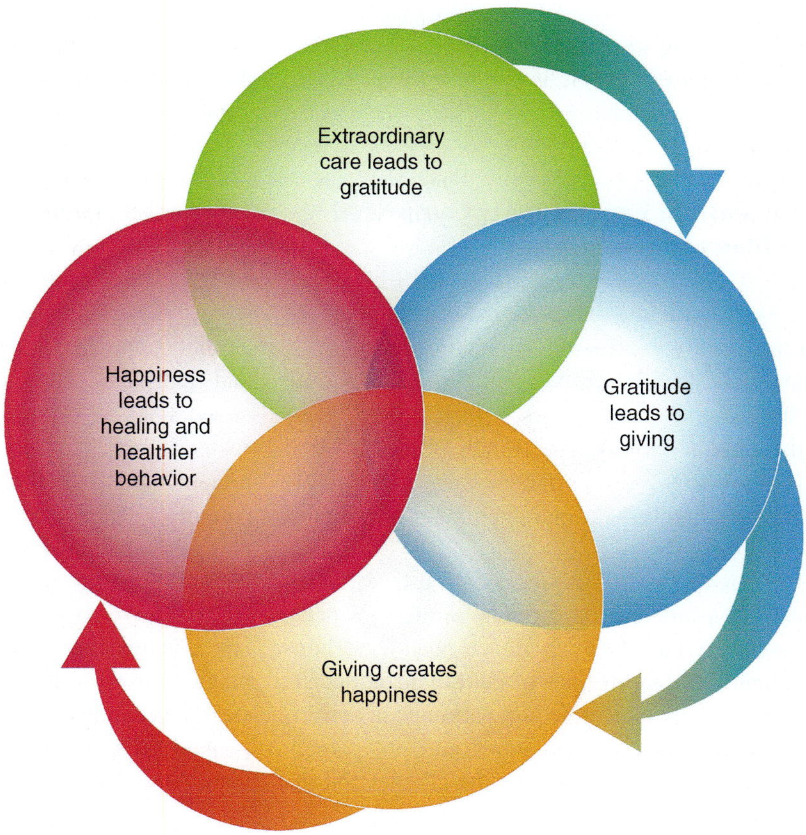

one better to paint the picture of your organization in the minds of others.

In the United States today, healthcare organizations rely on advertising, marketing, and other public relations strategies. Hospital advertising goals and results are as diverse as the organizations they tout and the communities they are trying to reach. Most hospitals focus on local markets and their most profitable services lines. Some cast their net further afield to a regional, national, or even international audience. Many in the latter category are often working to establish their brand and reputation on a broader scale from a status and recruitment perspective. And today's multiple channels on social media and digital marketing platforms make outreach to consumers and others more affordable, direct, and even personal, than ever.

Add to this mix "third-party" endorsements, accreditations, rankings, and ratings from myriad organizations, all using their own combination of publicly available data or data sourced by themselves or others.

Layered with traditional advertising and public relations, coupled with vibrant social and digital marketing programs, you have a cacophony that the general public is exposed to yet has no true way of deciphering.

The Patient Experience is Comprised of Many Touch Points

Clearly, patient experience is far more nuanced than merely expressing satisfaction or dissatisfaction with clinical outcomes alone. Everything the patient sees, hears, smells, and feels throughout hundreds of touch points in their journey affects and influences—both positively and negatively—the patient's total experience of care.

Patients do not experience healthcare vertically, within one department or unit; patients (and their families) experience healthcare horizontally, across all lines of the organization. So, while the team might be highly trained in delivering excellent clinical outcomes, patients' perceptions are influenced by both the clinical and the nonclinical, or service excellence, aspects of the care they experience throughout the continuum of care.

By definition, every touch point along the patient experience journey is important: the parking attendant or valet who ushers them into the organization; the housekeeper who cleans their room; the dietician who delivers their food; the sterile processing team that cleans the instruments used during their surgery; the nurses and doctors who directly administer care; the volunteer who delivers the flowers; the billing team that handles and processes bills, insurance, and payments; and so on.

Imagine the patient experience as a kind of relay race with a wooden baton (representing the patient experience) that is handed off from one care team member to another, mimicking the patient (and family member) journey through your organization. Smooth transitions keep the baton (and patient experience) intact. But, if the baton is dropped, it (and the patient experience) gets chipped or damaged. Of course, the goal is to have an intact baton cross the finish line. But, with so many handoffs and interactions (opportunities for positive and negative experiences), how do we keep that baton (and the experience) whole?

Connect to Purpose

In healthcare, everyone has a role on the care team. The challenge is that sometimes team members operate as if they are wearing blinders, and they are (consciously or unconsciously) encouraged to do just that. They become so focused on their specific job tasks that they remain blind to their role on the care team and the patient experience and the important role they play in the healing process. This is the real secret behind creating a culture that goes beyond HCAHPS—creating a culture of service excellence: connecting people to purpose. It's the magic ingredient that makes other organizations stand head and shoulders above others.

And speaking of a culture of service excellence, Disney is known for their culture of excellence and for delivering world-class experiences. One of their keys to success is that every one of their 65,000+ employees is connected to something beyond just their job tasks: they're connected to their purpose (which is to create happiness).

One of the most popular questions at Disney is "What time is the 3 o'clock parade?" It might seem like a ridiculous question, but consider what the guest is really asking. Disney cast members are trained to answer the question behind the question and then provide additional information. The guest really wants to know what time the 3 o'clock parade will come by HERE—the spot where they're standing right at that moment. If they're on Main Street now and the parade begins in Frontierland, it won't pass in front of them for about 20 min. Armed with this information, the cast member's answer can range from "Duh! It starts at 3 o'clock!" (not recommended) to "It starts at 3 p.m., but it won't be here until about 3:20. You'll want to save a spot early and stand over there to get great pictures with the castle in the background, and, oh by the way, here's a sticker so the princesses will invite your child to dance with them in the parade…." Clearly, this last option is connected to the employee's purpose—to create happiness. Imagine how delighted the guest is.

Now Translate This to Healthcare

A mother has just spent the night in the emergency room with her daughter, who is now stable and resting. The mom is tired and hungry and doesn't want to leave her sleeping daughter's bedside. The nurse tells her the doctor will be stopping by "soon." Still, the mother asks, "What time will the doctor be coming?" The question behind the question could be *I'm starving, and I want to know if I have time to grab a quick bite to eat so I don't miss the doctor … do I have time? Is there a place nearby to get a cup of coffee and a muffin?*

If the nurse's purpose is to provide compassionate care, the compassionate care the mom needs right now is some nourishment after a long night in the emergency room with a sick child.

People don't often say exactly what they mean, but if you apply the technique of looking for the question behind the question, you can raise the patient experience to the next level. Perception is shaped by the human side. If we don't get the human side right, patients (and their families) won't trust the clinical side.

Culture Shaping, Not Necessarily Culture Change

The saying "culture eats strategy for lunch" is true. No matter what strategy or tactics you employ to move the needle on patient experience, it's the culture—or as your employees might say "the way we do things around here"—that will override any temporary strategy you put forth.

To truly earn loyalty, moving the needle can't just be another thing that you do; it has to become who you are as an organization. As you shape your culture, intentionally, it has to be woven into your organizational DNA. Similar to the two basic strands of a human DNA chain, which gives instructions to each living cell to live a healthy life, each step of your patient experience must be composed of two integral parts: clinical quality and service quality. These two strands need to be woven together intentionally into all your processes and procedures, and then hardwired across every department, throughout the entire continuum of care. When employees learn to be intentional in delivering clinical quality with service quality, they learn that their job tasks are connected to a greater purpose to which the entire organization is aligned.

Many will be happy to hear that shaping an intentional culture, so to speak, is not necessarily about a complete culture "change," but about a culture transformation that identifies and releases the many strengths that already exist in your organization, rather than trying to impose another culture on it.

It is said that Michelangelo actually saw the shape of his sculptures in the raw material before him. If you were Michelangelo looking at your organization, most likely you see many amazing things about your organization and your culture (the great things that you all stand for and the way you all *want* to do things here.) But, they are imprisoned by the things that are not so good (the way we *don't want* to do things here and we won't stand for anymore). The key is to agree and shine a light on, release, or hardwire, recruit for, and celebrate, those things that are great, and together agree about the things that are not so great—those things that whittle away at the experience and the reason you work here—and contribute to the negative perceptions.

How to Shift a Culture?

What's the blueprint for success and the secret sauce for sustainability? For any intentionally designed culture to be successful and long lasting, it must grow organically, ideally through a true grassroots effort. It must be driven by patients and embraced by physicians, employees, and leaders with everyone working *together* as architects in its design and implementation. Culture change cannot be perceived as just another top-down initiative or flavor-of-the-year effort borrowed from a recent healthcare conference. Programs like these are a lot like artificial turf. When you first lay it down, it looks pretty good; it may even yield quick some results (aka the Hawthorne effect), but because it is not tied to who you are as an organization, employees feel like it's been imposed on them from up high. As a result, it never really takes root. It does not grow naturally. And, eventually it dies. But the initiative or program is not the only thing that dies in this process. So does employee trust, morale, and pride. So, involving key leaders and informal leaders in the design and the implementation process is critical because participation drives authorship. Authorship drives ownership. And ownership drives mutual accountability among the unit, division department, and workforce, even when the boss is not around (Fig. 39.6).

The real key to sustainability is ensuring every employee is working in concert—off the same set of sheet music, so to speak. When all members of the care team are using the same set of operational priorities and service recovery tools, are pointed toward the same common goal, and are being recognized for reflecting the culture in all that they do, the patient's perception of their experience is one of a seamless delivery of care.

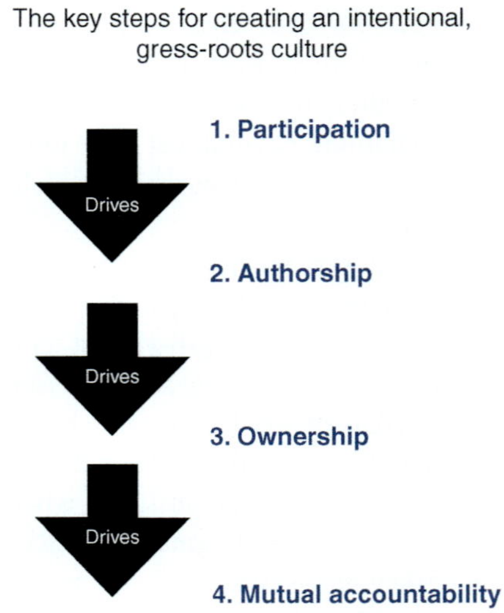

Fig. 39.6 Key steps for creating an intentional culture. (Courtesy of Integrated Loyalty Systems)

Conclusion

When Jake Poore (co-author of this chapter) was a teenager with a new driver's license, his grandmother asked him to drive her to the hospital for a procedure. Arriving early, his grandmother suggested they get a cup of coffee and a muffin to pass the time. At the cafeteria, she pulled out a food tray. Seeing that it was dirty, she set it aside and grabbed another one. Also, dirty. Finally, the third one she picked up was wet from having been washed recently, but it was clean. So, she wiped it dry and reached for the silverware. The first fork she grasped had food still stuck on it. So did the second one. And so did the third. Exasperated, his grandmother turned to him and said, "If they can't even clean the silverware, how do I know they've cleaned the tools they're going to use for my eye surgery?"

Perception is reality. Everything speaks because everything matters (remember the baton). Patients are experts at what they know (clean forks, damp trays, clean bathrooms, smile and eye contact). And then they'll use that information to judge us on what they don't know (quality of food, cleanliness of surgical instruments and surgical trays, capability, etc.) Their perception is their, and our, reality and, for the modern hospital, it matters.

References

1. Report to congressional committees: hospital value-based purchasing [Internet]. Washington, DC: United States Governmental Accountability Office; [cited 2018 June 29]. Available from https://www.gao.gov/assets/690/685586.pdf.
2. Helping patients cope with a traumatic event [Internet]. Atlanta: Centers for Disease Control and Prevention; [cited 2018 June 28]. What is a traumatic event?; [about 3 screens]. Available from: https://www.cdc.gov/masstrauma/factsheets/professionals/coping_professional.pdf.
3. westchesermedicalcenter.com [Internet]. Valhalla: Westchester Medical Center; c2018 [cited 2018 June 28]. The Caregiver Center; [about 2 screens]. Available from: https://www.westchestermedicalcenter.com/caregiver-center.
4. Understanding gratitude: the connection between healing and philanthropy [Internet]. Kennett Square: Gobel Group; c2017; [cited 2018 June 29]. Available from: https://gobelgroup.com/wp-content/uploads/2018/02/Understanding-Gratitude-Whitepaper.pdf.

Part V

The Human Benefits and Cost of Modern Hospital

Surgical Volunteerism as an Extension of Modern Hospital: Serving One Patient at Time and Building Bridges

40

Rifat Latifi

Introduction

Surgical volunteer missions (SVMs) have become a popular approach for reducing the burden of surgical disease worldwide. While these missions have been organized for many decades, newly published report by the Lancet Commission (LC) on Global Surgery adds more importance and weight to SVM. The LC reported that nearly 45% of the total estimated surgical cases worldwide are left unoperated upon each year, leaving more than 143 million people in low- and middle-income countries (LIMICs) without adequate surgical care [1]. Moreover, nearly two-thirds of the world's population do not have access to safe, affordable, and timely surgical care, with the majority being from low-income countries, versus only 15% from high-income countries [1, 2]. While two billion people are currently unable to undergo a necessary surgical procedure due to an insufficient surgical infrastructure including lack of surgeons, tens of millions each year face ruinous financial hardship when they are forced to pay for their own surgery and anesthesia [1, 3]. Surgical volunteer missions (SVMs) offer a flexible and often rapid response to the gaps in surgical care worldwide [4]. However, long-term results have not been studied, and although SVMs are nearly universally welcomed, their overall benefits have not been studied. There are a number of SVMs taking place worldwide, mostly from developed countries to low- and middle-income countries.

The exact number of missions taking place worldwide and number of patients that are being served are not known. Some of these volunteer missions are organized by different hospitals, are supported by governments, or are supported and organized by faith-based organizations. Other SVMs are based on emergency situations (i.e., disaster-response missions), are created in an ad hoc fashion from a single institution, or are formed from an existing roster of emergency volunteers. Irrespective of how the missions are organized and who conducts them, the goal of some missions is to lessen the burden of surgical conditions such as cataract, cardiovascular, plastic surgery, fistulae care, and other surgical services with clearly defined, well-planned, and executed mission goals [5–7]. The majority of SVMs address a variety of surgical problems, based on the expertise and composition of the surgical and anesthesia teams, as well as the infrastructure of the hospital of the country where the mission is taking place. What is not clear, however, is the long-term impact of SVMs; this is mainly due to the lack of data collection infrastructure and reporting of such data on these long-term impacts. The lack of surgical practice

R. Latifi (✉)
New York Medical College, School of Medicine, Department of Surgery and Westchester Medical Center, Valhalla, NY, USA
e-mail: rifat_latifi@nymc.edu; rifat.latifi@wmchealth.org

R. Latifi (ed.), *The Modern Hospital*, https://doi.org/10.1007/978-3-030-01394-3_40

guidelines on surgical volunteerism is another reason for lack of such data. In this chapter we will discuss major organizational topics that we believe would make SVM safe and effective way of lessening the burden of disease.

Surgical volunteer missions comprise a valuable approach for reducing the burden of surgical disease in countries with limited resources worldwide. As mentioned above such missions are organized worldwide, both in peace and during catastrophes, be it man-made (wars, conflicts) or natural disasters (earthquakes, volcano eruptions, mud sliding, and others). In one continuous single multispecialty surgical volunteer mission (SVM) (unpublished data), we analyzed the results of 1327 patients operated over 12 surgical missions (2006–2018), in one of the islands of Bohol in the Philippines (with a population of 1.3 million people) [8]. The surgical mission has been organized over the years by the same group of surgeons and local support system in the same hospital for 11 out of 12 missions (1 mission was organized in a governmental hospital). During the study period, 1327 operations were performed (842 females (63.4%) and 485 males (36.6%) (male-to-female ratio 0.59), mean age 37 ± 18 years). The majority of operations were for thyroid disease (31.6%), followed by hernia (17.3%), hysterectomies/salpingo-oophorectomies (12.2%), soft tissue tumors (9.9%), cleft lip/palate repairs (7.2%), breast (6.4%), gallbladder disease (4.7%), cataract (2.9%), parotid masses (1.4%), and others (6.4%). For each mission, there were an average 5.5 days of operating, performing a median of 105.5 (80–148) cases per mission.

During these missions, surgeons of various disciplines (general, plastic, otorhinolaryngologic, and gynecologic surgeons), anesthesiologists, nurse anesthetists, surgical and anesthesia residents, surgical nurses, surgical technologists, and other volunteers have joined for a week-long mission. This operation is supported by a number of organizations, the local government, and individuals from the community and a nongovernmental organization Gift of Life ™ Foundation for the Philippines. The latter screens and identifies patients in need of surgery. On the day of surgical team's arrival, as many as 200 patients in a single day are screened. After evaluating patients, each surgeon will schedule four to seven operations a day for six operative days (Sunday–Friday). In recent years, in order to facilitate the process, we have used store-and-forward telemedicine to evaluate patients in advance, in order to better prepare for the mission [8]. During the telemedicine session, the surgeon can identify patients and plan for surgery.

Five Critical Organizational Issues of Surgical Volunteer Missions

Surgical missions are complex by any stretch of imagination and have been shown to reduce the burden of surgical disease worldwide, but their organizational complexity has not been addressed adequately, and it is unclear if those who wish to undertake SVMs truly understand associated challenges and goes into sustainability of such missions. We have divided these challenging issues into five groups: (1) creation of the team; (2) patient selection; (3) case complexity; (4) cost of the mission; (5) quality of care and safety of surgical missions; (6) Informed Consent; (7) the overall efficiency of the SVM, and (8) Team Safety and safety of each member of the mission.

Surgical Volunteer Mission Team

The core and the soul of a surgical mission is the team, which consists of surgeons, anesthesiologists, nurses, and other volunteers. For successful SVM, volunteer organizations should partner with nongovernmental organizations (NGOs), private companies, and other governments with shared goals [6]. Once these alliances have been forged, partnerships with the local Ministries of Health or their departments should be made in order to form culturally sensitive and sustainable programs [7, 8]. In addition to surgeons, anesthesiologists, and surgical nurses, there is great variety among the individuals who can support a surgical team during a volunteer mission, depending on the nature of the mission. Surgical/scrub technologists, cardiopulmonary bypass perfusionists (when cardiac operations are performed), intensive care nurses, dietitians, dentists, speech pathologists, prosthetics, biomedical engineers, respiratory therapists, and various other medical specialists may be recruited. Pharmacists may also be useful members of the team for their abilities to store, compound, and counsel on medications [9]. During times when medical volunteers are faced with unfamiliar medications in labels they cannot confidently interpret, a pharmacist can clarify many questions [10].

Having support from a pathology and/or radiology department can significantly improve the diagnostic capabilities and overall quality of care [11]; however, most SVMs do not have a pathologist nor a radiologist on their teams. While in our mission, almost all thyroid or breast masses undergo some sort of pathology examination (fine needle aspiration or open biopsy), commonly patients cannot afford biopsy, and so they go undiagnosed.

Many volunteer missions rely on local nurses to assist with operations and other workers to provide translation services between the surgical team and the patients and staff. However, these informal interpreters are not guaranteed to understand complicated surgical procedures well enough to adequately convey the information to patients and ensure that the surgical consent is genuinely informed. In our case, a number of team members speak the local language, and the communication has not been an issue. However, in general, identifying potential interpreters early and then sending them to complete formalized training as medical interpreters has been shown to improve lines of communication [12]. When considering local team members, there should be an on-site coordinator, community physicians and healthcare staff, members from the hosting organization, a patient counselor, and potentially a lecture coordinator (if the mission is focused on education and training). A clear understanding by the local physicians and healthcare workers can better ensure their cooperation and support, particularly with referrals and prescreening of patients [13], as well as postoperative follow-up of these patients.

There are many ways to create a team, and the Operation Giving Back website [14] serves as an excellent platform to volunteer or to recruit members for your existing surgical mission. Diligent screening of potential personnel, however, is important. Many surgeons, especially after they retire, believe that there is still something in them that they would like to give back. We believe that a surgical mission is not the place for retired surgeons, unless they have retired early in their age and have maintained their surgical skills and surgical stamina and are up to date with surgical and medical knowledge. Often these retired surgeons show up in the middle of the mission (usually on their way to visiting their families if they are from that country or they do part vacation and part mission), perform perhaps one or two operations a day, and frankly are more of a burden to the mission than helpful. SVM should not be a mechanism to visit various countries around the world, even if it is happened to be your own country of origin. There should be no difference in the credentialing process between a surgical mission and the process that every surgeon undergoes before starting any new job. Also, SVM should not be used as a place where you learn or relearn a novel technique or a new operation; this is not ethical, and the leader of the mission should ensure that such things never occur. We must honor the trust that these patients bestowed upon us by providing them with the highest quality of care possible. This does not preclude a surgical or anesthesia resident from participating in these missions, provided they work directly under the supervision of a qualified attending. Finally, for surgical volunteer mission groups to provide safe and affordable care to patients in LIMICs, it is important to recognize the needs of the local area, as well as the limitations of the surgical team.

Patient Selection

Proper patient selection is of the utmost importance for the successful and optimal impact of the mission. Throughout the year, patients are identified from a large pool for potential operations, and then at the beginning of the mission, key surgeons of SVM perform the final selection of the patients and put together the full schedule for the week. One has to be cognizant that a patient or two may actually be removed from the schedule for whatever reason and new patients with more acute conditions may be placed on schedule. Therefore, some ability to be flexible is important.

A well-defined screening process for patients should be in place. Without such a process, the mission volunteers will likely be seeing many patients who have conditions that either do not require surgery or are too complicated to be adequately handled in the short timespan when the mission will be present [13, 15]. It may be frustrating to turn away patients because their condition has progressed beyond the scope of the mission, especially if the condition has a good prognosis if treated early, but the goal should be to help as many patients as possible [16].

Preoperative evaluation of surgical mission patients is a complex, time-consuming, and often chaotic process, because these evaluations typically require intense work by the operating team on the day of arrival at the mission site. Our group has found that low-cost telemedicine is a viable and secure alternative for preoperative evaluation of surgical mission patients [8]. It increases efficiency and optimizes the use of existing resources. More specifically, store-and-forward telemedicine (SAFT) helps ensure an accurate assessment of patients before the surgical team arrives, reduces on-site prescreening time, and decreases the number of surgical candidates on the waiting list. Previous results from our work described a 98% correlation rate between SAFT and in-person preoperative evaluations [8].

Case Complexity

Determining whether a case is too complex for the capabilities of the surgical volunteer team [17]. In our experience, we give priority to those patients with the largest and most deforming pathology (e.g., thyroid masses). The biggest and most difficult cases, however, should not be done on the first day of the mission, as there is a need for refining the team effectiveness, unless this team has worked together previously. One has to be sensitive to the distance that patients and their families had to travel to be seen and schedule those individuals from outlying areas earlier in the week to minimize their cost of lodging. An inundation of cases not related to surgical care is a common distraction, and even if the surgical mission is not advertised, subsequent mission years are bound to produce greater numbers of patients and family showing up to be evaluated than can be helped. It is not uncommon for parents of children who were turned away by previous missions and asked not to come back to return again the following year, often accompanied by additional individuals seeking care.

Not all patients are the same, even when dealing with an identical diagnosis. There are complex thyroid goiters or thyroid cancer, and there are smaller thyroid goiters. Defining clear selection criteria prior to the mission will treat patients more fairly and give everyone an equal survival chance [16]. What diagnoses and conditions are treated should be based entirely and exclusively on the experience and the expertise of the mission members. These selection criteria should be made clear to prospective patients and their families, and deviating from or neglecting these established criteria may create a sense of resentment by those being seen.

Many missions are organized together with local medical schools or faculties, and missions are deployed and implemented in a collaborative fashion. These are probably most effective missions, as far as training and creating local expertise. These short-term missions serve as good training for many local staff, who will be able to perform these procedures in future years, and therefore this approach is an investment in the sustainability of the local healthcare system. Often, such as in our own experience on the other hand, there are no residents or local faculty working with us. This local private expertise, however, is too expensive, and most of our patients cannot afford the surgery. In other situations, with simple cases being handled by local professionals, subsequent surgical volunteer missions can focus almost entirely on the more advanced cases. A clear focus regarding whether the surgical volunteer mission is primarily service-related or devoted to teaching is critical and should be established early [16, 17]. Telesurgery and telementoring are viable options to meet the needs of training, while still performing as many surgeries as possible during a surgical volunteer mission. However, this needs to be prepared well in advance and have the technical infrastructure in place, which commonly these hospitals cannot afford.

Time constraints and the volume of patients may require that each patient receives only one surgical procedure per visit, while other missions may mandate combining several related surgeries [18]. While trying to operate on as many patients as possible is a noble goal, focusing entirely on simple cases essentially ignores those with more complex conditions. This potential dilemma exemplifies the need for clearly defined criteria with respect to both patient selection and case complexity and should be based on team expertise and ability to care for these patients long after the mission has ended.

The Cost of the Mission

The cost of the mission is difficult to estimate if not impossible. While we have not done so, the cost of a mission should be done prospectively. While the main focus may be on serving as many patients as possible, having a member of volunteer mission who is dedicated to monitoring cost and outcomes would provide valuable information for future missions and has been dramatically absent from the literature. To avoid the impression that surgical volunteer missions are "paid vacations," many organizations require that volunteers travel at their own expense [8, 18]. In other cases, the logistics, housing, and meals may be handled by the host country or the mission organization, but it is important to confirm these details before you make the commitment to volunteer. In our case, each member of the mission pays her/his own expenses including travel, lodging, and other incidental expenses. When considering supplies for the surgical mission, sometimes it will be more cost-effective to partner with a regional funding source or even another volunteer organization than it would be to ship the needed supplies with the mission team. While we at OGBB have local partners who store and care for the surgical supplies, all materials are shipped from the USA to the Philippines.

The cost of the mission does not include only of the surgery (based on the local cost) but include the cost of travel and lodging of each member of the team, as well as all the surgical materials and the cost of shipping it to our mission. Several studies have documented the cost-effectiveness of individual surgical missions, focusing on particular specialties such as orthopedics [19], pediatric neurosurgery [20], and hernia repair [21, 22]. One recent systematic review of the cost-effectiveness of surgery in resource-poor countries suggests that a subset of surgical procedures are cost-effective or very cost-effective and quite comparable to other generally accepted medical mission priorities [23]. A second systematic review suggests that dedicated surgical centers demonstrated greater cost-effectiveness compared to short-term surgical volunteer missions, but inconsistent data collection and reporting in the literature by past surgical missions make any type of systematic review somewhat incomplete [24].

Quality of Care and Safety of Surgical Missions

Regardless of the location, clinical discipline, or mission focus, a surgical team must provide the same quality of care on a volunteer mission as they would provide in their home country [25] which is the highest possible quality of care. A surgeon should only perform the operations that is well prepared to perform; it is not the purpose of a surgical mission to allow a surgeon to attempt procedures that does not practice [26]. Surgical missions are not the place where primary surgeons come to learn or relearn surgical procedures. Given the wider variety of cases that a surgeon may see on a volunteer mission, one may wish to seek out some formalized training before embarking.

Surgery-related outcomes during volunteer missions should be subject to the same quality assessment and regulation as other core medical treatments [27]. There are few standardized surgical outcomes databases, and the ones that do exist are often specific to certain volunteer missions (e.g., Smile Train's global database for cleft lip and palate), but a lack of awareness of these databases makes it difficult to perform comparisons between surgical humanitarian missions [27]. The use of operating room checklists, such as those developed by the World Health Organization (WHO) [28], is useful in performing risk assessments and has been recommended by the Lancet Commission on Global Surgery [1]. The implementation of the WHO checklists is linked to lowered mortality and morbidity, but a checklist alone is not able to precisely track quality [29]. Some attempts have been made to standardize the care for surgical volunteer missions. These include adopting domestic standard policies, such as the Blue Cross/Shield's Blue Distinction criteria [25], or a survey-based standardized tool developed by Maki et al. to evaluate parameters of short-term medical missions including cost, efficiency, impact, preparedness, education, and sustainability [30]. To achieve high-quality care in low-resource settings, it is important to recognize the cultural differences that could impact the delivery of care [29]. While cultural competency training is deemed to be important, and it is recommended that it be taught to surgical residents, there is no standard curriculum offered [29].

Informed Consent

Despite the impressions of some that informed consent is somehow less important in developing countries, it is perhaps even more significant when operating in another country [28, 31]. While the use of formal written contracts may not be a part of many cultures, ensuring informed consent of the patient or their family should be a priority. This should be done by means of an official translator and ideally local physicians and nurses who are also fluent in [26] the language of the mission team. A related ethical issue involves the use of photographic and/or video records of patients taken during their medical treatment on surgical volunteer missions that are or could be included in their medical record. These individuals are invested with the same privacy protections as a US citizen under the Health Insurance Portability and Accountability Acts of 1996 (HIPAA). Therefore, it would be a good practice to develop a policy to obtain witnessed written or verbal consent for the use of such media [32]. One has to be particularly aware of HIPAA violations in the new social media age. Publication of patient information on private social media pages for whatever reason should be strongly discouraged and not used for advertisement of ones' "new skills" in order to attract new patients to a local practice.

Overall Mission Efficiency

Surgical mission may be stressful, and team cohesion may mitigate such stress [33] and make rather useful and often unforgiven experience. In today's era of organizing virtual conference calls, a face-to-face virtual meeting is easily accomplished and should be done before every SVM. Unfortunately, surgical volunteer mission teams don't have a lot of time to work together, which makes early planning and any opportunity for team building prior to the mission significant [34]. Team cohesion will likely form faster among small groups with similar norms and between those who work in close proximity to complete a common goal under an external pressure for some form of shared reward [34]. Such meeting or communication should be mandatory [35]. Vashdi et al. recommend using a briefing/debriefing learning model adapted by the military for surgical teams [36]. Others also recommend that physicians on any type of medical volunteer mission have deliberate team building training [37], in order to avoid ineffective communication, scarcity of resources, and lack of trust [38].

Cooperation is essential for effective team cohesion, and it only takes one uncooperative individual to erode team morale [38].

Safety of Surgical Missions

Ensuring the safety of team members is an obligation both of the team leader and of each individual. Irrespective of where the mission is taking place, one should avoid being alone and not to venture out at night. In our program, the local government makes sure that we are always accompanied by local security personnel to and from the hospital, as well as everywhere we go during the entire mission. Special measures should be taken in "hot zones" and in the disaster settings. A basic understanding of the history of a region where one plans to volunteer can help shape the context regarding matters of personal safety. The impression local communities have of medical missionaries may be influenced by longstanding historical factors including colonialism, war, and the interrelation of medical missions with religious organizations [39]. There are increased safety risks for any humanitarian worker if they are providing services in areas of conflict, and are not perceived as being completely impartial [40]. Increased tensions between countries and intergovernmental organizations can place humanitarian organizations in the precarious position of needing personal security to fulfill their humanitarian mission, while trying to remain neutral and apolitical [40, 41]. While planning your volunteer mission, register with the US State Department, and purchase a travel insurance policy that covers medical evacuation [42].

Most recently the American Academy of Pediatrics (AAP) Delivery of Surgical Care Subcommittee and American Pediatric Surgical Association (APSA) Global Pediatric Surgery Committee, with the American Pediatric Surgical Nurses Association, Inc. (APSNA) Global Health Special Interest Group, and the Society for Pediatric Anesthesia (SPA) Committee on International Education and Service generated consensus recommendations for STMs based on extensive experience with STMs. These are really very useful guidelines that should be adopted by others as well [43].

Among three distinct areas identified, travel and safety considerations are critical to success of the mission and include travel logistics, health tips and safety measures, tips on packing, bringing money with you and credit cards, technical advice on phone/Internet, and cultural sensitivity.

Recently, the healthcare workers who volunteer in conflict zones have been exposed to violence and death with increasing number [44]. Moreover, since 2012, there have been 2300 incidents of violence or threats of violence reported to the International Federation of the Red Cross (IFRC), though the IFRC suspects that many more go unreported [45]. The sheer number of death and injuries among healthcare workers in conflict countries is staggering [46].

The dashboard on attacks on healthcare worker of WHO shows that during 2014 and 2017, there were 1218 attacks, 1625 deaths, and 2348 injuries. Only during the 2017 there were 104 attacks, 64 deaths, and 59 injuries in 16 countries. Only for the first quarter the dashboard shows that there were already 221 deaths, 149 attacks, and 261 injuries on healthcare workers [46].

While these data are staggering, it is not possible to distinguish between volunteers from other countries who have come to provide aid to the region in conflict, or these are mainly local healthcare workers, who refused to leave their countries and region or hospitals where they practice beforehand. Working as a surgeon in conflicts and wars is complex, difficult, outright dangerous, yet rewarding and fulfilling [47], and hopefully those who are involved being bad guys or worse guys will think of international humanitarian law (IHL): the Geneva Conventions of 1949 for the protection of the sick and wounded and of those who care for them. Making combatants comply with IHL is a difficult task. War pathology will challenge even most experienced trauma surgeon.

In August of 2014, I took a young man who was shot in Syria and was transferred to Jordan in septic shock and his abdomen full of bile for re-exploration, frankly as Giannou describes as absolute urgency imposed by those who may be under the influence of "toxic cocktail" [47]. Luckily, I found a missed gallbladder injury from the bullet that has traversed the liver and into the duodenum. I did a cholecystectomy and washed his abdomen, and the patient did well.

Summary

Surgical volunteer missions are complex undertakings for everyone who participates. It is a wonderful way to help those who otherwise cannot afford surgical care. Surgeons embarking on these missions must understand their intricacies, and operating is perhaps the easiest of the all tasks involved. In the future, information regarding team creation, patient selection, provision of highest quality possible, and analysis of outcomes, including the cost of the mission, should be ensured, analyzed, and reported.

References

1. Meara JG, Leather AJM, Hagander L, et al. Global Surgery 2030: evidence and solutions for achieving health, welfare, and economic development. Lancet. 2015;386(9993):569–624.
2. Alkire BC, Raykar NP, Shrime MG, et al. Global access to surgical care: a modelling study. Lancet Glob Health. 2015;3(6):e316–e23.
3. Funk LM, Weiser TG, Berry WR, et al. Global operating theatre distribution and pulse oximetry supply: an estimation from reported data. Lancet. 2010;376:1055–61.
4. Casey KM. The global impact of surgical volunteerism. Surg Clin North Am. 2007;87(4):949–60.
5. Wallen TJ, Arnaoutakis GJ, Blenden R, Soto R. Programmatic changes to reduce mortality and morbidity in humanitarian congenital cardiac surgery. World J Pediatr Congenit Heart Surg. 2018;9(1):47–53.
6. Rapp DE, Colhoun A, Morin J, Bradford TJ. Assessment of communication technology and post-operative telephone surveillance during global urology mission. BMC Res Notes. 2018;11(1):149.
7. Walker ME, Chuang C, Moores CR, et al. The hand surgeon consultation improves patient knowledge in a hand surgery mission to Honduras. J Hand Surg Asian Pac Vol. 2018;23(1):11–7.
8. Latifi R, Mora F, Bekteshi F, Rivera R. Preoperative telemedicine evaluation of surgical mission patients: should we use it routinely? Bull Am Coll Surg. 2014;99(1):17–23.
9. Brown DA, Ferrill MJ. Planning a pharmacy-led medical mission trip, part 1: focus on medication acquisition. Ann Pharmacother. 2012;46(5):751–9.
10. Kobayashi MA. Evolution of a triage and flow process during a joint American-Chinese medical mission in Dali, Yunnan, China. J Emerg Nurs. 2011;37(4):394–8.
11. Naujokas A. Raising the quality of care during medical missions: a survey to assess the need for clinical and anatomic pathology services in international medical missions. Arch Pathol Lab Med. 2013;137:637–41.
12. Hasbun Avalos O, Pennington K, Osterberg L. Revolutionizing volunteer interpreter services: an evaluation of an innovative medical interpreter education program. J Gen Intern Med. 2013;28(12):1589–95.
13. Nguah S. Ethical aspects of arranging local medical collaboration and care. J Clin Ethics. 2014;25(4):314–6.
14. American College of Surgeons. Home page. Retieved from: www.operationgivingback.facs.org.
15. Latifi R, et al. Outcomes of 1,327 Patients Operated On Through Twelve Multispecialty Surgical Volunteerism Missions and Challenges that Every Volunteer Surgeon.
16. Eyal N. Pediatric heart surgery in Ghana: three ethical questions. J Clin Ethics. 2014;25(4):317–22.
17. Hollier LH Jr, Sharabi SE, Koshy JC, Schafer ME, O'Young J, Flood TW. Surgical mission (not) impossible–now what? J Craniofac Surg. 2010;21(5):1488–92.
18. MacIntosh RB, Herman LT, Shivapuja PK, Echeverri-Arguello RC. Volunteer cleft surgery in Colombia: an 18-year perspective. J Oral Maxillofac Surg. 2013;71(10):1742–51.
19. Chen AT, Pedtke A, Kobs JK, Edwards GS Jr, Coughlin RR, Gosselin RA. Volunteer orthopedic surgical trips in Nicaragua: a cost-effectiveness evaluation. World J Surg. 2012;36(12):2802–8.
20. Davis MC, Than KD, Garton HJ. Cost effectiveness of a short-term pediatric neurosurgical brigade to Guatemala. World Neurosurg. 2014;82(6):974–9.
21. Schillcutt SC, Clarke M, Kingsnorth A. Cost-effectiveness of groin hernia surgery in the Western Region of Ghana. Arch Surg. 2010;145(10):954–61.
22. Shillcutt SD, Sanders DL, Teresa Butron-Vila M, Kingsnorth AN. Cost-effectiveness of inguinal hernia surgery in northwestern Ecuador. World J Surg. 2013;37(1):32–41.
23. Chao TE, Sharma K, Mandigo M, Hagander L, Resch SC, Weiser TG, et al. Cost-effectiveness of surgery and its policy implications for global health: a systematic review and analysis. Lancet Glob Health. 2014;2(6):e334–e45.
24. Shrime M, Sleemi A, Ravilla T. Charitable platforms in global surgery: a systematic review of their effectiveness, cost-effectiveness, sustainability, and role training. World J Surg. 2015;39:10–20.
25. Dempsey KE, Ghazinouri R, Diez D, Alcantara L, Beagan C, Aggouras B, Hoagland M, Thornhill TS, Katz JN. Enhancing the quality of

international orthopedic medical mission trips using the blue distinction criteria for knee and hip replacement centers. BMC Musculoskelet Disord. 2013;14(275):1–16.
26. Precious DS. Important pillars of charity cleft surgery: the avoidance of "safari surgery". Oral Surg Oral Med Oral Pathol Oral Radiol. 2014;117(4):395–6.
27. Chu KM, Trelles M, Ford NP. Quality of care in humanitarian surgery. World J Surg. 2011;35(6):1169–72; discussion 73–4.
28. Holt G. Ethical conduct of humanitarian medical missions: I. Informed consent. Arch Facial Plast Surg. 2012;14(3):215–7.
29. Campbell A, Sullivan M, Sherman R, Magee WP. The medical mission and modern cultural competency training. J Am Coll Surg. 2011;212(1):124–9.
30. Maki J, Qualls M, White B, Kleefield S, Crone R. Health impact assessment and short-term medical missions: a methods study to evaluate quality of care. BMC Health Serv Res. 2008;8:121.
31. Aliu O, Corlew SD, Heisler ME, Pannucci CJ, Chung KC. Building surgical capacity in low-resource countries: a qualitative analysis of task shifting from surgeon volunteers' perspectives. Ann Plast Surg. 2014;72(1):108–12.
32. Holt G. Ethical conduct of humanitarian medical missions: II. Use of photographic images. Arch Facial Plast Surg. 2012;14(4):295–6.
33. Brown DB, Brown DL, Yocum CK. Planning a pharmacy-led medical mission trip, part 2: servant leadership and team dynamics. Ann Pharmacother. 2012;46:895–900.
34. Sundstrom E, De Meuse KP, Futrell D. Work teams: applications and effectiveness. Am Psychol. 1990;45(2):120–33.
35. Friedman DB, Improving Team DL. Structure and communication: a key to hospital efficiency. Arch Surg. 2004;139:1194–998.
36. Vashdi DR, Bamberger PA, Erez M, Weiss-Meilik A. Briefing-debriefing: using a reflexive organizational learning model from the military to enhance the performance of surgical teams. Hum Resour Manag. 2007;46(1):115–42.
37. Schwartz RW, Pogge C. Physician leadership: essential skills in a changing environment. Am J Surg. 2000;180:187–92.
38. Scarnati JT. On becoming a team player. Team Perform Manag Int J. 2001;7(1/2):5–10.
39. Dilger H. Claiming territory: medical mission, interreligious revivalism, and the spatialization of health interventions in urban Tanzania. Med Anthropol. 2014;33(1):52–67.
40. Eckenwiler L, Hunt M. Counterterrorism, ethics, and global health. Hast Cent Rep. 2014;44(3):12–3.
41. Karlsrud J, Felix da Costa D. Invitation withdrawn: humanitarian action, United Nations peacekeeping, and state sovereignty in Chad. Disasters. 2013;37(Suppl 2):S171–87.
42. Mettner J. Staying safe overseas. Minn Med. 2014;97(10):12–4.
43. Butler M, Drum E, Evans FM, et al. Guidelines and checklists for short-term missions in global pediatric surgery: recommendations from the American Academy of Pediatrics Delivery of Surgical Care Global Health Subcommittee, American Pediatric Surgical Association Global Pediatric Surgery Committee, Society for Pediatric Anesthesia Committee on International Education and Service, and American Pediatric Surgical Nurses Association, Inc. Global Health Special Interest Group. J Pediatr Surg. 2018;53(4):828–36. https://doi.org/10.1016/j.jpedsurg.2017.11.037. Epub 2017 Nov 15.
44. World Helath Organization (WHO). WHO condemns rising violence against health care workers, patients. Retrieved from: http://www.who.int/hac/events/HCWviolence/en/. Accessed 17 June 2018.
45. Klibanoff E. Medical workers in conflict zones have never faced greater risks. December 16th, 2014. NPR.com. Retrieved from: https://www.npr.org/sections/goatsandsoda/2014/12/16/371273053/medical-workers-in-conflict-zones-have-never-faced-greater-risks. Accessed 17 June 2018. World Health Organization (WHO). Attacks on Health Care DASHBOARD. Retrieved from: http://www.who.int/emergencies/attacks-on-health-care/dashboard2017-Q4.pdf?ua=1. Accessed 17 June 2018.
46. World Health Organization (WHO). Attacks on health care. Retrieved from: http://www.who.int/emergencies/attacks-on-health-care/en/.
47. Giannou C. A volunteer surgeon in war zones: experience of 35 years and a call to action. Current Trauma Rep. 2017;3(1):75–7.

41 The Human Cost of Modern Hospital and Healthcare

Rifat Latifi

Introduction

While the transformation in medicine and in particular surgery and care that we provide has improved patient outcome, in recent years, it has become obvious that this transformation has had a toll on practitioners, known nowadays as burnout. Coined by Dr. Herbert Freudenberger, the term *burnout* is defined as "the consequences of severe or prolonged stress and anxiety experienced by people working in the healing professions" [1].

Later this was further defined as "a syndrome of emotional exhaustion and cynicism that occurs frequently among individuals who do people work of some kind" [2].

In recent publication by JAMA surgery, this topic has rightly taken a center stage [3, 4]. More than half of US physicians are now experiencing professional burnout. Moreover, satisfaction with work-life balance also declined in physicians between 2011 and 2014 (48.5% vs 40.9%; $P < 0.001$ [5]. Substantial differences in rates of burnout and satisfaction with work-life balance were observed by specialty. In contrast to the trends in physicians, minimal changes in burnout or satisfaction with work-life balance were observed between 2011 and 2014 in probability-based samples of working US adults, resulting in an increasing disparity in burnout and satisfaction with work-life balance in physicians relative to the general US working population. Compared to 2011, burnout rates were higher for all specialties in 2014. In fact, nearly a dozen specialties experienced more than a 10% increase in burnout over those 3 years: family medicine (51.3% of physicians reported burnout in 2011 versus 63.0% in 2014), general pediatrics (35.3% versus 46.3%), urology (41.2% versus 63.6%), orthopedic surgery (48.3% versus 59.6%), dermatology (31.8% versus 56.5%), physical medicine and rehabilitation (47.4% versus 63.3%), pathology (37.6% versus 52.5%), radiology (47.7% versus 61.4%), and general surgery subspecialties (42.4% versus 52.7%) [5].

This is not new by any stretch of imagination. A paper published almost five decades ago [6] reviewed the international literature for the previous 75 years of suicide among physicians and reported that (1) suicide among physicians was high; (2) suicide among female physicians is higher than among male physicians; (3) physician suicide varies from country to country, with the highest rate among the Danes, the next among British, and the next among US physicians; (4) there is a high incidence of psychiatric morbidity, alcoholism, and drug addiction among physicians who suicide; (5) as in suicides among other groups, there are significant variable correlates of age,

R. Latifi (✉)
New York Medical College, School of Medicine, Department of Surgery and Westchester Medical Center, Valhalla, NY, USA
e-mail: rifat_latifi@nymc.edu; rifat.latifi@wmchealth.org

R. Latifi (ed.), *The Modern Hospital*, https://doi.org/10.1007/978-3-030-01394-3_41

gender, medical school affiliation, geographic residence, type of medical practice and specialty, the state of physical and emotional health, the use of alcohol and drugs, and professional and psychosocial factors; and (6) preventive action is both possible and desirable [6]. Since this paper was published, suicidal rate among Danish doctors has dropped significantly [7].

While there are many factors that have been identified as contributing to the raise of burnout and suicidal among physicians, in a recent cross-sectional study, 557 physicians found significant relationships between anhedonia and suicidal ideation or suicide attempts, even when significant variables or covariates were taken into account and, in particular, depressive symptoms [8]. These authors conclude that dissatisfaction, in particular in the workplace, should be explored as a strong predictor of suicidal ideation in physicians.

Burnout and Suicide Rate Among Surgeons and Surgery Residents

While, as seen from the Shanafelt et al. study (above study), all physicians are at risk, for obvious reasons, I will concentrate more on surgeons and surgery residents while of course respecting and absolutely not discounting the burnout among other healthcare providers. Mass media has made a note of this as well, and it is estimated that one million Americans lose their healthcare to suicide. There is a great chance that every one of us surgeons knew a surgeon who killed themselves at one point of our carrier. Personally I worked as a research fellow with an outstanding surgeon named Chuck Peters, MD, FACS, whose first page of the CV was one of the best I have ever seen since, who jumped to death of the 26th floor of St. Luke's Hospital in Houston, Texas, in 1988. I was devastated. He had some sport-related injuries that he was dealing with, but none of us thought that he may take it that far.

As a medical student in Pristina, I was the first one to find a classmate hanged in the pathology department in the basement. He was the best student in our class with average grade of 9.9 out of 10.

To this end, fast forward, almost 40 years later, a survey of 7905 participating surgeons in 2008 by Shanafelt et al. found that 6.3% or 1 of the 16 surgeons reported suicidal ideation (SI) during the previous 12 months [9]. Among individuals 45 years and older, SI was 1.5–3.0 times more common among surgeons than the general population ($P < 0.02$). However, only 130 surgeons (26.0%) with recent SI had sought psychiatric or psychological help, while 301 (60.1%) were reluctant to seek help due to concern that it could affect their medical license. The authors report that recent SI had a large, statistically significant adverse relationship with all three domains of burnout (emotional exhaustion, depersonalization, and low personal accomplishment) and symptoms of depression. Burnout and depression were independently associated with SI after controlling for personal and professional characteristics. Other personal and professional characteristics also related to the prevalence of SI.

In a most recent cross-sectional survey of 92 general residents and 55 attendings, the prevalence of burnout and risk of depression among general surgery residents were high (58 of 77 [75%] and 30 of 76 [39%], respectively) [10]. Residents and faculty members significantly underestimated the prevalence of burnout and depression but identified the same barriers to seeking treatment.

Forty-two residents (55%) had high emotional exhaustion and high depersonalization scores. Significant associations were revealed between high emotional exhaustion and high depersonalization scores (42 of 77 residents [55%]; $P < 0.001$) and high emotional exhaustion and low personal achievement scores (37 of 77 residents [48%]; $P = 0.005$).

This study is pretty alarming in more than one level. Of those with burnout, 28 of 58 (48%) were at elevated risk of depression ($P = 0.03$). Nine of 77 residents (12%) had suicidal ideation in the past 2 weeks. Most residents (40 of 76 [53%]) correctly estimated that more than 50% of residents had burnout, whereas only 13 of 56 attendings (23%) correctly estimated this prevalence ($P < 0.001$). Clearly, although the burnout has become a common understanding, in this study, authors report that 42 of 83 residents (51%) and 42 of 56 attendings (75%) underestimated the true prevalence of depression ($P = 0.002$). Sixty-six of 73 residents (90%) and 40 of 51 attendings (78%) identified the same top 3 barriers to seeking care for burnout: inability to take time off to seek treatment, avoidance or denial of the problem, and negative stigma toward those seeking care.

The reasons for surgeons' and other healthcare workers' burnout are complex and multiple. In the editorial at JAMA surgery following the above study, Patti, Schlottman, and Sarr [3] identified the following major causes of burnout: generation gap, electronic medical records, legal issues, recertification, mentoring, and personal wellness, and offer some broad advice on how to mitigate or eliminate altogether this significant problem.

Suicidal Among Healthcare Providers

The burnout syndrome is not isolated among surgeons and surgery residents, but it is very prevalent among anesthesiologist (up to 50%) [11–14], critical care physicians and nurses [15], nurses [16–22], emergency physicians [23], pediatricians, cardiac surgeon, internist, psychiatrist, and others.

The suicidal rate among physicians is higher than that of the general population. Physicians have higher rates of burnout, depressive symptoms, and suicide risk than the general population [24]. Physicians and trainees can experience high degrees of mental health distress and are less likely than other members of the public to seek mental health treatment. Physicians report several barriers to seeking mental healthcare, including time constraints, hesitancy to draw attention to self-perceived weakness, and concerns about reputation and confidentiality. An estimated 300–400 physicians die by suicide in the USA per year [25]. Not seeking or receiving mental health treatment compared with nonphysicians who took their lives even though depression was found to be a significant risk factor at approximately the same rate in both groups [26]. Moreover, the suicide rate among male physicians is 1.41 times higher than the general male population. And among female physicians, the relative risk is even more pronounced—2.27 times greater than the general female population.

In all, it is important to acknowledge and understand the high rates of burnout among clinicians and to take preventive measures against risk factors for burnout and suicide. Perhaps we need to remember a mundane rule that we have heard many times on an airplane: "to put the oxygen mask first on yourself before assisting others." We need to take care of ourselves and, in doing so, may become more helpful to others who are in the same position. The risk of anxiety, depression, stressed or broken relationships, substance dependence, and possibly suicide as a result of these stressors affects up to 75% of surgeons [27–35].

Postscriptum

Burnout, depression, and suicidal rate are serious healthcare problem that we need to understand, study, prevent, and treat all of them like any other disease. Those who are supposed to take care of the sick patient should be healthy themselves first and then be able to render help to others. When a popular actor or movie star or a television personality commits suicide, we all mourn, and rightly so. The nation mourns. When an old or young doctor or those in training, a medical student, a nurse, or any other healthcare personnel commits suicide, gets divorced, is drinking way too much and/or becoming alcoholic, starts looking for peace in drugs and alcohol, becomes obese, and simply does not take care of herself or himself, we do not hear much about it; we do not talk about it. It is a stigma. A taboo. Well, it is not any longer. It is not, and it should not be. We need not to condemn them but to understand why, to do a root cause analysis, and to come up with solutions. It is not that they are doing out of toxic success. It is not.

Suicide rates have been rising in nearly every state, according to the latest *Vital Signs* report by the Centers for Disease Control and Prevention (CDC). In 2016, nearly 45,000 Americans age 10 or older died by suicide. Suicide is the 10th leading cause of death and is one of just three leading causes that is on the rise [36]. The CDC report stated that "the most recent overall suicide rates (2014–2016) varied four-fold; from 6.9 per 100,000 residents per year in Washington, D.C. to 29.2 per 100,000 residents in Montana.

Across the study period, rates increased in nearly all states. Percentage increases in suicide rates ranged from just under 6 percent in Delaware to over 57 percent in North Dakota. Twenty-five states had suicide rate increases of more than 30 percent." And this increase is not only in the USA. It is across the entire world.

References

1. Freudenberger HJ. Staff burn-out. J Soc Issues. 1974;30(1):159–65. https://doi.org/10.1111/j.1540-4560.1974.tb00706.x.
2. Maslach C, Jackson SE. The measurement of experienced burnout. J Organ Behav. 1981;2(2):99–113. https://doi.org/10.1002/job.4030020205.
3. Patti GM, Schlotman F, Sarr MG. The problem of burnout among surgeons. JAMA Surgery. 2018;153:5.
4. Freischlag JA. Burnout and depression among general surgery residents image is everything—it alters perception. JAMA Surg . Published online May 02, 2018. https://doi.org/10.1001/jamasurg.2018.1003.
5. Shanafelt TD, et al. Changes in burnout and satisfaction with work-life balance in physicians and the general us working population between 2011 and 2014. Mayo Clin Proc. 2015;90(12):1600–13.
6. Ross M. Suicide among physicians. Psychiatry Med. 1971;2(3):189–98.
7. Nordentoft M. Prevention of suicide and attempted suicide in Denmark. Epidemiological studies of suicide and intervention studies in selected risk groups. Dan Med Bull. 2007;54(4):306–69.
8. Loas G, Lefebvre G, Rotsaert M, Englert Y. Relationships between anhedonia, suicidal ideation and suicide attempts in a large sample of physicians. Hashimoto K, ed. PLoS ONE. 2018;13(3):e0193619. https://doi.org/10.1371/journal.pone.0193619.
9. Shanafelt TD, Balch CM, Dyrbye L, Bechamps G, Russell T, Satele D, Rummans T, Swartz K, Novotny PJ, Sloan J, Oreskovich MR. Special report: suicidal ideation among American surgeons. Arch Surg. 2011;146(1):54–62. https://doi.org/10.1001/archsurg.2010.292.
10. Williford ML, Scarlet S, Meyers M, et al. Multiple-institution comparison of resident and faculty perceptions of burnout and depression during surgical training. JAMA Surg . Published online May 2, 2018. https://doi.org/10.1001/jamasurg.2018.0974.
11. Hyman SA, Shotwell MS, Michaels DR, et al. A survey evaluating burnout, health status, depression, reported alcohol and substance use, and social support of anesthesiologists. Anesth Analg. 2017;125(6):2009–18. https://doi.org/10.1213/ANE.0000000000002298.
12. Misiołek A, Gil-Monte PR, Misiołek H. Prevalence of burnout in Polish anesthesiologists and anesthetist nursing professionals: a comparative non-randomized cross-sectional study. J Health Psychol. 2017;22(4):465–74. https://doi.org/10.1177/1359105315604377. Epub 2016 Jul 9.
13. Barbosa FT, Eloi RJ, Santos LM, et al. Correlation between weekly working time and burnout syndrome among anesthesiologists of Maceió-AL. Braz J Anesthesiol. 2017;67(2):115–21. https://doi.org/10.1016/j.bjane.2015.06.001. Epub 2017 Jan 18.
14. Katz JD. The impaired and/or disabled anesthesiologist. Curr Opin Anaesthesiol. 2017;30(2):217–22. https://doi.org/10.1097/ACO.0000000000000423.
15. Fumis RRL, Junqueira Amarante GA, de Fátima NA, Vieira Junior JM. Moral distress and its contribution to the development of burnout syndrome among critical care providers. Ann Intensive Care. 2017;7(1):71. https://doi.org/10.1186/s13613-017-0293-2. Epub 2017 Jun 21.
16. Jiang H, Ma L, Gao C, Li T, Huang L, Huang W. Satisfaction, burnout and intention to stay of emergency nurses in Shanghai. Emerg Med J. 2017;34(7):448–53. https://doi.org/10.1136/emermed-2016-205886. Epub 2017 May 4.
17. Dall'Ora C, Griffiths P, Ball J, Simon M, Aiken LH. Association of 12 h shifts and nurses' job satisfaction, burnout and intention to leave: findings from a cross-sectional study of 12 European countries. BMJ Open. 2015;5(9):e008331. https://doi.org/10.1136/bmjopen-2015-008331.
18. Akman O, Ozturk C, Bektas M, Ayar D, Armstrong MA. Job satisfaction and burnout among paediatric nurses. J Nurs Manag. 2016;24(7):923–33. https://doi.org/10.1111/jonm.12399. Epub 2016 Jun 7.
19. Campana KL, Hammoud S. Incivility from patients and their families: can organisational justice protect nurses from burnout? J Nurs Manag. 2015;23(6):716–25. https://doi.org/10.1111/jonm.12201. Epub 2013 Dec 30.
20. Labrague LJ, McEnroe-Petitte DM, Gloe D, Tsaras K, Arteche DL, Maldia F. Organizational politics, nurses' stress, burnout levels, turnover intention and job satisfaction. Int Nurs Rev. 2017;64(1):109–16. https://doi.org/10.1111/inr.12347. Epub 2016 Dec 20.
21. Hunsaker S, Chen HC, Maughan D, Heaston S. Factors that influence the development of compassion fatigue, burnout, and compassion satisfaction in emergency department nurses. J Nurs Scholarsh. 2015;47(2):186–94. https://doi.org/10.1111/jnu.12122. Epub 2015 Jan 20. Review.

22. Hatch DJ, Freude G, Martus P, Rose U, Müller G, Potter GG. Age, burnout and physical and psychological work ability among nurses. Occup Med (Lond). 2018;68(4):246–54. https://doi.org/10.1093/occmed/kqy033.
23. Bragard I, Dupuis G, Fleet R. Quality of work life, burnout, and stress in emergency department physicians: a qualitative review. Eur J Emerg Med. 2015;22(4):227–34. https://doi.org/10.1097/MEJ.0000000000000194. Review.
24. American Foundation for Suicide Prevention. Healthcare professional burnout, depression and suicide prevention. 2018. Retrieved from: https://afsp.org/our-work/education/healthcare-professional-burnout-depression-suicide-prevention/. Accessed 3 June 2018.
25. Center C, Davis M, Detre T, et al. Confronting depression and suicide in physicians A consensus statement. JAMA. 2003;289(23):3161–6. https://doi.org/10.1001/jama.289.23.3161).
26. Gold KJ, Sen A, Schwentk TL. Details on suicide among U.S. physicians: data from the National Violent Death Reporting System. Gen Hosp Psychiatry. 2013;35(1):45–9. Published online 2012 Nov 2. https://doi.org/10.1016/j.genhosppsych.2012.08.005.
27. Bittner JG 4th, Khan Z, Babu M, Hamed O. Stress, burnout, and maladaptive coping: strategies for surgeon well-being. Bull Am Coll Surg. 2011;96(8):17–22. PubMed PMID: 22319907.
28. Balch CM, Freischlag JA, Shanafelt TD. Stress and burnout among surgeons: understanding and managing the syndrome and avoiding the adverse consequences. Arch Surg. 2009;144(4):371–6.
29. Balch CM, Shanafelt T. Combating stress and burnout in surgical practice: a review. Adv Surg. 2010;44:29–47. Review
30. Shanafelt TD, Oreskovich MR, Dyrbye LN, Satele DV, Hanks JB, Sloan JA, Balch CM. Avoiding burnout: the personal health habits and wellness practices of US surgeons. Ann Surg. 2012;255(4):625–33. https://doi.org/10.1097/SLA.0b013e31824b2fa0.
31. Joseph V. Sakran, Haytham Kaafarani, ; Nicolas J. Mouawad, and Heena P. Santry. When things go wrong. ACS Bull 2011; 96 (8); 13–16).
32. Luu S, Leung SO, Moulton CA. When bad things happen to good surgeons: reactions to adverse events. Surg Clin North Am. 2012;92(1):153–61. https://doi.org/10.1016/j.suc.2011.12.002. Epub 2011 Dec 27.
33. Wu A. Medical error: the second victim. The doctor who makes the mistake needs help too. BMJ. 2000;320:726–7.
34. Wallace JE, Lemaire JB, Ghali WA. Physician wellness: a missing quality indicator. Lancet. 2009;374(9702):1714–21.
35. Look FD. Leadership and medicine. Gulf Breeze: Fire Starter Publishing; 2009.
36. Centers for Disease Control and Prevention (CDC). Suicide rates rising across the U.S. June 7th, 2018. Retrieved from: https://www.cdc.gov/media/releases/2018/p0607-suicide-prevention.html. Accessed 17 June 2018.

Index

R. Latifi (ed.), *The Modern Hospital*, https://doi.org/10.1007/978-3-030-01394-3

O

P

Q

Printed by Printforce, the Netherlands